THERAPY FOR

DIABETES

MELLITUS

AND RELATED DISORDERS

FOURTH EDITION

Harold E. Lebovitz, MD, Editor

American Diabetes Association®

Cure • Care • Commitment®

Director, Book Publishing, John Fedor; *Associate Director, Professional Books,* Christine B. Charlip; *Editor,* Joyce Raynor; *Copyeditor,* Wendy Martin; *Proofreader,* Jennifer Gross; *Associate Director, Book Production,* Peggy M. Rote; *Composition,* Circle Graphics, Inc.; *Cover Design,* Koncept, Inc.; *Printer,* Port City Press, Inc.

Printed in the United States of America
1 3 5 7 9 10 8 6 4 2

The suggestions and information contained in this publication are generally consistent with the *Clinical Practice Recommendations* and other policies of the American Diabetes Association, but they do not represent the policy or position of the Association or any of its boards or committees. Reasonable steps have been taken to ensure the accuracy of the information presented. However, the American Diabetes Association cannot ensure the safety or efficacy of any product or service described in this publication. Individuals are advised to consult a physician or other appropriate health care professional before undertaking any diet or exercise program or taking any medication referred to in this publication. Professionals must use and apply their own professional judgment, experience, and training and should not rely solely on the information contained in this publication before prescribing any diet, exercise, or medication. The American Diabetes Association—its officers, directors, employees, volunteers, and members—assumes no responsibility or liability for personal or other injury, loss, or damage that may result from the suggestions or information in this publication.

∞ The paper in this publication meets the requirements of the ANSI Standard Z39.48-1992 (permanence of paper).

ADA titles may be purchased for business or promotional use or for special sales. To purchase this book in large quantities, or for custom editions of this book with your logo, contact Lee Romano Sequeira, Special Sales & Promotions, at the address below, or at LRomano@diabetes.org or call 703-299-2046.

American Diabetes Association
1701 North Beauregard Street
Alexandria, Virginia 22311

Library of Congress Cataloging-in-Publication Data

Therapy for diabetes mellitus and related disorders / editor, Harold E. Lebovitz.—4th ed.
    p. ; cm.
    Includes bibliographical references and index.
    ISBN 1-58040-187-2 (pbk. : alk. paper)
1. Diabetes–Treatment. 2. Diabetes—Complications—Treatment. I. Lebovitz, Harold E., 1931 - II. American Diabetes Association.
[DNLM: 1. Diabetes Mellitus—therapy. 2. Diabetes Mellitus—complications. WK 815 T398 2004]
RC660.T476 2004
616.4'6206—dc22

                                                    2004041071

Contents

Preface

The last 15 years have seen a worldwide rising tide of metabolic diseases triggered by changing lifestyles. Initially, this was manifested by an increase in type 2 diabetes in developing countries. It was appreciated that the emergence of the large population of individuals with type 2 diabetes in Japan, India, and the South Pacific region was associated with an increase in body weight from substandard levels to normal or slightly increased levels. Projections made in the mid-1990s estimated the worldwide population of individuals with diabetes would reach 221 million by 2010. As the 1990s progressed, it became clear that the world was in the midst of an obesity epidemic. Moving hand in hand with the obesity was an epidemic of insulin resistance, the metabolic syndrome, and type 2 diabetes. This cluster of metabolic diseases is occurring with progressively greater frequency in all populations and at a progressively younger age. For example, the number of individuals with diabetes in the U.S. increased ~60% during the 1990s. Today, in many communities, 25–40% of children presenting with diabetes are obese and have type 2 diabetes. The number of cases of diabetes worldwide is exceeding the earlier predicted numbers by tens of millions.

This epidemic will lead to marked increases in cardiovascular disease, end-stage renal disease, visual impairment, limb amputations, and mortality. The cost of providing so much health care for so many people has the potential to bankrupt the health care budgets of most countries.

Therefore, it is imperative to create strategies to delay or prevent the development of type 2 diabetes. It is equally important to have and to implement treatments that will diminish the development and reduce the severity of the complications of type 2 diabetes and insulin resistance. Fortunately, the creation of new strategies, pharmacological agents, and devices since the last edition of this manual provides promise of being able to achieve both goals. This fourth edition of *Therapy for Diabetes Mellitus and Related Disorders* provides both a concise overview of the new advances and an update of previously available information from leading experts around the world. Each expert was asked to focus specifically on the management aspects of his or her subject and to present a concise and practical approach. Each chapter represents accepted approaches to therapy and contains information that is generally consistent with the Clinical Practice Recommendations of the American Diabetes Association. Now is the time to apply the advances of the last 2 decades and win the battle against this metabolic epidemic and its devastating effects on the health of the world's population. This manual is part of the American Diabetes Association's efforts to help you engage in this battle.

Together with the American Diabetes Association, I thank the many contributors and Association staff who have put in so much effort and given so much of their time to make this edition possible.

Harold E. Lebovitz, MD
Editor

Introduction: Goals of Treatment

HAROLD E. LEBOVITZ, MD

D iabetes mellitus is one of the major public health issues facing the world in the 21st century. The prevalence of type 1 diabetes is increasing slowly, whereas that of type 2 diabetes is increasing explosively. Changing lifestyle, longer life expectancy, and rapid growth of ethnic and racial populations who have high prevalence rates of type 2 diabetes are likely to double the worldwide prevalence of diabetes by the year 2020. The human toll of diabetes can be estimated not only by medical statistics, which show it to be the leading cause of end-stage renal disease and new cases of visual loss in individuals <65 years old and a major cause of macrovascular disease, but also by the quantity of health care resources that are consumed to care for patients with diabetes. Table 1 tabulates estimated medical costs for diabetes in the United States in 2002. The average cost of caring for a patient with diabetes is ~2.4 times that of the average of other patients being cared for in the health care system. Much of the disability and costs associated with diabetes are related to the care of individuals afflicted with its chronic complications. The major tasks of the health care establishment today are to implement current treatments that we know will prevent or minimize the complications of diabetes and to further define and implement the new strategies that we know will prevent or delay the development of type 2 diabetes and its complications in individuals with genetic predispositions.

Since the publication of the first edition of this manual in 1991, remarkable advances in understanding and treating diabetes mellitus and its related disorders have occurred. Data from many studies have proven the importance of glycemic control in preventing or delaying microvascular and neuropathic complications of both type 1 and type 2 diabetes mellitus. The importance of blood pressure control and the unique benefits of angiotensin-converting enzyme inhibitors and angiotensin II receptor blockers in preventing microvascular and cardiovascular disease are now well established. The effect of statin drugs in reducing coronary artery disease events and mortality in patients with diabetes has been documented by many clinical trials. The rapid development of new types of therapeutic agents that aid in the management of all aspects of diabetes is truly remarkable. It is the task of this fourth edition to help health care professionals understand and apply these major advances to the care of their patients.

The ideal management of the individual with diabetes should ensure the following:

Table 1 Medical Costs for Diabetes: 2002

- 12.1 million diagnosed patients with diabetes (4.1% of U.S. population)
- Total direct medical costs: $91.8 billion
  - Inpatient hospital days (16.91 million), 43.9%
  - Nursing home days (82.35 million), 15.1%
  - Office-based visits (62.64 million), 10.9%
  - Medications (oral agents, insulin and supplies, all other), 19.1%
- Indirect costs (loss of work, disability, etc.): $40 billion

- Of the inpatient costs, 63% were for general medical conditions, 24% for cardiovascular problems, and 5% for diabetes.
- Diabetes patients use 8 more hospital days per year than nondiabetic patients.
- Diabetes patients cost 2.4 times more per year for health care than nondiabetic patients.
- The 4.1% diagnosed diabetic population costs 10.1% of the health care budget.

- no symptoms attributable to diabetes
- prevention of acute complications
- prevention of microvascular and neuropathic disease
- reduction in macrovascular disease risk to that of nondiabetic patients
- life expectancy equal to nondiabetic individuals

Whereas ideal management is not yet attainable, studies such as Steno 2, which showed remarkable reductions in both microvascular complications (risk reduction ~60%) and macrovascular complications (risk reduction 53%) in patients with type 2 diabetes by a strategy of intensive treatment of glycemia, blood pressure, lipids, and the procoagulant state, indicate that we are quite close. Figure 1 depicts the metabolic targets that were set for the Steno 2 study and the percentage of intensively treated and conventionally treated type 2 patients who achieved those goals during the 7 1/2-year study. The ongoing ACCORD (Action to Control Cardiovascular Risk in Diabetes) study, which is attempting to treat a very large cohort of patients with type 2 diabetes to even more rigorous metabolic goals, will show us how close we can come with aggressive use of our present tools.

Tables 2 and 3 summarize the American Diabetes Association's suggested levels of glycemic control and lipoprotein levels that have been shown to significantly decrease the risk of microvascular and macrovascular complications in both type 1 and type 2 diabetes patients.

Glycemic control that maintains plasma glucose values at <200 mg/dl (<11.1 mmol/l) will generally eliminate the symptoms of polydipsia, polyuria, polyphagia, weight loss, and increased fatigue. Maintaining plasma glucose levels at 150–165 mg/dl (8.3–9.2 mmol/l) is usually associated with a sense of well-being and good health. Preventing chronic microvascular and neuropathic complications and eliminating diabetes complications associated with pregnancy probably require normoglycemic or near-normoglycemic regulation. Minimizing macrovascular disease requires addressing all of the risk factors (e.g., smoking, hypertension, plasma triglycerides, and serum LDL and HDL cholesterol) as well as blood glucose control.

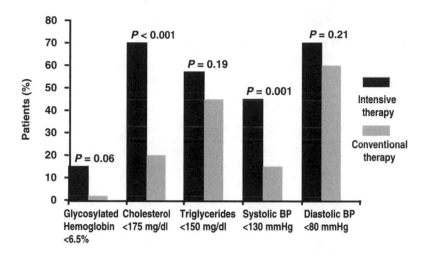

Figure 1 Percentage of patients in each group who reached the intensive treatment goals at a mean of 7.8 years. A total of 160 type 2 diabetes patients with microalbuminuria were randomized to intensive metabolic control or the ordinary control recommended by the Danish Diabetes society. The intensive targets are listed below each column, and the percentage of each group attaining those values for the 7 1/2 years of the study is provided for each column. The risk reductions for microvascular and macrovascular disease are given in the text. Reproduced with permission from Gaede et al. Copyright © 2003 Massachusetts Medical Society. All rights reserved.

Table 2 Recommendations for Glycemic Control

A1C	<7.0%*
Preprandial plasma glucose	90–130 mg/dl
Postprandial plasma glucose	180 mg/dl

Key concepts in setting glycemic goals are as follows:
- Goals should be individualized.
- Certain populations (children, pregnant women, and elderly) require special considerations.
- Less intensive glycemic goals may be indicated in patients with severe or frequent hypoglycemia.
- More stringent glycemic goals (i.e., a normal A1C, <6%) may further reduce complications at the cost of increased risk of hypoglycemia (particularly in individuals with type 1 diabetes).
- Postprandial glucose may be targeted if A1C goals are not met despite reaching preprandial glucose goals.

*Referenced to a nondiabetic range of 4.0–6.0% using a Diabetes Control and Complications Trial–based assay. A1C, glycated hemoglobin A1C.

Table 3 Recommendations for Lipid Control

LDL cholesterol	<100 mg/dl (<2.6 mmol/l)
HDL cholesterol	>40 mg/dl (>1.1 mmol/l) for men
	>50 mg/dl (>1.3 mmol/l) for women
Triglycerides	<150 mg/dl (<1.7 mmol/l)

Current NCEP/ATP III guidelines suggest that in patients with triglyceride, ≥200 mg/dl, the "non-HDL cholesterol" (total cholesterol – HDL cholesterol) be utilized. The goal is ≤130 mg/dl (≤1.45 mmol/l). From American Diabetes Association, 2004.

In defining glycemic treatment goals, alleviating symptoms and increasing the sense of well-being are realistic goals for all individuals with diabetes. Striving for goals to prevent chronic complications requires that

- the patient's life expectancy is at least 10–15 years more
- the patient does not already have significant chronic complications
- the patient does not have an illness that contraindicates intensive treatment
- the patient is willing and able to follow a regimen for intensive treatment

Blood pressure control and regulation of serum lipids in diabetes patients require somewhat different goals than in the nondiabetic population and are discussed in great detail in subsequent specific chapters.

BIBLIOGRAPHY

American Diabetes Association: Economic costs of diabetes in the U.S. in 2002. *Diabetes Care* 26:917–932, 2003

American Diabetes Association: Standards of medical care in diabetes (Position Statement). *Diabetes Care* 27 (Suppl. 1):S15–S35, 2004

Gaede P, Vedel P, Larsen N, Jensen GV, Parving HH, Pedersen O: Multifactorial intervention and cardiovascular disease in patients with type 2 diabetes. *N Engl J Med* 348:383–393, 2003

1. Diagnosis and Classification of Diabetes Mellitus

HAROLD E. LEBOVITZ, MD

A cardinal feature in preventing the complications of diabetes mellitus is early diagnosis. This is particularly important in type 2 or late-onset auto-immune type 1 diabetes because these disorders start with a relatively asymptomatic period that lasts as long as 5–10 years. About 30% of all people with type 2 diabetes in the United States are undiagnosed. Unfortunately, this relatively symptom-free undiagnosed period is not benign; ~50% of newly diagnosed patients with type 2 diabetes already have evidence of early chronic complications.

Diabetes mellitus is a group of metabolic disorders characterized by inappropriate hyperglycemia that results in chronic microvascular, neuropathic, and/or macrovascular disease. The difficult task is to define inappropriate hyperglycemia. Several task forces have struggled with this issue and have concluded that an inappropriate blood glucose is one that will lead to diabetic microvascular complications. Retinopathy was chosen as the primary complication because it is unique to diabetes, easy to quantify, and the most common chronic complication. Numerous studies have shown that a plasma glucose level of ≥200 mg/dl (≥11.1 mmol/l) 2 h after a glucose challenge is associated with the development of diabetic retinopathy within 5–10 years. In 1979, it was proposed (but not measured) that this corresponded to a fasting plasma glucose (FPG) of 140 mg/dl (7.8 mmol/l). This value has since been shown to be wrong. Several recent studies show that FPG levels between 120 and 130 mg/dl (6.7 and 7.2 mmol/l) are comparable to the 2-h post–glucose challenge level of 200 mg/dl (11.1 mmol/l) and are associated with the subsequent development of retinopathy.

These data have led to a new set of criteria for the diagnosis of diabetes (Table 1.1). Criteria 2 and 3 should be confirmed by repeat testing on a separate day. In redefining the criteria for the diagnosis of diabetes mellitus, it became necessary to define intermediate grades of glucose intolerance. Table 1.2 defines categories of glucose tolerance in terms of either FPG or 2-h post–glucose challenge levels. The reason for defining impaired fasting glucose (IFG) or impaired glucose tolerance (IGT) is that both degrees of glucose intolerance predict future development of diabetes and both are associated with insulin resistance and an increase in cardiovascular risk factors. Additionally, several studies have shown that the development of type 2 diabetes can be delayed by several years or more by identifying individuals with IGT and treating them by intensive lifestyle modification or pharmacological agents (see Chapter 19). The

Table 1.1 Criteria for the Diagnosis of Diabetes Mellitus

1. Symptoms of diabetes plus casual plasma glucose concentration ≥200 mg/dl (≥11.1 mmol/l): Casual is defined as any time of day without regard to time since last meal. The classic symptoms of diabetes include
   - polyuria
   - polydipsia
   - unexplained weight loss
   or
2. FPG ≥126 mg/dl (≥7.0 mmol/l): Fasting is defined as no calorie intake for at least 8 h.
   or
3. 2-h plasma glucose ≥200 mg/dl (≥11.1 mmol/l) during an oral glucose tolerance test: The test should be performed as described by the World Health Organization with a glucose load containing the equivalent of 75 g anhydrous glucose dissolved in water.

Criteria 2 and 3 should be confirmed by repeat testing on separate day. From American Diabetes Association, 2004.

IFG category has been very recently extended to include those individuals with FPG levels ≥100 mg/dl (≥5.6 mmol/l), and the normal range for FPG has been redefined as <100 mg/dl (<5.6 mmol/l).

The new diagnostic criteria do not create more people with a diagnosis of diabetes but make it easier to diagnose the large pool of undiagnosed individuals with diabetes by FPG rather than requiring an oral glucose tolerance test. For example, the total diabetes prevalence in U.S. adults 40–74 years old is 14.26%. Undiagnosed diabetes patients who would be detected by a 2-h postglucose load, plasma glucose ≥200 mg/dl (≥11.1 mmol/l), is 6.34%. Approximately two-thirds (4.35%) of them are detected by an FPG ≥126 mg/dl (≥7.0 mmol/l). Only one-third (2.35%) are detected by an FPG ≥140 mg/dl (≥7.8 mmol/l).

The new classification of patients with diabetes is based on etiology (Table 1.3). The new classification eliminates the terms insulin-dependent and non–insulin-dependent and replaces them with type 1 and type 2 diabetes.

Type 1 diabetes is that characterized by absolute insulin deficiency. Most of these patients have immune-mediated destruction of their β-cells, but a few have an unknown or idiopathic process that leads to β-cell loss.

Table 1.2 Categories of Glucose Tolerance

FPG	2-h postload plasma glucose (oral glucose tolerance test)
■ Normal: <100 mg/dl (<5.6 mmol/l) ■ IFG: ≥100 mg/dl (≥5.6 mmol/l) and <126 mg/dl (<7.0 mmol/l) ■ Diabetes: ≥126 mg/dl (≥7.0 mmol/l)	■ Normal: <140 mg/dl (<7.8 mmol/l) ■ IGT: ≥140 mg/dl (≥7.8 mmol/l) and <200 mg/dl (<11.1 mmol/l) ■ Diabetes: ≥200 mg/dl (≥11.1 mmol/l)

From American Diabetes Association, 2004.

Table 1.3 Classification of Diabetes Mellitus

Type 1 diabetes
- Immune-mediated
- Idiopathic

Type 2 diabetes
- May range from predominantly insulin-resistant to predominantly insulin-deficient

Other specific types
- Genetic defects of β-cell function
- Genetic defects in insulin action
- Diseases of endocrine pancreas
- Endocrinopathies
- Drug- or chemical-induced
- Infections
- Uncommon forms of immune-mediated diabetes
- Other genetic syndromes sometimes associated with diabetes

Gestational diabetes

From American Diabetes Association, 2004.

Type 2 diabetes is the classic form, with varying degrees of insulin resistance and relative insulin secretory deficiency. The etiology is unknown. It can occur in both children and adults and is frequently associated with obesity. Known causes of diabetes fall into the category "other specific types," which includes the various forms of maturity-onset diabetes of the young (MODY). Gestational diabetes remains the fourth category, and its definition remains unchanged.

BIBLIOGRAPHY

American Diabetes Association: Diagnosis and classification of diabetes mellitus (Position Statement). *Diabetes Care* 27 (Suppl. 1):S5–S10, 2004

Dr. Lebovitz is Professor of Medicine at the State University of New York Health Science Center at Brooklyn, Brooklyn, NY.

2. Genetic Counseling for Autoimmune Type 1 Diabetes

George S. Eisenbarth, MD

DIAGNOSIS

Autoimmune type 1 diabetes mellitus can occur at any age. Approximately 50% of individuals develop the disorder before age 40 years, but another 50%, including relatives of patients, develop the disease as adults. The oldest anti-islet autoantibody (AIAA)-positive patient we have followed to diabetes was aged 69 years at diabetes onset. It is generally thought that most children developing type 1 diabetes have the immune-mediated form of diabetes (type 1A). With recent improvements in the ability to diagnose autoimmune diabetes and advances in genetic analysis of diabetes, it is clear that autoimmunity as the cause of childhood diabetes can vary from a major to a minor factor, depending on ethnicity, associated diseases, and, obviously, family history.

As illustrated in Table 2.1, not all diabetes in children is autoimmune type 1A. Approximately 50% of African-American and Hispanic-American children presenting with diabetes do not have autoimmune diabetes. These individuals lack AIAAs, a major subset has a BMI >25 kg/m^2 (~25%), many have the most protective DQB1 HLA allele (~20% DQB1*0602), and many have insulin-resistant syndromes. African-American children often have what has been termed *type 1.5* diabetes or *Flatbush* diabetes. Despite an episode of ketoacidosis, these individuals are often able to discontinue insulin for prolonged periods before again requiring insulin therapy. The best-characterized nonautoimmune forms of diabetes in childhood are maturity-onset diabetes of the young (MODY)-2, MODY-1, and MODY-3. MODY-2 is often a mild form of diabetes with normal fasting blood glucose. MODY-2 results from a mutation in the glucokinase gene. MODY-3 can be confused with type 1 diabetes, is inherited as an autosomal-dominant trait, and is caused by mutations in the hepatic nuclear factor (HNF) gene 1α. MODY-1 results from a mutation in HNF-4α. MODY-3 is currently the most frequently defined form of MODY, but patients develop this disorder as both children and adults. The most common forms of nonautoimmune diabetes in children are probably caused by none of the currently identified mutations, but rather are probably variants of type 2 diabetes and are polygenic in origin.

Table 2.1 Differential Diagnosis of Autoimmune Diabetes in Childhood

Characteristics	Likely Diagnosis	Diagnostic Tests
Non-Hispanic Caucasian	90% autoimmune DM	Autoantibody positive, high-risk HLA
Hispanic American	50% not autoimmune DM, diabetes etiology unknown	Autoantibody negative
African American	50% not autoimmune DM, diabetes etiology unknown	Autoantibody negative
Transient hyperglycemia	"Stress" hyperglycemia	Autoantibody negative, normal IVGTT
DM + deafness/maternal inheritance	Mitochondrial DM	Autoantibody negative, mitochondrial gene analysis
MODY family history	MODY-2, MODY-3, etc.	Autoantibody negative, glucokinase, HNF gene sequence
DM + diabetes insipidus	DIDMOAD syndrome	Autoantibody negative, characteristic syndrome

DIDMOAD, diabetes insipidus, diabetes mellitus, optic atrophy, deafness; DM, diabetes mellitus.

ASSOCIATED AUTOIMMUNE DISORDERS

The most important genetic counseling information that can be currently offered to families with type 1A diabetes is that individuals with autoimmune diabetes and their relatives are at increased risk for a series of organ-specific autoimmune disorders. Most of these disorders can be effectively treated. Table 2.2 lists several of the most common associated diseases, the diseases most important to diagnose, and screening tests.

Celiac Disease

Celiac disease is one of the most common associated diseases and is often asymptomatic in patients with type 1A diabetes. Celiac disease is primarily associated with the high-risk HLA alleles DR3, DQA1*0501, and DQB1*0201. Tests for transglutaminase autoantibodies (formerly anti-endomysial autoantibodies) are both highly specific and sensitive. Given the finding of high-titer transglutaminase autoantibodies, follow-up intestinal biopsy usually confirms the diagnosis of celiac disease. With avoidance of gluten, the intestinal mucosa heals and autoantibodies disappear. When celiac disease is asymptomatic, the decision to screen and ultimately to treat the disease often relates to the long-term conse-

Table 2.2 Type 1A–Associated Autoimmune Disorders

Disorder	Patients (%)	Relative of Patient with Type 1 Diabetes (%)	Screening Test
Celiac disease	5.4	2.6	Transglutaminase autoantibody
Graves' disease	0.5–2.0	?	Sensitive TSH assay
Hypothyroidism	1.4–5.0	?	Sensitive TSH assay
Addison's disease	0.5	?	Anti–21-hydroxylase autoantibody
Pernicious anemia	1.4	?	Serum B12
Type 1 diabetes	NA	5	AIAAs

quences of the disorder, which can include both osteoporosis and intestinal malignancies (both of which have been reported to be prevented by dietary therapy). Because the levels of transglutaminase autoantibodies fluctuate, it is important to biopsy individuals close to the time of confirmation of high levels of autoantibodies. A test for transglutaminase autoantibodies on the day of biopsy is recommended to aid evaluation.

Graves' and Addison's Disease

Graves' disease and Addison's disease are both also highly associated with HLA DR3. In patients with type 1A diabetes, Addison's disease is most often found in individuals with the highest-risk HLA genotypes, HLA DR3 and DR4. Of the patients with type 1A diabetes, 2% have autoantibodies reacting with the enzyme 21-hydroxylase, a major adrenal autoantigen. Approximately 25% of 21-hydroxylase autoantibody–positive patients have Addison's disease on initial testing, and more progress to overt disease during follow-up. Because of the rarity of Addison's disease, it is often a missed diagnosis. In a patient with type 1A diabetes, a distinctive sign of Addison's disease is decreasing insulin dosage and recurrent hypoglycemia. Increasing insulin sensitivity can precede hyperpigmentation. If untreated, Addison's disease is fatal. The therapy is relatively simple with oral replacement of glucocorticoids.

To detect both Graves' disease and hypothyroidism, we determine serum thyrotropin (thyroid-stimulating hormone [TSH]) with a sensitive assay to detect both high (hypothyroidism) and low (Graves' disease) levels of TSH. Antithyroid autoantibodies appear to be more frequent than progression to overt thyroid disease. With hypothyroidism and type 1 diabetes, Addison's disease should be excluded before thyroid hormone replacement, for fear of exacerbating the Addison's disease.

Pernicious Anemia

Pernicious anemia is usually diagnosed late in life (often beyond the 6th decade). In patients with type 1A diabetes, pernicious anemia appears earlier in life. The major irreversible effect of pernicious anemia is loss of proprioception and vibratory sensation, which can occur in the absence of anemia (especially in patients receiving vitamin supplements). Screening for serum B12 followed by a Schilling test is usually adequate for diagnosis, although serum B12 levels can be low-normal with disease. Therapy for pernicious anemia consists of injections of vitamin B12.

Autoimmune Syndromes

There are three autoimmune syndromes associated with type 1A diabetes: XPID (X-linked polyendocrinopathy, immune dysfunction, and diarrhea), APS-I (autoimmune polyendocrine syndrome type I), and APS-II (autoimmune polyendocrine syndrome type II). Diagnosis of each syndrome of associated autoimmune disorders requires specialized follow-up and treatment. The mutated genes responsible for XPID (Surfy gene) and APS-I (AIRE [autoimmune regulator]) are known. Neonates with the XPID syndrome present with overwhelming autoimmunity and will die unless they receive a bone marrow transplant. Patients with APS-I present often in infancy with mucocutaneous candidiasis followed by Addison's disease and hypoparathyroidism. They often develop asplenism and require infectious prophylaxis, follow-up for multiple autoimmune disorders, and aggressive treatment for oral candida with associated oral cancers (see "Type 1 Diabetes: Cellular, Molecular, and Clinical Immunology" at www.barbaradaviscenter.org).

RISK OF TYPE 1A DIABETES

Type 1A diabetes occurs in 1 in 300 children. However, this is probably an underestimate of the total prevalence; adults with the autoimmune form of diabetes can now be diagnosed through AIAA assays. Table 2.3 shows the genetic risk of developing type 1A diabetes according to family history of diabetes. The highest risk for type 1A diabetes occurs in the identical twin of a patient with type 1 diabetes. With long-term follow-up, we have observed that ~50% of monozygotic twins who were initially discordant for diabetes progress to type 1A diabetes. In a combined series from the U.S. and Great Britain, almost half of initially discordant twins who developed diabetes became concordant for diabetes >5 years after the diagnosis in their twin. The incidence of diabetes in the second twin is highest within 10 years of onset of diabetes in the first twin and declines steadily, but some monozygous twins develop diabetes decades after the first twin. The risk of diabetes for the second monozygous twin is influenced by the age at which the first twin developed diabetes (falling to <5% for index twins with onset after age 25). Even in Japan, a country with one of the lowest prevalences of type 1 diabetes, the risk to an identical twin is similar to that in the U.S.

Why offspring of a mother with type 1 diabetes have a lower risk of diabetes than offspring of a father with type 1 diabetes is unknown. Generally, the risk to

Table 2.3 Empiric Risk of Type 1A Diabetes

Relative with Type 1 Diabetes	Modifying Factor	Risk of Diabetes (%)
Identical twin	Age at onset in first twin: If >25 yr of age, risk is <5%	50
Father	HLA DR3/DR4(DQ8): Risk is ~25%	6
Mother	HLA DR3/DR4(DQ8): Risk is ~25%	2
Sibling	HLA DR3/DR4(DQ8): Risk is ~50%	5
First-degree relatives	HLA DR3 and DR4(DQ8)	20
	HLA DR3 or DR4(DQ8)	5
	HLA DR2 with DQB1*0502	5
	HLA DR2 with DQB1*0602	<0.2

a sibling of a patient with type 1A diabetes in childhood is ~1 in 20. Risk within a family is greatly influenced by HLA alleles of chromosome 6, particularly HLA DR and DQ alleles, with the dominant effect associated with DQ. DQ molecules consist of two chains, an α- and a β-chain, both of which are polymorphic in their amino acid sequence. DR molecules also consist of an α- and a β-chain, but only the β-chain gene is polymorphic for DR genes. Each different polymorphic amino acid sequence is assigned a unique number. Thus, DR molecules can simply be described with one number for their β-chain gene (e.g., DRB1*0301 [DR3]), whereas both α- and β-chains must be specified for DQ molecules (e.g., DQA1*0501,DQB1*0201). The highest-risk genotype for type 1A diabetes consists of the common DR3 haplotype with the highest-risk DR4 haplotype (DQA1*0301,DQB1*0302 [with DRB1*0401, 0402, or 0404 but not 0403]).

In addition to being associated with risk for type 1A diabetes, HLA alleles are associated with protection from diabetes. In particular, DQA1*0102,DQB1*0602 provides dominant protection from type 1A diabetes in all populations studied to date. In most populations, this protective haplotype is present in ~20% of the general population and <1% of children with type 1A diabetes. The protection is not absolute, and, in particular, adults with type 1 diabetes have DQB1*0602 more often than children. DRB1*1401 and DQA1*0201,DQB1*0301 are also strongly protective.

Some HLA DQ alleles are rare in the general U.S. population, but when present in families with type 1 diabetes, they may confer high diabetes risk. Such alleles include DQA1*0102,DQB1*0502 and DQA1*0401,DQB1*0402. Although most reviews do not list these molecules as high-risk alleles because only a small percentage of patients with type 1A diabetes express them, they confer a risk of diabetes similar to the DR3 or DR4 haplotypes within families. DQB1*0402 has aspartic acid at position 57 of its DQB chain (Asp57 positivity was reported to correlate with protection from diabetes). In evaluating HLA DQ alleles for their "diabetogenicity," Table 2.4 lists various alleles in order of decreasing transmission to diabetic offspring from a parent with the specified allele and high-risk HLA DQ alleles on the other chromosome (i.e., DQA1 *0301,DQB1*0302). A 50% transmission to the child with diabetes would indicate that an HLA allele is as diabetogenic as the high-risk DQ allele DQA1*0301,DQB1*0302. The number of parents with the given allele in Table 2.4 provides information on the population frequency of the allele. For example, 13% of parents had the DQB1*0602 protective allele with DQB1*0302 on their second HLA chromosome, and this allele was never transmitted to their diabetic offspring (0/59). The gradation of risk for diabetes and the complexity (with so many alleles) suggests that genetic counseling on the basis of HLA alleles requires caution.

A large study in Denver is evaluating the presence at birth of DR and DQ alleles from cord blood in the general population. Of ~10,000 births, 2.4% of children express the highest-risk genotype (DR3/4 [DQB1*0302]). Such children may comprise ~40% of all children developing type 1 diabetes and have an absolute risk of diabetes of ~6% (similar to having a father with type 1 diabetes). In contrast, for children with a first-degree relative with type 1A diabetes (father or sibling), the risk of diabetes is >25% if the child has both DR3 and DR4 (DQB1*0302). For such children, autoantibodies frequently appear in the first 2 years of life, and DR3/4 heterozygosity is associated with an earlier age at diabetes development.

Table 2.4 Transmission of Specified DQ Alleles to a Child with Diabetes from a Parent Whose Other DQ Haplotype Is DQA1*0301,DQB1*0302

HLA-DQ Alleles	Percent Transmitted	Number of Parents with Allele
A1*0501,B1*0201	54	79
A1*0301,B1*0201	50	4
A1*0102,B1*0502	46	15
A1*0401,B1*0402	40	15
A1*0102,B1*0604	33	24
A1*0101,B1*0501	26	61
A1*0301,B1*0301	23	26
A1*0201,B1*0201	11	54
A1*0501,B1*0301	8	51
A1*0103,B1*0603	5	21
A1*0301,B1*0303	0	4
A1*0201,B1*0303	0	24
A1*0101,B1*05031	0	20
A1*0102,B1*0609	0	6
A1*0102,B1*0602	0	59

Adapted from Kawaskai et al. 1997.

GENETIC, IMMUNOLOGICAL, AND METABOLIC TESTS

Genetic

The primary genetic test currently associated with defining risk for type 1A diabetes or aiding in its diagnosis is typing for DR and DQ alleles. The finding of DQA1*0102,DQB1*0602 in an individual thought to have type 1A diabetes should point to other causes of diabetes or autoimmune syndromes where HLA alleles may have less influence. Approximately 10% of relatives of patients with type 1A diabetes express DQB1*0602 with its greatly reduced risk for type 1A diabetes. In addition, ~7% of cytoplasmic islet cell autoantibody (ICA)-positive relatives of patients with type 1A diabetes express DQB1*0602. Despite expression of cytoplasmic ICA, these relatives have a low risk of progression to type 1A diabetes, and most of these relatives express only a single biochemical AIAA. High risk for type 1A diabetes is usually associated with the expression of multiple biochemical autoantibodies. There are too few relatives with DQB1*0602 who express multiple biochemical autoantibodies to currently assess their risk of progression to diabetes.

More than 14 additional loci associated with diabetes risk have been reported, but each has small effects and many are likely to be false-positive associations. A polymorphism 5' of the insulin gene contributes ~10% of the familial aggregation of type 1A diabetes. The diabetes protective polymorphism is associated with greater insulin messenger RNA in the thymus, potentially increasing tolerance to the key autoantigen insulin.

Immunological

The best predictor of risk for type 1A diabetes is the expression of multiple AIAAs (Table 2.5). This is a rapidly developing field. In the past 10 years, a series of specific islet autoantigens have been identified and sequenced. Reliable and convenient autoantibody assays for these autoantigens are now available. The standard autoantibody test for type 1A diabetes was the cytoplasmic ICA test, which used frozen sections of human pancreas. This test is difficult to standardize and measures some but not all of the autoantibodies that can be determined with biochemical autoantibody testing. The test still has specific research roles (especially in identification of additional unknown autoantigens). Generally, given a combination of testing for glutamic acid decarboxylase (GAD)-65, ICA512/IA-2, and insulin autoantibodies, testing for cytoplasmic ICA is of limited utility. More than 90% of individuals with typical autoimmune insulin-dependent diabetes express one or more of the three biochemical autoantibodies (each assay set with specificity >99th percentile).

Among relatives at risk for type 1A diabetes, the highest risk is associated with expression of more than one of the biochemically defined autoantibodies. Figure 2.1 illustrates the risk of diabetes relative to autoantibody expression among a series of first-degree relatives of patients with type 1 diabetes. Adding the assay for cytoplasmic ICA to the determination of biochemical autoantibodies runs the risk that a single biochemical autoantibody (e.g., GAD65) may result in ICA positivity, suggesting that a relative may have two antibodies (ICA and

Table 2.5 Major β-Cell Autoantigens Associated with Immune-Mediated Type 1 Diabetes

Autoantigen	Positive (%)	Comment
Insulin	49–92	>90% children <5 yr old, autoantibody positive
GAD	84	Low risk as single antibody
ICA512/IA-2	74	Highly specific for type 1
Phogrin/IA-2β	61	Usually a subset IA-2

GAD65) when he or she has only one. The form of ICA reacting only with GAD65 has been termed *restricted* or *selective* ICA and is associated with a lower risk of progression to diabetes than is nonrestricted ICA, which is usually associated with expression of multiple autoantibodies.

Most of the other autoantigens and putative autoantigens that have been identified are either relatively uncommon or the assay for autoantibodies is incon-

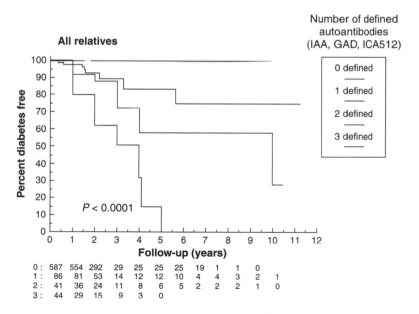

Figure 2.1 Progression of first-degree relatives to diabetes strongly depends on the number of biochemical autoantibodies expressed. From Verge et al. 1996.

venient. The autoantigen phogrin, or IA-2β, is related to ICA512/IA-2, and most (>95%) of IA-2β–positive sera are detectable as ICA512/IA-2 positive. Several large studies indicate that the expression of multiple autoantibodies in the general population approximates the risk for type 1 diabetes.

Caveats of autoantibody testing include the following:

- Variation exists in the sensitivity and specificity of assays. Particularly wide variation is found between different assays for cytoplasmic ICAs. GAD65 autoantibody enzyme-linked immunosorbent assays (ELISAs) are relatively poor, and insulin ELISAs are of little use. AIAA fluid-phase radioassays are easy to perform. Most assays produce labeled autoantigens by transcribing and translating DNA of relevant clones in vitro. These assays are usually performed in a semiautomated 96-well format.
- Insulin autoantibodies cannot be measured after insulin therapy. Within weeks, and certainly within a month, of the institution of insulin therapy, insulin antibodies are produced.
- Expression of insulin autoantibodies is inversely correlated with the age at onset of type 1A diabetes. Thus, this assay is particularly sensitive for children developing type 1A diabetes before age 12 years. However, with excellent insulin autoantibody assays, ~50% of adults developing diabetes also express such antibodies.
- Autoantibodies usually develop sequentially, and the first autoantibody often appears before 3 years of age. In some individuals, the first or subsequent autoantibodies can develop in late adulthood; hence, repetitive testing is necessary.
- The prognostic significance of even multiple autoantibodies in the presence of the protective allele DQB1*0602 is unknown.
- Although most individuals stably express autoantibodies for years to decades before the development of diabetes, as many as 10% of young children may transiently express a single autoantibody.

Metabolic

Loss of first-phase insulin secretion during an intravenous glucose tolerance test (IVGTT) usually precedes the development of type 1A diabetes by several years. Fasting insulin and insulin levels 1 and 3 min after a glucose infusion are typically measured. There is a wide variation in insulin secretion among normal individuals, but patients developing type 1A diabetes often have responses below the first percentile of normal (<48 µU/ml). Normal first-phase insulin secretion in a patient recovering from transient hyperglycemia is one of the best indications that the hyperglycemia will only be transient. Children <8 years old have lower first-phase secretion than adults, particularly on their first IVGTT. Given the variability of the test, at least two tests should be obtained to confirm an abnormality. Among multiple islet autoantibody–positive individuals, the level of insulin release inversely correlates with the approximate time to diabetes.

APPLICATIONS

Physicians caring for patients with type 1A diabetes should make patients and their relatives aware of the symptoms and signs of both type 1 diabetes and associated autoimmune disorders. We generally screen patients every 2 years for the disorders listed in Table 2.1.

Over the next 5 years, the diagnosis of autoimmune type 1 diabetes and other genetic diabetes syndromes will probably play a role in deciding therapy and assessing prognosis for these multiple diabetic disorders. An initial screening of new-onset patients for islet autoantibodies will help discern the subset of children who do not have type 1 diabetes as well as identify adults with type 2 diabetes who have the autoimmune form. With sensitive and specific radioassays for autoantibodies reacting with biochemically characterized autoantibodies, the presence of a single autoantibody would be consistent with autoimmune diabetes.

For children with mitochondrial mutations, associated neurological disorders should be sought (e.g., hearing impairment). With identification of MODY mutations, familial analysis and early diabetes diagnosis will be facilitated. Children with "mild" diabetes caused by glucokinase mutations may require no therapy or respond to oral agents.

Individuals with transient hyperglycemia, where the question concerns the risk of progression to permanent diabetes, can be distinguished on the basis of expression of autoantibodies and whether first-phase insulin secretion on an IVGTT is normal.

An individual being considered as a living kidney donor for a relative with type 1A diabetes should be evaluated for expression of AIAAs and for metabolic function. When possible, relatives donating a kidney should lack high-risk characteristics.

Parents often request HLA typing to assess risk of autoimmune diabetes in siblings of a child with type 1A diabetes. If DQB1*0602 is present in a nondiabetic child, the parents can be reassured that the risk of type 1A diabetes approaches that of the general population (1 in 300). DQB1*0602 is present in ~10% of siblings of patients with type 1A diabetes. The benefit of such testing probably does not justify HLA typing outside of research studies.

With developments in in vitro fertilization and embryo transfer, the question has arisen whether DNA-based typing for diabetes risk of early-stage embryos should be considered. For example, would a family consider selecting embryos with DQB1*0602 or that lack DR3 and DR4? Although DQB1*0602 protects from autoimmune diabetes, it is a high-risk allele for multiple sclerosis.

Determination of biochemical autoantibodies can identify individuals at risk for type 1A diabetes among family members and the general population. A caveat is that expression of a single autoantibody is often associated with a low risk for progression to type 1A diabetes. Expression of no autoantibodies can be reassuring, but autoantibodies can appear later in life. The major benefit of identification of autoantibodies should be the prevention of severe disability or death at presentation in ketoacidosis. This is estimated to occur in ~1 in 200 children presenting with diabetes in the general population. The cons of such testing are potential anxiety and the potential for decreased insurability with "disease" detection. The best rationale for such screening is potential participation in a trial for the prevention of type 1A diabetes. First- and second-degree relatives of patients in the U.S. can be screened for expression of autoantibodies without charge as part of the program by calling 1-800-HALT-DM1.

BIBLIOGRAPHY

Cox NJ, Wapelhorst B, Morrison VA, Johnson L, Pinchuk L, Spielman RS, Todd JA, Concannon P: Seven regions of the genome show evidence of linkage to type 1 diabetes in a consensus analysis of 767 multiplex families. *Am J Hum Genet* 69:820-830, 2001

Diabetes Prevention Trial–Type 1 Diabetes Study Group: Effects of insulin in relatives of patients with type 1 diabetes mellitus. *N Engl J Med* 346:1685–1691, 2002

Eisenbarth GS (Ed.): *Type 1 Diabetes: Cellular, Molecular, and Clinical Immunology.* Available at www.barbaradaviscenter.org

Eisenbarth GS, Gottlieb P: Immunoendocrinopathy syndromes. In *Williams Textbook of Endocrinology.* 10th ed. Larsen PR, Kronenberg H, Melmed S, Polonsky KS, Eds. Philadelphia, W.B. Saunders, 2003, pp. 1763–1776

Falorni A, Nikoshkov A, Laureti S, Grenback E, Hulting A, Casucci G, Santeusanio F, Brunetti P, Luthman H, Lernmark A: High diagnostic accuracy for idiopathic Addison's disease with a sensitive radiobinding assay for autoantibodies against recombinant human 21-hydroxylase. *J Clin Endocrinol Metab* 80:2752–2755, 1995

Kawaskai E, Noble J, Erlich H, Mulgrew CL, Fain P, Eisenbarth G: Transmission of DQ haplotypes to patients with type 1 diabetes. *Diabetes* 41:1971–1973, 1997

Nepom GT: Genetic markers in IDDM: the MHC. In *Prediction, Prevention, and Genetic Counseling in IDDM.* Palmer JP, Ed. Chichester, U.K., Wiley, 1996, pp. 19–26

Pugliese A, Eisenbarth GS: Human type I diabetes mellitus: genetic susceptibility and resistance. In *Type I Diabetes: Molecular, Cellular, and Clinical Immunology.* Eisenbarth GS, Lafferty KJ, Eds. New York, Oxford University Press, 1996, pp. 134–152

Rewers M, Bugawan TL, Norris JM, Blair A, Beaty B, Hoffman M, McDuffie RS Jr, Hamman RF, Kligensmith G, Eisenbarth GS, Erlich HA: Newborn screening for HLA markers associated with IDDM: Diabetes Autoimmunity Study in the Young (DAISY). *Diabetologia* 39:807–812, 1996

Saukkonen T, Savilahti E, Reijonen H, Ilonen J, Tuomilehto-Wolf E, Akerblom HK: Coeliac disease: frequent occurrence after clinical onset of insulin-dependent diabetes mellitus. *Diabet Med* 13:464–470, 1996

She J: Susceptibility to type I diabetes: HLA-DQ and DR revisited. *Immunol Today* 17:323–329, 1996

Verge CF, Gianani R, Kawasaki E, Yu L, Pietroapolo M, Jackson RA, Chase HP, Eisenbarth GS: Prediction of type I diabetes in first-degree relatives using a combination of insulin, GAD, and ICA512bdc/IA-2 autoantibodies. *Diabetes* 45:926–933, 1996

Dr. Eisenbarth is the Executive Director of the Barbara Davis Center for Childhood Diabetes and a Professor at the University of Colorado Health Sciences Center, Denver, CO.

3. Gestational Diabetes Mellitus

THOMAS A. BUCHANAN, MD

DEFINITION AND PREVALENCE

G estational diabetes mellitus (GDM) is defined as glucose intolerance of any severity that has its onset or is first recognized during pregnancy. In essence, GDM occurs in women without known abnormalities of glucose whose circulating glucose concentrations are sufficiently high to impart some increase in perinatal risk to their infants. GDM also occurs in women who themselves are at increased risk for having or developing diabetes when they are not pregnant. The prevalence of GDM varies according to the diagnostic criteria used and the ethnicity of the patient population. When the criteria of the American Diabetes Association (see below) were applied to a Toronto cohort composed predominantly of white women, all of whom had 3-h oral glucose tolerance tests, the prevalence of GDM was 7%. Prevalence rates will likely be higher in ethnic and racial groups in the general population who have higher background rates of diabetes and impaired glucose tolerance.

SCREENING AND DIAGNOSIS

GDM almost never causes symptoms. Accordingly, the American Diabetes Association recommends screening all pregnant women to assess their risk for GDM and testing at-risk individuals' glucose tolerance. The process involves three steps:

1. Evaluate the patient for clinical characteristics that are associated with high, average, or low risk of glucose intolerance.
2. Among women with high or average clinical risk factors for GDM, perform a simple glucose challenge to distinguish women with little or no risk from women with some risk.
3. In the women with some risk, perform a more complicated glucose challenge test to determine whether the individual has GDM.

Specific aspects required for implementation of these three steps are summarized in Tables 3.1 and 3.2.

Table 3.1 Screening for GDM

Clinical Risk Assessment*		
Risk Category	**Clinical Characteristics**	**Recommended Screening**
High risk (any sufficient)	Marked obesity Diabetes in first-degree relatives Personal history of glucose intolerance Prior macrosomic infant Current glycosuria	Blood glucose screening at initial antepartum visit or as soon as possible thereafter; repeat at 24–28 wk if not already diagnosed with GDM by that time
Average risk	Fits neither low- nor high-risk profile	Blood glucose screening between 24 and 28 wk gestation
Low risk (all required)	Age <25 yr Low-risk ethnicity† No diabetes in first-degree relatives Normal prepregnancy weight and pregnancy weight gain No personal history of abnormal glucose levels No prior poor obstetrical outcomes	Blood glucose screening not required

Blood Glucose Screening‡		
Test§	50 g oral glucose challenge, measure serum or plasma glucose 1 h later	
Preparation	None (can be done any time of day)	
Interpretation	Glucose cut point‖	Fraction of women with positive test¶	Sensitivity for GDM¶
	≥140 mg/dl (≥7.8 mmol/l)	14–18%	~80%
	≥130 mg/dl (≥7.2 mmol/l)	20–25%	~90%

Adopted from the summary and recommendations of the 4th International Workshop-Conference on GDM and American Diabetes Association, 2004.
*Performed at initial antepartum visit.
†Ethnicities other than Hispanic, African, Native American, South or East Asian, Pacific Islander, or indigenous Australian, who have increased rates of GDM.
‡Women with very-high-risk clinical characteristics may proceed directly to measurement of fasting glucose or to a diagnostic oral glucose tolerance test (OGTT) (see Table 3.2).
§Performed in patients with high or average clinical risk characteristics.
‖Venous serum or plasma glucose measured by certified clinical laboratory.
¶May vary with ethnicity and with diagnostic OGTT used.

Table 3.2 Diagnosis of GDM

Probable Preexisting Diabetes			
Serum or plasma glucose			
After overnight fast	≥126 mg/dl (≥7.0 mmol/l)		
Random*	≥200 mg/dl (≥11.1 mmol/l)		

GDM			
Procedure	Glucose cut points†		
100-g, 3-h OGTT‡	Time (h)	Glucose (mg/dl)	Glucose (mmol/l)
	Fasting	95	5.3
	1 h	180	10.0
	2 h	155	8.6
	3 h	140	7.8

Data are based on the recommendations of the 4th International Workshop-Conference on GDM.
*Venous serum or plasma glucose measured by certified clinical laboratory; two or more values that meet or exceed cut points are required for diagnosis.
†Outside of formal glucose challenge testing.
‡The glucose cut points for the 75-g, 2-h OGTT are identical to the fasting, 1-h, and 2-h values of the 100-g, 3-h OGTT, and two or more values are required to meet or exceed the cut points for diagnosis.

PATHOPHYSIOLOGY

The Mother

All forms of hyperglycemia result from an imbalance between tissue insulin requirements and the ability of pancreatic β-cells to meet those requirements. GDM is no exception. Physiological studies in several ethnic groups indicate ~50% lower β-cell compensation for insulin resistance in women with GDM compared with women who maintain normal glucose levels in pregnancy. Causes of the β-cell defect in GDM are as varied as the causes of β-cell defects underlying hyperglycemia in other settings. A minority of women have evidence for evolving type 1 diabetes (i.e., circulating antibodies to pancreatic islet cells or antigens). The frequency is highest in populations with the highest rates of type 1 diabetes but does not appear to be >20% in any population (and <5–10% in most). Causes of β-cell dysfunction vary among women without evidence for β-cell autoimmunity. Some have specific genetic problems affecting β-cells, such as genetic variants that also cause maturity-onset diabetes of the young (MODY). Most others have clinical (obesity) and physiological (insulin resistance and poor β-cell compensation) characteristics that suggest evolving type 2 diabetes. At least two studies have shown that women with GDM and characteristics suggesting evolving type 2 diabetes do not have a fixed limitation in insulin secretion. Rather, they can increase or decrease their secretion in response to changes in insulin resistance. They do so, however, at a different glucose set point than normal women. More importantly, the set point changes over time as women with prior GDM lose β-cell function and develop diabetes. Recent evidence from Hispanic women at risk for type 2 diabetes indicates that declining β-cell function is caused or worsened by the high secretory demands placed on β-cells by chronic insulin resistance. Treatment of insulin resistance can preserve β-cell function and delay or prevent diabetes.

The variability in pathophysiology means that clinicians should view GDM not as one disease, but as a montage of virtually all diseases that can cause hyperglycemia. Clinical management during pregnancy is generally aimed at enhancing insulin secretion, which is poor in all patients. Ideally, management after pregnancy should be tailored to the specific disease process(es) causing hyperglycemia and subsequent diabetes in each patient. At the present time, those processes can only be assessed crudely by patients' clinical characteristics. Lean patients of European descent should raise a suspicion of evolving type 1 diabetes. Testing for autoimmune markers of type 1 diabetes can confirm the suspicion. Patients with a strong family history of young-onset diabetes should suggest MODY. No specific interventions have been shown to delay or prevent diabetes in such patients. Obese patients or patients with other evidence for insulin resistance should suggest typical type 2 diabetes, which itself may prove to be a number of diseases when genetic etiologies are worked out. Treatment of insulin resistance after pregnancy appears to reduce the risk of type 2 diabetes in such patients (see below).

The Infant

Development in a diabetic environment can have effects on the human fetus that range from major birth defects and late-term death to mild increases in adiposity. In general, the more severe complications are associated with glycemia in the range of preexisting diabetes (Table 3.2), which is present in a minority of women whose hyperglycemia is first diagnosed during pregnancy. More often, hyperglycemia in GDM is mild and associated with an increased risk of increased fetal size and adiposity. The best evidence suggests fetal overnutrition and hyperinsulinemia as mediators of the excessive growth. The risk of perinatal trauma increases with fetal size, especially at very high birth weights, and cesarean deliveries are often performed to reduce that risk. Unfortunately, there is now good evidence that the diagnosis of GDM per se raises cesarean delivery rates in the absence of increased fetal size. Two important concepts are often overlooked in the antepartum management of GDM. First, the risk of fetal overnutrition increases slowly and continuously with rising maternal glucose levels. Second, different fetuses grow differently in response to the same glucose levels. Thus, there are no true thresholds of glucose that distinguish pregnancies at high risk from pregnancies at low risk for glucose-related perinatal complications. In fact, over the range of glucose levels most often encountered in women with GDM, only a minority of infants are at risk for complications related to maternal hyperglycemia.

In addition to perinatal complications, maternal GDM has been associated with unexpectedly high rates of obesity and abnormalities of glucose tolerance in children and adolescents. The relative contributions of genetics versus exposure to the intrauterine environment of GDM have not been worked out precisely, although it appears that both factors may play a role in the childhood problems.

ANTEPARTUM METABOLIC MANAGEMENT

General Approach

Given the highly variable relationship between fetal growth and related complications on the one hand and maternal glucose levels on the other, the general goal of management of GDM during pregnancy should be to achieve glucose levels that are appropriate to minimize the risk of perinatal complications in each individual pregnancy. This general goal can be achieved by either *1*) treating all women to a glucose level that, on average, results in good perinatal outcomes or *2*) tailoring interventions that modify maternal glucose to the growth pattern of the individual baby. The two approaches are not completely exclusive of one another. For example, glucose measurements can be used to define pregnancies with very high (i.e., in need of metabolic interventions) or very low (no need for intervention) perinatal risks based on glucose alone. Fetal growth characteristics can then be used in the intermediate risk group to identify pregnancies with increased fetal risk that also need intervention despite relatively mild hyperglycemia.

Nutrition Therapy

Diet is often stated to be the cornerstone of therapy for GDM. Nonetheless, there is a paucity of sound scientific evidence based on optimization of perinatal outcomes on which recommendations for dietary management can be based. A standard diet in the third trimester of pregnancy should provide 30–32 kcal/kg body weight. Modifications that lower glucose levels in the mother are *1*) restriction to ~25 kcal/kg body weight for overweight patients, *2*) restriction of carbohydrate to ~40% of calories, and *3*) a focus on complex rather than simple carbohydrates. The only one of these approaches that has been shown to improve perinatal outcomes is the restriction of carbohydrates to ~40% of calories. Nonetheless, all three approaches can be combined to form the basis for general dietary recommendations. Medical nutrition therapy, in which individualized nutritional prescriptions are used to achieve clinical goals (e.g., glucose levels), is a sound approach to dietary management in GDM.

Monitoring Effectiveness of Therapy

The effectiveness of nutrition therapy and/or the need for additional interventions can be assessed in two ways: *1*) by measuring blood glucose concentrations in the mother and *2*) by measuring fetal size and growth patterns. Measurement of blood glucose concentrations can take two general forms: measurements performed in an office or clinic by certified laboratory methods (very accurate but cannot be done often) and self-measurement by the patient (not as accurate but can be done several times each day). If the general approach to management is based solely on maternal glucose levels, than all patients will need to perform glucose self-monitoring to assess whether they are achieving glycemic targets that are, on average, associated with a low risk of perinatal complications. The optimal timing and frequency of monitoring have not been determined. Some studies support a focus on postprandial monitoring, whereas others report good perinatal outcomes when the focus is on premeal monitoring. In reality, the timing of measurements and the glycemic goals together determine average glycemia, which is probably most important to the fetus. Goals recommended by the American Diabetes Association for pre- and postmeal glucose values in women managed according to glycemia alone appear in Table 3.3.

Management that takes into account fetal growth characteristics can be based on laboratory glucose measurements performed at 1- to 2-week intervals combined with assessment of fetal growth. Women who maintain fasting glucose levels of ≥105 mg/dl after initiation of nutrition therapy are at a sufficient risk of fetal complications to warrant intensification of metabolic management, usually with insulin. Women with lower fasting glucose levels can continue nutritional management until ~30 weeks' gestation, at which time fetal ultrasound is performed to measure the abdominal circumference. Pregnancies in which the abdominal circumference is below the 70th percentile for gestational age are at low risk for excessive growth; the mothers can continue nutrition therapy. Pregnancies in which the fetal abdominal circumference is ≥70th percentile are the ones at risk for growth-related complications. These patients should have intensified management, again usually with insulin. When insulin is started, patients should also begin glucose self-monitoring. Glycemic goals can be lowered below those recommended when management is based on maternal glycemia alone (Table 3.3), because there is little, if any, risk of inducing growth retardation by strict glucose control when the baby is already somewhat large.

Intensification of Treatment

Patients in whom maternal glycemia and/or fetal growth indicate a risk of excessive growth despite nutritional treatment should have intensification of their metabolic management. The standard approach and the one for which there is the best evidence of improving fetal outcomes is addition of exogenous insulin. No one regimen has been proven optimally effective, and regimens should be tailored to meet glycemic goals (Table 3.3). Starting doses can be based on observed insulin

---

Table 3.3 Glucose Targets for Antepartum Management of GDM

Approach	Self-Monitored Blood Glucose (mg/dl)*	Self-Monitored Plasma Glucose (mg/dl)*
Maternal glycemia alone†		
Fasting and before meals	≤95	≤105
1 h after meals	≤140	<155
2 h after meals	≤120	≤130
Fetal growth plus maternal glycemia‡		
Fasting and before meals	≤80	≤90
2 h after meals	≤110	≤120

*Refers to product information to determine which type of measurement a given meter makes.
†Adapted from the American Diabetes Association Clinical Practice Recommendations, 2003.
‡For pregnancies identified as at-risk for excessive fetal growth on the basis of ultrasound measurement of abdominal circumference.

requirements in pregnant women, which average 0.6–1.0 units/kg depending on the stage of gestation (i.e., requirements rise during pregnancy). Combinations of intermediate- or long-acting preparations with short- or rapid-acting preparations have been useful to reach glucose targets and improve fetal outcomes. Insulin requirements often fall dramatically at delivery; at the same time, glucose goals become less strict. Thus, insulin can be stopped at delivery to allow reassessment of maternal glucose levels.

Other approaches that have been used to intensify metabolic management include aerobic exercise and glyburide, which does not appear to cross the human placenta in appreciable quantities. Exercise (e.g., 45 min of exercise at ~50% of maximal aerobic capacity three times a week) has been shown to lower maternal glucose levels over 4–6 weeks. Effects on fetal outcomes are not well studied. Glyburide (2.5–20 mg/day) has been reported to achieve glucose control and perinatal outcomes similiar to insulin in one study of women whose glucose levels indicated a need for intensification of metabolic management.

OBSTETRIC MANAGEMENT

Assessment of Fetal Well-Being

The obstetric care provider is generally responsible for determining the mode and frequency of testing of fetal well-being. Several tests exist, and no single approach is superior. The most widely used approaches are as follows:

- *Fetal activity determinations (kick counts):* The patient notes each perceived fetal movement for a specific time interval each day or notes the amount of time that passes before a predetermined number of movements have occurred each day. A decline in the number of movements or an increase in the time it takes to attain the appropriate number of movements prompts the need for one of the tests described below. Fetal activity determinations have a high likelihood of false-positive results, but the test costs nothing and is convenient for the patient.
- *Contraction stress test:* If at least three uterine contractions occur within 10 min, a fetal monitor can be used to evaluate the fetal response to those contractions. Recurrent late decelerations of the fetal heart rate are evidence of fetal compromise. If contractions are not occurring spontaneously, some specialists may use an oxytocin challenge. This test may become abnormal earlier than many of the other tests and, hence, is considered particularly sensitive.
- *Nonstress test:* The fetal monitor is placed, and the patient notes fetal movements. The presence of accelerations of the fetal heart rate in conjunction with fetal movements denotes fetal well-being.
- *Biophysical profile:* This test combines the nonstress test with ultrasound determination of fetal movement, tone, breathing, and amniotic fluid volume. It is sensitive and specific but requires an ultrasound unit and an experienced operator plus a fetal monitor.

Hypertension in pregnancy is defined as a systolic blood pressure of >140 mmHg or a diastolic blood pressure of >90 mmHg on at least two occasions at least 6 h apart. Complications such as hypertension, inadequate diabetes control, or a previous perinatal loss dictate that testing begin sooner and/or be performed more frequently.

Timing and Mode of Delivery

GDM is not of itself an indication for cesarean delivery before 38 completed weeks of gestation. Prolongation of pregnancy beyond 38 completed weeks has been associated with an increase in rates of large-for-gestational-age infants without reducing cesarean delivery rates. Thus, delivery during the 38th week is recommended unless other obstetrical considerations dictate otherwise. Most women can maintain serum or plasma glucose levels <120 mg/dl during labor and delivery without exogenous insulin. In those who cannot, continuous intravenous insulin may be used to lower glucose levels and reduce the risk of neonatal hypoglycemia.

MANAGEMENT AFTER PREGNANCY

The Mother

Nutritional management during breast-feeding should continue as prescribed during pregnancy. Any pharmacological treatments for diabetes can be stopped at delivery to allow reassessment of maternal glycemia in the hospital and, if the mother is not clearly diabetic at that time, at a follow-up visit 1–2 months after delivery. All women with GDM are at increased risk for diabetes, although the type may vary. No data are available on effective diabetes preventatives for women with evidence of autoimmune β-cell dysfunction (evolving type 1 diabetes). Because their course can be relatively rapid, follow-up should be relatively frequent (e.g., at 6-month intervals) for women with clinical characteristics that suggest type 1 diabetes and/or evidence of immunity directed against β-cells (e.g., antibodies to glutamic acid decarboxylase, known as anti-GAD antibodies). Most women have clinical features suggestive of a risk for type 2 diabetes (especially obesity). Current evidence suggests that interventions directed at reducing insulin resistance can delay or prevent diabetes. Regular exercise and weight loss, metformin, and thiazolidinedione drugs have all been effective in this regard. Women should be encouraged to exercise and, if they are overweight, to lose weight. They should be evaluated at least annually for diabetes, but probably more frequently. Rising glucose levels are indicative of progression toward diabetes and should indicate more aggressive efforts at treatment of insulin resistance to prevent diabetes. Because conception of another pregnancy in the presence of even mild diabetes can increase the risk of congenital malformations in the infant, patients should practice effective family planning to ensure that glycemia can be evaluated and optimized before any additional pregnancies. Low-dose combination oral contraceptives do not appear to increase the risk of diabetes after GDM.

The Child

No standard approach to evaluation and management of children of women with prior GDM has been established. Because these children may be at increased risk of obesity and diabetes at a relatively young age, they should have regular assessment of growth and development and be encouraged to pursue behaviors that minimize obesity. Children who are overweight should have regular assessment of glucose levels as well. The role of pharmacological treatment to prevent or delay diabetes in children has not been studied.

BIBLIOGRAPHY

American Diabetes Association: Diagnosis and classification of diabetes mellitus (Position Statement). *Diabetes Care* 27 (Suppl. 1):S5–S10, 2004

American Diabetes Association: Gestational diabetes mellitus (Position Statement). *Diabetes Care* 27 (Suppl. 1):S88–S90, 2004

Buchanan TA, Kjos SL, Schafer U, Peters RK, Xiang A, Byrne J, Berkowitz K, Montoro M: Utility of fetal measurements in the management of gestational diabetes mellitus. *Diabetes Care* 21:B99–B106, 1998

Buchanan TA, Xiang AH, Peters RK, Kjos SL, Marroquin A, Goico J, Ochoa C, Tan S, Berkowitz K, Hodis HN, Azen SP: Preservation of pancreatic β-cell function and prevention of type 2 diabetes by pharmacological treatment of insulin resistance in high-risk Hispanic women. *Diabetes* 51:2796–2803, 2002

Expert Committee on the Diagnosis and Classification of Diabetes Mellitus: Report of the Expert Committee on the Diagnosis and Classification of Diabetes Mellitus. *Diabetes Care* 20:1183–1197, 1997

Jovanovic L, Pettitt DJ: Gestational diabetes mellitus. *JAMA* 286:2516–2518, 2001

Kjos SL, Peters RK, Xiang A, Schaefer U, Buchanan TA: Hormonal choices after gestational diabetes: subsequent pregnancy, contraception and hormone replacement. *Diabetes Care* 21 (Suppl. 2):B50–B57, 1998

Metzger BE, Coustan DR, the Conference Organizing Committee: Summary and recommendations of the 4th International Workshop-Conference on Gestational Diabetes. *Diabetes Care* 21 (Suppl. 2):B161–B167, 1998

Dr. Buchanan is Professor of Medicine, Obstetrics and Gynecology, and Physiology and Biophysics, and Director of the General Clinical Research Center at the University of Southern California Keck School of Medicine in Los Angeles, CA. He is also attending physician at the Los Angeles County—University of Southern California Medical Center.

4. Management of Pregnant Women with Diabetes

E. Albert Reece, MD, MBA, PhD, Carol Homko, RN, PhD, CDE, and Lois Jovanovic, MD

PRECONCEPTIONAL METABOLIC CONTROL AND CONGENITAL MALFORMATIONS

The prevalence of congenital anomalies among children of women with diabetes (except for women with gestational diabetes) is 4 to 10 times higher than that among children of their nondiabetic counterparts. Glycated hemoglobin determinations made at the time of conception and by the end of the first trimester show that the frequency of malformations correlates with the degree of glycemic control rather than with the patient's White's classification.

Evidence suggests that the maternal metabolic milieu has a direct influence on embryogenesis during a critical and vulnerable developmental period. Normalization of blood glucose in the preconceptional period and the maintenance of normal glycemic control throughout this critical phase of organogenesis result in a reduced prevalence of anomalies.

Intensive insulin treatment in periconceptional women improves glycemic control. The goal of preconceptional counseling is to achieve glycemic control before conception.

MANAGEMENT OF UNCOMPLICATED PREGNANT WOMEN WITH TYPE 1 OR TYPE 2 DIABETES

From a management perspective, women with type 1 or type 2 diabetes can be classified into two groups, according to the presence or absence of diabetic vasculopathy. The first group includes White's classes A, B, and C, and the second group consists of classes D, F, FR, and H. The fundamental differences in the management of the two groups are that patients in the second group have advanced disease, requiring more intense evaluation and surveillance, because advanced disease places the pregnancy at a greater risk for both maternal and fetal complications.

The third-trimester mean maternal blood glucose level correlates linearly with the perinatal mortality rate. Other complications associated with maternal hyperglycemia include neonatal hypoglycemia, macrosomia, hyperbilirubinemia, hypocalcemia, erythrocytosis, and respiratory distress syndrome. Therefore, the major management goal of these pregnancies is to achieve and maintain euglycemia.

The recommended management approach for diabetic pregnancy and labor is outlined in Table 4.1 and includes the following:

- Blood glucose levels should be monitored at least four to seven times a day (e.g., before and after each meal and at bedtime) throughout the course of pregnancy.
- Blood glucose goals during pregnancy are 60–90 mg/dl (3.3–5.0 mmol/l) before meals and <120 mg/dl (<6.7 mmol/l) after meals.
- An early ultrasound examination should be performed to date the pregnancy and to establish growth parameters against which future examinations can be compared.
- At 18–22 weeks, all pregestational patients with diabetes should receive a level 2 ultrasound and fetal echocardiogram to rule out malformations.
- Patients should be seen for clinical evaluation every 1–2 weeks (depending on degree of glucose control) until 34 weeks, after which they should be seen weekly.
- Nonstress tests and/or biophysical profiles should be done weekly beginning between 32 and 34 weeks' gestation.
- Because of maternal or fetal indications such as preeclampsia, placenta previa, or poor glycemic control, fetal lung maturity studies should be undertaken for women in poor glucose control or with poor dating when elective delivery is planned.

Table 4.1 Management of Uncomplicated Pregnant Diabetes Patients

White's Classes B and C

- Self-monitoring of blood glucose (four to seven times daily)
- Biweekly visits until 34 wk, then weekly
- Ultrasound: level 2 at ~20 wk, then follow up every 4–6 wk
- Glycated hemoglobin A1C monthly
- Daily fetal movement counts
- Nonstress test at 32–34 wk, then weekly
- Ophthalmologic evaluation, follow up according to findings
- 24-h urine, initially and in each trimester, for protein and CrCl

White's Classes D–FR

- Above, plus electrocardiogram initially; uric acid, liver function test, fibrinogen, fibrin split product determinations; may repeat in each trimester

Delivery time

- Classes A and B: ≤42 wk gestation (if in good glycemic control)
- Classes C–FR: at term or pulmonary maturity

Labor

- Blood glucose to be maintained at ≤90 mg/dl (≤5.0 mmol/l)
- Intravenous normal saline solution to be started at a rate of 7 ml/h and insulin and/or glucose solutions to be administered based on hourly blood glucose checks

Nutrition Recommendations

Pregnancy normally demands an additional intake of 300–400 kcal/day above basal requirements. No further additional calories are required for pregnant women with diabetes. Nutrition recommendations should be determined based on an individualized nutrition assessment. Monitoring blood glucose levels, urine ketones, appetite, and weight gain can be a guide to developing and evaluating an appropriate meal plan and to making adjustments to the meal plan. Weight loss diets should not be prescribed. Three meals a day with one or two snacks are usually sufficient for patients with type 1 diabetes. Snacks may be omitted for patients with type 2 diabetes. A weight gain of 22–30 lb is considered acceptable, with 2–4 lb in the first trimester and 0.5–1 lb per week thereafter.

Exercise

The risk-benefit ratio of either occasional or regular exercise in pregnant women with type 1 or type 2 diabetes is unknown. Pregnancy generally is not a time for a woman who was previously sedentary to initiate strenuous activity. However, active women can continue to do similar activities during pregnancy. General guidelines for exercise during pregnancy are listed in Table 4.2. Exercise should not be prescribed for patients with uterine bleeding, antecedent hypertension, pregnancy-induced hypertension, macrovascular or microvascular disease, autonomic dysfunction, or lack of counterregulatory mechanisms. Supervision is necessary with the prescription of exercise to pregnant women with diabetes.

Insulin

A basal/bolus injection program should be designed for all pregnant diabetic women. In general, two-thirds of the total dose for the day is given in the morning, in a 2:1 ratio of intermediate- to short-acting insulin (e.g., NPH:regular). The remaining third is given before dinner in a 1:1 ratio as short-acting before dinner and NPH at bedtime. This regimen allows for smoother control of fasting blood glucose levels during overnight fasting. Occasionally, patients need to be treated with short-acting insulin before each meal and with intermediate-acting insulin at bedtime.

Table 4.2 Exercise Guidelines for Pregnant Women with Diabetes

- Gradually increase exercise intensity and duration
- Perform recommended exercises: upper-body exercises, swimming, walking
- Monitor blood glucose levels frequently
- Adjust insulin dose and food intake as indicated
- Be aware of the risks of late post-exertional hypoglycemia
- Palpate uterus for contractions
- Carry source of glucose and diabetes identification

New rapid-acting insulin analogs with peak insulin action 1–2 h after injection offer the potential for improved postprandial glucose control and are being increasingly used during gestation. Most studies have demonstrated improved metabolic control with less hypoglycemia and increased patient satisfaction when compared with regular insulin. Few clinical trials to date have been reported using insulin analogs in type 1 or type 2 pregnant women.

Insulin can also be administered continuously through the use of battery-operated pumps, which deliver insulin at a defined rate. Although insulin pumps most closely resemble the physiological insulin secretion of the pancreas, clinical studies have failed to show any significant advantages over multiple daily injections in terms of fetal outcome, mean blood glucose, glycated hemoglobin, or mean amplitude of glycemic excursion. Adverse effects of insulin pump therapy include hypoglycemia and ketosis.

Hypoglycemia. Both chemical and clinical hypoglycemic episodes occur during the course of pregnancy and are believed to result, in part, from intensive insulin treatment aimed at achieving good glycemic control. Insulin clamp studies demonstrate a blunted counterregulatory hormone response in patients with diabetes who experience multiple hypoglycemic episodes. Hypoglycemia has been associated with teratogenic effects in rat offspring; however, there are no clinical data to confirm any potential teratogenic effect of hypoglycemia on human fetuses.

Ketosis. The presence of ketone bodies denotes a state of cellular starvation due to hypoglycemia or to a relative lack of insulin with concomitant hyperglycemia. Ketoacidosis has been associated with a 30–60% fetal mortality rate. Ketonemia may have an adverse effect on neurological development in the fetus. Therefore, ketosis should be vigorously treated and prevented.

MANAGEMENT OF PREGNANT WOMEN WITH DIABETES WITH VASCULOPATHY

Evidence of vascular complications places pregnant women with diabetes in a higher risk category for both maternal and fetal morbidity and mortality. The primary cause of maternal death among pregnant women with diabetes is no longer diabetic ketoacidosis but cardiorenal complications. Similarly, fetal mortality is significantly higher in diabetes patients with vasculopathy than in patients without vasculopathy. Although many organs can be affected by diabetic vascular complications, the kidneys, eyes, and heart are associated with the most significant clinical consequences.

Diabetic Nephropathy

Diabetic nephropathy (White's class F) is one of the most critical complications affecting the outcome of pregnancy and is the leading cause of death in diabetes patients <40 years old. It is characterized by proteinuria (positive reading on Albustix, >300 mg/24-h collection), hypertension, reduced glomerular filtration rate, and end-stage renal disease. Its prevalence rises sharply after 10–15 years of diabetes. Because of the increase in glomerular filtration rate observed and the decreased tubular reabsorption of protein in pregnancy, the diagnosis of diabetic nephropathy in pregnancy is based on a value of >300–500 mg urinary protein per day during the first half of the pregnancy.

The physician caring for the pregnant woman with diabetic nephropathy should be interested in knowing whether pregnancy will alter the course of the renal damage and how the renal involvement will affect the pregnancy. The amount of proteinuria may increase during pregnancy (because of the combination of factors mentioned above) and subsides after delivery. On the other hand, the expected rise in creatinine clearance (CrCl) in pregnancy is only observed in one-third of patients. Whether tighter glycemic control allows for the normal expected rise in CrCl is unknown. The presence of hypertension is associated with heavier proteinuria, lower CrCl, mild azotemia, and poorer neonatal outcomes. The perinatal impact of diabetic nephropathy is outlined in Table 4.3.

The risks of preterm labor, stillbirth, neonatal death, and fetal distress are significantly increased among patients with diabetic nephropathy. However, with contemporary means of evaluation and treatment, perinatal survival in this group can exceed 90% if fetuses are delivered at or after 36 weeks with documentation of lung maturity.

Management should begin before conception with adequate counseling and glycemic control defined as A1C <6.5%. Assessment of kidney function, including a 24-h urine collection every trimester to determine CrCl and the rate of protein excretion, is recommended. Treatment of hypertension is indicated; however, experience with antihypertensive drugs in pregnant diabetes patients is limited. The drugs of choice include methyldopa, arteriolar vasodilators, and β-blockers. Angiotensin-converting enzyme inhibitors have been used in the nonpregnant state but are contraindicated in pregnancy. However, calcium-channel blockers, such as diltiazem, have been shown to decrease excess protein excretion and have not been associated with an increased risk of congenital malformations.

The presence of kidney failure, defined as CrCl <30 ml/min, or creatinine >5 mg/dl (>442 mmol/l), constitutes a particular management problem for patients with diabetic nephropathy. If such patients are seen in a preconception

---

Table 4.3 Perinatal Outcome of Class F Diabetes Patients Compared with Nonnephropathic Pregnant Diabetes Patients

■ No higher prevalence of spontaneous abortions	■ Preterm delivery labor: 25%
■ No higher prevalence of congenital malformations	■ Fetal distress: 30%
■ Increased prevalence of intrauterine growth restriction: 15 vs. 2.2%	■ Superimposed pregnancy-induced hypertension: 40–60%
■ Risk of stillbirth: higher than in diabetes patients without kidney disease	■ Respiratory distress syndrome: 23 vs. 8% of diabetes patients without kidney disease
■ Risk of neonatal death: twice that of diabetes patients without kidney disease	■ Neonatal jaundice: 36 vs. 20%
	■ 3% of babies have developmental problems in childhood; most do well

clinic and are seriously contemplating becoming pregnant, they should be advised to consider kidney transplantation or dialysis before pregnancy. On the other hand, if kidney failure develops during pregnancy, peritoneal dialysis or hemodialysis may be used. Patients with uncontrollable hypertension should be advised against conception.

Retinopathy

Class R diabetes includes pregnant patients with diabetic retinopathy. There are essentially two types of diabetic retinopathy: background diabetic retinopathy, which is nonproliferative, and proliferative diabetic retinopathy. Proliferative diabetic retinopathy is the most frequent cause of blindness among patients with type 1 diabetes, whereas macular edema is the primary cause for patients with type 2 diabetes.

Diabetic retinopathy can progress rapidly over short periods. Recent evidence suggests that there is an increased risk for both the development and progression of retinopathy during pregnancy especially when the glycemia is rapidly normalized. Risk factors for progression include the status of retina at conception, the degree of hyperglycemia, and the duration of diabetes. Therefore, patients with diabetes should have a complete ophthalmologic evaluation at the beginning of pregnancy. Follow-up visits or treatments should be scheduled according to the findings. Although there is no contraindication for laser photocoagulation in pregnancy, not enough data are available regarding the safety of fluorescein use in pregnancy.

Coronary Artery Disease

White's class H diabetes is defined as the presence of coronary artery disease (CAD) in pregnant diabetes patients. CAD occurs more commonly at a younger age and with greater severity in diabetes patients than in nondiabetic patients. Patients are defined as class H if they have a history of myocardial infarction (MI) or angina or if they develop these complications during pregnancy. Particular problems in the diagnosis of class H diabetes result from the inability of most pregnant patients to complete a standard stress-tolerance test. Additionally, neither radioisotopes nor angiography may be used safely to confirm the diagnosis. Therefore, clinicians must rely on signs and symptoms of advanced disease such as angina or MI to diagnose CAD in pregnancy. There are few data regarding the outcome of pregnancy in diabetes patients with CAD. Patients with angina seem to have had better prognoses than patients whose pregnancies were complicated by either a history of MI or the development of MI during pregnancy.

If CAD is diagnosed before pregnancy, patients should be advised against pregnancy. Patients may elect to undergo bypass surgery to improve their overall medical condition. When CAD is first diagnosed during pregnancy, however, management should depend on whether the patient presents with angina or MI.

Patients with angina can be treated with selective β-blockers. In addition, although the use of calcium-channel blockers in pregnancy has not been tested, they may be an appropriate therapeutic choice. MI during pregnancy presents a particularly difficult management problem. The coexistence of pregnancy and

MI is stressful; patients are at an increased risk of dying if they undergo surgery within 3–6 months after MI. This 3- to 6-month period is likely to overlap with the end of the pregnancy. Should the patient require a cesarean section for obstetric indications, the same risk applies. No recommendations can be made as to whether the termination or continuation of pregnancy is preferable.

BIBLIOGRAPHY

American Diabetes Association: *Medical Management of Pregnancy Complicated by Diabetes*. Alexandria, VA, American Diabetes Association, 2000

Bhattacharyya A, Brown S, Hughes S, Vice PA: Insulin lispro and regular insulin in pregnancy. *QJM* 94:255–260, 2001

Chew EY, Mills JL, Metzger BE, Remaley NA, Jovanovic L, Knopp RH, Conley M, Rand L, Simpson JL, Holms LB, Aarons JH, and The NICHD-DIEP: Metabolic control and progression of retinopathy. *Diabetes Care* 18:631–637, 1995

Gordon M, Landon M, Samuels P, Hissrich S, Gabbe S: Perinatal outcome and long-term follow-up associated with modern management of diabetic nephropathy. *Obstet Gynecol* 87:401–409, 1996

Gordon MC, Landon MB, Boyle J, Stewart KS, Gabbe SG: Coronary artery disease in insulin-dependent diabetes mellitus of pregnancy (class H): a review of the literature. *Obstet Gynecol Surv* 51:437–444, 1996

Homko CJ, Khandelwal M: Glucose monitoring and insulin therapy during pregnancy. *Obstet Gynecol Clin N Am* 23:47–74, 1996

Homko CJ, Reece EA: Ambulatory management of the pregnant woman with diabetes. *Clin Obstet Gynecol* 41:584–596, 1998

Jovanovic L, Peterson CM: *DeNovo* hypothyroidism in pregnancies complicated by type 1 diabetes and proteinuria: a new syndrome. *Am J Obstet Gynecol* 159:441–446, 1988

Jovanovic L, Peterson CM: Insulin and glucose requirements during the first stage of labor in insulin-dependent diabetic women. *Am J Med* 75:607–612, 1983

Jovanovic L, Peterson CM: Maternal milk and plasma glucose and insulin levels: studies in normal and diabetic subject.

Jovanovic L, Peterson CM, Reed GF, Metzger BE, Mills JL, Knopp RH, Aarons JH: Maternal postprandial glucose levels and infant birth weight: the Diabetes in Early Pregnancy study. The National Institute of Child Health and Human Development—Diabetes in Early Pregnancy Study. *Am J Obstet Gynecol* 164:103–111, 1991

Jovanovic-Peterson L, Peterson CM: Exercise and nutritional management of diabetes during pregnancy. *Clin Obstet Gynecol* 23:75–85, 1996

Kimmerle R, Heinemann L, Delecki A, Berger M: Severe hypoglycemia incidence and predisposing factors in 85 pregnancies of type I diabetic women. *Diabetes Care* 15:1034–1037, 1992

Kitzmiller JL, Buchanan TA, Kjos S, Combs CA, Ratner RE: Preconception care of diabetes, congenital malformations, and spontaneous abortions. *Diabetes Care* 19:514–541, 1996

Kitzmiller JL, Gavin LA, Gin GD, Jovanovic L, Main EK, Zigrang WD: Preconceptional care of diabetes: glycemic control prevents congenital anomalies. *JAMA* 265:731–736, 1991

Klein BEK, Moss SE, Klein R: Effect of pregnancy on progression of diabetic retinopathy. *Diabetes Care* 13:34–40, 1990

Reece EA, Coustan DR (Eds.): *Diabetes Mellitus in Pregnancy.* New York, Churchill-Livingston, 1995

Reece EA, Homko CJ, Wu YK: Multifactorial basis of the syndrome of diabetic embryopathy. *Teratology* 54:171–182, 1997

Reece EA, Leguizamon G, Homko C: Pregnancy performance and outcomes associated with diabetic nephropathy. *Am J Perinat* 15:413–421, 1998

Rosenn B, Midovnik M, Combs A, Khoury J, Siddiqi TA: Glycemic thresholds for spontaneous abortion and congenital malformations in insulin-dependent diabetes mellitus. *Obstet Gynecol* 84:515–520, 1994

Sadler TW, Hunter ES III: Hypoglycemia: how little is too much for the embryo? *Am J Obstet Gynecol* 157:190–193, 1993

White P: Diabetes mellitus in pregnancy. *Clin Perinatol* 1:331–347, 1974

Dr. Reece is Vice Chancellor and Dean of the University of Arkansas College of Medicine, Little Rock, AR. Dr. Homko is a Nurse Manager at the General Clinical Research Center, a Research Assistant Professor in the Department of Medicine, and a Diabetes Nurse Specialist in the Department of Obstetrics, Gynecology, and Reproductive Sciences at Temple University School of Medicine, Philadelphia, PA. Dr. Jovanovic is Director and Chief Scientific Officer, Sansum Diabetes Research Institute, Santa Barbara, CA.

5. Antepartum and Intrapartum Obstetric Care

DAVID A. SACKS, MD

The best time to begin antepartum care of a woman who has diabetes mellitus is before conception. Both practically and ethically, the woman who has diabetes or who is at substantial risk for developing diabetes in pregnancy should be aware of the additional risks to her life and to that of her unborn child. She should also be aware of the additional diabetes-related workload imposed during her pregnancy (e.g., strict attention to diet, exercise, and glucose monitoring; increased frequency of visits for antepartum testing). She should discuss with her employer the schedule changes necessary for maintenance of health during pregnancy (e.g., allocation of time for snacks, glucose checks, and insulin administration). For all the foregoing reasons, pregnancy for the woman with diabetes should ideally be both intended and planned. Patient preparation for pregnancy should include a frank discussion about and provision of information on family planning, including materials and medications. Ideally, such education should begin at puberty or when diabetes is first diagnosed during a woman's reproductive years. Practically speaking, because a woman's first encounter with her obstetrician/gynecologist often occurs after conception, the burden for conveying this information to the woman with type 1 or type 2 diabetes, impaired glucose tolerance, or a previous occurrence of gestational diabetes most often falls to her generalist, internist, endocrinologist, or pediatric/adolescent specialist. Clearly, this burden may be shared with a perinatologist or obstetrician/gynecologist who is knowledgeable about the care of diabetes during pregnancy. In the interest of brevity, only the additional obstetric care required during pregnancy for a woman who has diabetes will be discussed. A discussion of general obstetric care may be found in standard texts.

PREPARING FOR PREGNANCY

The maternal metabolic milieu before conception may affect both maternal and fetal health. The development of congenital malformations and progression of maternal diabetic ophthalmopathy may be affected by the degree of maternal glycemic control in the weeks immediately preceding pregnancy. Some medications taken for glycemic control or control of vascular complications of diabetes should be replaced by others, particularly during the period of organogenesis.

Congenital Malformations

Birth defects are a major cause of perinatal morbidity and mortality in pregnancies complicated by diabetes. The frequency of major birth defects among infants of diabetic mothers (IDMs) (6–10%) is three to six times that of infants of nondiabetic mothers. Induction of malformations likely takes place from the third to the sixth week after conception, which is the period when organ differentiation takes place. There is a positive relationship between maternal glucose concentrations early in gestation and the incidence of both major malformations and the number of organ systems affected. Although diabetic embryopathy may be found in a number of organ systems, neural tube defects, cardiovascular anomalies, renal anomalies, and caudal dysgenesis appear with disproportionate frequency among IDMs.

Several theories have been explored regarding the mechanisms of development of congenital defects in IDMs. Whereas maternal hyperglycemia is an obvious candidate teratogen, other possible causative elements include β-hydroxybutyrate, somatomedin inhibitors, free oxygen radicals, zinc, branched-chain amino acids, and disordered metabolism of myoinositol and arachidonic acid. Laboratory evidence suggests that maternal hyperglycemia results in disturbed expression of genes that regulate cellular development via a number of different pathways. The final common pathway appears to be programmed cell death (apoptosis). Preimplantation (fertilization to blastocyst) embryopathy has been demonstrated in a murine model. At the blastocyst stage, downregulation of the GLUT1, -2, and -3 transporters resulting in intra-embryonic free glucose has been demonstrated in response to maternal hyperglycemia. Also demonstrated was an increased expression of *Bax*, a preapoptotic protein synthesized at the blastocyst stage. Postimplantation embryopathy may be due to hyperglycemia-induced defective signaling within the yolk sac. A cascade of molecules, that transcribe information from the plasma membrane to the cell nucleus via different pathways has been demonstrated. In the presence of hyperglycemia, downregulation of transcription factors (kinases) involved in cell survival (e.g., ERKs, AKT, and *Pax3*), as well as activation of transcription factors leading to apoptosis (e.g., PKC, p38MAPK, and JNKs), has been described. Death of 60% of the cell mass results in fetal loss or reabsorption. Malformations likely result from the loss of fewer cells within a defined developing organ system (e.g., neural tube or cardiovascular). Respectively, these have been proposed as mechanisms for the increased incidence of miscarriages and malformations in pregnancies of women with diabetes who exhibit hyperglycemia early in pregnancy. Variations in the incidence of both adverse pregnancy outcomes are likely a function of the timing and duration of exposure to maternal hyperglycemia as well as of the actual maternal glucose concentration.

Although evidence is sparse, there does appear to be a glycemic threshold for both spontaneous abortions and congenital malformations. Among women with type 1 diabetes, a median first trimester premeal glucose of ≥120 mg/dl (6.7 mmol/l) was associated with both outcomes. Among women whose diabetes was first diagnosed during pregnancy, a fasting glucose of ≥120 mg/dl (6.7 mmol/l) at the time of diagnosis was also found to be the threshold above which the risk of major malformations increased. Clinical evidence suggests that a program of normalization of glucose before conception will reduce the incidence of major fetal malformations to that of nondiabetic women.

Because human organogenesis begins at the time when the woman first notes missed menses (5 weeks after the onset of the last menstrual period) and is completed 3 weeks thereafter, it seems prudent to assess glycemic control before suspension of the family planning method being used by the woman at risk for early gestational hyperglycemia (i.e., individuals who have type 1 or type 2 diabetes, who had gestational diabetes in a previous pregnancy, or who have impaired glucose tolerance or impaired fasting glucose). Normalization of glucose during the preconception period is virtually risk free, except in women who have type 1 diabetes. For these type 1 patients, the risk of hypoglycemia over an uncertain duration of time before conception must be balanced against the risk of developing fetal malformations. Given the existing evidence, targeting an average premeal glucose of <120 mg/dl and a glycated hemoglobin A1C <1% above the normal range until conception is achieved seems reasonable.

An alternative or ancillary strategy of attempting prevention of congenital anomalies involves dietary supplementation for women of reproductive age. In laboratory animals, reduction in hyperglycemia-induced malformations has been affected by supplementation with myoinositol, arachidonic acid, prostaglandins, and antioxidants (e.g., vitamin E). In addition, a current recommendation for all women of reproductive age is to supplement their diets with 0.4 mg folic acid both before conception and throughout the first trimester. It is also recommended that women who have had babies with neural tube defects take 4 mg/day folic acid during the same time period. Whether either dose decreases the incidence of diabetes-related neural tube defects in humans has not yet been established.

Retinopathy

Diabetic retinopathy can be separated into two broad classifications: baseline (nonproliferative) and proliferative. The earliest ophthalmologic findings related to diabetes include capillary basement membrane thickening and a diminution of pericytes. Microaneurysms then develop in capillary walls at sites previously reinforced by pericytes. These microaneurysms have a variable progression, with some hyalinizing and disappearing and others rupturing and hemorrhaging. Over a period of years, hard exudates, which consist of lipoproteins leaked from microaneurysms into the outer retina, may appear. The exudates and leaked plasma thicken the macula. The resultant macular edema is the primary cause of decreased vision in diabetes patients. Further progression in retinopathy occurs when terminal arterioles thicken and veins become tortuous and their basement membranes thicken. Cotton/wool (soft) exudates appear as a result of infarction of nerve fibers. Extensive areas of nonperfusion may be revealed on examination. Progression in diabetic retinopathy takes the course of neovascularization, with proliferation of vessels from existing veins into the disc or other parts of the retina. Of all the subsequent retinal changes, including fibrosis, gliosis, vitreous hemorrhage, and retinal detachment, the latter two pose a major threat to vision.

Although the independent effect of pregnancy on the development and progression of diabetic eye disease is unclear, pertinent relationships have been demonstrated. The better that maternal glycemia is controlled immediately preceding the pregnancy or during the early part of pregnancy, the less likely the development or progression of retinopathy. The most important predictor of the development or severity of diabetic eye disease is the duration of diabetes. The worse the retinopathy is at the start of pregnancy, the more likely its progression. Less than 15% of women who have no positive retinal findings at the start of pregnancy will develop them in the course of pregnancy, and the development of proliferative retinopathy among these women is extremely rare. The coexistence of hypertension greatly increases the risk of worsening retinopathy during pregnancy. Postulated reasons for progression of retinopathy during pregnancy include the growth hormone–like effect of human placental lactogen as well as increases in other angiogenic factors. A decrease in pregnancy-associated retinal blood flow that is significantly greater in pregnant women with diabetes than in nondiabetic pregnant women may worsen preexisting retinal ischemia. After delivery, some pathologic changes will regress. Overall, pregnancy does not appear to have a deleterious effect on the long-term progression of diabetic retinopathy.

A dilated retinal examination before conception is advisable, as is the treatment of proliferative retinopathy that may be discovered. Women with any degree of retinopathy should be advised that their retinopathy may progress during pregnancy and that they should have periodic dilated retinal examinations during their pregnancies. They should also be aware that proliferative retinopathy may be treated during the course of pregnancy, should it develop.

Nephropathy

Incipient diabetic nephropathy is most often noted ≥5 years after the diagnosis of type 1 diabetes and at any time after diagnosis of type 2 diabetes. Early histological changes include an increase in glomerular size and glomerular capillary surface area accompanied by an increase in glomerular perfusion. Hyperfiltration, characterized by a glomerular filtration rate (GFR) >150 ml/min, accompanied by microalbuminuria (30–300 mg/day) are the hallmarks of this development. Over the next 3–7 years, particularly among individuals in poor glycemic control, the glomerular basement thickens and the mesangium expands. This stage is characterized by a continued increase in GFR as well as exercise-induced proteinuria and the development of hypertension. Overt nephropathy histologically appears as hyalinization of arterioles, further thickening of the glomerular basement membrane, mesangial expansion, and the development of (usually diffuse) glomerulosclerosis. GFR declines and hypertension increases. End-stage renal disease is characterized by a markedly decreased GFR (<10 ml/min and/or a serum creatinine level ≥3 mg/dl) and is often accompanied by a decline in protein excretion. Hypertension often worsens.

Two therapeutic strategies have been advanced to avert diabetic nephropathy. One is the maintenance of good glycemic control. The second is the use of angiotensin-converting enzyme (ACE) inhibitors such as captopril, enalapril, and lisinopril. In addition to their antihypertensive effect, this class of drugs has been shown to prevent progression of diabetic nephropathy. ACE inhibitors exhibit a number of deleterious fetal effects when used from late in the first trimester to early in the second trimester. Likely because of decreased fetal renal arterial perfusion caused by the drug, fetal renal failure and oligohydramnios have been reported. Concomitants of oligohydramnios include pulmonary hypoplasia, limb contractures, craniofacial defects, calvarial hypoplasia, renal tubular dysplasia, and fetal growth retardation. Because of the indefinite duration of the preconception period as well as the fact that the undesired fetal effect of ACE inhibitors does not become manifest until after confirmation of pregnancy, the woman taking a drug of this class is well advised to continue it until pregnant, and then, in concert with her physician, discontinue it and/or substitute another antihypertensive as needed.

Because of the changes in renal physiology that normally accompany it, pregnancy might be thought to exacerbate or induce diabetic nephropathy. In normal pregnancy, by mid-trimester, the GFR increases by 40–100%. Perhaps because of either an increased GFR or a decreased tubular absorption, proteinuria normally increases. Hypertension, which usually promotes the progression of diabetic renal disease, is found in up to 20% of pregnancies among women who have diabetes. However, in several studies, pregnancy has not been found to cause the development or enhance the progression of either incipient nephropathy or end-stage renal disease. In contrast, pregnancy may accelerate the progression of pre-existing overt nephropathy (serum creatinine ≥1.4 mg/dl). Fetal outcome is largely governed by maternal hypertension. The presence of hypertension, either ante-dating or developing during pregnancy, carries with it the risks of fetal growth retardation and both spontaneous and iatrogenic prematurity.

The foregoing considerations indicate that preconception assessment of GFR, protein excretion, and blood pressure will aid in the counseling and treatment of women who have diabetes and are considering pregnancy. Individuals whose renal function is normal and/or who have incipient nephropathy may be reassured that pregnancy likely will not cause the development or progression of kidney damage. Individuals who have overt nephropathy should be cautioned that pregnancy may promote the progression of their diabetes-related renal failure. Data regarding pregnancy in women with diabetes who have had renal transplants or who undergo renal dialysis are sparse and are frequently combined with data of women whose renal disease stems from causes other than diabetes. Available evidence suggests that transplant rejection occurs in <10% of pregnant women and that immunosuppressive drugs appear not to be associated with specific malformations. Pregnant women who have undergone dialysis and/or renal transplants do, however, have an increased incidence of hypertension and preterm delivery.

Hypertension

The background risk for pregnancy-induced hypertension or preeclampsia is about 5%. In women who have type 1 diabetes, the incidence averages 16% in the absence of nephropathy and 51% in its presence. Factors positively associated with preeclampsia include nulliparity, duration of diabetes, poor glycemic control before 20 weeks, proteinuria ≥190 mg/24 h, and nephropathy. While the overall incidence of hypertension during pregnancy among women with type 2 diabetes is similar to that of women with type 1 diabetes, the relative incidence of preeclampsia is less among the former. The insulin resistance of pregnancy augments the intrinsic insulin resistance that characterizes type 2 diabetes. It has been postulated that the consequent maternal hyperinsulinemia results in vascular smooth muscle hypertrophy as well as left ventricular hypertrophy. Insulin also stimulates norepinephrine release and augments transmembrane calcium influx in smooth muscle, thus increasing vascular tone.

The goal of management of hypertension during pregnancy is to prevent its major complications (e.g., cerebrovascular bleeding) while maintaining sufficient systemic maternal blood pressure to adequately sustain fetal oxygenation and nutrition. Whereas the ideal blood pressure for the woman who has diabetes and hypertension is unknown, the target blood pressure of 130/80 mmHg proposed for nonpregnant women seems reasonable during pregnancy also. Adjusting blood pressure before pregnancy not only affords the opportunity to gradually adjust medications, but also to eliminate those that have teratogenic potential and those with which there is little experience during pregnancy. Because there are no randomized controlled trials of drugs given during organogenesis in humans, the antihypertensives used during pregnancy are those with which the greatest amount of experience has been reported. Included among these antihypertensive agents are α-methyldopa, labetalol, and hydralazine. Because the calcium-channel blockers diltiazem and verapamil have been found to retard the progression of diabetic nephropathy as efficiently as ACE inhibitors, they may be reasonable alternatives to ACE inhibitors.

Glycemic Control

In an attempt to prevent or minimize the previously mentioned glycemia-related maternal and fetal pregnancy complications, the same or similar maternal glycemic target values are advised during the preconceptional period as throughout pregnancy (Table 5.1). Although there is much published experience during

---

Table 5.1 Preconception Evaluation and Preparation for Pregnancy for the Woman Who Has Diabetes

Evaluation	Preparation
1. Dilated retinal examination	1. Provision of family-planning information and material until best glycemic control is achieved
2. Blood pressure, cardiovascular, and neurological examination	
3. Renal function tests (e.g., 24-h urine creatinine clearance and protein)	2. Change from oral hypoglycemic agents to insulin
4. Thyroid-stimulating hormone	3. Suggested glycemic goals (plasma glucose)
5. Glycated hemoglobin A1C	▪ Before breakfast: 60–90 mg/dl (3.3–5.0 mmol/l)
6. Electrocardiogram	▪ Before lunch, supper, and bedtime snack: 60–90 mg/dl (3.3–5.0 mmol/l)
	▪ 1 h after meals: <120 mg/dl (<6.7 mmol/l)
	▪ 2:00–6:00 a.m.: 60–90 mg/dl (3.3–5.0 mmol/l)
	4. Control hypertension; discontinue ACE inhibitors (see text)

pregnancy with intermittently injected intermediate- (e.g., NPH) and short-acting (e.g., regular) insulins, there is little experience with some of the insulin analogs and with some of the newer methods of insulin administration. In addition, women with type 2 diabetes may present for care having taken oral hypoglycemic agents.

Insulin lispro, an ultra short-acting insulin, may decrease the frequency of biochemical and severe clinical hypoglycemia in some pregnant women with diabetes. Compared with regular insulin, lispro may also improve overall glycemic control. Although disparate findings have been reported regarding the influence of lispro on maternal diabetic retinopathy and fetal congenital malformations, most evidence suggests neither beneficial nor detrimental effects of this insulin analog on other maternal or perinatal outcomes. Only one randomized controlled trial of the use of lispro during pregnancy in subjects with pregestational diabetes has been reported. There were 33 patients in that study, and randomization was not performed until week 15 of pregnancy. Given the minimum amount of experience with lispro during pregnancy, a conservative strategy would be to limit its use either before or during pregnancy to those women who cannot achieve glycemic goals using conventional insulin regimens and/or those whose glycemic control is achieved at the price of severe hypoglycemia.

Insulin glargine, an analog that provides a continuous depot of insulin, has been reported in rats and rabbits to not be teratogenic. In humans, one case has been reported in which its substitution for other insulin regimens after the 14th week of pregnancy resulted in a decrease in nocturnal hypoglycemia, with no major untoward maternal or perinatal effects. More data are necessary to determine the safety of glargine during pregnancy.

The few publications concerning the use of the insulin pump in pregnancy suggest that maternal and perinatal outcomes as well as maternal glycemic control are not significantly different compared with those of women using multiple-dose insulin therapy. In contrast with the latter, use of the insulin pump requires that patients be highly compliant with dose adjustment, diet, and frequent self-monitoring of blood glucose. A potential advantage of the pump is avoiding extremes of glucose concentrations by adjusting insulin administration to match diet, activity, and self-monitoring of blood glucose measurements in an ongoing fashion. Disadvantages include the potential for pump malfunction and injection site infections, both of which may contribute to rapid development of poor glycemic control.

In nonrandomized studies, the insulin-sensitizing drug metformin has been used to induce ovulation and prevent spontaneous abortion in women with polycystic ovary syndrome. When used throughout pregnancy, metformin has also retarded insulin resistance, insulin secretion, and the development of gestational diabetes in women with polycystic ovary syndrome. However, one retrospective study found a higher incidence of preeclampsia and third-trimester fetal death among pregestational and gestational diabetic women treated with metformin compared with women treated with either sulfonylureas or insulin (Hellmuth et al.). Pending the outcome of a randomized controlled trial, the use of metformin in pregnancy for the treatment of diabetes cannot be recommended at this time.

Only one randomized controlled trial of a sulfonylurea (glyburide) has been reported. In that study, the drug was first given after the 11th week to gestationally diabetic women. There were no significant differences in maternal or perinatal outcomes between the group treated with glyburide and the group treated with insulin. Thus, this drug's known safety in pregnancy is limited to use in gestational diabetes and only after the period of organogenesis.

EARLY PREGNANCY TO THE END OF THE SECOND TRIMESTER

Testing

At the time pregnancy is confirmed, a sonogram should be performed to confirm dates. This will assist in the planning of other maternal and fetal tests that are time sensitive. A second ultrasound examination should be planned during the second trimester, after the fetus is developed enough to enable visualization of sonographically detectable anomalies and early enough to allow the patient to consider the options of pregnancy termination, in-utero treatment, or fetal surgery. Fetal echocardiography and triple-marker screening should also be made available, because malformations of the cardiovascular and central nervous systems comprise a large percentage of the anomalies found among IDMs (Table 5.2). The patient and her family should understand that despite biochemical and sonographic testing, a substantial proportion of fetal anomalies may not be detected before birth.

Glycemic Control

It is virtually axiomatic that normal maternal glucose values should be targeted during pregnancy for the woman who has pre-diabetes and gestational diabetes. A comprehensive program of diet, exercise, and insulin should be used to achieve maternal glycemic goals. The rationale for normalizing glucose during this phase of pregnancy is that of optimizing nutritional programming of fetal growth. Unfortunately, the findings of studies that have attempted to determine normal values during pregnancy have not been uniform; hence, the definition of "normal" remains problematic. As a practical point, for most women with diabetes, the same glucose target values that were used in preparation for conception may be applied throughout pregnancy (Table 5.1). A rationale for this practice is supplied by data from a study of diet- and insulin-controlled gestationally diabetic women tested in the second and third trimesters. Those women whose mean (pre- and postprandial) glucose concentrations fell below 87 mg/dl (4.8 mmol/l) had an increased proportion of small-for-gestational-age neonates; those women whose mean glucose was >104 mg/dl (>5.8 mmol/l) had an increased proportion of large-for-gestational-age babies.

A caveat should be inserted regarding the universal application of the glycemic targets presented in Table 5.1. The normal initial physiological response to hypoglycemia is the release of glucagon. The accompanying epinephrine release is responsible for the autonomic symptoms (i.e., perspiration, palpitations, and tremors) that alert the patient to hypoglycemia and of impending unconsciousness. Patients who have type 1 diabetes often have defective glucagon and epinephrine responses to hypoglycemia. During pregnancy, attempted normalization of maternal glucose may lower the threshold for release of these counterregulatory hormones. Therefore, pregnant women who have type 1 diabetes are at increased risk of unpredictable, sudden, severe hypoglycemia and hypoglycemic unawareness. Although the fetal consequences of maternal hypoglycemia are unclear, maternal seizures, coma, and serious injury due to accidents have been reported. One study found equivalent clinical outcomes (e.g., shoulder dystocia, cesarean delivery, large-for-gestational-age infants, and neonatal hypoglycemia) for women with type 1 and type 2 diabetes, despite the fact that the mean premeal glucose throughout pregnancy was 110 mg/dl (6.1 mmol/l) for type 1 patients and 97 mg/dl (5.4 mmol/l) for type 2 patients. Thus, targeting glucose values during pregnancy that are higher than those presented in Table 5.1 for women who have type 1 diabetes might decrease the incidence of maternal hypoglycemia while not compromising fetal or maternal care.

THIRD TRIMESTER

Efforts during the third trimester are focused on minimizing fetal and neonatal risks. The risks of fetal mortality and of each morbidity may have different maternal glycemic thresholds. Practical considerations require that a single set of maternal glycemic target values be used that are consistent with the minimization of risk of fetal mortality and most perinatal morbidities. With the caveat previously expressed for women who have type 1 diabetes, adherence to the same glycemic goals used earlier in pregnancy seems reasonable (Table 5.1). Selected perinatal problems unique to the woman with diabetes will now be presented. A discussion of the routine aspects of care during the third trimester may be found in standard obstetrics texts.

Fetal Mortality

While great strides have been made in the prevention of fetal mortality in pregnancies complicated by diabetes, an increased frequency of fetal demise unassociated with congenital malformations is still reported among infants of women with type 1 diabetes, type 2 diabetes, and gestational diabetes. A number of factors unique to pregnancy in women with diabetes have been postulated as predisposing to fetal demise. These include thickening of chorionic villi, impeding nutrient and oxygen exchange; fetal insulin-induced visceromegaly, creating increased oxygen and nutrient demands and subsequent metabolic acidosis; and the effects of diabetes-related vasculopathy and/or hypertension, which may also affect the intrauterine milieu. Normalizing the concentration of maternal nutrients therefore remains a cornerstone of fetal therapy during pregnancy.

Although unsupported by definitive evidence of prevention of fetal demise, antepartum testing is widely used in the management of insulin-treated diabetes. Nonstress testing, contraction stress testing, modified and unmodified biophysical testing, and fetal kick counts are widely used. Umbilical artery Doppler studies may be useful in the management of suspected intrauterine growth retardation. A current recommendation is that once- or twice-weekly antepartum testing be initiated starting between 32 and 34 weeks unless additional indications for testing exist. In the latter instance, testing as early as 26–28 weeks may be appropriate.

Fetal Macrosomia

Fetal macrosomia is likely the most frequently investigated and most controversial clinical endpoint in the study of diabetes in pregnancy. No universally accepted definition of this entity exists. Although easily committed to memory, a definition using an absolute birth weight (e.g., 4,000 or 4,500 g) fails to consider the influence of gestational age. Defining a big baby as "large for gestational age" (i.e., >90th percentile birth weight for gestational age) controls for this variable but fails to consider the unique distribution of subcutaneous fat and visceromegaly that often distinguishes the infant of the mother with diabetes. Maternal hyperglycemia has been shown to have an independent positive relationship with fetal macrosomia. Other maternal variables (e.g., age, parity, ethnicity, and prepregnancy weight) are also independent predictors of fetal macrosomia. The relative influence of each of these variables on birth weight is unclear. However, because maternal glycemia is an easily measurable variable that can be controlled during this phase of pregnancy, prudence dictates continued maintenance of maternal glycemic control for the duration of pregnancy.

DELIVERY

Timing of Delivery

The avoidance of fetal demise and the prevention of excessive fetal growth and its concomitants (shoulder dystocia and labor arrest disorders) are the two major rationales offered to support consideration of delivery before the spontaneous onset of labor. In the only randomized controlled trial investigating planned induction of labor for women who have diabetes, birth weights of infants delivered at 38 weeks were significantly lower than birth weights of infants whose mothers were managed expectantly. The three cases of shoulder dystocia were confined to the expectantly managed group. However, there was no difference in cesarean delivery rates between the two groups.

For individuals considering delivery before the spontaneous onset of labor, amniocentesis was previously a routine procedure to ensure that the risk of surfactant-deficient neonatal respiratory distress (RDS) was absent. The combination of the rarity of RDS after 37 weeks, accurate sonographic confirmation of gestational age (Table 5.2), and the availability of an armamentarium of neonatal treatments for RDS suggests that amniocentesis at term (and the accompanying risks) can be avoided in pregnancies of women in good glycemic control.

Maternal indications, such as severe preeclampsia, and fetal indications, such as preterm premature rupture of membranes and/or premature labor, occasionally dictate the necessity of delivery remote from term. A common practice in such instances is to attempt tocolysis (e.g., with magnesium sulfate) and to inject the mother with β-methasone or dexamethasone in an effort to decrease the risk of RDS. Maternal hyperglycemia and ketoacidosis have been reported even in nondiabetic women who have received steroids for this indication. Factors such as the probability of RDS at the given gestational age as well as amniotic fluid assessment for fetal pulmonary maturity should be considered before steroids are

Table 5.2 Evaluation and Care During the First Two Trimesters

Evaluation	2. Triple-marker screen at 16–18 wk
1. Ultrasound	**Treatment**
■ At first visit for dating	1. Diet
■ At 15–20 wk for fetal anatomical survey	2. Insulin
■ Fetal echocardiogram	

Content of Table 5.1 also applies if patient first presents for pregnancy-related care after conception.

administered. Pregnant women with diabetes deemed to be candidates for steroid treatment, especially women who have type 1 diabetes, require extremely close observation of glucose concentrations and frequent adjustment of insulin dosage (Table 5.3). The proposal has been made to empirically augment the insulin dose at the time of administration of β-methasone for women who have type 1 diabetes.

Route and Method of Delivery

Likely because of the increased distribution of truncal and upper-torso sub-cutaneous fat, when matched by birth weight, IDMs have a higher risk of shoulder dystocia than infants of nondiabetic mothers. In addition, the incidence of shoul-

Table 5.3 Preparation for and Management of Delivery

1. Consideration of amniocentesis if
   - Poor glycemic control
   - Remote from term
2. If steroids administered, close observation and control of maternal glycemia for up to 24 h after the last dose, e.g.,
   - Maternal glycemia checks every 1–2 h
   - IV: D_5LR (5% dextrose in lactated Ringers solution) at 125 ml/h
   - IV piggyback insulin with adjustments pending maternal glycemia checks
3. For elective delivery
   - On evening before delivery
     - Usual intermittent-dose insulin and meal plan until midnight
     - Only water by mouth after midnight
     - If using intermittent insulin dosing,

do not take any after midnight
   - If using continuous subcutaneous insulin infusion, do not program morning bolus
   - On day of delivery
     - Blood glucose before starting IV
     - IV: D_5LR at 125 ml/h
     - Continuous IV piggyback insulin starting at 1.0 units/h
     - Check blood glucose hourly until within desired range (e.g., 70–120 mg/dl), then every 2–4 h
     - Pending glucose results, adjust IV insulin infusion up or down from prior dose by 0.2 units/h
4. If patient presents in labor and has taken her insulin that day, manage as in "On day of delivery" above, except check glucose hourly.

der dystocia increases with increasing birth weight. Both ultrasound and manual estimates of fetal weight carry a large margin of error. One cohort study in which fetuses whose sonographically estimated weight was ≥4,250 g had a cesarean delivery before the onset of labor did find a reduction in shoulder dystocia, but at the price of an increased cesarean rate. In addition, nearly half of infants delivered by cesarean section weighed <4,250 g. A current recommendation based on consensus and expert opinion is to not consider planned cesarean delivery for women with diabetes unless the estimated fetal weight exceeds 4,500 g.

Induction of labor has been used in the management of women who have diabetes. The availability of cervical ripening agents, measured intravenous oxytocin administration, and electronic fetal heart rate monitoring makes this an attractive option for delivery before the spontaneous onset of labor. However, it must be noted that among women who experience both spontaneous and induced labor, there is a higher incidence of cesarean delivery if the mother has diabetes than if she does not. The suggestion has been made that the mere knowledge that the patient has diabetes predisposes the obstetrician toward this route of delivery.

The administration of insulin and intravenous dextrose during labor or cesarean delivery requires careful planning and observation. Whereas intraoperative management of fluid and insulin is primarily the responsibility of the anesthesiologist, responsibility for maintenance of maternal glucose concentrations during labor falls on the shoulders of the obstetrician. An approach to the preparation for and management during delivery is presented in Table 5.3. It must be noted that the ideal maternal glucose concentration in the period immediately preceding delivery is not clearly established. However, experience suggests that neonatal hypoglycemia is more closely correlated with maternal glucose concentrations during the intrapartum period than earlier in pregnancy. Maternal hyperglycemia results in fetal hyperglycemia and hyperinsulinemia. Once out of the hyperglycemic maternal milieu, the hyperinsulinemic neonate may drop his or her blood glucose to concentrations <30 mg/dl within 30 min of cord clamping. Sample target glucose values that have been associated with minimized neonatal hypoglycemia are found in Table 5.3.

POSTPARTUM

Immediate Postpartum Period

Even in the face of intravenous glucose administration, maternal glucose has a tendency to fall (often to the nondiabetic range) in the hours immediately after delivery. Because women who have gestational or type 2 diabetes are not prone to ketoacidosis, maintenance of tight glycemic control for the first 24–36 h after delivery is likely not warranted. On the other hand, glycemic control for the woman who has type 1 diabetes during this time period may be problematic. Resumption of intravenous insulin may be considered for the woman who has type 1 diabetes and who is not being fed (e.g., immediately after cesarean delivery). Resuming either intermittent-dose or continuous subcutaneous (pump) insulin beginning at a dose equal to two-thirds the prepregnancy dose is a reasonable approach once regular feedings are resumed.

Breast-feeding is to be encouraged for all women who have diabetes. Besides benefiting their babies, breast-feeding may help lower maternal blood glucose. The potential for baby's hypoglycemia is a theoretical concern if a nursing mother takes oral hypoglycemic agents. Therefore, when medication is required for glycemic control in the breast-feeding mother, insulin use should be considered.

Before Discharge

Because ovulation may resume before the traditional 6-week postpartum visit, a frank discussion with the patient about her family-planning alternatives is advised. Some contraceptives (e.g., injectable agents, pills, and barrier methods) may be started within the first 3–4 weeks after delivery, whereas insertion of the intrauterine device probably should not be done before a 4- to 6-week postpartum visit. Advice should be given to control glucose before discontinuing the family-planning method to minimize the risk of hyperglycemia-associated birth defects with a subsequent pregnancy.

For the woman with pregestational diabetes, a visit with the physician who now assumes responsibility for her diabetes care should be arranged before discharge. A woman who had gestational diabetes should have a glucose tolerance test just before her postpartum visit. At that visit, the results of the glucose tolerance test should be reviewed. Referral to the appropriate caregivers should be made for the woman found to have any degree of glucose intolerance. The now-normoglycemic woman who had gestational diabetes should be encouraged to have her blood glucose evaluated regularly (e.g., annually). All overweight women should be encouraged to enroll in a weight reduction program.

CONCLUSION

The comments and suggestions made in this chapter are based on both published data and clinical experience. It is hoped that they will serve as useful guidelines in the antepartum and intrapartum care of the pregnant woman who has diabetes.

BIBLIOGRAPHY

American College of Obstetricians and Gynecologists: *Antepartum Fetal Surveillance.* ACOG Practice Bulletin No. 9. Washington, DC, American College of Obstetricians and Gynecologists, 1999

American College of Obstetricians and Gynecologists: *Guidelines for Perinatal Care.* 5th ed. Elk Grove Village, IL, and Washington, DC, American Academy of Pediatrics and American College of Obstetricians and Gynecologists, 2002

Hellmuth E, Damm P, Molsted-Pedersen L: Oral hypoglycaemic agents in 118 diabetic pregnancies. *Diabet Med* 17:507–511, 2000

Langer O, Berkus MD, Huff RW, Samueloff A: Shoulder dystocia: should the fetus weighing greater than or equal to 4000 grams be delivered by cesarean section? *Am J Obstet Gynecol* 165:831–837, 1991

Langer O, Conway DL, Berkus MD, Xenakis EM, Gonzales O: A comparison of glyburide and insulin in women with gestational diabetes mellitus. *N Engl J Med* 343:1134–1138, 2000

Okun N, Verma A, Mitchell BF, Flowerdew G: Relative importance of maternal constitutional factors and glucose intolerance of pregnancy in the development of newborn macrosomia. *J Matern Fetal Med* 6:285–290, 1997

Reece EA, Homko CJ: Why do diabetic women deliver malformed infants? *Clin Obstet Gynecol* 43:32–45, 2000

Rosenn BM, Miodovnik M: Glycemic control in the diabetic pregnancy: is tighter always better? *J Matern Fetal Med* 9:29–34, 2000

Rosenn BM, Miodovnik M: Medical complications of diabetes mellitus in pregnancy. *Clin Obstet Gynecol* 43:17–31, 2000

Rosenn B, Miodovnik M, Combs CA, Khoury J, Siddiqi TA: Glycemic thresholds for spontaneous abortion and congenital malformations in insulin-dependent diabetes mellitus. *Obstet Gynecol* 84:515–520, 1994

Wong SF, Chan FY, Cincotta RB, Oats JJN, McIntyre HD: Routine ultrasound screening in diabetic pregnancies. *Ultrasound Obstet Gynecol* 19:171–176, 2002

Dr. Sacks is the Director of the Division of Maternal-Fetal Medicine, Department of Obstetrics and Gynecology, Kaiser Foundation Hospital, Bellflower, CA, and a Clinical Professor at the Department of Obstetrics and Gynecology, Keck School of Medicine, University of Southern California, Los Angeles, CA.

6. Infants of Mothers with Diabetes

Mark R. Mercurio, MD, and Richard A. Ehrenkranz, MD

Approximately 0.2–0.3% of all pregnancies are complicated by overt diabetes, and gestational diabetes develops in an additional 1–5% of pregnancies. Because diabetes in pregnancy is associated with significant perinatal mortality and morbidity, this is clearly an important clinical entity. Common neonatal and fetal problems associated with infants of diabetic mothers (IDMs) are listed in Table 6.1.

PATHOGENESIS

The etiology of fetal and neonatal complications related to maternal diabetes is multifactorial and not completely understood. It is generally accepted that maternal hyperglycemia leads to fetal hyperglycemia, which in turn eventually causes fetal hyperinsulinism. Fetal hyperinsulinism leads to macrosomia with selective organogenesis, leading to problems such as cardiomyopathy and septal hypertrophy. After delivery, the hyperinsulinism can precipitate an abrupt fall in serum glucose unless the interrupted placental supply of glucose is replaced by an alternative glucose source. Hyperinsulinism can also delay pulmonary maturation, and as a result, IDMs are at increased risk for respiratory distress syndrome (RDS) until near term.

Congenital malformations, which account for most of the increased mortality and severe morbidity in IDMs, may be related to increased delivery of glucose and other metabolic substrates across the placenta. Because organogenesis occurs

Table 6.1 Common Fetal and Neonatal Problems Associated with Diabetic Pregnancy

■ Congenital anomalies	■ Macrosomia	■ Hypocalcemia
■ Stillbirth	■ Cardiomyopathy and/or	■ Hyperbilirubinemia
■ Late-gestational death	septal hypertrophy	■ Shoulder dystocia
■ Intrauterine growth	■ Respiratory distress	■ Birth trauma
restriction	■ Polycythemia	■ Renal vein thrombosis
■ Prematurity	■ Hypoglycemia	

in the first 8 weeks of gestation, long before the fetal pancreas can produce insulin, hyperinsulinism is unlikely to contribute to this problem.

Decreased placental blood flow secondary to maternal vascular disease (White's classification R and F) can be a causative factor in intrauterine growth restriction, which may be seen in the more severe cases of overt (preexisting) maternal diabetes.

NEONATAL PROBLEMS AND MANAGEMENT

Obtaining a full maternal history is important, including White's classification and intrapartum maternal blood glucose level and management (e.g., insulin infusion and glucose-containing intravenous fluids). The newborn examination should include evaluation for macrosomia, congenital anomalies, stigmata of growth restriction, and an accurate gestational age assessment. Table 6.2 lists characteristics of infants who should be evaluated and treated in a special-care nursery. In addition, there is evidence that infants with disproportionate macrosomia are at greater risk for acidosis, severe hypoglycemia, and hyperbilirubinemia.

Birth Injury/Asphyxia

Macrosomic infants are at risk for asphyxia and birth injury secondary to difficult delivery. Although these infants may have significant macrosomia, the brain (and therefore the head) is not markedly enlarged, placing the infant at higher risk for shoulder dystocia. Therefore, delivery should take place where trained personnel are available and preparations can be made to deal with a potentially distressed infant.

Hypoglycemia

Within 30–90 min after birth, a newborn's plasma glucose will fall, partly related to cessation of maternal glucose transfer. In the IDM, it is more likely to fall to an abnormally low level because of the persistence of fetal hyperinsulinism. Although it is agreed that significant hypoglycemia can lead to serious neurological morbidity (and rarely mortality) in the newborn, there is no clear

Table 6.2 Indications for Evaluation and Treatment in the Newborn Intensive Care Unit

▪ All infants of insulin-dependent diabetic mothers	−Birth weight <2 kg
	−Weak suck
▪ Infants of gestational diabetic mothers with any of the following complicating factors:	−Tachypnea
	−Risk factors for sepsis
	−Hypothermia
−Preterm birth (<37 wk)	−Poor tone
−Jitteriness	−5-min Apgar score <6
−Tachycardia	−Bradycardia

consensus on the precise definition of hypoglycemia for this age-group. A study of normal full-term newborns from the 1980s, still one of the best and most frequently referenced, indicates that values as low as the high 30s (mg/dl) may be within normal limits in the first hours of life. Although the exact threshold for hypoglycemia is somewhat unclear, it is nevertheless necessary to establish a glucose level below which the asymptomatic newborn requires intervention. Recommendations for this operational threshold in recent years have ranged from 35 mg/dl (2.0 mmol/l) to 45 mg/dl (2.5 mmol/l). We recommend an operational threshold for hypoglycemia in all asymptomatic newborns of 40 mg/dl (2.2 mmol/l), and our recommended management of IDMs reflects an effort to maintain plasma glucose at or above this level. Although a lower threshold for hypoglycemia has previously been used for preterm compared with full-term newborns, there is not adequate evidence to support this practice, and most physicians do not currently recommend it.

Blood glucose measurements depend on factors such as hematocrit, type of sample (plasma, serum, or whole blood), and method of analysis. The rapid reagent-strip methods have a high variance and poor reproducibility, particularly at levels <50 mg/dl (<2.8 mmol/l). A rapid glucose oxidase reagent-strip method for screening should be confirmed by a laboratory glucose determination when an abnormal screening value is obtained. However, treatment should not be delayed while awaiting laboratory confirmation.

The flow diagram in Fig. 6.1 represents one approach to monitoring and responding to blood glucose values in IDMs. Note that this algorithm, and the operational threshold of 40 mg/dl (2.2 mmol/l), are intended for asymptomatic newborns at risk for hypoglycemia. For symptomatic patients, particularly those with signs of hypoglycemia, a higher threshold (45–50 mg/dl [2.5–2.8 mmol/l]) is appropriate. Furthermore, once a patient has demonstrated evidence of significant hypoglycemia requiring intravenous therapy, it is recommended that the glucose level be kept ≥50 mg/dl (2.8 mmol/l). Because a rapid infusion of glucose to treat hypoglycemia may lead to rebound hypoglycemia, such therapy should always be followed by a constant infusion of an intravenous dextrose solution.

Respiratory Distress

Respiratory symptoms may develop in the IDM and may be caused by polycythemia, congestive heart failure, hypoglycemia, sepsis, asphyxia, meconium aspiration, transient tachypnea of the newborn, or RDS. The IDM is known to have delayed lung maturation and inhibition of surfactant production. RDS has been described in IDMs where the amniotic fluid lecithin-sphingomyelin ratio is mature (>2:1) and the phosphatidyl-glycerol is absent. Although it is important to determine the primary cause of the respiratory symptoms, treatment of respiratory distress remains largely supportive.

Congenital Malformations

Initial stabilization should be followed by close examination for congenital malformations. The child born to a mother with preexisting diabetes is at increased risk for malformations such as cardiac anomalies (ranging from severe

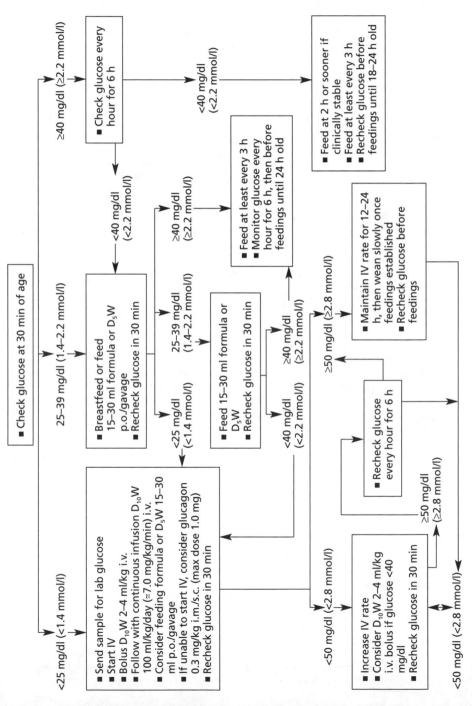

Figure 6.1 Management of asymptomatic hypoglycemia. D₅W, 5% dextrose solution; D₁₀W, 10% dextrose solution.

congenital heart disease to the more common septal hypertrophy), renal anomalies, neural tube defects, and gastrointestinal anomalies. Caudal regression syndrome, which involves hypoplasia of the sacrum and lower extremities, is far more common in IDMs than in infants of nondiabetic mothers, but the overall incidence of this syndrome remains quite low.

The incidence of significant congenital anomalies is increased in overt (pre-existing) maternal diabetes but not in gestational diabetes. This is consistent with causation early in pregnancy, during the period of organogenesis. The frequency of these anomalies can be reduced in overt diabetes by beginning careful diabetic control before conception and maintaining it early in the pregnancy.

Hypocalcemia

Hypocalcemia is defined by a total serum calcium level of <7 mg/dl (<1.75 mmol/l) or ionized Ca <3.5 mg/dl (<0.88 mmol/l). As many as 50% of IDMs may have hypocalcemia. If the patient is asymptomatic, it is probably not necessary to monitor calcium levels or to treat with supplemental calcium. Symptoms such as jitteriness, irritability, seizures, hypotonia, or decreased myocardial contractility indicate that serum calcium levels should be tested. In addition, serum calcium levels should be tested in infants requiring intravenous glucose for hypoglycemia.

Treatment consists of 1–2 ml/kg i.v. calcium gluconate 10% solution, administered initially as a slow infusion, with monitoring of heart rate. This could be followed by 100 mg/kg every 6 h until the hypocalcemia corrects or until total parenteral nutrition including calcium begins. Alternatively, many prefer a continuous infusion of 300–800 mg/kg/day of calcium gluconate, because this may be more effective than intermittent boluses in maintaining an adequate serum calcium level. If hypocalcemia is a persistent problem, hypomagnesemia should be investigated and corrected if necessary.

Polycythemia

Polycythemia is common in IDMs. Treatment consists of a reduction exchange transfusion to lower the hematocrit to 55%. The procedure should be done over 30 min. The volume to be exchanged is calculated by the following formula:

Exchange volume (ml) = [(Hct − 55)/Hct] × weight (kg) × (80–100 ml/kg),

where Hct is the starting hematocrit, and 80–100 ml/kg reflects the blood volume of a baby per kilogram of body weight. Reduction exchange transfusion should be performed if the central Hct is ≥70 in any newborn and for an Hct of 65–69 if there are clinical signs of hyperviscosity (e.g., persistent hypoglycemia). Symptomatic patients with an Hct of 60–64 may also be considered for this procedure.

Hyperbilirubinemia

Hyperbilirubinemia usually results from an exaggerated physiological jaundice, but pathological causes must be excluded. Breast-feeding, though generally the optimum nutrition for most newborns, may exacerbate hyperbilirubinemia. Evidence suggests the diabetic mother's breast milk contains significantly higher concentrations of β-glucuronidase, which may increase enterohepatic circulation of bilirubin. Treatment with phototherapy is almost always sufficient.

Renal Vein Thrombosis

When the symptoms of hematuria, signs of acute kidney failure, and a palpable renal mass are present, especially in the IDM, renal vein thrombosis is likely. Once suspected, a renal ultrasound with Doppler is indicated to confirm the diagnosis.

BIBLIOGRAPHY

Ballard JL, Rosenn B, Khoury JC, Miodovnik M: Diabetic fetal macrosomia: significance of disproportionate growth. *J Pediatr* 122:115–119, 1993

Cordero L, Landon M: Infant of the diabetic mother. *Clin Perinatol* 20:635–648, 1993

Cornblath M, Hawdon JM, Williams AF, Aynsley-Green A, Ward-Platt MP, Schwartz R, Kalhan SC: Controversies regarding definition of neonatal hypoglycemia: suggested operational thresholds. *Pediatrics* 105:1141–1145, 2000

Cornblath M, Ichord R: Hypoglycemia in the neonate. *Semin Perinatol* 24:136–149, 2000

Cowett RM, Loughead JL: Neonatal glucose metabolism: differential diagnosis, evaluation, and treatment of hypoglycemia. *Neonatal Netw* 21:9–19, 2002

Kalhan SC, Parimi PS: Diabetes in pregnancy: the infant of a diabetic mother. In *Neonatal-Perinatal Medicine.* Fanaroff AA, Martin RJ, Eds. St. Louis, MO, Mosby, 2002, p. 1357–1364

Koh THHG: Glucose and the newborn baby: sweet justice? *J Paediatr Child Health* 32:281–284, 1996

Koh THHG, Vong SK: Definition of neonatal hypoglycemia: is there a change? *J Paediatr Child Health* 32:302–305, 1996

Lindsay CA: Pregnancy complicated by diabetes mellitus. In *Neonatal-Perinatal Medicine.* Fanaroff AA, Martin RJ, Eds. St. Louis, MO, Mosby, 2002, p. 277–286

Lucas A, Morley R, Cole TH: Adverse neurodevelopmental outcome of moderate neonatal hypoglycemia. *Br Med J* 297:1304–1308, 1988

Schwartz RP: Neonatal hypoglycemia: how low is too low? *J Pediatr* 131:171–172, 1997

Sirota L, Ferrera M, Lerer N, Dulitzky F: Beta-glucuronidase and hyperbilirubinaemia in breast fed infants of diabetic mothers. *Arch Dis Child* 67:120–121, 1992

Sperling MA, Menon RK: Infant of the diabetic mother. *Curr Ther Endocrinol Metab* 5:372–376, 1994

Srinivasan G, Pildes RS, Cattamanchi G, Voora S, Lillien LD: Plasma glucose values in normal neonates: a new look. *J Pediatr* 109:114–117, 1986

Warshaw JB: Infant of the diabetic mother. In *Oski's Pediatrics: Principles and Practice*. McMillan JA, DeAngelis CD, Feigin RD, Warshaw JB, Eds. Philadelphia, Lippincott, 1999, p. 356–358

Weintrob N, Karp M, Hod M: Short- and long-range complications in offspring of diabetic mothers. *J Diabetes Complications* 10:294–301, 1996

Dr. Mercurio is Associate Clinical Professor of Pediatrics at Yale University School of Medicine, Attending Neonatologist at Lawrence and Memorial Hospital, and Attending Neonatologist at Yale-New Haven Children's Hospital. Dr. Ehrenkranz is Clinical Director, Newborn Special Care, Yale-New Haven Children's Hospital, and Professor of Pediatrics and Obstetrics and Gynecology at Yale University School of Medicine, New Haven, CT.

7. Diabetic Ketoacidosis in Children

FRANCINE KAUFMAN, MD

Diabetic ketoacidosis (DKA) is a common occurrence in pediatric patients with diabetes. At presentation, 25–40% of subjects with type 1 diabetes have DKA, and in established patients, there are ~10–20 episodes of DKA that require hospitalization per 100 patient-years. In addition, in pediatric subjects with type 2 diabetes, 33% have ketonuria and 5–10% have ketoacidosis at diagnosis, with even higher rates described in African-American youth.

DKA is a major source of morbidity and mortality, with 1–2% of patients developing fatal or near-fatal cerebral edema, a complication of DKA and its treatment almost unique to children. As a result, there are aspects of the treatment of DKA that are different in children than in adults, particularly with regard to the rate and composition of initial fluids. The prevention of DKA, however, should be the goal, because despite meticulous attention to its treatment, morbidity and mortality still occur. Hence, DKA accounts for two-thirds of overall childhood diabetes mortality.

DEFINITION

DKA is characterized by the following:

- hyperglycemia with blood glucose usually >300 mg/dl (>17 mmol/l)
- ketonemia with total ketones (β-hydroxybutyrate [βOHB] and acetoacetate) in serum >3 mmol/l
- acidosis with blood pH <7.3 or serum bicarbonate <15 meq/l
- hyperosmolar dehydration with serum osmolality >320 mmol/l

Pure lactic acidosis (blood lactate >7 mmol/l), salicylate ingestion, and non-ketotic hyperglycemic coma should be distinguished from DKA. Occasionally, DKA can occur with near-normoglycemia. Vomiting and poor intake along with continued insulin therapy induce this condition. Hyperosmolar coma can occur in very young children, children with Down's syndrome or significant developmental delay, and adolescents with type 2 diabetes. Nonketotic hyperosmolar coma has been associated with mortality, particularly in obese adolescents at the onset of type 2 diabetes.

PATHOPHYSIOLOGY AND PRESENTATION

The metabolic derangements of DKA result from absolute or relative insulin deficiency amplified by an increased action of the counterregulatory hormones catecholamine, glucagon, cortisol, and growth hormone.

In new-onset patients, signs and symptoms of near-absolute insulin deficiency are often not recognized before the development of DKA. Children and teens presenting to the emergency department with altered level of consciousness should have a fingerstick glucose obtained immediately to determine if diabetes and DKA are present. Individuals presenting with signs and symptoms of the flu should be questioned about antecedent weight loss and polyuria. Failure to consider the diagnosis of diabetes leads to a delay in its diagnosis and a higher incidence of DKA at presentation. In established cases of diabetes, DKA is due to inappropriate sick-day management, intercurrent illness, physical and psychological stress, pump failure, and advertent or inadvertent skipping of insulin doses. Awareness that vomiting is almost universally associated with DKA mandates that, when emesis begins, blood glucose and urine or blood ketones should be tested immediately. If levels are compatible with DKA, immediate action must be taken and contact with the diabetes health care team established so that the safe reversal of early DKA can take place at home.

Normally, insulin is secreted with feeding, and the high-insulin state is associated with anabolism, whereas the fasting low insulin state is associated with catabolism. Increased counterregulatory hormones compound and accelerate the catabolic state. Acting in concert, these hormones do the following:

- increase glucose production by glycogenolysis and gluconeogenesis (catecholamines, glucagon)
- impair glucose utilization by antagonizing the effects of insulin (catecholamines, cortisol, growth hormone)
- mobilize fatty acids by lipolysis (catecholamines, glucagon, growth hormone)
- induce ketogenesis with accumulation of the organic acids βOHB and acetoacetic acid (glucagon)

Excessive production and diminished use of these metabolites lead to hyperglycemia. Polyuria due to osmotic diuresis occurs when the renal threshold of ~180 mg/dl (~10 mmol/l) is exceeded. Osmotic diuresis is associated with electrolyte depletion (Table 7.1). Vomiting occurs and dehydration rapidly progresses. Accumulating organic acids lead to metabolic acidosis with some lactic acidosis from poor perfusion and/or sepsis. Coma is the result of hyperosmolarity (>320 mmol/l) and not of acidosis.

CLINICAL MANIFESTATIONS

Clinical manifestations of ketoacidosis include the following:

- signs of dehydration: delayed capillary refill, postural changes of blood pressure and pulse, dry mucous membranes

Table 7.1 Treatment Approach for Patients with DKA

- Initial approach: in the emergency department
  - Obtain and monitor vital signs, including blood pressure, on all patients.
  - Do a bedside glucose determination to determine glucose level, then monitor at 30- to 60-min intervals.
  - Assess the degree of hydration and mental status.
  - Obtain a urine sample for glucose and acetone; continue to monitor every void.
  - Draw blood for electrolytes, blood urea nitrogen, venous pH, and complete blood cell count.
  - Start an intravenous line and give 10 ml/kg normal saline over 30–60 min.
  - Bolus bicarbonate therapy is contraindicated.
- Begin therapy
  - Use 0.45–0.66% normal saline for maintenance (at a rate of 1.5 maintenance fluid requirements [1,500–2,000 ml/m²]) plus replacement of dehydration over 36–48 h (>2 yr of age: 30 ml/kg for mild deficit, 60 ml/kg for moderate deficit, and 90 ml/kg for severe deficit; <2 yr of age: 50 ml/kg for mild deficit, 100 ml/kg for moderate deficit, and 150 ml/kg for severe deficit).
  - Begin an insulin drip of regular insulin at 0.1 units/kg/h within 2 h of fluid resuscitation (for younger children, the mildly ill, or within 6 h of subcutaneous dose, use 0.05–0.08 units/kg/h).
  - Add potassium chloride at 3–5 meq/kg/24 h to intravenous fluids; potassium phosphate is not standard but may be used for half of potassium dose.
  - Follow laboratory parameters, electrolytes, and pH every 1 h until pH is >7.2, then every 2–4 h, then every 4–6 h.
  - Add dextrose to the intravenous fluids: 5% glucose when the blood glucose level is between 250 and 300 mg/dl and 10% glucose when the blood glucose level is between 180 and 200 mg/dl. Target fall in blood glucose level to 80–100 mg/dl/h.
  - Consider obtaining a urine microscopy/culture, chest X-ray, blood culture, and throat culture.
  - Assess known patients for noncompliance, infection, and trauma.

- signs of acidosis: deep-sighing respirations (Kussmaul) in an attempt to blow off carbon dioxide, shortness of breath, chest pain due to accessory muscle exhaustion
- results of vomiting, dehydration, and hyperosmolality: abdominal pain mimicking pancreatitis or an acute surgical abdomen
- results of counterregulatory hormone release: elevated leukocyte count to 15,000–20,000/mm³
- signs of hyperosmolality: progressive obtundation and loss of consciousness related to the degree of evolving hyperosmolality; serum osmolality calculated as mosM = 2(Na + K)meq/l + glucose (mg/dl)/18

CAVEATS

- The degree of sodium loss may be overestimated because of the presence of hyperlipidemia and hyperglycemia. For each increase in glucose of 100 mg/dl (5.5 mmol/l), serum sodium may be decreased by

~2 meq/l (formula: corrected Na = serum Na + serum glucose mmol/l – 100 mg/dl (5.5 mmol/l)/18). An increase in corrected serum sodium is a goal of therapy.

$$\text{Corrected sodium} = \text{measured sodium} + 1.6 \times \frac{\text{plasma glucose (mg/dl)} - 100}{100}$$

$$= \text{measured sodium} + 1.6 \times \frac{\text{plasma glucose (mmol/l)} - 5.5}{5.5}$$

- Serum potassium may be normal, but total-body potassium is commonly depleted. During acidosis, intracellular potassium moves to the extracellular compartment and may be lost in urine or vomitus. Hyperkalemia in DKA is therefore uncommon unless renal shutdown has occurred. In contrast, hypokalemia may develop rapidly after treatment is initiated because the provision of insulin in the presence of hyperglycemia and the correction of acidosis promote the return of potassium to the intracellular compartment. Hypokalemia may be life-threatening in its predilection for cardiac arrhythmias; therefore, provision of potassium and monitoring of its plasma concentration is paramount in treating DKA.
- Ketone bodies may cause spurious elevation in creatinine values in some assays. Urine and blood ketone tests measure different metabolites: urine ketone tests measure acetoacetate, and blood ketone tests measure βOHB. Because βOHB is the predominant ketone body in DKA, urine measurement may give false-negative results. The concentration of βOHB is 4- to 10-fold higher than that of acetoacetic acid at initial presentation. With correction of acidosis, the βOHB is oxidized back to acetoacetate and is now measured. Hence, physicians should not be misled by the persistence of a strong ketone reaction as long as the patient manifests evidence of clinical and biochemical improvement in acidosis.
- Ketoacidosis takes longer to correct than hyperglycemia. Therefore, insulin therapy should not be discontinued if ketoacidosis has not cleared, even if glucose concentrations are approaching 300 mg/dl (17 mmol/l). Glucose should be provided in the intravenous solutions because the provision of substrate in the form of intravenous glucose and insulin will reverse ketogenesis.
- The provision of excessive chloride is almost inevitable and usually presents no problem, although it can lead to hyperchloremic acidosis in the recovery phase of ketoacidosis. The provision of some of the potassium deficit as potassium phosphate has certain theoretical and possible practical benefits. Potassium acetate has also been used. Acetate provides substrate to correct acidosis.

MANAGEMENT

Table 7.1 outlines the management approach to DKA, which includes correcting hyperglycemia, dehydration, and electrolyte disturbances using intravenous fluids, electrolytes, and insulin. Treatment protocols for adults advocate more rapid and aggressive reversal of DKA than what is recommended for children.

- The initial management is usually begun in the emergency department with isotonic saline. Recommendations vary from 10 to 20 ml/kg of isotonic saline during the first hour, followed by repeat boluses if the patient remains in hypovolemic shock.
- The patient should then be transferred to an appropriate inpatient unit—likely an intensive care unit, where the goal of treatment is to gradually correct the metabolic disturbances of the patient over the ensuing 36–48 h (Table 7.2).
- Within 2 h of presentation, intravenous insulin treatment at a dosage of 0.1 units/kg/h should be begun. A lower dosage of 0.05–0.08 units/kg/h should be considered for children <2 years of age, for those who have had prior insulin administration, and for those mildly ill. Hourly bedside blood glucose determinations help achieve the goal of lowering glucose by 50–100 mg/dl/h. As the glucose levels start to fall, 5 or 10% dextrose is added to the infusion to avoid rapidly lowering the glucose level and to help stabilize blood glucose concentrations between 150 and 200 mg/dl within the first 12–24 h. Maximal substrate (10% dextrose) and intravenous insulin will reverse ketogenesis, halt hepatic glucose production, and facilitate peripheral glucose uptake.
- 0.45–0.66% saline is given for maintenance fluids at a rate of 1,500 ml/m² per 24 h to which the calculated fluid deficit is added to correct dehydration in 36–48 h.
- Patients with DKA have total-body potassium depletion. This depletion can be corrected by infusing potassium chloride at 3 meq/kg/day, started after the patient is transferred. Potassium levels drop during the first 12–24 h concomitant with correction of acidosis and as potassium enters the cells. Potassium infusion often needs to be increased to maintain serum levels >3.5 meq/l. In severe hypokalemia, a cardiac monitor should be used to assess the development of U waves and arrhythmia. If the patient requires >4–5 meq/kg/day, half of the infusion can be given as potassium phosphate and/or acetate.
- The use of bolus bicarbonate in DKA is contraindicated. Hydration and insulin therapy alone will correct the acidosis; bolus bicarbonate places the patient at risk for paradoxical central nervous system acido-

Table 7.2 Criteria for Admission to the Intensive Care Unit

▪ pH <7.2	▪ Prior administration of excess fluids with rapid dropping of glucose level
▪ Age <2 yr	
▪ Unconscious or other neurological symptoms	▪ Low corrected serum sodium
	▪ Administration of bolus bicarbonate
▪ Blood glucose >800–1,000 mg/dl (>43–55 mmol/l)	

sis, cardiac arrhythmias, and hyperosmolality. If used, it should be given at a rate of 40–80 mmol/l over at least 2 h. Rechecking the pH level after the initial provision of a bolus of fluids may document a change in pH sufficient to make further treatment unnecessary.

- Close monitoring of the status of the patient must occur. Obtain hourly bedside blood glucose levels (laboratory values are required if blood glucose is >600 mg/dl). Record accurate input and output of fluid, along with urine glucose, ketones, and specific gravity, with each void. Observe electrolytes and acid-base status at 2-h intervals initially, then at 4- to 6-h intervals. Follow clinical progress and neurological status. Mannitol is available so that it can be rapidly administered at the first sign of neurological deterioration.

COMPLICATIONS

Electrolyte Changes

Inappropriate levels of serum electrolytes, particularly hyperkalemia and hypokalemia, hypophosphatemia, and hypocalcemia, from too vigorous use of phosphate replacement can be avoided by scrupulous monitoring and appropriate adjustment of the electrolyte composition. If acidosis is not resolved, check the composition of the insulin mixture to ensure that an error in dilution has not occurred. If no error is identified and the acidosis is not resolved despite appropriate fluids and insulin, consider the coexistence of severe sepsis causing lactic acidosis and that certain bacteria possess insulin-degrading enzyme activity.

Cerebral Edema

Cerebral edema is the gravest complication of DKA. It occurs in 1–2% of DKA episodes, and the rates of morbidity and mortality are high. The onset is usually within 6–12 h after the initiation of treatment, and the warning signs include headache, lethargy, incontinence, seizures, pupillary changes, decreasing heart rate, and increasing blood pressure (Table 7.3). Retrospective studies have suggested that cerebral edema is associated with fluid administration in excess of 4 l/m^2/24 h or >50 ml/kg over the first 4 h of treatment. In a recent multicenter study, 61 children who developed symptomatic cerebral edema associated with DKA were compared with 181 randomly selected children with DKA and 174 children with DKA, matched for age, new-onset versus known case, initial pH, and initial serum glucose concentration. As given in Table 7.4, multivariate statistical methods showed that children with DKA-related cerebral edema had lower initial PCO$_2$ values and higher serum urea nitrogen concentrations than the control groups. A lesser rise in serum sodium concentration during treatment was seen in children with cerebral edema, although it is unclear whether this was due to therapy itself or to a physiological response to cerebral injury. The administration of bicarbonate bolus was also associated with the development of cerebral edema, suggesting that bicarbonate therapy, for the most part, is contraindicated in children with DKA.

Table 7.3 Signs, Symptoms, and Treatment of Cerebral Edema

Signs and symptoms

In children <10 yr old (especially children <5 yr old), anticipate possible clinical cerebral edema after 4–6 h of treatment. Remember that many children have some change in affect or increase in irritability. For example:

- Headache
- Change in consciousness level/response
- Unequal dilated pupils
- Delirium
- Incontinence
- Vomiting
- Bradycardia

Treatment

- Treat on clinical basis rather than waiting on imaging.
- Reduce intravenous infusion rate.
- Give mannitol 1 g/kg i.v. (or 10–20 g/m^2). Repeat in 2–4 h.
- Consider intubation.

The pathophysiological basis for the development of cerebral edema is incompletely understood. This complication can occur despite meticulous attention to these or any other guidelines. Patients have developed cerebral edema before the institution of treatment. Computed tomography of the head suggests that most patients with DKA have some evidence of raised intracranial pressure due to narrow ventricles during therapy, which then widen when the patient recovers. Individuals experienced in the treatment of DKA in children recognize that most children experience some mild transitory change in affect, state of alertness, or irritability during the course of treatment. Only a few of these patients manifest clinical cerebral edema, which is more common in children <5 years of age and includes the symptoms outlined in Table 7.3. Usually, these are patients with new-onset diabetes whose clinical manifestations occur several hours after the institution of therapy and after clinical and biochemical indexes have suggested improvement. The symptoms and signs of raised intracranial pressure (e.g., headache, deterioration in conscious state, bradycardia, papilledema, development of fixed dilated pupils, and occasionally polyuria secondary to diabetes insipidus) should alert the physician to the existence of this potentially fatal complication. Although the use of magnetic resonance imaging indicates that some children have cerebral thrombosis or infarction in addition to cerebral edema, early intervention with intravenous mannitol, reduction of the intravenous infusion rate, and the institution of hyperventilation are indicated. The diagnosis of cerebral edema remains a clinical diagnosis. Reliance on confirmatory imaging may cause a fatal delay. The dose of mannitol is 10–20 g/m^2 i.v., repeated after 2–4 h if necessary. When instituted promptly (before coma), these measures can be lifesaving and may avoid neurological sequelae. In the case of severe cerebral edema, the use of high-dose dexamethasone therapy should be considered.

The most efficient way to decrease the incidence of cerebral edema is by the prevention of DKA through early diagnosis of diabetes and avoidance of recurrent episodes of DKA by effective patient/family education and support. Recurrent episodes of DKA in a child, particularly an adolescent, should be viewed as a sign that there is inappropriate supervision in the home environment or that the treatment regimen needs to be radically altered.

Table 7.4 Multivariate Association Between Predictive Variables and Cerebral Edema in Children with Cerebral Edema versus Matched Control Subjects

Variable	Relative Risk	95% CI	P
Sex	0.6	0.3–1.4	0.27
Age (per 1-yr increase)	0.9	0.6–1.3	0.53
Initial serum sodium (per increase of 5.8 mmol/l)	0.7	0.5–1.02	0.06
Initial serum glucose (per increase of 244 mg/dl)	1.4	0.5–3.9	0.58
Initial serum urea nitrogen (per increase of 9 mg/dl)	1.8	1.2–2.7	0.008
Initial partial pressure of arterial carbon dioxide (per decrease of 7.8 mmHg)	2.7	1.4-5.1	0.002
Initial serum bicarbonate concentration (per increase of 3.6 mmol/l)	1.2	0.5–2.6	0.73
Rate of decrease in serum glucose during therapy (per decrease of 190 mg/dl/h)	0.8	0.5–1.4	0.41
Rate of increase in serum bicarbonate during therapy (per increase of 3 mmol/l/h)	0.8	0.5-1.1	0.15
Rate of increase in serum sodium during therapy (per increase of 5.8 mmol/l/h)	0.6	0.4–0.9	0.01
Treatment with bicarbonate	4.2	1.5-12.1	0.008
Rate of infusion of intravenous fluid infusion (per increase of 5 ml/kg body weight/h)	1.1	0.4–3.0	0.91
Rate of infusion of sodium (per increase of 0.6 mmol/kg/h)	1.2	0.6–2.7	0.59
Administration of insulin bolus	0.8	0.3–2.2	0.62
Rate of infusion of insulin (per increase of 0.04 units/kg/h)	1.2	0.8–1.8	0.30

Adapted from Glaser et al. 2001.

BIBLIOGRAPHY

Felner EI, White PC: Improving management of diabetic ketoacidosis in children. *Pediatrics* 108:735–740, 2001

Finberg L: Why do patients with diabetic ketoacidosis have cerebral swelling, and why does treatment sometimes make it worse? *Arch Pediatr Adolesc Med* 150:785–786, 1996

Glaser N, Barnett P, McCaslin I, Nelson D, Trainor J, Louie J, Kaufman F, Quayle K, Roback M, Malley R, Kupperman N, for the Pediatric Emergency Medicine Collaborative Research Committee of the American Academy of Pediatrics: Risk factors for cerebral edema in children with ketoacidosis. *N Engl J Med* 344:264–269, 2001

Harris G, Fiordalisi I: Physiologic management of diabetic ketoacidemia: a 5-year prospective pediatric experience in 231 episodes. *Arch Pediatr Adolesc Med* 148:1046–1052, 1994

Harris GD, Fiordalisi I, Harris WL, Mosovich LL, Finberg L: Minimizing the risk of brain herniation during treatment of diabetic ketoacidemia: a retrospective and prospective study. *J Pediatr* 117:22–31, 1990

Kaufman FR, Halvorson M: The treatment and prevention of diabetic ketoacidosis in children and adolescents with type 1 diabetes mellitus. *Pediatr Ann* 28:576–582, 1999

Krane EJ, Rockoff MA, Wallman JK, Wolfsdorf JI: Subclinical brain swelling in children during treatment of diabetic ketoacidosis. *N Engl J Med* 312:1147–1151, 1985

Mahoney C, Vlcek B, Del Aguila M: Risk factors for developing brain herniation during diabetic ketoacidosis. *Pediatr Neurol* 21:721–727, 1999

Marcin JP, Glaser N, Barnett P, McCaslin I, Nelson D, Trainor J, Louie J, Kaufman FR, Quayle K, Roback M, Malley R, Kuppermann N: Factors associated with adverse outcomes in children with diabetic ketoacidosis-related cerebral edema. *J Pediatr* 141:793–797, 2002

Muir A: Cerebral edema in diabetic ketoacidosis: a look beyond rehydration. *J Clin Endocrinol Metab* 85:509–513, 2000

Rosenbloom AL: Intracerebral crises during treatment of diabetic ketoacidosis. *Diabetes Care* 13:22–33, 1990

Rosenbloom AL, Hanas R: Diabetic ketoacidosis (DKA): treatment guidelines. *Clin Pediatr* 35:261–266, 1990

Sperling MA: Diabetic ketoacidosis. *Pediatr Clin North Am* 31:591–610, 1984

Dr. Kaufman is Professor of Pediatrics at the Keck School of Medicine at the University of Southern California and Head of the Center for Diabetes, Endocrinology and Metabolism at Childrens Hospital Los Angeles in Los Angeles, CA.

8. Type 1 Diabetes in Children

WILLIAM V. TAMBORLANE, MD, PATRICIA M. GATCOMB, RN, BSN, CDE,
MARY SAVOYE, RD, CD-N, CDE, AND JOANN AHERN, APRN, MSN, CDE

The adequacy of diabetes care received during childhood may be the most important factor determining whether patients develop the late degenerative complications of diabetes. On the other hand, the rapid physiological and psychosocial changes that occur during childhood and adolescence make these patients the most difficult to manage.

INITIATION OF TREATMENT

Most children with newly diagnosed type 1 diabetes should be admitted to the hospital for initiation of treatment. The diagnosis of type 1 diabetes in a child is a major shock and crisis for the family, who requires time for adjustment and healing. The hospital provides a safe environment for this process to begin. Usually, 2–3 days of hospitalization are necessary to accomplish basic diabetes education and initiation of treatment. A comprehensive day treatment program staffed by a multidisciplinary diabetes team can provide a suitable alternative to hospitalization in newly diagnosed patients who are not in ketoacidosis.

INSULIN THERAPY

The aim of insulin replacement in the treatment of type 1 diabetes is to simulate the fluctuations in plasma insulin levels that are normally seen in nondiabetic individuals (see Chapter 24). However, in the face of the severe insulin deficiency that characterizes type 1 diabetes in youth and practical considerations of acceptability and compliance, the ability to simulate normal insulin profiles may be more limited in young patients. A generally acceptable compromise for newly diagnosed children is a two-injection/day regimen consisting of a mixture of human intermediate-acting (NPH or lente) and short-acting (regular or Humalog) insulin at a total dose of ~1.0–1.5 units/kg/day. Two-thirds of the total is given in the morning before breakfast and one-third as a predinner dose. The starting prebreakfast dose is usually divided in a 2:1 ratio of intermediate- to short-acting insulin, as is the predinner dose. Because of the more rapid onset and shorter duration of action of human NPH and lente, relatively more intermediate- and less short-acting insulin may ultimately be needed. This can be accomplished in the initial dosage-adjustment period by preferentially increasing the doses of intermediate-acting insulin until adequate control of the prebreakfast and predinner plasma glucose levels are achieved. Extra short-acting insulin should then be added, if needed, for control of prelunch and bedtime glucose levels.

Early in the course of the disease, many children go through a "honeymoon" or partial remission phase. This phase is usually heralded by dropping blood glucose levels. At this stage, the evening dose of intermediate-acting insulin should be reduced if nocturnal hypoglycemia is a problem, because residual endogenous insulin secretion helps regulate the fasting glucose level. Most patients also require a reduction in their morning mixture and predinner short-acting insulin. However, evidence supports the concept of aggressive insulin therapy during the early stages of the disease. Such treatment may play an important role in helping to preserve residual β-cell function months or even years after diagnosis, which will in turn facilitate achievement of good diabetes control.

The overall goals of treatment of type 1 diabetes in children and adolescents have changed substantially over the years. The treatment regimen should still be adjusted to minimize symptoms of hypoglycemia and hyperglycemia and promote normal growth and development. With intensive education, independence and self-management can be maximized to reduce the adverse psychosocial effects of this chronic disease. On the other hand, increasing effort is directed toward maintaining blood glucose profiles as close to normal as possible. Steadily increasing doses of insulin are required to meet these aims for several reasons:

- Weight and calorie intake increase with age.
- Residual endogenous insulin secretion declines after the honeymoon period so that most children and adolescents are totally insulin deficient after having had type 1 diabetes for 2–3 years.
- Hormonal and physiological changes of puberty may themselves induce a state of relative insulin resistance.

As a result, the average daily insulin dose in children with long-standing diabetes is ~1 unit/kg body weight, and doses of 1.5–3 units/kg body weight may be required by well-controlled adolescents. These changes in the treatment program are best accomplished by frequent alterations made by the parents or patients themselves with review by the health care provider on at least a 3-month basis. Frequent telephone contact is also helpful.

There are two types of day-to-day adjustments of insulin doses. In patients on two injections/day, small adjustments in the prebreakfast and predinner doses of short-acting insulin can be made if the blood glucose value is outside the target range. If glucose levels are high before breakfast and/or dinner, adjustments in the intermediate- or long-acting insulin are made. Patients and parents should be taught to look for patterns of hyperglycemia or hypoglycemia that indicate a need for adjustment of the usual dose. Dosage changes of 5–10% at a time are usually recommended.

INTENSIFIED INSULIN THERAPY IN CHILDREN AND ADOLESCENTS

More aggressive insulin treatment with a combination of long-acting (ultralente or Lantus), intermediate-acting (lente/NPH), and short-acting (regular or Humalog) insulin; three to four injections/day; or continuous subcutaneous insulin infusion (CSII) with a portable pump can provide means to more closely simulate normal insulin profiles and avoid some of the problems with the standard two-shot schedule. A major problem with twice-daily injections is that the peak of the predinner intermediate-acting insulin may coincide with the time of minimal insulin requirement (i.e., 2:00–4:00 a.m.). Subsequently, insulin levels fall off when basal requirements are increasing (i.e., 4:00–8:00 a.m.). This situation can be avoided if long-acting insulin is used either alone or in combination with an intermediate- and/or short-acting insulin. A three-injection schedule—mixed short- and intermediate-acting insulin at breakfast, only short-acting insulin at dinner, and intermediate-acting insulin at bedtime—may also effectively compensate for these problems. Adding long-acting insulin to the morning injection can help cover late-afternoon snacks (after school) and keep predinner glucose levels normal. Alternatively, long-acting insulin can replace basal insulin and short-acting insulin given with each meal (see Chapter 24). Adherence and compliance issues have been the major obstacles that have limited the use of complex multiple-dose regimens in children. Use of convenience devices such as insulin pens may be helpful.

CSII has also been used sparingly in young patients with type 1 diabetes in the past. There are several problems specific to CSII therapy, particularly in children. It is sometimes difficult to get the personnel at nursery schools, day care programs, or elementary schools to help deliver the bolus doses that must be taken before meals. Young children need help delivering these doses, even when the parent has told them how much to give. This is resolved by working closely with nursery schools, day care programs, and elementary schools. Children are given an insulin-to-carbohydrate ratio that is kept in the pump case or more recently, programmed into the pump along with the correction dose, and the nurse, principal, or director also has one to help the child give the bolus and make corrections for high blood glucose readings. Parents count the carbohydrates and put a card in the lunch bag or send it with the child if he or she is having a hot lunch. Once the school personnel realize that delivering the bolus dose is simple, they are usually very cooperative.

Because only short-acting insulin is used with CSII, any interruption of the flow can lead to ketosis if not corrected swiftly. The solution to this problem lies in meticulous care of the infusion system and frequent blood glucose measurements (at least four times per day, before meals, and bedtime). CSII offers a very attractive alternative to multiple daily injections for children of all ages.

Intensified insulin therapy takes more effort and commitment on the part of patients and their parents, and much support is required from the treatment team. Nevertheless, the results of the Diabetes Control and Complications Trial (DCCT) indicate that such an effort is worth the investment in terms of reduced risk of microvascular complications. In the adolescent subset of patients 13–18 years of age at entry into the DCCT, intensive therapy delayed the onset and slowed the progression of diabetic retinopathy and nephropathy by 60–70%, similar to its effects in adults (see Chapter 26). The benefits of intensive treatment in adolescents appear to outweigh the increased risk of hypoglycemia that accompanies such treatment. It is necessary to extrapolate from this information that, because they will have diabetes for many years, young children should also be treated intensively to reduce the risks of complications. Prepubertal children do develop microalbuminuria, meaning that control matters at the onset of diagnosis.

MONITORING GLUCOSE CONTROL

Self-Monitoring of Blood Glucose

Self-monitoring of blood glucose (SMBG) represents one of the most important advances in diabetes management. To be helpful, SMBG must be performed accurately and frequently, and the results must be interpreted correctly. The parent or child must be taught what a normal blood glucose value is so that he or she understands the glucose target, the degree to which levels should be expected to vary, and what the relationship is between blood glucose and diet, insulin, and exercise.

All patients should perform at least four blood tests daily (before each meal and at bedtime) and record them in a logbook. These data are used to make ongoing adjustments to the insulin regimen. Waning enthusiasm for performing blood testing may result in less frequent monitoring or even falsification of SMBG data. This is more of a problem in children and adolescents than in adults with diabetes, and it remains a formidable obstacle impeding achievement of targeted levels of glycemic control. It is therefore essential to involve children or adolescents in their own care and constantly remind them why this is such an important component of their treatment.

Glycated Hemoglobin A1C Levels

Glycated hemoglobin A1C (A1C) levels should be obtained regularly (every 3 months) because they provide an index of glucose control over the preceding 4- to 8-week period. Measurement of A1C complements SMBG by providing a relatively simple way to independently and objectively assess diabetes control. Discrepancies between SMBG and A1C results are more commonly due to problems with the former than with the latter. A1C levels in the normal range are difficult to achieve in children and adolescents, except during the honeymoon period. When patients and parents have the ability to frequently contact a diabetes expert by phone, the chances of achieving normal A1C levels are greatly increased. Even in adults with type 1 diabetes enrolled in intensive treatment programs, A1C values usually hover around or are modestly above the upper limit of normal. Because the DCCT results indicate that the rate of progression of retinopathy is correlated with mean A1C levels, successful efforts in lowering A1C values should be accompanied by a corresponding decrease in the risk of onset and/or progression of such complications.

DIET

Dietary guidance for children with type 1 diabetes requires careful instruction and frequent reinforcement. Involvement of a registered dietitian who is knowledgeable about and comfortable working with children is strongly recommended (see Chapter 17). A meal plan should be based on the child's usual food intake and used as a basis for incorporating insulin therapy into typical eating and exercise patterns. The success of the nutritional program may ultimately depend on the degree to which the meal planning is individualized and tailored to well-established eating patterns in the family and how well the child and parents understand carbohydrate counting. If understood by both parent and child, adjustments in insulin can be made more readily. Moreover, flexibility can be enhanced if blood glucose–monitoring results are used to evaluate the impact of change in dietary intake. As with other aspects of the treatment regimen, we preach consistency of carbohydrate intake and teach how to adjust for deviations from the usual intake.

EXERCISE

Regular exercise and active participation in organized sports has positive implications concerning the psychosocial and physical well-being of young patients (see Chapter 18). Aerobic endurance exercise is preferred over weight lifting and other activities that involve straining and increased systemic blood pressure. Patients should be advised that different types of exercise may have different effects on blood glucose levels. For example, sports that involve short bursts of intensive exercise (e.g., hockey) may increase rather than decrease blood glucose levels. On the other hand, long-distance running and other prolonged activities are more likely to lower blood glucose levels.

Patients and parents should be warned that exercise may have a prolonged effect for up to 24 h. Some children and adolescents remain euglycemic during exercise but become hypoglycemic hours later; therefore, it is important to check glucose levels frequently when beginning a new exercise—even once in the middle of the night.

At some centers, patients are discouraged from exercising if they are hyperglycemic (i.e., have a blood glucose level >240 mg/dl [>14 mmol/l]). This is because, in someone who is underinsulinized, glucose will rise with exercise because a certain amount of insulin is needed for glucose to enter the muscles. If the high glucose occurs because the child has skipped an insulin dose, he or she should not exercise. If the hyperglycemia is merely food related and there is sufficient circulating insulin, it is safe and even beneficial to exercise. Exercise should be encouraged unless the patient is insulin deficient, not feeling well, or ketotic.

ROUTINE OUTPATIENT CARE

Children and adolescents with type 1 diabetes should be routinely referred to a diabetes center that uses a multidisciplinary team knowledgeable and experienced in the management of young patients. This team should ideally consist of a pediatric diabetologist, nurse educators, dietitians who are certified diabetes educators, social workers, psychologists, and exercise physiologists, and referral resources for ophthalmology, neurology, nephrology, and other problems.

During the first few weeks after diagnosis, patients and parents should maintain close follow-up with the treatment team. This is a critical period for the child and parent to learn the principles of adjusting insulin dosage and overall diabetes self-management. The parent or older child should be in daily telephone contact with the clinician. Clinical well-being, monitoring results, and the effect of changes in diet and exercise should be reviewed. The patient's thoughts about changes in the insulin regimen should be sought before making recommendations. The timing of phone calls should be prearranged and ideally made to the same clinician each day. Usually within 1–2 weeks, the children (and parents) will feel more confident and should be able to make their own insulin adjustments.

Subsequently, regular follow-up on a 2- to 3-month basis is recommended for each patient. The main purpose of these visits is to ensure that the patient is achieving the primary treatment goals of normal growth in the absence of significant symptomatic complaints related to hyperglycemia or hypoglycemia. In addition to serial measurements of height and weight, particular attention should be paid to monitoring of blood pressure and examinations of the thyroid and injection sites. Limited mobility of the joints of the fingers in association with waxy thickening of the skin can indicate increased susceptibility to the microvascular complications of type 1 diabetes. Signs and symptoms referable to diabetes complications are sought. Such surveillance is complemented by laboratory tests to measure lipids and thyroid levels annually. Urine should be checked for microalbumin, and a dilated eye exam should be performed on an annual basis after 5 years' duration. Tissue transglutaminase should be obtained annually to check for celiac disease, since this disease is becoming more common in individuals with diabetes. Routine outpatient visits provide an opportunity to review glucose monitoring and to adjust the treatment regimen. Follow-up advice and support should be given by the registered dietitian, diabetes nurse specialist, and mental health professional.

HYPOGLYCEMIA

The nonphysiological nature of conventional insulin replacement and relatively large insulin doses required by children and adolescents, defective glucagon responses, irregularities in diet and exercise, unreliability of blood glucose monitoring, and other problems contribute to the vulnerability of young patients to severe reductions in plasma glucose. Severe hypoglycemia is a more common problem in patients striving for strict glycemic control with intensive treatment regimens. In adolescents and adults in the DCCT, the risk of severe hypoglycemia was threefold higher in intensively treated patients than in conventionally treated patients. On the other hand, brisk epinephrine responses are commonly observed in children with poorly controlled diabetes, even when plasma glucose falls into the normal range, which can confuse the clinical assessment of hypoglycemic symptoms and emphasizes the need for accurate blood glucose monitoring.

Treatment of a mild to moderate reaction consists of at least 15 g carbohydrate (60 kcal) (e.g., orange juice, regular soda, glucose tablets). If the child is on an insulin pump, only 8 g carbohydrate is required. Candy bars or special treats are not recommended because they do not raise glucose quickly enough because of the fat content. Also, children may pretend to be hypoglycemic to get these types of treats, so it is important to find a way to incorporate these foods into their usual treatment plan. Children should carry glucose tablets to treat hypoglycemia efficiently and effectively. Friends should also be aware of how to treat low blood glucose levels. The child should not walk to the nurse's office while hypoglycemic. Glucose should be checked in the classroom or treatment should be given without verification.

Proper insulin and dietary adjustments should be made to prevent further hypoglycemia. Parents must be taught how to inject glucagon for treatment of more severe reactions. They can also administer a quick glucose solution (e.g., honey, glucose gel, cake icing) to the lips and cheeks.

SICK-DAY GUIDELINES

Children with intercurrent illnesses such as infections or vomiting should be closely monitored for elevations in blood glucose levels and ketonuria. On sick days, blood glucose should be checked every 2–4 h, and urine should be checked for ketones every 3–4 h. Supplemental doses of short- or intermediate-acting insulin (0.1–0.3 units/kg) should be given every 2–4 h for elevations in glucose and ketones. If the patient uses an insulin pump and large or moderate ketones are present, the patient must change the site, double the correction bolus, and enter a temporary basal rate of double the usual basal for 3 h. This can usually be managed at home. Adequate fluid intake is essential to prevent dehydration. Fluids such as Gatorade, flat soda, clear soups, popsicles, and gelatin water are recommended to provide some electrolyte and carbohydrate replacement. If vomiting is persistent and ketones remain large after several supplemental insulin doses, arrangements should be made for parenteral hydration. Recurrent episodes of ketonuria and vomiting are usually the result of missed insulin doses or overall poor metabolic control.

BIBLIOGRAPHY

Ahern JA, Boland EA, Doane R, Ahern JJ, Rose P, Vincent M, Tamborlane WV: Insulin pump therapy in pediatrics: a therapeutic alternative to safely lower HbA1c levels across all age groups. *Pediatric Diabetes*, 3:10–15, 2002

Ahern JA, Grey M: New developments in managing children with insulin-dependent diabetes mellitus. *J Pediatr Health Care* 10:161–166, 1996

Ahern JA, Tamborlane WV: Steps to reduce the risks of severe hypoglycemia. *Diabetes Spectrum* 10:39–41, 1997

Boland E, Ahern JA: The use of CSII in a young adolescent with diabetes mellitus. *Diabetes Educ* 23:52–54, 1997

DCCT Research Group: The effect of intensive treatment of diabetes on the development and progression of the diabetic complications in adolescent subjects in the Diabetes Control and Complications Trial. *J Pediatr* 125:177–188, 1994

Sperling MA: Diabetes mellitus. In *Clinical Pediatric Endocrinology.* Kaplan SA, Ed. Philadelphia, Saunders, 1990, p. 127–164

Tamborlane WV, Ahern JA: Insulin dependent diabetes in children. In *Current Therapy of Endocrinology and Metabolism.* 6th ed. Bardin WC, Ed. Philadelphia, Mosby-Yearbook, 1997, p. 413–418

Tamborlane WV, Amiel SA: Hypoglycemia in the treated diabetic patient: a risk of intensive insulin therapy. *Endocrinol Clin North Am* 21:313–327, 1992

Dr. Tamborlane is Professor of Pediatrics at Yale University School of Medicine, New Haven, CT. Ms. Gatcomb, Ms. Savoye, and Ms. Ahern are members of the Yale Type 1 Diabetes Treatment Team.

9. Psychosocial Adjustment in Children with Type 1 Diabetes

BARBARA J. ANDERSON, PHD, JOSEPH I. WOLFSDORF, MD, AND ALAN M. JACOBSON, MD

Daily treatment of children with diabetes affects and intrudes on everyday behavior in the family, alters family routines, and affects relationships among family members. How the family handles these intrusions determines the effectiveness with which childhood diabetes is managed. This chapter addresses these issues from a developmental perspective by examining the changing tasks of different-aged children and their families.

CRISIS AT DIAGNOSIS

The diagnosis of diabetes in a child or adolescent hurls the parent from a secure and known reality into a frightening and foreign world. At diagnosis, they grieve the loss of their healthy child and cope with such normal distress reactions as shock, disbelief and denial, fear, anxiety, anger, and extreme blame or guilt. However, while grieving, parents are expected to acquire an understanding of the disease and behavioral skills to manage the illness at home and to assist the child in achieving acceptable blood glucose control.

Parents should receive the emotional support required to begin coping with the emotional distress and not be overwhelmed by unrealistic expectations from a well-meaning diabetes treatment team (Table 9.1). Parents must find a sense of balance after the diagnosis and should be encouraged to progress at their own pace, with emotional support offered by a staff member or another parent.

Table 9.1 Recommendations for the Diabetes Treatment Team at Diagnosis

- Give the parent time to "grieve the diagnosis."
- Limit guidelines to basic skills.
- Keep to a minimum the number of medical staff providing information and treatment.
- Include both parents, in some fashion, in the diabetes education program.
- Encourage, in single-parent families, another adult (e.g., a grandparent or neighbor) to support the parent.

DIABETES AND CHILD DEVELOPMENT

Diabetes presents family members with the task of being sensitive to the balance between the child's need for a sense of autonomy and mastery of self-care activities and the need for ongoing family support and involvement. The struggle to balance independence and dependence in relationships between the child and family members presents a long-term challenge and raises different issues for families at different stages of child and adolescent development. Focusing on normal developmental tasks at each stage of the child's growth and development provides the most effective structure with which to address this concern.

INFANTS AND TODDLERS WITH DIABETES (0–3 YEARS OLD)

At this earliest stage of child development, the parent is the only appropriate patient with respect to diabetes management. Researchers have identified several problems facing parents of infants and toddlers with diabetes (Table 9.2).

Children diagnosed before age 5 years may be at risk for specific subtle cognitive deficits caused by recurrent severe hypoglycemic episodes. This relates to difficulties in administering and adjusting the small insulin doses needed by most infants and toddlers, as well as the preverbal child's inability to recognize and communicate symptoms of hypoglycemia.

At this stage of development, two important aspects of care are 1) how treatment responsibilities are shared between parents and 2) the prevention of severe hypoglycemic episodes. The primary developmental task during infancy is to achieve a stable, trusting relationship between infant and primary care provider.

The central task of the child from age 1 to 3 years is to establish an initial sense of mastery over the world. Toddlers do not have the cognitive skills to understand why cooperation with the intrusive, sometimes painful, procedures of the diabetic regimen is needed. Thus, injections or fingersticks for blood glucose monitoring may become battlegrounds when the toddler resists and will require significant emotional stamina by the parent.

PRESCHOOLERS AND EARLY-ELEMENTARY SCHOOLCHILDREN WITH DIABETES (4–7 YEARS OLD)

Nursery school, day care, or kindergarten may represent the first arena in which both parents and children face the social consequences of diabetes, including the need to educate others about the disease (Table 9.2). Thus, separation problems that often appear in children this age may be heightened in the child with diabetes.

Children who are 4–7 years old are beginning to use cause-effect thinking. Thus, the young child with diabetes may blame himself or herself for having the disease or see injections and restrictions as punishments. Youngsters with diabetes at this age may benefit from informal contact and group interactions with other children with diabetes.

Table 9.2 Challenges Facing Parents and/or Children with Diabetes

Parents of infants and toddlers (0–3 yr old)

- Monitoring diabetes control and avoiding hypoglycemia
- Establishing a meal schedule despite the child's normally irregular eating patterns
- Coping with the very young child's inability to understand the need for injections
- Managing the conflicts with older siblings that result from unequal sharing of parental attention

Preschoolers and early-elementary schoolchildren (4–7 yr old)

- Mastering separation from the family and adapting to the expectations of teachers
- Blaming self for having diabetes; regarding injections and restrictions as punishments
- Educating school personnel, coaches, and scout leaders about diabetes (parents)

Later-elementary schoolchildren (8–11 yr old)

- Engaging in a wide range of activities with peers
- Learning about the benefits of intensive diabetes management (child and parents)

- Becoming involved in diabetes self-care tasks (selecting snacks, selecting and cleaning injection sites, and identifying symptoms of low blood glucose) while sustaining parent involvement in major tasks

Early adolescence (12–15 yr old)

- Integrating physical changes into self-image and body image
- Acknowledging that the young teenager is on the threshold of becoming an adult (parents)
- Renegotiating parents' and young adolescents' roles in taking responsibility for diabetes management in the face of physiological changes caused by puberty, which complicate matters
- Fitting in with the peer group
- Maintaining good glycemic control while concerned about possible weight gain

Later adolescence (16–19 yr old)

- Making decisions regarding post–high school plans
- Living more independently of parents
- Strengthening relationships with fewer friends
- Assuming more independent responsibility for health and health care

---

At this stage of development, parents continue to be the primary recipients of diabetes education and to interact with the health care team. However, the child's increasing motor coordination and cognitive skills enable him or her to become a more involved partner in diabetes self-care tasks. Children can select appropriate snacks, select and clean injection sites, and begin to identify symptoms of low blood glucose. The goal is for elementary school–aged children to be positively drawn into their own care without premature and unrealistic expectations for independence while parental control and supervision continue.

LATER-ELEMENTARY SCHOOLCHILDREN (8–11 YEARS OLD)

The preadolescent child forms close friendships with children of the same sex, strives to gain approval from this peer group, and seriously begins to evaluate himself or herself by comparing abilities to those of peers. Children with diabetes, in the process of making these social comparisons, need to develop a strong positive self-image. In fact, preadolescent children with diabetes with adjustment problems may often be overlooked because they are not overtly rebellious and hostile, but rather are overdependent on family members and withdrawn from peers. Participation and positive self-image are key concepts at this age, and health care providers should emphasize to parents the importance of the child with diabetes participating in a wide range of activities with peers.

Parents should focus diabetes education on realistic blood glucose goals and safety guidelines for prevention of hypoglycemia. That is, parent and child should be ready to increase monitoring of blood glucose and plan ahead for additional snacks with extra activity.

It is important to continue emphasizing the long-term benefits of continued diabetes care. Children this age can check blood glucose levels and give injections on occasion without supervision. Health care providers should negotiate more directly with the child concerning issues and problems with diabetes rather than talking solely to the parents.

EARLY ADOLESCENCE (12–15 YEARS OLD)

At this stage of development, dramatic changes typically occur in five areas:

- physical development
- family dynamics
- school experiences
- cognitive development
- social networks

During all of these normal changes of early adolescence, the change in balance of responsibility for diabetes management tasks continues between the child and the family. It is common for families to change their expectations of the young adolescent and frequently "turn over" responsibility for diabetes management. However, physiological changes of puberty, which are associated with insulin resistance in both nondiabetic and diabetic adolescents, can complicate this transition. Reduced sensitivity to insulin probably contributes significantly to the difficulty experienced by many young adolescents in achieving optimal glycemic control.

If the diabetes care regimen makes a teen stand out from the peer group, conflicts can arise. Some teenagers may stop their self-care and try to prove they are "normal." Others may use diabetes as an excuse to withdraw. Many who never before hid their diabetes may now refuse to talk about it with friends.

Young teenagers have an increasing cognitive ability to analyze themselves and the world around them and do not accept authority, but rather examine, criticize, and question. This growing ability leads many teenagers with diabetes to a new sensitivity about their disease (e.g., for the first time, they may vent their anger about having diabetes at parents). Parents and health care professionals frequently overestimate the teenager's conceptual understanding of diabetes. Parents also can overestimate the adolescent's ability to follow through with diabetes care tasks without immediate positive reinforcement and support, mistakenly assuming that long-term good health will provide motivation for adherence to the diabetes treatment plan.

Diabetes can further threaten the young teenager's self-confidence. Fluctuating blood glucose levels that defy control contribute to younger teenagers feeling uneasy in their bodies. Insulin reactions, injections, and blood glucose monitoring can further undermine the child's ability to feel attractive or normal. Concerns about body image must be taken seriously by parents and health care providers. For example, a problem seen frequently in young adolescent girls who are distressed about weight gain is a dramatic increase in blood glucose levels. When adolescent girls are worried about their weight, and parents and the health care team focus exclusively on good control, many patients begin to secretly reduce their insulin and thereby purge calories and lose weight. This self-destructive behavior is a form of bulimia nervosa, and this diabetes-specific eating disorder may cause repeated hospitalizations for diabetic ketoacidosis in adolescent girls.

Because puberty causes such physiological barriers to controlling blood glucose and because of the psychological and social vulnerabilities of this age, parents should continue involvement in and supervision of insulin administration and blood glucose testing throughout early adolescence. Negotiation of continued support and supervision is critical even if the young adolescent initially rejects it. Likewise, parents should recruit participation from the child even if the notion is rejected initially. Negative family interactions surrounding diabetes management contribute to compliance and metabolic control problems in adolescents with diabetes. The key is that both adolescents and parents must redefine their roles and renegotiate a balance of responsibility for diabetes that is acceptable to both parties.

Families should also be encouraged to change their pattern of relationships with diabetes health care providers. Young teenagers often have issues (e.g., concerns about sexuality) that they do not feel comfortable discussing in front of parents. Thus, health care providers should begin seeing parents and young teenagers individually and sequentially.

Both young adolescents and their parents may benefit from contact with other families coping with similar struggles. Diabetes camps often provide an important forum for peer identification, and peer-group educational and support programs may be helpful for both children and parents.

LATER ADOLESCENCE (16–19 YEARS OLD)

As growth and change decrease and stabilize, so do conflicts over diabetes self-care. The central developmental tasks of the older adolescent are outlined in Table 9.2.

Some older teenagers with diabetes who feel overwhelmed with the pressures of high school and the need to plan for the future may ignore their self-care. When peer relationships are insecure or schoolwork seems beyond their abilities, some teenagers may use their diabetes to avoid the conflicts at school. Some older teenagers with poor metabolic control reflect a chronic unmet need for more family support for self-care tasks. Poor control in a teenager can be a reflection of chaos and dysfunction at home. In these instances, more (not less) parental involvement may be needed. Family counseling can help parents and teenagers negotiate adjustments.

Table 9.3 Families Benefiting from Additional Psychosocial Support

- All families at the time of diagnosis
- Single-parent families
- Families in which another member has a serious chronic physical illness (includ-ing diabetes) or mental illness (includ-ing a learning disability)
- Families with infants and toddlers with type 1 diabetes

Conflicts over friendships are the primary cause of alienation between parents and teenagers. This is especially true when issues of alcohol and drugs, safety (driving), and sexual activity are raised. Older teenage girls (and their parents) should be educated about the importance of good metabolic control before conception and about the difficulties of managing a diabetic pregnancy.

During this stage of development, growth and the upheaval of puberty slow and insulin needs stabilize. Many older adolescent girls continue to be concerned about weight gain caused by insulin dose increases and a meal plan that provides significantly more calories than needed to meet the requirements of accelerated growth. Patients should be evaluated for insulin manipulation whenever poor metabolic control remains unexplained in an adolescent girl concerned about her weight. More gradual separation from medical providers is not a sign of psychological problems or overdependence. Expectations are that the older adolescent can manage diabetes with less parental involvement; however, each family situation must be assessed individually.

REFERRAL TO A MENTAL HEALTH PROFESSIONAL

Several types of families should be considered high risk and may benefit from additional psychosocial support resources and more frequent appointments with the health care team (Table 9.3). Similarly, several warning signals are used to identify a child (Table 9.4) or family (Table 9.5) for whom mental health intervention is required.

Table 9.4 Risk Factors Related to Individual Children

Children and their families should be referred for counseling if any one of the following is present:

- Failure to master the tasks of normal child or adolescent development
- Identification of the child/adolescent as a "problem" by the legal system or school (extended school absences, school failure)
- Serious depression, anxiety, learning disability, or other severe mental disorder
- Inability to show age-appropriate cooperation with the tasks of diabetes care
- More than one diabetes-related hospitalization for unexplained causes during a 1-yr period
- Weight loss and chronic hyperglycemia (elevated A1C), especially in adolescent girls

A1C, glycated hemoglobin A1C.

Table 9.5 Risk Factors Related to the Entire Family

Family therapy is recommended if any one of the following problems is present:

- Prolonged intense conflict between parent and child over division of responsibilities for diabetes care tasks
- Life crisis, such as divorce or death of family member, that causes severe grief reactions within family
- Suspicion of child sexual/physical/emotional abuse or neglect, which should also be reported immediately to state legal authorities

BIBLIOGRAPHY

Amiel SA, Sherwin RS, Simonson DC, Lauritano AA, Tamborlane WV: Impaired insulin action in puberty: a contributing factor to poor glycemic control in adolescents with diabetes. *N Engl J Med* 315:215–219, 1986

Anderson B, Coughlin C, Goldberg E, Laffel L: Comprehensive, family-focused outpatient care for very young children living with chronic disease: lessons from a program in pediatric diabetes. *Children's Services: Social Policy, Research, and Practice* 4:235–250, 2001

Anderson BJ, Ho J, Brackett J, Finkelstein D, Laffel L: Parental involvement in diabetes management tasks: relationships to blood glucose monitoring adherence and metabolic control in young adolescents with insulin-dependent diabetes mellitus. *J Pediatr* 130:257–265, 1997

Jacobson AM: Psychological care of patients with insulin-dependent diabetes mellitus. *N Engl J Med* 334:1249–1253, 1996

Rydall AC, Rodin GM, Olmsted MP, Devenyi RG, Daneman D: Disordered eating behavior and microvascular complications in young women with insulin-dependent diabetes mellitus. *N Engl J Med* 336:1849–1854, 1997

Wolfsdorf JI: Improving diabetes control in adolescents with type 1 diabetes. In *Practical Psychology for Diabetes Clinicians.* 2nd ed. Anderson B, Rubin R, Eds. Alexandria, VA, American Diabetes Association, 2002, p. 149–160

Wolfsdorf JI, Anderson BJ, Pasquarello C: Treatment of the child with diabetes. In *Joslin's Diabetes Mellitus.* 13th ed. Kahn CR, Weir GC, Eds. Philadelphia, Lea & Febiger, 1994, p. 530–551

Dr. Anderson is Associate Professor of Pediatrics at Baylor College of Medicine, Houston, TX. Dr. Wolfsdorf is Associate Professor of Pediatrics at Harvard Medical School, Boston, MA. Dr. Jacobson is Professor of Psychiatry at Harvard Medical School and Senior Vice President at the Joslin Diabetes Center, Boston, MA.

10. Psychosocial Aspects in Adults

LAWSON R. WULSIN, MD, ALAN M. JACOBSON, MD,
AND MARK F. PEYROT, PhD

ORIGIN OF PSYCHOSOCIAL COMPLICATIONS

Diabetes itself does not cause specific psychiatric illness or changes in personality beyond the general effect of chronic illness, which increases the risk for psychiatric disorders. However, particular subgroups of the diabetic population are at risk for developing psychosocial complications. Women with type 1 diabetes mellitus seem to have a higher prevalence of eating disorders (e.g., anorexia nervosa and bulimia), and those with long-standing diabetes and major medical complications have a higher prevalence of symptoms of depression and anxiety. The estimated prevalence of major depression in patients with diabetes is 20%, which is double the prevalence in individuals without chronic disease. Depression is associated with poorer glycemic control, and recovery from depression is associated with improvements in glycemic control. The mechanism for depression's contribution to hyperglycemia is not established but may include the well-documented alterations in the autonomic regulation of catecholamines and cortisol during a major depressive episode. Depression is also associated with an increased risk for diabetes complications, so good management of diabetes includes the management of comorbid depression.

Stress

Stress is one of many factors that may interfere with glycemic control. Two pathways, one behavioral and one humoral, mediate the effect of stress on glucose levels. Stress may cause the person to change key behaviors that upset self-care habits, e.g., increased alcohol intake or decreased exercise. Alternatively, stress hormones (e.g., catecholamines and cortisol) directly alter glucose levels in response to stress.

Barriers to Self-Care

Psychological and social factors influence a patient's success in adhering to any prescribed self-care regimen (Table 10.1). Rubin and Peyrot (2001) have documented that patients often have beliefs about diabetes that are inconsistent with

---

Table 10.1 Barriers to Self-Care

Patient attitudes and beliefs that affect self-care	Psychosocial factors affecting self-care
▪ Anticipating an early cure ▪ Believing that self-care regimen is too difficult ▪ Believing that treatment is unlikely to improve or control health problems	▪ Stressful events in a patient's life ▪ Development of new complications ▪ Availability and quality of social support for the patient ▪ Psychiatric problems unrelated to the patient's diabetes ▪ Health care provider's approach to medical care

---

provider perspectives. Several medical problems can be reliable indicators of psychosocial barriers (Table 10.2).

Detection of Psychosocial Factors

The framework that favors early detection of complicating psychosocial factors is an effective working relationship with the patient and regular monitoring visits. Periodically, examine the patient's psychological functioning by asking open-ended questions (Table 10.3):

- Ask patients to describe any stressful events or situations.
- Determine whether patients have adequate social and family support.
- Ask about problems concerning mood, anxiety, and sense of well-being.
- Ask young women who might be at risk for eating disorders whether they have skipped insulin doses, dieted excessively, eaten in binges, or vomited.
- Engage the patient, and at times the family, in monitoring behaviors or events in addition to glucose levels.

Because depression is common and detrimental, all patients with diabetes should be screened for depression initially and at times of illness progression. The Beck Depression Inventory or the PHQ-9 are useful screening and monitoring measures for depression.

Inquiries along these lines collect practical information that guide interventions and build the collaborative alliance. Over time, this alliance may lead to bet-

---

Table 10.2 Medical Problems Indicating Psychosocial Barriers to Diabetes Control

▪ Recurrent hypoglycemia ▪ Frequent episodes of ketoacidosis	▪ Very high glycated hemoglobin levels ▪ Brittle diabetes

Table 10.3 Open-Ended Questions for Patients with Self-Care Problems

Practitioners should ask for the patient's perception regarding the following:

- Importance of glycemic control
- Feasibility of adhering to a prescribed diet
- Importance of self-monitoring of blood glucose
- Susceptibility to developing complications
- Efficacy of treating complications
- Reasonableness of practitioner's recommendations and expectations

ter glycemic control by helping the patient address such self-care barriers as low motivation, preconceived judgments about treatment, and fears about diabetes.

THERAPY

Table 10.4 summarizes the major principles of effective glycemic control when psychosocial factors impair that control. The first six steps are behavioral and focus on accomplishing a goal; the latter two steps recognize the importance of maintaining a strong long-term working relationship. Changing behavior to improve adherence is a complex task requiring assessment of readiness for change, tailoring interventions to the patient's stage of readiness, and motivating patients to take the appropriate next steps for behavior change. This process has been well described in *Changing for Good* by Prochaska et al. (1994).

A systematic approach to glycemic control following these principles may require a considerable initial investment of time and energy from the patient and clinician. The physician or diabetes educator should coordinate the effort,

Table 10.4 Guidelines for Improving Adherence to Diabetes Regimens

- Give specific instructions, written and oral, about who will do what, tailored to the patient's specific needs and situation.
- Train the patient and family in the skills necessary for the regimen and monitoring.
- Monitor self-care behaviors in several ways by several people.
- Increase the frequency of self-care behaviors with reminders.
- Reinforce or reward steps toward adherence to the regimen.
- Begin with small tasks and achievable goals; shape behaviors with successive revisions of the plan or contract as short-term goals are met.
- Meet the patient at the level of effort the patient is prepared to make.
- Avoid chastising patients when they fail to achieve a goal; instead, revise the goal or the approach.

From Wulsin and Jacobson 1988.

delegating responsibilities to the appropriate people and communicating the current plans to all involved. All team members can be helpful in carrying out the plan once it has been developed.

Diabetes self-help support groups are effective resources for patient education and for improving adherence to regimens.

The treatment of comorbid depression is essential to good diabetes management. Cognitive behavioral therapy and selective serotonin reuptake inhibitors have been shown to be effective in resolving depressive episodes as well as improving glycemic control. Exercise also can have the twin benefit of reducing depression and improving physical health.

REFERRAL TO A SPECIALIST

The practitioner will need to identify, for possible referral, mental health professionals who are knowledgeable about diabetes and who can serve as collaborators in treating the patient. The following individuals may need to be referred to a specialist:

- patients who have had two or more episodes of severe hypoglycemia or diabetic ketoacidosis without obvious causes in 1 year
- patients whom you find frustrating
- patients with comorbid psychiatric disorders that complicate the management of diabetes

BIBLIOGRAPHY

Anderson RJ, Freedland KE, Clouse RE, Lustman PJ: The prevalence of comorbid depression in adults with diabetes: a meta-analysis. *Diabetes Care* 24:1069–1078, 2001

Bradley C: Psychological aspects of diabetes. In *The Diabetes Annual.* Vol. 1. Alberti KGMM, Krall LP, Eds. New York, Elsevier, 1985, p. 374–388

Jacobson AM, Hauser S, Anderson B, Polonsky W: Psychosocial aspects of diabetes. In *Joslin's Diabetes Mellitus.* 13th ed. Kahn C, Weir G, Eds. Philadelphia, Lea & Febiger, 1994, p. 431–450

Kroenke K, Spitzer R, Williams JBW: The PHQ-9: validity of a brief depression severity measure. *J Gen Intern Med* 16:606–613, 2001

Lustman PJ, Clouse RE, Griffith LS, Carney RM, Freedland KE: Screening for depression in diabetes using the Beck Depression Inventory. *Psychosom Med* 59:559–560, 1997

Prochaska, James O, Norcross, John C, DiClemente, Carlo C: *Changing for Good: A Revolutionary Six-Stage Program for Overcoming Bad Habits and Moving Your Life Positively Forward.* New York, Avon Books, 1994

Rubin RR, Peyrot M: Psychological issues and treatments for people with diabetes. *J Clin Psychol* 57:457–478, 2001

Wulsin LR, Jacobson AM: Management of stress and glycemic control in diabetes. *Intern Med Specialist* 9:100–116, 1988

Dr. Wulsin is an Assistant Professor of Psychiatry at the University of Cincinnati, Cincinnati, OH. Dr. Jacobson is a Professor of Psychiatry at Harvard Medical School and Senior Vice President at the Joslin Diabetes Center, Boston, MA. Dr. Peyrot is a Professor of Sociology at the Center for Social Research, Loyola College, Baltimore, MD.

11. Diabetic Ketoacidosis and Hyperosmolar Hyperglycemic State in Adults

SAUL GENUTH, MD

DIABETIC KETOACIDOSIS

Diabetic ketoacidosis (DKA) occurs in 2–5% of patients with type 1 diabetes per year. Death due to failure of or delay in diagnosis, complications associated with treatment (such as hypokalemia), or precipitating comorbid conditions such as sepsis still occur in 1–10% of DKA patients, depending on treatment circumstances and locale. The pathophysiology of DKA is presented in Chapter 7.

DIAGNOSIS

Any person presenting with the following should have an immediate screening of blood or urine glucose and urine ketones:

- coma
- shock
- dehydration
- respiratory distress
- any other evidence of major illness

If this simple rule is followed, new-onset cases of diabetes that present in DKA should never be missed.

Any known diabetes patient with nausea or vomiting, abdominal pain, central nervous system (CNS) depression, shortness of breath, fever, localized signs of infection, or unexplained blood glucose >250 mg/dl (>14 mmol/l) is a candidate for DKA. This group includes adults at any age, normal weight or obese. Urine ketones (Ketostix or Acetest tablets) should be checked at once. A negative, trace, or small reaction virtually excludes DKA with the rare exception of the patient in uremia or with a high "reduced state" in his or her liver from alcohol intoxication or lactic acidosis. Direct measurement of blood β-hydroxybutyrate, the major ketoacid, is becoming increasingly available in the chemistry laboratory or by fingerstick at the bedside. This measurement will confirm or deny DKA in ambiguous cases where the acetoacetate level is not elevated enough. A moderate or large urine ketone reaction or blood β-hydroxybutyrate ≥3 mmol/l at home raises the possibility of existing or impending DKA. If vomiting cannot be controlled and fluid intake ensured at home and/or if ketosis does not promptly diminish with extra insulin, the patient must be examined. Clinical evidence of dehydration and acidosis suggests DKA:

- decreased skin turgor or eyeball pressure
- dry mucous membranes
- hypotension
- tachycardia
- tachypnea
- Kussmaul respirations

Laboratory confirmation is obtained by the values shown in Table 11.1, with some exceptions. The plasma bicarbonate concentration may be misleadingly higher than expected or even normal if the patient has coexisting chronic respiratory acidosis from pulmonary disease. Conversely, the blood pH may be misleadingly higher than expected or even normal if there is a concurrent metabolic alkalosis due to diuretic ingestion, excessive mineralocorticoid action, or extreme loss of gastric fluids. Occasionally, plasma glucose may be <250 mg/dl (<14 mmol/l) in a patient with diabetes who has ingested large amounts of alcohol and/or starved. Measured plasma sodium averages 130 meq/l, but when corrected for the plasma glucose level, it is usually in the normal range.

$$\text{Corrected sodium} = \text{measured sodium} + 1.6 \times \frac{\text{plasma glucose (mg/dl)} - 100}{100}$$

$$= \text{measured sodium} + 1.6 \times \frac{\text{plasma glucose (mmol/l)} - 5.5}{5.5}$$

Plasma potassium averages 5.2 meq/l but can be <3.5 or >6 meq/l on occasion. Plasma blood urea nitrogen (BUN) and creatinine tend to be slightly elevated because of reduced renal blood flow. An extremely high potassium level may be seen with accompanying renal failure or adrenal insufficiency.

Table 11.1 Typical Laboratory Findings in DKA

	Average	Range
Plasma glucose	600 mg/dl (33 mmol/l)	200–2,000 mg/dl (11–110 mmol/l)
Plasma β-hydroxybutyrate (mmol/l)	14	4–20
Plasma HCO_3^- (meq/l)	10	4–18
Blood pH	7.15	6.80–7.30
Pco_2 (mmHg)	20	14–30
Plasma anion gap ($Na^+ - [Cl^- + HCO_3^-]$) (meq/l)	29	16–35

All of the above should be carried out until the patient is stable, glucose levels are maintained at 150–250 mg/dl (8–14 mmol/l), and acidosis is largely reversed. An intensive care setting is preferred.

Body fluid losses can be estimated by subtracting the admission weight from a recently known dry weight. Hypotension suggests at least 10% dehydration. A precipitating infection is not excluded by a normal body temperature and should be assiduously sought. Meningeal signs call for computed axial tomography scan or magnetic resonance imaging of the head followed by a lumbar puncture. Necrotic lesions in the nasal turbinates suggest mucormycosis. Rectal and pelvic examinations should not be deferred because disorders such as appendicitis, pelvic inflammatory disease, diverticulitis, or cholecystitis may be the cause of the patient's abdominal pain. The urine sediment should be checked for evidence of urinary tract infection or gram-negative sepsis. Pulmonary infection should be routinely excluded by a chest X ray, and an acute silent myocardial infarction in older adults or in patients with type 1 diabetes for >15 years should be excluded by electrocardiogram (ECG).

Treatment

An intensive care unit (ICU) is the preferred setting for treatment of DKA. This is especially necessary for the more severe cases, i.e., individuals with HCO_3^- ≤10 meq/l, pH ≤7.20, 4.0 > K^+ ≥6.0 meq/l; hypotension despite rapid volume repletion; renal failure or oligo-anuria; CNS dysfunction; heart failure; age ≥65 years; or a concurrent comorbid condition such as sepsis that usually requires admission to an ICU. When an ICU is not available, an attending physician or resident should personally monitor the patient's progress frequently until the acidosis is broken and the patient is "out of the woods." An appropriate monitoring scheme is shown in Table 11.2.

The essential components of metabolic therapy are insulin administration, fluid replacement, and potassium repletion (Table 11.3). Bicarbonate, phosphate, and magnesium administration is not routinely required but may be needed or advantageous in certain situations.

Insulin. Short-acting (regular) insulin should always be used. Lispro insulin or insulin aspart can be expected to also be effective if regular insulin is unavailable. Intermediate-acting (NPH and lente) insulins are not suitable and should only

Table 11.2 Monitoring Patients with DKA

- Weight: admission and every 6–12 h
- Fluid intake and output: every 1–2 h (Foley catheter if incontinent)
- Blood pressure, pulse, respirations, mental status: every 1–2 h
- Temperature: every 8 h
- Blood (fingerstick) or plasma (laboratory) glucose: every 1–2 h
- Plasma K^+: every 2–4 h
- Plasma Na^+, chloride, and serum ketones: every 4 h

- Arterial blood pH, Pco_2, Po_2: admission; repeat as needed until arterial pH >7.0–7.1
- Plasma phosphate, Mg^{2+}, Ca^{2+}: admission; if low, repeat every 4 h; otherwise, every 8–12 h
- Urine for ketones: every voiding
- ECG: admission; repeat if follow-up plasma K^+ abnormal or unavailable
- Complete blood count, BUN, creatinine, urinalysis, appropriate cultures, chest X-ray: admission

Table 11.3 Essential Components in Treatment of DKA

Insulin	
Insulin	■ Subsequently, 0.45% saline at 150–300 ml/h
■ 10 units short-acting (regular) insulin/h by continuous intravenous infusion	■ Add 5% glucose when plasma glucose reaches 250 mg/dl (14 mmol/l)
■ Increase 2- to 10-fold if no response by 4 h	**K+**
■ Decrease to 1–2 units/h when acidosis is corrected	■ 10–20 meq/h when plasma K+ <6.0, ECG normal, urine flow documented
Fluids	■ 40–80 meq/h when plasma K+ <3.5 or if bicarbonate is given
■ 2–3 liters 0.9% saline over first 3 h	

be used as a temporizing measure if DKA occurs in isolated circumstances where short-acting insulin is unavailable. Whenever possible, short-acting insulin should be administered as a continuous intravenous infusion in a starting dose of 10 units or 0.1 units/kg/h via pump. If this is not feasible, 10 units/h i.m. or s.c. short-acting insulin is a satisfactory substitute. An initial bolus of 10 units i.v., although not essential, guarantees an immediate therapeutic level of insulin while the rest of the treatment regimen is being prepared. Lower doses than these should not be used at the outset, and higher initial doses offer no advantage.

In response to insulin, plasma glucose should fall at an average rate of 75 mg/dl/h. If no response has occurred by 4 h, an unusual degree of insulin resistance may be present. The dose of short-acting insulin should then be raised to 20–100 units/h i.v., with the higher doses being given for more extreme hyperglycemia and sicker patients. The dose should be further doubled every 2 h until plasma glucose definitely declines. The effectiveness of insulin therapy should also be demonstrated within 4–8 h by an increase in plasma bicarbonate, and/or a decrease in the plasma anion gap, and a decrease in plasma ketones or β-hydroxybutyrate level (if available). It is not necessary to monitor arterial pH routinely, but it should be rechecked if there is evidence of an inadequate response to insulin, if sodium bicarbonate has been administered (see below), or if coexisting pulmonary disease complicates the acid-base picture. Consultation with a diabetologist is strongly recommended if there is insulin unresponsiveness, insulin allergy, an admission pH <7.0, or coma.

Once plasma glucose has reached 250 mg/dl (14 mmol/l), glucose should be added to the replacement fluids. This addition permits continued administration of insulin to abolish ketosis completely while protecting the patient from hypoglycemia. The insulin dose may be reduced when plasma bicarbonate has risen to 18 meq/l, the anion gap has decreased to 15 meq/l, plasma ketones and urine ketones have virtually disappeared, arterial pH has risen to 7.30, or β-hydroxybutyrate has decreased to 1.0 mmol/l. Plasma ketones may persist because some β-hydroxybutyrate is converted to acetoacetate during the recovery phase. Two units per hour intravenously is usually a satisfactory insulin dosage—along with 5% glucose at 100–150 ml/h (5–7.5 g glucose/h)—with which to maintain plasma glucose at 150–250 mg/dl (8–14 mmol/l) and prevent recurrent ketoacidosis.

Once the patient is judged capable of reliable oral intake, the insulin infusion should be stopped. For practical reasons, this is best done the morning after admission. Before stopping the insulin infusion, it is vital to administer 4–10 units s.c. short-acting insulin. It is a common mistake not to do so on the grounds that plasma glucose is satisfactory at that point. However, ketosis often recurs if subcutaneous insulin is not administered until prominent hyperglycemia returns. In patients with previously known diabetes and no precipitating stress, their usual morning dose of intermediate- or long-acting insulin can also be given with the short-acting insulin. In new-onset patients, 20 units intermediate-acting insulin is a reasonable addition to the short-acting insulin, if desired.

Fluids. The initial goal of fluid therapy is to restore circulating volume and protect against cerebral, coronary, or renal hypoperfusion. In this phase, isotonic fluid is needed. Generally, 0.9% saline is used, although Ringer's lactate without glucose is also satisfactory. One liter should be administered in the first 30–60 min, followed by a second liter in the ensuing hour. In patients who are initially hypotensive or with estimated 10% dehydration, a rapid third liter of isotonic fluid is advisable. Frank shock may call for a colloidal volume expander such as plasma.

The second objective of fluid therapy is to replace total-body and intracellular losses, and this objective is achieved more slowly. Because total sodium and water losses are approximately in half-isotonic proportions, 0.45% saline is logical. Once plasma glucose reaches 250 mg/dl (14 mmol/l), 5% glucose in 0.45% saline, 0.2% saline, or water should be administered. This choice is guided by the plasma sodium level, which should rise as plasma glucose falls, and by the patient's cardiac status. Measured or even corrected plasma sodium levels reaching 150 meq/l or a history of congestive heart failure indicate the need for more hypotonic fluids. The optimal rate of fluid replacement after circulatory volume has been initially stabilized cannot be stated categorically because it will vary with the original degree of dehydration, with renal or cardiac function, and with time into treatment. The range of rates is 150–500 ml/h. This should be tapered until an overall positive balance of 6 liters on average is achieved. In the average case, fluid repletion is completed in 12–24 h. In mild cases of DKA, handled in an emergency room setting, 6–8 h may suffice.

It is vital to document that a cumulative positive balance is occurring by comparing fluid intake with output every 1–2 h. Urine flow can remain 100–200 ml/h until plasma glucose has declined to 250 mg/dl (14 mmol/l). In addition, there may be continuing gastrointestinal fluid losses or excessive ventilatory fluid losses due to fever. Plasma sodium should be checked to ensure that it is gradually increasing as plasma glucose falls. If this is not happening, there may be excessive administration of free water, which may increase the risk of clinically significant cerebral edema.

Potassium. Nothing in the treatment of DKA requires more care and finesse than potassium replacement. Deaths have resulted from hypokalemia and, more rarely, from hyperkalemia. The average deficit of potassium is ~5 meq/kg body weight. If the patient has lain undiagnosed in coma from DKA or has delayed seeking treatment for 24 h, the deficit can reach 500–1,000 meq. Despite the body potassium losses, plasma potassium on admission is usually normal or increased. Values <4.0 meq/l indicate unusually large losses and require frequent subsequent plasma potassium measurement. The objective of therapy is simple:

Maintain plasma potassium of at least 3.5–4.0 meq/l at all times.

This should prevent hypokalemic death from cardiac arrhythmia or respiratory arrest until DKA is reversed. Total potassium repletion by the intravenous route is not necessary; it is completed later when oral intake is resumed.

Plasma potassium begins to decline as soon as insulin starts to act. Therefore, potassium should be administered from the outset, after insulin, unless the initial plasma level is >5.5 meq/l or oligo-anuria is demonstrated by bladder catheterization. If plasma potassium cannot be rapidly ascertained, a normal pretreatment ECG will exclude life-threatening hyperkalemia. Potassium should be administered continuously at a beginning rate of 10–30 meq/h (not necessarily equivalent to 10–30 meq/l intravenous fluid). The lower the initial plasma potassium, the higher the rate should be. If hypokalemia is present at the outset or if bicarbonate is given, 40–80 meq/h may be needed initially. In the first 12 h, 150–250 meq potassium is generally administered.

One practical recommendation is to administer potassium according to the plasma level with the following concentrations in the replacement fluids: K^+ >5.0, no potassium; K^+ 4.0–5.0, 20 meq/l; K^+ 3.0–4.0, 30–40 meq/l; K^+ <3.0, 40–60 meq/l. However, following any guideline by rote should never substitute for monitoring plasma potassium and using individual judgment according to patient circumstances.

Preferably start with potassium chloride. Later, some potassium may be given as the phosphate to reduce the chloride load. Each 1 mmol/l potassium phosphate provides ~1.5 meq potassium. Serial ECGs can help track potassium status: flattened or inverted T waves and the appearance of U waves indicate hypokalemia; tall symmetrical T waves, a widened QRS complex, and loss of P waves indicate hyperkalemia. However, discrepancies and misinterpretations can occur; therefore, it is always best to measure plasma potassium directly (Table 11.2).

Bicarbonate. Treatment with bicarbonate is not essential to and does not increase the rate of recovery from hyperglycemia or hyperketonemia. The acidosis of DKA will be corrected in due time by insulin inhibition of ketogenesis. Therefore, the routine administration of alkali in all cases is not recommended. Furthermore, giving bicarbonate has the demonstrated disadvantage of significantly increasing the risk of hypokalemia and the theoretical disadvantages of decreasing tissue oxygen delivery and CNS pH.

However, in some instances, metabolic acidosis per se may be so severe or directly deleterious that it warrants emergency amelioration (Table 11.4). When buffering reserve is dangerously low, as indicated by a pH level <7.0 or a plasma bicarbonate level <5.0 meq/l, a slight increase in acid production or decrease in ventilation can result in lethal acidosis. Rarely, hyperkalemia is severe enough on admission to require immediate reversal by bicarbonate. If acidosis blunts vasoconstrictor responsiveness to catecholamines, dangerous hypotension can persist despite vigorous fluid replacement. Severe acidosis can also compromise cardiac output, leading to pulmonary edema and lactic acidosis, or it can impair ventilation, superimposing respiratory acidosis. Rarely, non–anion gap hyperchloremic

---

Table 11.4 Indications for Considering Bicarbonate Therapy

- pH <7.0 or HCO_3^- <5.0 meq/l
- Hyperkalemia (K^+ >6.5 meq/l)
- Hypotension unresponsive to fluid replacement
- Severe left ventricular failure
- Respiratory depression
- Late hyperchloremic acidosis

---

acidosis of sufficient severity to warrant alkali treatment develops late in the course of DKA.

If it is decided that any of these circumstances requires directly attacking the acidosis, sodium bicarbonate should be administered promptly to a defined end point. Doses of 50–100 meq in 250–1,000 ml 0.45% saline can be administered in 30–60 min. Arterial pH should be rechecked after each 50–100 meq administered, and bicarbonate treatment should be continued until the pH has reached at least 7.10. To prevent hypokalemia, an extra 10 meq potassium chloride should accompany each dose of bicarbonate unless hyperkalemia was the original indication for alkali treatment.

Phosphate and magnesium. Although plasma levels of phosphate and magnesium are usually normal or elevated on admission, body stores of both are somewhat depleted by DKA. This becomes evident as insulin administration regularly produces hypophosphatemia, often to levels <1.5 mg/dl, and a less dramatic fall in plasma magnesium. However, clinical consequences of these changes are seldom observed, and prospective studies of routine phosphate supplementation have shown no particular benefit. Still, some physicians deem it wise to correct, or at least attenuate, hypophosphatemia by administering potassium phosphate in doses of 1–2 mmol phosphate/kg body weight i.v. over 6–12 h. If rhabdomyolysis, CNS deterioration, cardiac dysfunction, or hemolysis parallel the initial fall in plasma phosphate, then phosphate therapy as described is definitely indicated. Plasma calcium should then be monitored carefully, because hypocalcemia and even tetany have occurred with phosphate therapy. Magnesium is indicated when ventricular arrhythmias occur that are not accounted for by hypokalemia. Doses of 10–20 meq i.v. magnesium should be given over 30–60 min as emergency therapy in the form of 2.5–5.0 ml 50% magnesium sulfate diluted in 100 ml fluid. The need for additional doses is determined by ECG monitoring.

HYPEROSMOLAR HYPERGLYCEMIC STATE

Hyperosmolar hyperglycemic state (HHS) should probably not be considered a specific syndrome but rather one end of the spectrum of severe metabolic decompensation in diabetes. In the pure case, HHS is differentiated from DKA by the absence of significant ketosis and by the pres-ence of higher average levels of plasma glucose and osmolarity. By definition, plasma glucose should be >600 mg/dl (>33 mmol/l), and osmolarity should be >320 mOsm/kg in HHNS. By these osmolar criteria, ~50% of all cases of extreme diabetic decompensation are due to HHS. However, in 35% of these cases, acidosis (pH <7.30) is also present. This may be due to accompanying lactic acidosis or uremia but also occasionally indicates significant accumulation of ketoacids. The distinction between pure and mixed cases of HHS is of little practical importance because the main elements of therapy are similar in both.

HHS is responsible for ~1/1,000 hospital admissions. It occurs predominantly in adults over age 50 years and almost exclusively in patients with type 2 diabetes, 35% of whom were previously undiagnosed. In one survey, 40% of patients had accompanying infection, 38% had been on diuretics, and 28% were living in nursing homes. Mortality rates in various series range from 12% to 42%. Death is associated with age >70 years, nursing home residency, higher plasma osmolarity, and higher plasma sodium but not with higher plasma glucose or anion gap. These results emphasize the key pathogenetic features of HHS. Ketosis is relatively suppressed, perhaps by more available endogenous insulin and by hyperosmolarity itself, compared with DKA. However, losses of total-body water, especially relative to total-body sodium, are greater than those in DKA. This is probably due to a combination of age and dementia-related diminished thirst, decreased renal urine concentrating ability, and the absence of ketosis-associated vomiting as a warning sign of decompensation. In turn, the greater degree of dehydration causes more prerenal reduction in glomerular filtration rate and secondarily raises plasma glucose to even higher levels than usually seen in DKA.

HHS is more insidious in nature, and patients typically come to medical attention later and sicker. Precipitating conditions can include otherwise silent myocardial infarction, pancreatitis, sepsis, stroke, and an array of drugs (glucocorticoids, diuretics, phenytoin, β-blockers, and Ca^{2+}-channel blockers). CNS findings range from confusion to complete coma, but in contrast to DKA, patients can also present with generalized or focal seizures, myoclonic jerking, and reversible hemiparesis.

Diagnosis

HHS should be suspected in any elderly person with or without diabetes who exhibits acute or subacute deterioration of CNS function and is severely dehydrated. Blood pressure is low or lower than expected if the patient is known to have hypertension. Either hyperthermia or hypothermia may be present. A fingerstick blood glucose above the readable range of any test strip or meter suggests HHS. Average plasma values on admission are

- glucose 1,000 mg/dl (55 mmol/l)
- osmolarity 360 mOsm/kg
- sodium 140 meq/l
- BUN 65 mg/dl (23 mmol/l)
- creatinine 3.0 mg/dl (265 μmol/l)
- potassium 4.9 meq/l
- anion gap 23 meq/l

Arterial pH is usually >7.30 but may be decreased by accompanying metabolic or respiratory acidosis.

Management

An intensive care setting is even more necessary for HHS compared with DKA because of older-aged patients, more precarious volume status, greater CNS dysfunction, comorbidities, and the threat of thromboses.

Fluids. The most critical element in the management of HHS is the choice of replacement fluid and its rate of administration. As noted above, both the total losses of fluid and the proportion represented by free water are usually greater in HHS than in DKA. The average admission plasma sodium is 10 meq/l higher in HHS, despite a greater degree of hyperglycemia. Furthermore, the degree of CNS abnormality in HHS correlates best with the level of hyperosmolarity, which reflects intracellular dehydration. Therefore, rehydrating brain cells is of great therapeutic importance. On the other hand, overhydrating brain cells can also impair their function. This may be a risk during treatment of HHS, because animal studies suggest that brain cells respond to hypotonic dehydration by increasing intracellular osmoles such as myo-inositol, taurine, and betaine. The benefit of this response is to diminish the amount of water that must leave brain cells to maintain osmolar equilibrium in the face of rising plasma osmolarity. However, if these intracellular osmoles persist while plasma glucose is being rapidly reduced with treatment, they can stimulate overcorrection of CNS dehydration because they attract extra water back into the brain cells.

Such considerations may explain why many patients with HHS do not completely recover their baseline CNS function until a considerable time after plasma glucose has decreased to <300 mg/dl (<17 mmol/l). In some instances, it is because of continued hyperosmolarity, as revealed by very high plasma sodium (Fig. 11.1). This can result from inadequate free-water replacement and may be aggravated by persistent renal losses of free water as kidneys recover from functional impairment due to severe prior dehydration. In other instances, slow CNS recovery may occur because of too-rapid correction of hyperosmolarity, as would be indicated by development of a low plasma sodium level when plasma glucose declines.

As in DKA, the initial objective of fluid therapy is to immediately raise the circulating volume. Hence, 1 liter of 0.9% saline should be administered in the first 30 min. If the patient remains hypotensive, a second liter of 0.9% saline should be given in the next 30–60 min. Thereafter, all fluids should ordinarily be hypotonic. The ensuing 2–3 liters should be 0.45% sodium chloride infused at ~500 ml/h. This rate may be slowed thereafter, but ultimately as much as 12 liters positive fluid balance may be required over 24–36 h to restore normal body fluid content. When plasma glucose has declined to 250–300 mg/dl (14–17 mmol/l), 5% glucose should be added to 0.45% sodium chloride. If plasma sodium exceeds 150 meq/l at this point, 5% glucose in 0.2% sodium chloride or in water is indicated. The rate of fluid administration must be guided by body weight, urine output, kidney function, and presence or absence of pulmonary congestion and jugular venous distention. In patients with prior congestive heart failure or renal insufficiency or in patients with acute kidney failure secondary to HHS, catheter monitoring of central venous pressure is also indicated. Most important, the

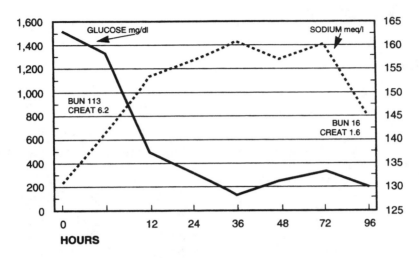

Figure 11.1 Plasma glucose and Na+ levels during treatment of hyper-osmolar coma. CREAT, creatinine.

patient's neurological status must be observed frequently. Failure to show any improvement may indicate inadequate rates of fluid replacement or of reduction in plasma osmolarity. Regression after initial improvement may indicate too rapid a reduction in plasma osmolarity. A slow but steady improvement in CNS function paralleling a gradual decline in plasma osmolarity is the best evidence that fluid management is satisfactory.

Other therapy. Insulin should be infused at an initial rate of 10 units/h i.v., as in DKA. Although fluid repletion itself has a major impact on hyperglycemia, it should not be relied on as the sole therapy of HHS. On the other hand, rapidly lowering plasma glucose by giving insulin without adequate fluids is also dangerous, because water will shift into cells and temporarily lower circulating volume and perfusion of vital organs. Once plasma glucose has reached 250–300 mg/dl (14–17 mmol/l), the insulin infusion can be reduced to 1–2 units/h. This infusion should be adjusted to maintain plasma glucose around the recommended level until rehydration has been accomplished. Subcutaneous insulin should be started after recovery from HHS, as it is in DKA treatment. However, because patients with HHS almost always have type 2 diabetes, they may be subsequently tried on sulfonylurea drugs, other oral drugs, or diet alone if they achieve normoglycemia with small doses of insulin.

Potassium repletion is also necessary in HHS. Although potassium losses are less well established in HHS, they may be lower than in DKA because of less acidosis and vomiting or higher than in DKA if a severe osmotic diuresis persisted for a long time before treatment was begun. Because initial oliguria is more common in HHS, potassium may not be needed at the outset and the rates of administration should be more cautious (e.g., 10–20 meq/h). Bicarbonate is not needed unless there is severe lactic acidosis (see Chapter 12). Phosphate and magnesium can be given as in DKA and for similar reasons. Overall monitoring of the patient should be conducted essentially as outlined in Table 11.2.

COMPLICATIONS OF DKA AND HHS

Persistent Vomiting

Nasogastric suction is helpful to prevent aspiration pneumonia. Stomach contents often test positive for occult blood, but significant blood loss requiring investigation or transfusion is unusual.

Infection

Appropriate antibiotics for pulmonary, genitourinary tract, abdominal, soft tissue, or CNS infection should be given intravenously to ensure that they reach the bloodstream promptly. Amphotericin is specifically indicated for mucormycosis. Sepsis is a grave complication, the signs of which may overlap with those of DKA or HHS. A greatly elevated serum C-reactive protein or interleukin-6 level suggests sepsis and a poor prognosis. In febrile patients who appear very ill or are hypotensive, obtain blood cultures and treat with an antibiotic regimen that covers the common gram-positive and gram-negative organisms as well as pseudomonas and anaerobes.

Acute Kidney Failure

Severe volume depletion and/or papillary necrosis may lead to secondary kidney failure. Anuria on admission or persistent oliguria despite rehydration calls for nephrological consultation.

Rhabdomyolysis

Rhabdomyolysis can occur in HHS patients with especially elevated plasma osmolarity and creatinine. It can also occur in DKA associated with phosphate deficiency. Rhabdomyolysis increases the mortality rate in HHS and should be treated vigorously with fluids and bicarbonate.

Acute Respiratory Distress Syndrome

Tachypnea, after acidosis is corrected, calls for a repeat chest X-ray. A "shock-lung" or "white-out" picture requires positive-pressure oxygen, central venous pressure monitoring, and more cautious fluid replacement.

Disseminated Intravascular Coagulation

The picture of multiple thromboses and/or bleeding, accompanied by thrombocytopenia, low fibrinogen levels, prolonged prothrombin time and partial thromboplastin time, and the presence of circulating fibrin products is characteristic of disseminated intravascular coagulation (DIC). Therapy with heparin is usually indicated. In elderly patients without DIC but with a history of venous thrombosis, pulmonary embolism, or congestive heart failure, prophylactic low-dose heparin (5,000 units s.c. every 12 h) should be considered.

PREVENTION OF DKA AND HHS

Clear instructions should be given to always test blood glucose and urine ketones at home when symptoms of diabetic decompensation or intercurrent illness appear. The physician or nurse should be called immediately for vomiting, when blood glucose is >500 mg/dl (>28 mmol/l), or when blood glucose is >250 mg/dl (>14 mmol/l) and urine ketones are moderate or large. In turn, the physician and/or nurse should maintain constant (every 2–4 h) telephone or office contact with the patient either until extra insulin, fluids, anti-emetics, etc., have aborted development of DKA or HHS or until a decision to hospitalize the patient is made. If extra insulin is given at bedtime because of acute hyperglycemia and/or ketosis, the patient must set an alarm and check blood glucose and urine ketones 4 h later. If levels remain dangerously high, the physician must be called again. A routine instruction to "call back in the morning" is not an adequate response to the threat of DKA or HHS.

BIBLIOGRAPHY

Adrogue HJ, Wilson H, Boyd AE, Suki WN, Eknoyan G: Plasma acid-base patterns in diabetic ketoacidosis. *N Engl J Med* 307:1603–1610, 1982

Berger W, Keller U: Treatment of diabetic ketoacidosis and non-ketotic hyperosmolar diabetic coma. *Ballieres Clin Endocrinol Metab* 6:1–22, 1992

Brandenburg M, Dire D: Comparison of arterial and venous blood gas values in the initial emergency department evaluation of patients with diabetic ketoacidosis. *Ann Emerg Med* 31:449–465, 1998

Carrol P, Matz R: Uncontrolled diabetes mellitus in adults: experience in treatment of diabetic ketoacidosis and hyperosmolar nonketotic coma with low-dose insulin and a uniform treatment regimen. *Diabetes Care* 6:579–585, 1983

DeFronzo RA, Matsuda M, Barrett EJ: Diabetic ketoacidosis: a combined metabolic-nephrologic approach to therapy. *Diabetes Metab Rev* 2:209–238, 1994

Ennis E, Kreisberg R: Diabetic ketoacidosis and the hyperglycemic hyperosmolar syndrome. In *Diabetes Mellitus: A Fundamental and Clinical Text*. 3rd ed. LeRoith D, Taylor S, Olefsky J, Eds., Philadelphia, Lippincot, Williams & Wilkins, 2004, p. 627–642

Fisher JN, Kitabchi AE: A randomized study of phosphate therapy in the treatment of diabetic ketoacidosis. *J Clin Endocrinol Metab* 57:117–180, 1983

Foster DW, McGarry JD: The metabolic derangements and treatment of diabetic ketoacidosis. *N Engl J Med* 309:159–169, 1983

Genuth S: Diabetic ketoacidosis and hyperglycemic hyperosmolar coma. In *Current Therapy in Endocrinology and Metabolism.* 6th ed. Wayne Bardin C, Ed. St. Louis, MO, Mosby, 1997, p. 438–446

Gogos CA, Giali S, Paliogianni F, Dimitracopoulos G, Bassaris HP, Vagenakis AG: Interleukin-6 and C-reactive protein as early markers of sepsis in patients with diabetic ketoacidosis or hyperosmosis. *Diabetologia* 44:1011–1014, 2001

Lever E, Jaspan JB: Sodium bicarbonate therapy in severe diabetic ketoacidosis. *Am J Med* 75:263–268, 1983

Marinac J, Mesa L: Using a severity of illness scoring system to assess intensive care unit admissions for diabetic ketoacidosis. *Crit Care Med* 28:2238–2241, 2000

Matz R: Hyperosmolar nonacidotic uncontrolled diabetes: not a rare event. *Clin Diabetes* 6:25, 30–37, 46, 1988

May ME, Young C, King J: Resource utilization in treatment of diabetic ketoacidosis in adults. *Am J Med Sci* 306:287–294, 1993

Soler NG, Bennet MA, Dixon K, Fitzgerald M, Malins J: Potassium balance during treatment of diabetic ketoacidosis with special reference to the use of bicarbonate. *Lancet* 2:665–667, 1972

Wachtel TJ, Silliman RA, Lamberton P: Prognostic factors in the diabetic hyperosmolar state. *J Am Geriatr Soc* 35:737–741, 1987

Westphal S: The occurrence of diabetic ketoacidosis in non-insulin-dependent diabetes and newly diagnosed diabetic adults. *Am J Med* 101:19–24, 1996

Wiggam MI, O'Kane MJ, Harper R, Atkinson AB, Hadden DR, Trimble ER, Bell PM: Treatment of diabetic ketoacidosis using normalization of blood β-hydroxybutyrate concentration as the endpoint of emergency management: a randomized controlled study. *Diabetes Care* 20:1347–1352, 1997

Dr. Genuth is a Professor of Medicine at Case Western Reserve University, Cleveland, OH.

12. Lactic Acidosis

STEPHEN C. CLEMENT, MD

Lactic acidosis (LA) usually results from inadequate oxygen delivery or use in patients with serious underlying diseases but can also occur in disorders without obvious tissue hypoperfusion. LA is the most common form of metabolic acidosis in hospitalized patients. Regardless of cause, the accumulation of lactic acid indicates that the balance between lactate production and use has been disturbed.

CLASSIFICATION OF LA

A modest elevation in blood lactate concentration (usually <5.0 meq/l) can occur without changes in blood pH and may represent an increased set point for lactate, such as occurs with some hypermetabolic states. In contrast, true LA, in which elevated blood lactate (usually ≥5.0 meq/l) is associated with significant hemodynamic and metabolic decompensation, usually has a lowered blood pH. The most widely used classification divides LA into two broad categories: type A, associated with disorders in which there is reduced O_2 delivery (DO_2), and type B, which is not associated with reduced DO_2 (Table 12.1).

Type A LA

Type A LA is much more common than type B LA and forms the basis for most of the understanding of LA biochemistry. Type A LA occurs when DO_2 is inadequate to meet the metabolic demands of tissues, resulting in tissue hypoxemia and anaerobic glycolysis. Systemic shock and regional hypoperfusion, hypoxemia, anemia severe enough to reduce DO_2, and CO intoxication are examples of LA related to decreased DO_2. Vigorous exercise, seizures, and severe asthma are examples of type A LA, where tissue O_2 demand outstrips supply. With type A, the hemodynamic abnormalities of mismatched supply and demand precede and lead to the LA.

Type B LA

Type B LA develops in settings in which there is no clinical evidence for reduced DO_2 to tissues. It has been further divided into subcategories related to

Table 12.1 Some Causes of LA

Type A (clinical evidence of inadequate O$_2$ delivery)
■ Shock (septic, cardiogenic, hypovolemic)
■ Severe hypoxemia or anemia
■ Status post cardiopulmonary bypass
■ CO poisoning
 	
Type B (no clinical evidence of inadequate O$_2$ delivery)
■ B$_1$ (associated with underlying disease)
 –Diabetes mellitus
 –Liver disease
 –Malignancy
 –Sepsis
 –AIDS
■ B$_2$ (due to drugs/toxins)
	–Biguanides
	–Ethanol/methanol
	–Nucleoside reverse transcriptase inhibitors
	–Ethylene/propylene glycol
	–Acetaminophen
	–Salicylates
	–Cyanide
	–Nitroprusside
	■ B$_3$ (due to congenital defects in gluconeogenesis or pyruvate oxidation)
	 –Deficiency of:
	  □ Glucose-6-phosphatase
	  □ Pyruvate carboxylase
	  □ Fructose-1,6-diphosphatase
	  □ Pyruvate dehydrogenase
	  □ Oxidative phosphorylation

underlying disease (type B$_1$), drugs or toxins (type B$_2$), and inborn errors of metabolism (type B$_3$). Although some cases of type B LA may have occult tissue hypoperfusion, many occur without evidence for primary DO$_2$ problems. There are several causes of type B LA.

Diabetes mellitus. Lactate metabolism is abnormal in diabetes. LA occurring in the setting of diabetes, even with diabetic ketoacidosis, is rare. When it does occur in association with diabetes, it is usually the result of reduced DO$_2$ and/or tissue hypoxia related to severe volume contraction, myocardial dysfunction, or sepsis. Therefore, when LA is present in patients with diabetes, underlying causes for LA related to reduced DO$_2$ should be found.

Liver disease. An association between liver disease and altered lactate metabolism is expected because of the central role of the liver in lactate homeostasis. LA is frequently seen in patients with serious liver disease, and acidemia may be masked because of coexistent metabolic and respiratory alkaloses. Basal blood lactate concentrations appear to be normal in these patients, but clearance of infused lactate may be prolonged by ~20%. Thus, although basal lactate production and use are matched, any condition that increases production of lactate may result in hyperlactatemia and LA due to impaired hepatic clearance. Shunting of lactate around the liver via collateralization (e.g., in cirrhotic patients) may play a role in reducing lactate use by the liver.

Malignancy. LA is associated with malignant disease, most commonly with uncontrolled leukemia (usually lymphocytic, rarely myelocytic), lymphoma, and less commonly with solid tumors (most often with associated hepatic or bone marrow metastasis). The mechanism is not completely understood, although the LA in malignancy has most often been attributed to overproduction via glycolysis by tumor cells. Underutilization (e.g., reduced clearance) has also been proposed as a mechanism for tumor-associated LA, often with almost complete replacement of the liver with malignant cells. Both overproduction and underutilization probably occur in LA associated with malignancy. Again, inadequate tissue DO_2 (e.g., sepsis, volume depletion, or cardiac dysfunction) is still the most common cause of LA in cancer patients and must be evaluated and treated aggressively.

Sepsis. Sepsis is common and often associated with hyperlactatemia and/or LA. Both type A and type B LA can occur in sepsis. Type A LA clearly occurs in the setting of septic shock because of a marked vasodilation of systemic vessels, varying degrees of myocardial depression, and most often, a reduction in intra-vascular volume. This acute shock state, identified clinically by a marked reduction in systemic vascular resistance, severe hypotension, and systemic signs of reduced DO_2, is easily diagnosed. As in any other form of shock with acidemia, confirming the presence of elevated blood lactate is unnecessary diagnostically, at least initially, because therapy would be immediately directed toward improving DO_2 and tissue perfusion. Depending on myocardial dysfunction and depression, volume status, and degree of initial volume resuscitation, patients with sepsis have a normal or high cardiac output and therefore normal DO_2 with significant LA. Depending on the underlying pathophysiology, this type B LA is probably related to occult tissue hypoperfusion or, in contrast, to an isolated or coexistent cellular metabolic defect, which alters lactate metabolism and produces hyper-lactatemia and acidosis independent of tissue hypoperfusion.

Biguanides. Of the various drugs/toxins implicated in causing LA, the biguanides are of considerable interest to the physician caring for patients with diabetes. Metformin, a biguanide currently available for the treatment of type 2 diabetes, has been associated with LA in ~0.03 cases/1,000 patient-years of exposure (see Chapter 20). Reported cases of LA occurred primarily in patients with renal insufficiency and/or other concomitant medical conditions associated with poor renal perfusion, poor tissue perfusion, or hypoxia. These conditions include congestive heart failure, chronic obstructive lung disease, or old age ($\geq$80 years old). Patients who have substantial liver disease are also at risk because of their impaired ability to clear lactate. The mechanism for metformin-associated LA is unclear. Biguanides bind to mitochondrial membranes and inhibit aerobic metabolism. This inhibition is thought to induce a shift from aerobic to anaerobic metabolism, causing increased lactate production. Metformin has only minimal binding to mitochondrial membranes compared with phenformin (a biguanide that is no longer in use).

Acquired immunodeficiency syndrome. Nucleoside analog reverse transcriptase inhibitors have been implicated in causing a type B form of LA. The mechanism of this adverse effect is unknown but is thought to be mediated by mitochondrial toxicity. The degree of acidosis is usually mild but has been reported to be associated with life-threatening acidosis.

D-Lactic acidosis. D-Lactic acidosis typically occurs in a patient who has undergone a small bowel resection or jejunoileal bypass. Bacterial overgrowth in the remaining intestine metabolizes carbohydrate to D-lactic acid, a form of lactic acid that is not measurable with the usual lactate assay and is only slowly metabolized in humans. The syndrome presents as an altered mental status, an anion-gap metabolic acidosis, a normal lactate level, and an improvement after oral intake of food is discontinued. The diagnosis is confirmed by finding high levels of D-lactate in the urine and/or serum.

DIAGNOSIS OF LA

The measurement of lactate in the setting of obvious clinical shock with acidemia may be unnecessary to aid in diagnosis. However, in the absence of clinical signs of hypoperfusion or when an unexplained anion-gap acidosis exists, particularly in a critically ill patient, an elevated blood lactate concentration may allow for the diagnosis of LA and indicates that a search for occult tissue hypoperfusion should be undertaken.

A blood lactate concentration of >5 meq/l and a pH of <7.35 constitute the criteria for defining LA in which false-positive and false-negative diagnoses would be minimized. LA frequently occurs in association with disorders in which dynamic acid-base disturbances are common (e.g., the metabolic alkalosis of liver disease or hyperventilation related to early sepsis or mechanical ventilation). The initial pH may be normal or near normal, thus masking a significant acidemia.

TREATMENT

The cornerstone of therapy for LA is treatment of the underlying and predisposing disorders (Table 12.2). Although such therapy is essential for survival, poor outcome relates to both the seriousness of the associated primary disorder and to the inability to specifically treat LA.

Optimization of Do_2

In addition to therapy for the underlying disorder, another treatment approach is optimization of Do_2. Beyond clinically obvious shock, which should be dealt with swiftly and aggressively, many critically ill patients enter a clinical and biochemical gray zone. These patients may have mild to moderate hyperlactatemia (2–5 meq/l) with or without associated acidosis. Because noninvasive assessment of Do_2 and Vo_2 in these patients is relatively inaccurate and maintenance of Do_2 and consumption at supranormal levels reduces subsequent failure of multiple organ systems and improves survival, the use of hemodynamic monitoring and a trial to determine whether an occult perfusion defect and supply dependency exist is important for further therapeutic decisions in these patients with hyperlactatemia.

Acidosis has undesirable clinical effects, including

- significant adverse effects on the cardiovascular system
- reduced cardiac contractility, cardiac output, systemic blood pressure, and heart rate

Table 12.2 Treatment of LA

1. Correct perfusion.	4. Initiate dialysis if LA due to a drug
2. Maximize tissue O_2 delivery.	(i.e., metformin).
3. Treat any underlying sepsis.	

- decreased hepatic and renal blood flow
- impaired responsiveness to endogenous and exogenous catecholamines
- increased susceptibility to ventricular arrhythmias

These deleterious effects, which generally occur at pH <7.2, would further decrease tissue DO_2 and worsen the developing LA.

The use of bicarbonate as a buffering agent is controversial, and its use has undergone intense scrutiny recently. Because of the large quantities of bicarbonate usually required, hypernatremia, hyperosmolality, and volume overload can become significant problems, especially in the setting of already reduced flow, poor renal perfusion, and reduced renal secretion of sodium and water.

There may be adverse effects directly related to bicarbonate therapy that may be of considerable clinical importance and largely unmanageable. The administration of sodium bicarbonate increases production of CO_2, which rapidly diffuses into the myocardial cell, causing a decrease in intracellular pH and worsening myocardial function. The reduced contractility and cardiac output that occurs might be of great potential importance in settings where CO_2 removal is a problem (e.g., ventilatory failure or during resuscitation).

Furthermore, bicarbonate may have a detrimental effect on lactate production, probably related to the effect of pH on phosphofructokinase activity, which increases dramatically as pH increases from 6.8 to 7.2. Thus, bicarbonate administration might increase phosphofructokinase activity, stimulating lactate production and possibly nullifying any potential benefit.

Because of the potential adverse effects of intravenous bicarbonate therapy, an alternative agent, Carbicarb, has generated interest. Carbicarb is a mixture of Na_2CO_3 and $NaHCO_3$ that buffers similarly to $NaHCO_3$ but without the net generation of CO_2. Although animal studies suggest a benefit of Carbicarb over $NaHCO_3$, human studies are lacking.

Hemodialysis is indicated therapy for LA caused by some drugs or toxins. For example, for metformin-associated LA, metformin has a clearance of up to 170 ml/min under good hemodynamic conditions. For this drug, prompt hemodialysis is recommended to correct the acidosis and remove the accumulated metformin. Such management often results in prompt reversal of symptoms and in recovery.

Dichoroacetate, an experimental drug, has received attention as a possible treatment for lactic acidosis. However, randomized controlled trials have failed to show clinical benefit compared to standard therapy, and the drug is not recommended for treatment of lactic acidosis.

BIBLIOGRAPHY

Buchalter SE, Crain MR, Kreisberg R: Regulation of lactate metabolism in vivo. *Diabetes Metab Rev* 5:379–391, 1989

Cohen RD, Woods HF: *Clinical and Biochemical Aspects of Lactic Acidosis.* Boston, MA, Blackwell, 1976

Forsythe S, Schmidt G: Sodium bicarbonate for the treatment of lactic acidosis. *Chest* 117:260–267, 2000

Kreisberg RA: Lactic acidosis: an update. *J Intensive Care Med* 2:76–84, 1987

Luft FC: Lactic acidosis update for critical care clinicians. *J Am Soc Nephrol* 12:S15–S19, 2001

Madias NE: Lactic acidosis. *Kidney Int* 29:752–774, 1986

Mizock BA: Lactic acidosis. *Disease-a-Month* 35:235–300, 1989

Narins RG, Cohen JJ: Bicarbonate therapy of organic acidosis: the case for its continued use. *Ann Intern Med* 106:615–618, 1987

Stacpoole PW: Lactic acidosis: the case against bicarbonate therapy. *Ann Intern Med* 105:276–279, 1986

Uribarri J, Oh MS, Carroll HJ: D-lactic acidosis: a review of clinical presentation, biochemical features and pathophysiologic mechanisms. *Medicine* 77:73–82, 1998

Dr. Clement is Director of the Diabetes Center and Associate Professor at the Georgetown University Medical Center, Washington, DC.

13. Role of Diabetes Education in Patient Management

MARTHA M. FUNNELL, MS, RN, CDE,
AND ROBERT M. ANDERSON, EdD

Recent advances in knowledge, therapies, and technology have greatly enhanced our ability to effectively care for patients with diabetes. In spite of these advances, people with diabetes still experience less than optimal blood glucose levels as well as acute and long-term complications. Health care professionals are often frustrated by their patients' inability to make changes in their behavior, and people with diabetes sometimes feel that they are "just a blood sugar number" to their providers. Clearly, there is a gap between the promise and the reality of diabetes care. One of the keys to closing the gap is effective diabetes self-management.

DIABETES SELF-MANAGEMENT

Diabetes self-management refers to all of the activities in which patients engage to care for their illness; promote health; augment physical, social, and emotional resources; and prevent long- and short-term effects from diabetes. Education is the essential first step in becoming an effective self-manager. Traditional views of diabetes self-management education (DSME) were based on information transfer and compliance or adherence. Based on recent evidence, DSME has evolved to recognize the right and responsibility of patients to make decisions and set self-selected goals that make sense within the context of their lives. The purpose of providing DSME is to help patients make informed decisions and evaluate the costs and benefits of those choices.

Whereas patients need a comprehensive understanding of diabetes, its effect on their lives, and how to change behavior, it is unreasonable to think that a one-time educational intervention will be adequate to manage diabetes for a lifetime. Self-management support is the ongoing assistance patients need from health care professionals, the community, family and friends, and other relevant organizations to make informed self-management decisions and to make and sustain behavioral changes. It incorporates the provision of the needed intellectual, behavioral, emotional, psychosocial, and tangible resources to enable patients to manage their illness effectively. Strategies for providing self-management support include the following:

- Assess patient self-management knowledge, behaviors, confidence, and barriers.
- Incorporate effective behavior-change interventions and ongoing support from family, peers, and professionals.
- Incorporate strategies to help patients cope with the demands of diabetes.
- Ensure collaborative care planning and problem solving by a team.

DSME AND SUPPORT

Recent reviews and meta-analysis have indicated that DSME is effective in improving metabolic and psychosocial outcomes, at least in the short term. More time with the educator increases the effect. In addition, DSME interventions that integrate the physiological, behavioral, and psychosocial aspects of diabetes are more effective than programs that focus strictly on knowledge. Table 13.1 summarizes recent findings related to DSME.

DSME is increasingly available through group programs often offered by hospitals or community-based organizations. Programs that achieve Recognition from the American Diabetes Association (ADA) by meeting standards for process, structure, and outcomes are eligible to receive reimbursement from the Center for Medicare and Medicaid Services. ADA Recognition certifies that the program both meets quality standards and can be reimbursed for its services.

Essential content areas (Table 13.2) have been defined in the Standards for Diabetes Self-Management Education, developed by key diabetes organizations. These content areas were written in behavioral terms to maximize creativity on the part of the educator and allow programs to match instruction and methodology to the culture, literacy, and other needs of their target populations. The information provided is based on an individual assessment of needs and learning style. Evaluation of the effectiveness of DSME is based on patient achievement of self-selected behavior change goals, metabolic measures, and other outcomes.

Table 13.1 Recent Evidence for DSME

- DSME is effective for improving psychosocial and health outcomes.
- DSME is effective for patients with type 2 diabetes, especially in the short term.
- Traditional knowledge-based DSME is essential but not sufficient for sustained behavior change.
- No single strategy or programmatic focus shows any clear advantage, but interventions that incorporate behavioral and affective components are more effective.
- DSME has evolved from primarily didactic interventions into more theoretically-based empowerment models.
- Effective DSME is tailored to the patient's preferences and social and cultural situations.
- DSME is most effective when coupled with appropriate care and reinforcement by all health care professionals.

Table 13.2 Recommended DSME Content Areas

- Describe the diabetes disease process and treatment options.
- Incorporate appropriate nutritional management.
- Incorporate physical activity into lifestyle.
- Use medications (if applicable) for therapeutic effectiveness.
- Monitor blood glucose and urine ketones (when appropriate), and use the results to improve control.
- Prevent, detect, and treat acute complications.
- Prevent (through risk-reduction behavior), detect, and treat chronic complications.
- Set goals to promote health, and solve problems for daily living.
- Integrate psychosocial adjustment to daily life.
- Promote preconception care, management during pregnancy, and gestational diabetes management (if applicable).

PROVISION OF DSME AND SUPPORT

Any health care professional who provides diabetes education is a diabetes educator. A certified diabetes educator (CDE) is a health care professional who has specialized knowledge and practical experience in diabetes education and has passed an examination developed by the National Certification Board for Diabetes Education. Board-Certified–Advanced Diabetes Managers (BC-ADM) are advanced practice nurses, dietitians, or pharmacists who have passed an examination developed by the American Nurses Credentialing Center.

ROLE OF THE PROVIDER IN SELF-MANAGEMENT EDUCATION AND SUPPORT

Based on the Chronic Disease Model developed and tested by Wagner et al. (2001), successful management of a chronic illness requires actively involved patients working in partnership with a proactive practice team. Thus, effective diabetes care occurs at both the individual and system levels. Whereas it is unrealistic to expect providers to provide comprehensive DSME in the context of a busy practice, they do have an essential role to play in both of these arenas.

Starting at the time of diagnosis, providers need to provide key messages about diabetes and its treatment. Key messages include the following:

- All types of diabetes are serious.
- Diabetes can be managed.
- Effective self-management is essential for positive outcomes.
- A collaborative partnership between the patient, the patient's family, and the health care team is essential for successful diabetes care.

It is also useful to discuss the roles of the patient and the provider in diabetes care. Because chronic illness care differs from acute care, many patients will not have experienced working in partnership with their health care team. It is important to stress that the person with diabetes is the primary decision-maker and is responsible for the daily care of diabetes. It takes the provider's knowledge about diabetes combined with the expertise of the patients about their own goals and priorities to create a truly workable care plan. A plan that is not working is not a negative reflection on either the patient or the provider but simply needs to be revised.

Providers also need to stress the importance of DSME for successful self-management and offer referral to Recognized DSME programs and registered dietitians. Patients value physician opinions and recommendations. Providers need to let patients know that DSME is a wise investment in their future health and will provide the knowledge they need to make informed decisions as they care for themselves each day.

Providers can also acknowledge how difficult it is to live with diabetes and provide reinforcement for the education that has been provided based on feedback from the patient and the DSME program. Although most practices cannot offer comprehensive DSME, practitioners can take advantage of teachable moments that present during any patient encounter. For example, pointing out at-risk areas during a foot examination or making the link between heart disease and diabetes when reviewing lab results are powerful educational moments. Specific strategies that can be used with individual patients are listed in Table 13.3.

Table 13.3 Effective Provider-Based Strategies for Self-Management Support

- Stress the seriousness of diabetes.
- Stress the importance of DSME.
- Stress the importance of the patient's role in self-management.
- Offer referral to a Recognized DSME program and registered dietitian.
- Reinforce education provided in the DSME program.
- Begin each visit with an assessment of the patient's concerns, questions, and progress toward metabolic and behavioral goals.
- Address patient-identified fears and concerns.
- Assess patients' opinions about home blood glucose monitoring results and other laboratory and outcome measures.
- Review and revise the diabetes care plan as needed based on both the patients' and providers' assessment of its effectiveness.
- Provide ongoing information about the costs and benefits of therapeutic and behavioral options.
- Take advantage of teachable moments that occur during each visit.
- Establish a partnership with patients and their families to develop collaborative goals.
- Provide information about behavior change and problem-solving strategies.
- Assist patients to solve problems and overcome barriers to self-management.
- Support and facilitate patients in their role as self-management decision-makers.
- Abandon traditional dysfunctional models of care (e.g., adherence and compliance).

Physicians can not only ensure that individual patients receive DSME, but can also design their practices to facilitate ongoing self-management support. Although DSME and support work best when provided by a team of health care professionals, the team does not need to work in the same setting or in traditional roles. Better use of technology allows "virtual" teams to work and communicate effectively with each other and with patients. Table 13.4 lists strategies shown to be effective in facilitating self-management education and support in a variety of practice settings.

CONCLUSION

All types of diabetes are serious and can result in acute and long-term complications that diminish both the quality and length of patients' lives. Patients make multiple decisions each day that directly affect their outcomes, and they experience the consequences of their daily choices and self-care efforts. The key to closing the gap between the promise and reality of diabetes care is through the development of collaborative relationships and patient-centered practices to support our patients' self-management efforts. Effective DSME recognizes the patient's role as a collaborator, decision-maker, and expert on his or her own life and provides ongoing self-management support. DSME can help relieve the burden of diabetes care on your practice by helping patients to become informed, active participants in their own care. Staff members of a Recognized DSME program can become a valuable resource for you, your patients, and your staff. You can find an ADA Recognized DSME program in your area at www.diabetes.org. You can find a diabetes educator in your area at www.aadenet.org.

Table 13.4 Effective Practice-Based Strategies for Self-Management Support

- Use continuous quality improvement to develop, implement, maintain, and enhance DSME and improve practice.
- Link patient self-management support with provider support (e.g., systems changes, patient flow, and logistics).
- Supplement self-management support with information technology.
- Incorporate self-management support into practical interventions, coordinated by nurse case managers or other staff members.
- Create a team with other health care professionals in your system or area with additional experience or training in the clinical, educational, and behavioral or psychosocial aspects of diabetes care.
- Replace individual visits with group or cluster visits to provide efficient and effective self-management support.
- Assist patients to select one area of self-management on which to concentrate that can be reinforced by all team members.
- Create a patient-centered environment that incorporates self-management support from all practice personnel and is integrated into the flow of the visit.

BIBLIOGRAPHY

Anderson RM, Funnell MM: The role of the physician in patient education. *Pract Diabetol* 9:10–12, 1990

Funnell MM, Anderson RM: The problem with compliance in diabetes. *JAMA* 284:1709, 2000

Funnell MM, Anderson RM, Burkhart NT, Gillard ML, Nwanko R: *101 Tips for Diabetes Self-Management*. Alexandria, VA, American Diabetes Association, 2002

Glasgow RE, Funnell MM, Bonomi AE, Davis C, Beckham V, Wagner EH: Self-management aspects of the Improving Chronic Illness Care Breakthrough series: implementation with diabetes and heart failure teams. *Ann Behav Med* 24:80–87, 2002

Mensing C, Boucher J, Cypress M, Weinger K, Barta P, Hosey G, et al.: National standards for diabetes self-management education. *Diabetes Care* 23:682–689, 2000

National Diabetes Education Program: *Team Care: Comprehensive Lifetime Management for Diabetes*. Bethesda, MD, National Institutes of Health and the Centers for Disease Control and Prevention, 2001

Norris SL, Lau J, Smith SJ, Schmid CH, Engelgau MM: Self-management education for adults with type 2 diabetes: a meta-analysis on the effect on glycemic control. *Diabetes Care* 25:1159–1171, 2002

Wagner EH, Glasgow RE, Davis C, Bonomi AE, Provost L, McCulloch D, et al.: Quality improvement in chronic illness care: a collaborative approach. *Jt Comm J Qual Improv* 27:63–80, 2001

Ms. Funnell is a clinical nurse specialist and diabetes educator and Dr. Anderson is an educational psychologist and professor of medical education at the Michigan Diabetes Research and Training Center, Division of Endocrinology and Metabolism, Department of Internal Medicine, and the Department of Medical Education, University of Michigan, Ann Arbor, MI.

The authors were supported in part by grant number NIH5P60 DK20572 and 1 R18 0K062323-01 from the National Institute of Diabetes and Digestive and Kidney Diseases of the National Institutes of Health.

14. Monitoring Diabetes Mellitus

NATHANIEL G. CLARK, MD, MS, RD

Monitoring metabolic status in diabetes mellitus is critical to patient safety and a necessary element of self-management. The past two decades of clinical research resulted in major advances in monitoring, including the development and refinement of methods for self-monitoring of blood glucose (SMBG) and for measurement of chronic glycemia with glycated protein assays (glycated hemoglobin A1C [A1C]). The Diabetes Control and Complications Trial (DCCT) demonstrated the beneficial effects of intensive therapy in delaying the onset and slowing progression of long-term complications in type 1 diabetes. The DCCT established blood glucose and A1C goals for type 1 diabetes therapy and the requirement to perform blood glucose self-tests and periodic A1C tests as part of intensive therapy regimens. The United Kingdom Prospective Diabetes Study demonstrated similar results in newly diagnosed patients with type 2 diabetes. Therefore, comparable benefits of intensive management with a goal of achieving near-normal glucose levels in patients with either type 1 or type 2 diabetes have been demonstrated. Finally, recent studies have demonstrated that treatments targeted at meeting postprandial glucose goals are associated with improved outcomes in gestational diabetes. Furthermore, the demonstrated import of tight control in those planning pregnancy, the need to avoid hypoglycemia, and other practical considerations with regard to self-management dictate the need for monitoring guidelines. The relative lability of blood glucose profiles (and risks of hypoglycemia) in type 1 diabetes compared with type 2 diabetes requires more complex treatment and monitoring schedules.

MEASUREMENT OF GLUCOSE

The measurement of glucose levels, either laboratory based or patient performed, represents the most common means of assessing metabolic control in diabetes. Modern enzymatic (hexokinase or glucose oxidase) methods provide rapid, reliable, and accurate measurements. Serum and plasma levels as measured in most clinical laboratories and by most blood glucose meters are noted to be ~10–15% higher than simultaneous whole-blood levels. Therefore, care must be taken in interpreting the results of a particular test to determine the normal range.

Glucose oxidase–impregnated strips, read with a meter, provide patients with the opportunity to self-monitor. A list of products available for SMBG and their features can be found in the American Diabetes Association's Buyer's Guide to Diabetes Supplies, an annual supplement found in *Diabetes Forecast*. SMBG does require a bit of manual dexterity, cooperation, and intelligence. With available equipment and established patient education techniques, there are few people who cannot successfully monitor blood glucose at home. These meters come in a wide variety of shapes and sizes (from pens to cards to small boxes). Most have a memory for previous results, and some have sophisticated features such as allowing results to be downloaded to a computer and then graphically displayed. Some also allow the user to record medication doses and symptoms. Some strips require significantly smaller sample volumes than others, which may be an advantage for patients who have difficulty obtaining an adequate drop of blood. Similarly, some meters draw the sample in by capillary action, whereas others allow the user to smear the blood sample on the strip instead of applying a hanging drop as well as redosing the strip if an inadequate volume of blood is applied to the strip initially. As a result, some meters are clearly much easier for patients with various physical or cognitive impairments to use than others. Several can be adapted to voice synthesizers, which provide audio output of results. The use of an automated lancing device for fingersticks is recommended; several models are available, and some are more suited for children, frequent monitoring, and the squeamish. The biggest expense of SMBG is the strips. It is generally possible for most patients to get a meter heavily discounted or for free. The role of the diabetes educator in helping patients determine which meter meets their needs and the role of vendors in minimizing the financial repercussion of SMBG are critical in making this technique as widely and appropriately applied as possible. Unfortunately, a patient's socioeconomic circumstance often is the critical issue for many and too often determines whether SMBG is practical. Recent changes in federal and state insurance regulations are making SMBG a covered benefit for most insured patients.

Urine glucose measurements are not recommended. They are only an indirect semiquantitative reflection of blood glucose levels. Urine tests are blind to blood glucose levels below the renal threshold (generally 180–220 mg/dl [10–12.2 mmol/l]) and thus are incapable of distinguishing between blood glucose values in the normal to hypoglycemic range.

Type 1 Diabetes

Type 1 diabetes can be characterized by frequent, major fluctuations in blood glucose levels. Therefore, blood glucose monitoring is the method of choice for type 1 diabetes. Although intermittent office- or laboratory-based glucose assays may be useful in specific instances, labile glucose profiles in type 1 diabetes make sporadic measurements difficult to interpret. Isolated measurements may not be representative of values at other times or on other days. In addition, isolated measurements correlate poorly with the average level of glycemic control. Therefore, sporadic office-based glucose measurements are of limited value.

The logical method of monitoring type 1 diabetes is SMBG along with periodic A1C testing (see MEASUREMENT OF CHRONIC GLYCEMIA below). Table 14.1 describes the more commonly used regimens. The frequency of SMBG is predicated on the intensity and goals of the treatment regimen. The DCCT results

Table 14.1 SMBG in Type 1 Diabetes

Level of Treatment	Goals of Therapy	Expected A1C (%)	Time of Testing				
			Pre-breakfast	Pre-lunch	Pre-dinner	Pre-bedtime	Other*
Intensive (appropriate for most patients with type 1 diabetes)	Near-normal glucose levels Avoid complications	Goal <7; generally <8	X	X	X	X	X
≥3 injections/ day or insulin pump							
Frequent insulin dose self-adjustments							
Minimal							
2 injections/ day, gener-ally split-mixed	Avoid symptoms of hypoglycemia	Rarely <8; generally <9	As often as possible				
Frequent dose adjust-ments not made							

Insulin-treated patients with type 2 diabetes usually require minimal monitoring, consistent with their simple insulin injection regimen and overall greater glycemic stability.
*More frequent tests performed on sick days or when ketonuria is present, with changes in exercise or meal patterns, on travel days, or when hypoglycemia is suspected or imminent. Blood glucose levels 1–2 h postprandially may identify postprandial glycemic excursions that can be specifically targeted for treatment. Intensively treated patients should perform a test at midsleep (generally around 3:00 a.m.) on a weekly basis.

support intensive therapy as the treatment of choice for most patients with type 1 diabetes. Intensive treatment regimens (continuous subcutaneous insulin infusion with pumps or more than three daily injections) with glucose goals that approximate the nondiabetic range are associated with an increased risk for hypoglycemia, occasionally severe. To adjust insulin doses and to prevent hypoglycemia, frequent blood glucose monitoring is required. In the DCCT, a minimum requirement of four daily glucose tests (preprandial and bedtime) was implemented. In addition, 90-min postprandial tests were performed when A1C tests did not reach the normal range despite preprandial blood glucose levels in the target range (70–120 mg/dl [3.9–6.7 mmol/l]). A weekly 3:00 a.m. (or midsleep) blood glucose measurement was also required as a safety check to guard against unrecognized nocturnal hypoglycemia. A value <65 mg/dl (<3.6 mmol/l) required a repeat midsleep test the next day; if the repeat value was the same, the insulin regimen was adjusted.

Most patients with type 1 diabetes will benefit from intensive therapy; therefore, it is probably the most appropriate treatment regimen with which to initiate therapy. However, some patients are not interested in intensifying their regimen, and rare patients are incapable of following the more complex treatment algorithms associated with intensive management. Less intensive treatment regimens may include less frequent injections and self-monitoring. For example, patients treated with minimal treatment regimens, designed mainly to prevent symptomatic hyperglycemia and ketosis with two daily insulin injections, require less frequent monitoring. Here, the goal of monitoring is to prevent hypoglycemia and to adjust insulin on sick days.

Type 2 Diabetes

Blood glucose profiles are more stable in type 2 diabetes than in type 1 diabetes. Although SMBG has not been demonstrated to change outcomes in type 2 diabetes management in clinical trials, when evaluated in isolation, many diabetes self-management training programs have helped reduce complications (e.g., the DIGAMI and Kumamoto studies). In all of these programs, SMBG is an integral part of the process, suggesting that SMBG along with A1C testing is at least a component of effective therapy. The frequency and type of monitoring of diabetes therapy should be determined in consultation with the patient, taking into account the nature of the patient's diabetes, the overall treatment plan and goals, and the patient's abilities. Intermittent measurements (laboratory or office) of fasting or random blood glucose may suffice in stable non–insulin-treated type 2 diabetes patients but really do not provide a robust understanding of the level of overall glycemic control, as previously discussed.

SMBG is particularly recommended for all type 2 diabetes patients on insulin or sulfonylureas because it allows for the identification of minimal and/or asymptomatic episodes of hypoglycemia. It is well recognized that recurrent mild or asymptomatic hypoglycemia is a very strong risk factor for severe hypoglycemia. Although severe hypoglycemia is relatively rare in type 2 diabetes, it can have devastating consequences, such as trauma, self-injury, or a change in the perceived ability for a patient to continue to live independently as a result of confusion or loss of consciousness. Also, it is essential to have patients critically assess the nature of any hypoglycemic symptoms that occur during the day. Many patients are fearful or overconcerned about hypoglycemia and routinely consume extra calories when they are hungry, sweaty, nervous, upset, etc., because they believe that they are hypoglycemic. Monitoring with symptoms generally documents that most symptoms in patients with type 2 diabetes are not related to hypoglycemia and should not be treated with calories.

Timing of SMBG will vary depending on the diabetes therapy. Patients should not get into the habit of only checking at one particular time of day. The highest blood glucose of the day for some patients will be in the morning and that for others will be before bed. Particularly in early diabetes, gestational diabetes, and well-controlled diabetes, monitoring 1–2 h after meals allows patients to assess the effect of their lifestyle and pharmacological efforts in controlling postprandial glucose levels, which are usually the only glycemic abnormality present. Monitoring and thus targeting therapy at just one time of day could leave the patient with a less-than-ideal overall response to therapy. Some providers have patients concentrate initially on premeal glucose levels. If the A1C level is still not at target and the premeal glucose levels reach the mid- to low-100s, patients are encouraged to check 1- to 2-h postprandial glucose levels. This process may demonstrate the effects of lifestyle issues on glycemia and allow patients to identify how moderate changes in meal plan, activity, and medications have a significant impact on glycemic control.

The frequency of glucose monitoring needs to be matched to individual patient needs and treatment. Many clinicians ask patients to monitor at least once a day, varying before breakfast, lunch, dinner, or at bedtime, as well as with any hypoglycemic symptoms. Others ask intensively insulin-treated patients to monitor with an intensity similar to that described for patients with type 1 diabetes. Some ask for sets of glycemic readings more infrequently (e.g., fasting and 1 h after the biggest meal). In the subset of patients who achieve stable blood glucose levels, it is generally appropriate to decrease the frequency of SMBG to a few times a week. It is critical that SMBG be frequent enough that both patient and provider have a good understanding of both the adequacy of the treatment regimen and the stability of glycemic control.

SMBG RECORD KEEPING

It has been widely assumed that the benefits of SMBG stem from the effect of putting patients in a situation in which they can be in control of their own therapy. If patients are aware of the glycemic targets associated with the outcomes they seek, SMBG provides the ability for them to critically evaluate their response to therapy and to ensure themselves that they are reaching their goals. In this process, it is essential that patients and practitioners agree on acceptable glycemic targets, the frequency and pattern of SMBG, and a plan for interpreting and acting on the results obtained. To this end, it is generally useful for patients to keep a daily diary of their SMBG results, not only so that they can periodically assess their results but also so that they can share them with the health care team. Intermittently recording food intake, activity, symptoms, and doses of anti-diabetes medication simultaneously provides the patient and health care team with a better understanding of the factors that influence the level of glycemic control. Patients must have well-established plans for action based on the results they obtain. Unfortunately, many patients faithfully perform daily or more frequent SMBG, record the results as instructed, and only discuss them with their health care team at quarterly or semiannual visits despite inadequate control. Unless SMBG results are entirely within agreed-to targets, they should be communicated and reviewed at least monthly with a member of the health care team by phone, fax, mail, e-mail, or an interim visit to trigger changes in therapy as the need arises.

MEASUREMENT OF CHRONIC GLYCEMIA (A1C TEST)

Recognition that minor hemoglobin fractions, representing glycated adducts, increase in diabetic patients proportional to the average blood glucose over the preceding 2–3 months led to the development of the glycohemoglobin assay. Glycohemoglobin is expressed as a percentage of total hemoglobin (i.e., the fraction of total hemoglobin that has glucose attached). Depending on the assay method and laboratory used, the test may be called glycohemoglobin, glycated hemoglobin, glycosylated hemoglobin, hemoglobin A, or hemoglobin A1C. Although the different measurements all have different nondiabetic ranges, the results of all assay methods, when properly performed, correlate closely with each other (Table 14.2). Efforts to standardize these methods, making them traceable to the DCCT, continue. The term A1C should be used regardless of the specific lab test performed to make the understanding of this important test clearer to patients. Clinicians should become familiar with the assays used in their clinical laboratory, the factors that can interfere with them, and their nondiabetic range and should be vigilant for changes in the assay used by the laboratories they use. Laboratories should report the A1C result regardless of which assay was used, and these should be referable to the DCCT assay.

A1C testing may be used to assess the effects of changes in therapy made 4–12 weeks earlier. It should not be used to determine the need for short-term changes in treatment. Blood glucose levels, generally from SMBG, are still the best means by which hour-to-hour and day-to-day changes in insulin management can be determined. Furthermore, health care providers have learned not to rely solely on SMBG results, because the measurements are subject to errors in technique and the records are subject to errors of omission and commission.

Certain conditions and interfering substances affect A1C results depending on the assay method used. Any condition that increases erythrocyte turnover (e.g., bleeding, pregnancy, splenectomy, or hemolysis) will spuriously lower A1C concentration in all assays. In addition, hemoglobinopathies (e.g., sickle-cell trait or disease, or hemoglobin C or D) will falsely lower A1C results when hemoglobins

Table 14.2 Glycated Hemoglobin Assay (A1C Test)

- Measures average level of glucose over preceding 2–3 mo
- Provides objective index correlated with risk of complications not provided by other measures
- Different assay methods measure different fractions; must check non-diabetic range for each assay
- Correlate results to DCCT assay
- Interfering factors (e.g., sickle-cell hemoglobin and other hemoglobinopathies) may affect measurement, depending on method

- May be used to validate accuracy of SMBG; discrepancy between SMBG levels and A1C suggests inaccurate SMBG results or the need to alter times when SMBG is performed
- Optimal frequency not certain, but 2–4 assays/yr are necessary to determine efficacy of management and complement SMGB in type 1 diabetes; in stable type 2 diabetes, 2 assays/yr should suffice

are separated by nonspecific methods based on charge, solubility, and size. Other conditions (e.g., uremia, high concentrations of fetal hemoglobin, high aspirin doses [usually >10 g/day], or high concentrations of ethanol) may falsely increase A1C levels.

Measurement of other glycated proteins, such as albumin or serum proteins, has been proposed as another means of determining average glucose control. These methods, including measurement of serum fructosamine, reflect a shorter period (~2–3 weeks) of average glucose control than glycohemoglobin as a result of the shorter half-life of serum proteins compared with hemoglobin. The shorter period of average glycemia reflected by the measurement of glycated serum proteins limits their overall utility similarly to the situation for single glucose determinations. Measuring serum proteins does provide theoretical advantages in situations where the overall response to a recent (2- to 3-week) change in therapy is necessary. However, although A1C does reflect glycemic control over 2–3 months, the result is time weighted in that the level of glycemic control over the past month is a much greater determinant of the result than the previous months. Therefore, the A1C test is somewhat useful in assessing trends in response to therapy over a period as short as 1 month.

In general, well-controlled patients with type 2 diabetes on stable therapeutic regimens who perform SMBG should have their A1C determined at least twice a year. More frequent monitoring of A1C (quarterly) should be useful in assessing the response to therapy in patients with unstable courses or changes in therapy. Patients with type 1 diabetes should have A1C measurements performed quarterly.

MEASUREMENT OF URINE AND BLOOD KETONES

Patients with type 1 diabetes are ketosis prone, whereas patients with type 2 diabetes are generally ketosis resistant. Because ketoacidosis may be associated with gastrointestinal symptoms indistinguishable from gastroenteritis, patients and physicians should be particularly attentive to such symptoms and test ketones if they occur. In addition, patients with type 1 diabetes should test ketones if their SMBG indicates blood glucose levels consistently >300 mg/dl (>16.7 mmol/l). It is now possible to test blood ketones, along with blood glucose, with a portable meter.

BIBLIOGRAPHY

American Diabetes Association: Postprandial blood glucose (Consensus Statement). *Diabetes Care* 24:775–778, 2001

American Diabetes Association: Self-monitoring of blood glucose (Consensus Statement). *Diabetes Care* 17 (Suppl. 1):81–86, 1994

American Diabetes Association: Standards of medical care in diabetes (Position Statement). *Diabetes Care* 27 (Suppl. 1):S15–S35, 2004

American Diabetes Association: Tests of glycemia in diabetes (Position Statement). *Diabetes Care* 27 (Suppl. 1):S91–S93, 2004

deVeciana M, Major CA, Morgan MA, Asrat T, Toohey JS, Lien JM, Evans AT: Postprandial versus preprandial blood glucose monitoring in women with gestational diabetes mellitus requiring insulin therapy. *N Engl J Med* 333:1237–1241, 1995

Diabetes Control and Complications Trial Research Group: Implementation of treatment protocols in the Diabetes Control and Complications Trial. *Diabetes Care* 18:361–376, 1995

Diabetes Control and Complications Trial Research Group: The effect of intensive diabetes management on long-term complications in insulin-dependent diabetes mellitus. *N Engl J Med* 329:977–986, 1993

Faas A, Schellevis FG, van Eijk JTM: The efficacy of self-monitoring of blood glucose in NIDDM subjects: criteria-based review of the literature. *Diabetes Care* 20:1482–1486, 1997

Malmberg K, Ryden L, Efendic S, Herlitz J, Nicol P, Waldenstrom A, Wedel H, Welin L, on behalf of the DIGAMI Study Group: Randomized trial of insulin-glucose infusion followed by subcutaneous insulin treatment in diabetic patients with acute myocardial infarction (DIGAMI study): effects on mortality at 1 year. *J Am Coll Cardiol* 26:57–65, 1995

Ohkubo Y, Kishikawa H, Araki E, Isami S, Motoyoshi S, Kojima Y, et al.: Intensive insulin therapy prevents the progression of diabetic microvascular complications in Japanese patients with non-insulin-dependent diabetes mellitus: a randomized prospective 6-year study. *Diabetes Res Clin Pract* 28:103–117, 1995

Sacks DB, Bruns DE, Goldstein DE, MacLaren NK, McDonald JM, Parrott M: Guidelines and recommendations for laboratory analysis in the diagnosis and management of diabetes mellitus. *Diabetes Care* 25:750–786, 2002

U.K. Prospective Diabetes Study (UKPDS) Group: Intensive blood glucose control with sulphonylureas or insulin compared with conventional treatment and risk of complications in patients with type 2 diabetes (UKPDS 33). *Lancet* 352:837–853, 1998

Dr. Clark is the National Vice President for Clinical Affairs for the American Diabetes Association.

15. Rationale for Management of Hyperglycemia

Harold E. Lebovitz, MD

The principles involved in managing hyperglycemia in patients with diabetes mellitus are outlined in Table 15.1. Each patient should have an initial assessment to define the appropriate glycemic goal for his or her treatment program. Diabetes education in a structured program supervised by a qualified diabetes educator is essential for every patient with diabetes. Without adequate education, patients will not be able to self-monitor blood glucose, understand their disease, comply with their treatment program, or take appropriate action to minimize complications. Intervention is initiated with lifestyle modification and, when necessary to achieve the glycemic control target, with the addition of pharmacological agents. Changes in the therapeutic program are guided by the results of self-monitoring of blood glucose and glycated hemoglobin A1C (A1C) measurements.

Data from recent intervention studies in both type 1 and type 2 diabetes patients indicate that early initiation of intensive hyperglycemic management has profound long-term beneficial effects in reducing microvascular complications. The pathogenetic effects of the level of hyperglycemia on the microvascular system persist for many years. This effect of the "memory" of the microvascular system for its history of glycemic control is noted in the remarkable delay between the time at which intensive glycemic control is achieved and the time at which the rate of development of microvascular complications begins to decrease. In the Diabetes Control and Complications Trial (DCCT), this delay was about 3–4 years, and in the United Kingdom Prospective Diabetes Study, it was about 9 years. The most definitive proof of this effect is being shown in the EDIC (Epidemiology of Diabetes Interventions and Complications) study, which is the long-term follow-up of individuals who had been in the DCCT. At the conclusion of

Table 15.1 Principles of Glycemic Control

- Initiate the treatment program when hyperglycemia is first diagnosed.
- Define the appropriate target goal.
- The target goal should be near normoglycemia if possible.

- Diabetes education is essential.
- Monitor glycemic control.
- Initiate lifestyle modification.
- Use stepwise and combination pharmacological therapy.

the DCCT protocol, all of the patients were sent back to their primary care health facilities for continuing care. A substantial cohort of the individuals agreed to return to their DCCT research center yearly for continued monitoring for vascular complications. During the 7 years of follow-up, the mean A1C of the previously intensively treated group (mean A1C 7.2%) increased and has averaged 8.0%. In contrast, the mean A1C of the control cohort (mean A1C 9.0%) decreased and has averaged 8.0%. Despite the equal glycemic control over the last 4–5 years, the rate of development and progression of clinical retinopathy and nephropathy in the previously intensively treated cohort is less than one-third that of the previous control cohort.

Hyperglycemia in patients with diabetes mellitus results from a combination of overproduction and underutilization of glucose. In establishing a rational approach to the management of hyperglycemia, it is important to understand the dominant influences in the patient for whom the strategy is being developed.

Patients who are absolutely insulin deficient (e.g., those with type 1 diabetes or surgical removal or destruction of the pancreas) must receive insulin replacement therapy as the main therapeutic agent. None of the available oral antidiabetic agents can effectively ameliorate hyperglycemia in the absence of endogenous insulin.

Patients in whom hyperglycemia results from an imbalance between insulin secretory function and peripheral insulin sensitivity, as occurs in type 2 diabetes, are excellent candidates for initiation of nonpharmacological therapies that reduce insulin secretory requirements (diet) or increase peripheral insulin effectiveness (exercise, weight loss). If these measures do not result in the target glycemic control, pharmacological agents whose primary actions are to reduce postprandial glycemic excursions (α-glucosidase inhibitors), increase peripheral glucose utilization (thiazolidinediones), decrease hepatic glucose production (metformin), or increase β-cell insulin secretory function (sulfonylureas, repaglinide, or nateglinide) are indicated.

In most patients with type 2 diabetes, insulin secretory capacity decreases with time, and patients who were well controlled on one or more oral agents will lose their glycemic control. At that stage, addition of an intermediate-acting or basal insulin at bedtime or conversion to a multiple insulin injection regimen is probably necessary.

The degree of metabolic control achieved with initial dietary management of newly diagnosed type 2 diabetes patients is useful in defining an initial approach to treatment. Fasting plasma glucose (FPG) and A1C levels during treatment define when changes in therapy are indicated.

During hyperinsulinemic or normoinsulinemic phases of type 2 diabetes (FPG <150 mg/dl [8.3 mmol/l]), dietary management alone or combined with monotherapy with an β-glucosidase inhibitor, nateglinide, metformin, or a thiazolidinedione is likely to be very effective in normalizing glycemia. As insulin secretory function decreases (FPG 150–225 mg/dl [8.3–12.5 mmol/l]), β-glucosidase inhibitors, nateglinide, thiazolidinediones, and diet become less effective, and metformin, sulfonylureas, or repaglinide are more likely to be useful in controlling glycemia. Progressive insulin secretory deficiency (FPG 225–275 mg/dl [12.5–15.3 mmol/l]) will require combinations of oral agents and eventually insulin as part of the management strategy to control glycemia.

Going directly from dietary management to insulin treatment seems plausible, but problems of excessive weight gain, severe episodes of hypoglycemia, and lack of treating insulin resistance and the components of the metabolic syndrome are significant concerns. Additionally, available data indicate that, in most patients, a carefully constructed management scheme with combinations of oral agents is just as effective as multiple insulin injections during the first several years of treatment of type 2 diabetes.

An important issue in starting a treatment regimen for type 2 diabetes patients is the effect that hyperglycemia itself has on inhibiting insulin secretion and impairing insulin action. This so-called glucose toxicity effect suggests that oral agents that might be effective in controlling glycemia at modest levels of hyperglycemia by increasing insulin secretion or improving insulin action could be ineffective at higher levels of hyperglycemia. Treatment of such patients with insulin for a few days to reduce the marked hyperglycemia may make the patient more responsive to subsequent treatment with oral agents.

BIBLIOGRAPHY

Diabetes Control and Complications Trial Research Group: The effect of intensive treatment of diabetes on the development and progression of long-term complications in insulin-dependent diabetes mellitus. *N Engl J Med* 329:977–986, 1993

The Writing Team for the Diabetes Control and Complications Trial/ Epidemiology of Diabetes Interventions and Complications Research Group: Effect of intensive therapy on the microvascular complications of type 1 diabetes mellitus. *JAMA* 287:2563–2569, 2002

Lebovitz HE: Oral therapies for diabetic hyperglycemia. *Endocrinol Metab Clin North Am* 30:909–933, 2001

Lebovitz HE: Treating hyperglycemia in type 2 diabetes: new goals and strategies. *Cleve Clin J Med* 69:809–820, 2002

Turner R, Cull C, Holman R: United Kingdom Prospective Diabetes Study 17: a 9-year update of a randomized controlled trial of the effect of improved metabolic control on complications in non-insulin-dependent diabetes mellitus. *Ann Intern Med* 124:136–145, 1996

UK Prospective Diabetes Study 7: Response of fasting plasma glucose to diet therapy in newly presenting type II diabetic patients. *Metabolism* 39:905–912, 1990

UK Prospective Diabetes Study Group: Intensive blood-glucose control with sulphonylureas or insulin compared with conventional treatment and risk of complications in patients with type 2 diabetes (UKPDS 33). *Lancet* 352:837–853, 1998

UK Prospective Diabetes Study Group: Effect of intensive blood glucose control with metformin on complications in overweight patients with type 2 diabetes (UKPDS 34). *Lancet* 352:854–865, 1998

Yki-Jarvinen H: Glucose toxicity. *Endocr Rev* 13:415–431, 1992

Yki-Jarvinen H, Kauppila M, Kujansuu E, Lahti J, Marjanen T, Niskanen L, Rajala S, Ryysy L, Salo S, Seppala P, et al.: Comparison of insulin regimens in patients with non-insulin-dependent diabetes mellitus. *N Engl J Med* 327:1426–1433, 1992

Dr. Lebovitz is Professor of Medicine at the State University of New York Health Science Center at Brooklyn, Brooklyn, NY.

16. Medical Nutrition Therapy

ANNE DALY, MS, RD, CDE, AND MARGARET A. POWERS, MS, RD, CDE

Medical nutrition therapy (MNT) is an essential component of comprehensive diabetes care and management. Within 6–12 weeks of initiating MNT, glycated hemoglobin A1C (A1C) levels often decrease 1–2%. Additionally, MNT is effective in lowering blood pressure and improving one's lipid profile. With such a clinically significant treatment tool available, why do so many health care professionals not encourage its full use? Perhaps it is because they are unaware of the effectiveness of MNT. Perhaps some think it is too hard to follow a "diet." Perhaps a referral process for MNT has not been established. Perhaps health care professionals or their patients do not believe they can receive reimbursement for MNT. This chapter will address these issues so that your patients can receive the full benefit of MNT.

OVERVIEW OF MNT

The ultimate goal of diabetes nutrition therapy is for people with diabetes to be comfortable and confident in making daily food choices that contribute to improved metabolic status. This goal is achieved through the development of a personalized food plan that incorporates an individual's favorite foods and typical eating patterns. Additionally, counseling and coaching about behavioral strategies particular to the individual support the achievement of short- and long-term goals related to the food plan.

Table 16.1 lists the goals of MNT. Because 75% of deaths in individuals with diabetes are attributed to cardiovascular disease, it is critical that the focus of care be expanded beyond glycemic control. That is why the first goal encompasses the ABCs of diabetes care—managing A1C, Blood pressure, and Cholesterol. Nutrition therapy is the first-line therapy for managing elevations in each of these areas and heightens the effectiveness of medication when it is necessary. Table 16.2 highlights the effectiveness of MNT.

Thus, diabetes medications support the food plan and should be prescribed to correspond with eating times and food patterns. The medication should not force an individual to eat at inappropriate or unusual times. The fact that the medication needs of individuals with type 2 diabetes become more complex as their diabetes progresses is typical and should be expected. Combinations of oral agents are eventually needed, with 40–60% of patients requiring insulin. Continuous

---

Table 16.1 Goals of MNT

1. Attain and maintain optimal metabolic outcomes.
   - Blood glucose goals in a normal range to reduce risk for diabetes complications
   - Blood pressure levels to reduce risk for vascular disease
   - Lipid levels to reduce risk for macrovascular disease

2. Prevent, delay, or treat nutrition-related complications: obesity, dyslipidemia, cardiovascular disease, hypertension, and nephropathy.
3. Improve health through healthy food choices and physical activity.
4. Address individual nutrition needs.

---

reliance on MNT alone, or MNT and one diabetes agent, to achieve glycemic control may be poor care. As medication therapy advances, MNT needs to continue and may also need to advance.

Tables 16.3 and 16.4 outline MNT principles for type 1 and type 2 diabetes. Table 16.5 summarizes new nutrition paradigms based on the 2004 nutrition recommendations.

DIABETES PREVENTION

Key clinical research, including the Diabetes Prevention Program (DPP), concludes that the incidence of type 2 diabetes can be decreased by 58% in at-risk individuals. The success of such programs depends on the implementation of

---

Table 16.2 MNT Effectiveness in Diabetes Patients

Glycemic control

- ~1% decrease in A1C in newly diagnosed type 1 diabetes patients (10–12% decrease)
- ~2% decrease in A1C in newly diagnosed type 2 diabetes patients (22% decrease)
- ~1% decrease in A1C with an average 4-yr duration of type 2 diabetes (12% decrease)
- 50–100 mg/dl decrease in fasting plasma glucose
- Outcomes will be known by 6 wk to 3 mo

Lipids (7–10% saturated fat, 200–300 mg cholesterol intake)

- 10–13% decrease in total cholesterol (24–32 mg/dl)

- 12–16% decrease in LDL cholesterol (18–25 mg/dl)
- 8% decrease in triglycerides (15–17 mg/dl)
- Without exercise, HDL cholesterol decreases by 7%; with exercise, no decrease

Hypertension

- 2,400 mg sodium: 5 mmHg decrease in systolic blood pressure and 2 mmHg decrease in diastolic blood pressure in hypertensive patients

Table 16.3 Principles of Nutrition Therapy for Type 1 Diabetes

- Integrate insulin with individual eating and lifestyle.
- Conventional therapy: synchronize food with insulin; eat at consistent times; teach types of foods and portion sizes.
- Intensive therapy: adjust insulin to fit food intake, physical activity, lifestyle factors.
- Use self-monitored blood glucose results to adjust meal plan and insulin doses.
- Monitor potential weight gain with intensive therapy.
- Monitor blood glucose, A1C, lipids, blood pressure, and microalbuminuria.

lifestyle structured intervention programs (Table 16.6). These programs emphasize reduced fat and energy intake, regular physical activity, and regular participant contact. The interventions are well defined and available via the Internet at www.dpp.org.

The DPP intensive lifestyle participants achieved:

- a mean weight loss of 7% after 1 year and maintained a 5% weight loss at 3 years
- a mean level of physical activity of 208 min/week at 1 year and 189 min/week at 3 years

Dietitians were involved in the many facets of the study and were integral to achieving the reduction in new cases of diabetes.

Involving dietitians in the care of individuals at risk for developing diabetes will support the above study results. Individuals at risk include those described in Chapter 19. Special attention can be given to children who are overweight and women who had gestational diabetes. Children pose difficult challenges that involve public health and school policy issues. Diabetes care providers may need to become involved in these issues to ensure access to appropriate food and activity throughout the day.

Table 16.4 Principles of Nutrition Therapy for Type 2 Diabetes

- Focus on glucose, blood pressure, and lipid goals.
- Modify fat intake.
- Improve food choices.
- Space intake of carbohydrate foods throughout day.
- Increase physical activity.
- If obese, modify calories for moderate weight loss.
- Monitor blood glucose, A1C, blood pressure and lipids.
- Add and advance diabetes medication therapy, as needed.

Table 16.5 The Old Versus the New Nutrition Paradigm

Outdated Nutrition Advice	Updated Nutrition Advice
MNT was a calculated ADA diet (calories and percentage of macronutrients).	There no longer is an ADA diet that applies to all individuals with diabetes. An ADA diet can only be defined as an individualized food/meal plan based on assessment, therapy goals, and use of approaches that meet the patient's needs. Diet sheets or a one-time "diet instruction" rarely is sufficient to change eating habits. For people to make lifestyle changes that result in positive clinical outcomes, both education and counseling, especially in the areas of nutrition and physical activity, and support over time are required.
Weight loss was encouraged.	Weight loss is typically a helpful but not essential treatment for improving blood glucose. Weight loss may be a barrier for individuals who have tried multiple times to lose weight unsuccessfully. It is often possible to improve glucose control by changing food habits without weight loss. For those who are already at or below an appropriate weight, weight loss is not a treatment goal.
Standard treatment included 1–2 visits.	Frequent contact with individualized goal setting and implementation plans recommended.
Ideal body weight was used as the goal, and this goal often required a weight loss of 40–50 lb (18–23 kg).	Weight loss of 5–10% of current weight is proven effective to reduce health risk. Long-term follow-up to improve or maintain eating behaviors and increase physical activity.
Sugars and sweets were forbidden because they were believed to be more rapidly digested and absorbed and to cause blood glucose levels to go higher than starches.	Evidence from many clinical studies has demonstrated that sugars do not increase glycemia more than isocaloric amounts of starch. Therefore, the total amount of carbohydrate eaten is more important than the source of the carbohydrate.
Protein was recommended because it was believed to slow the absorption of carbohydrates and to prevent hypoglycemia.	Ingested protein does not slow the absorption of carbohydrate nor does adding protein prevent late-onset hypoglycemia or assist in the treatment of hypoglycemia.
Chromium and vitamin E were often recommended to improve blood glucose or lipid levels.	If individuals are not deficient in a micronutrient, supplements are unlikely to be beneficial. It is difficult to determine who is and who is not deficient in chromium. Supplementation with vitamin E has not been shown to be beneficial in the intervention trials.
"When diet and exercise fail," add medications: at this point, there was no need to pay attention to lifestyle.	Type 2 diabetes is a progressive disease, and MNT should always be part of the diabetes care plan. β-cells fail, not diet and exercise.

ADA, American Diabetes Association

Table 16.6 Components of a Structured Lifestyle-Change Program

- Calorie intake deficit achieved through calorie counting and/or fat gram counting, with strict attention to portion control
- Increased physical activity
- Individual goal setting

- Specific plan making
- Individual and/or group sessions
- Standardized curriculum
- Follow-up contact during weight-maintenance phase

INITIATING THERAPY

Nutrition therapy must be goal directed and individualized according to a person's usual food intake and lifestyle. It is not appropriate to prescribe a precise caloric intake or a precise distribution of food. It may take several visits to develop and refine the food plan, and more visits may be required for the patient to learn how to maintain the plan in a variety of situations and to incorporate a variety of food choices (see Table 16.7 for time frames for nutrition intervention). Modifying eating patterns is not a simple procedure, yet reasonable, achievable goals can be set and successfully met with the guidance of a skilled counselor. When initiating or adjusting MNT, blood glucose monitoring frequency should increase to guide changes in food intake, activity, and medications, when prescribed. More frequent blood glucose monitoring also helps determine whether changes to the food plan are necessary or if adjusting another therapy is more appropriate.

The five primary nutrition messages that apply to most people with diabetes are as follows:

1. Eat similar amounts of carbohydrate throughout the day each day (e.g., eat similar amounts at breakfast from day to day).
2. Practice portion control by measuring your food to become more aware of how much you are eating and to be able to eat similar amounts of carbohydrate.
3. Decrease fat by reducing portion sizes of high-fat foods, choosing foods prepared with less fat and using less fat as spreads and sauces.

Table 16.7 Time Frames for Nutrition Intervention

Initial workup/assessment (can be part of group DSMT)	Follow-up for therapy evaluation, adjustment, and education
■ 1–2 h, one to two appointments	■ As needed
	■ With lifestyle and life-cycle changes
Self-management education (can be part of group DSMT)	■ Minimum follow-up for children every 3–6 mo; for adults, every 6–12 mo
■ Biweekly or monthly sessions for 2–4 mo, 30–60 min each	■ Intensive therapy requires 4–6 visits a year plus phone contact
■ Daily/weekly phone calls with self-monitored blood glucose records, as needed	

4. Add physical activity to your day to total 30 min of activity each day.
5. Be at a healthy weight or, if overweight and interested in losing weight, lose about 10 lb and observe how your blood glucose, blood pressure, and/or cholesterol improves.

There are many details to understand in order to make these behavioral changes. Simply stating them to a patient will not promote adherence. The education process described below will help your patients achieve these goals.

OBESITY TREATMENT

The U.S. has experienced epidemics of both obesity and diabetes in the last decade. Approximately 36% of people diagnosed with diabetes have a BMI ≥30 kg/m², which classifies them as obese. Risk for developing diabetes increases from a BMI as low as 22. The relative risk for diabetes increases by approximately 25 percent for each additional unit of BMI over 22. Obesity increases insulin resistance and may aggravate hyperlipidemia and hypertension. Aggressive intervention is warranted to treat obesity in patients diagnosed with diabetes as well as individuals with pre-diabetes, or those with one or more risk factors for developing diabetes. Long-term weight maintenance poses a major challenge. Structured, intensive lifestyle-change programs (Table 16.6), similar to those used in the DPP, produce more successful weight loss and weight maintenance than conventional treatment consisting of one initial visit to the registered dietitian (RD), followed by two follow-up visits.

Recent nutrition recommendations encourage setting goals for a reasonable body weight, defined as a weight that the patient confirms as being achievable and sustainable. Baseline calorie needs depend on height, weight, the need for weight loss or gain, and usual activity/exercise patterns.

Diabetes in obese, inactive children has become a major concern and takes special skill in treating so as to not create eating disorders or a negative attitude toward health care. Encouraging physical activity and a well-balanced food plan that maintains weight is often a goal. Counseling support may be necessary to supplement other interventions.

Nonpharmacological Treatment of Obesity

Assessing patient readiness is an important first step to successful weight management. Readiness means that a patient is interested in weight reduction, understands that weight management is a lifelong commitment, and is willing to do what is appropriate and necessary to support success. Selection of weight-reduction treatment options can be based on health risk (Table 16.8).

Pharmacological Treatment of Obesity

Pharmacological agents for obesity can be a useful adjunct to, but not a substitute for, the necessary changes in food intake and physical activity. The effectiveness of any pharmacological intervention depends on its use with appropriate nutrition intervention, increased physical activity, and lifestyle change.

Table 16.8 Selected Weight-Reduction Treatment Options Based on Health Risk

Health Risk	Based Solely on BMI (kg/m²)	Adjusted for Comorbid Conditions and/or Risk Factors	Treatment Options Available
Minimal	<25		Healthful eating
			Increased physical activity
Low	25 to <27	<25	All the above plus moderate calorie deficit
Moderate	27 to <30	25 to <27	All the above plus low-calorie diet
High	30 to <35	27 to <30	All the above plus pharmacotherapy
Very high	35 to <40	30 to <35	All the above plus very-low-calorie diet
Extremely high	≥40	≥35	All the above plus surgical intervention

Pharmacological intervention is recommended for use only in clients with a BMI ≥27 kg/m² in the presence of a comorbid condition and ≥30 kg/m² when no comorbid condition is present (see Chapter 17).

NUTRITION EDUCATION PROCESS

Nutrition education involves a continuous four-step process.

1. **Assessment:** An initial diet history, food and blood glucose records, medications taken, laboratory values, lifestyle, readiness to change, and the ability to grasp information are assessed.
2. **Goal setting:** Client and health care providers agree on reasonable, measurable goals that are consistent with overall diabetes management. Communicating with other health care team members at team meetings, in the medical record, during clinic sessions, or on the telephone is helpful to share and compare assessments, goals, and impressions about a client's needs and abilities.
3. **Intervention:** No single strategy or method of nutrition intervention can be recommended because various methods have been tested and demonstrated to facilitate attainment of nutrition goals. During initial phases of education (survival), simplified resources are recommended. Subsequently, more complex approaches may be appropriate. Commonly used nutrition interventions are listed in Table 16.9. Use of various nutrition interven-

Table 16.9 Nutrition Intervention Options

	Level of Care	
Initial	**Continuing**	**Intensive**
Basic nutrition guidelines	Carbohydrate counting	Carbohydrate counting using insulin-to-carbohydrate ratios
Healthy food choices		
Food-guide pyramid	Exchange Lists: basic	Exchange Lists: advanced
First step in diabetes meal planning	Calorie counting	Structured lifestyle-change program
	Lifestyle changes	Medically supervised very-low-calorie diets
Carbohydrate counting: basic	Fat counting	

tions provides greater flexibility and choices to the person with diabetes and is especially useful for those who have been discouraged or frustrated by previous nutrition instruction methods. The different nutrition interventions have distinctive and varying characteristics of structure and complexity. The choice of a food plan depends on both the dietitian's experience with different strategies and which approach best meets the individual needs of the client.

4. **Evaluation:** Evaluation is a continuous process of observing metabolic outcomes and client perceptions of how things are going, as well as designing additional education and support services to meet instructional and lifestyle needs.

Follow-up educational sessions with the dietitian focus on various topics such as food composition, food labeling, shopping, recipe adaptations, and eating in restaurants. Dietitians guide patients in using food records in conjunction with blood glucose records to observe patterns in blood glucose control. A problem-solving approach is used to analyze individual blood glucose responses to food, activity, and medications. Patients are then able to make adjustments in food intake and/or insulin dosage to maintain target blood glucose levels. Algorithms for food, medication, and activity can be developed to help manage diabetes on a daily basis. Small careful steps over weeks or months help move the client toward nutrition goals. Follow-up sessions by the dietitian can be accomplished via clinic visits and telephone conversations to facilitate problem solving. Family members and significant others should be involved in the nutrition education process and are encouraged to follow the same healthy lifestyle recommendations as the person with diabetes.

Contact with a dietitian is recommended at least twice per year (Table 16.7) to monitor metabolic parameters and assess the appropriateness and effectiveness of the nutrition therapy. When patients experience lifestyle changes such as schedule changes, marriage, divorce, change of job or home, or pregnancy, nutrition therapy should be reviewed. If nutrition therapy goals are not met, changes can be made in the overall diabetes care and management plan. See Table 16.10 for the top five reasons to refer a patient to a dietitian.

WHO SHOULD PROVIDE MNT?

The complexity of nutrition issues requires a coordinated team effort, including the person with diabetes. To achieve nutrition goals, the American Diabetes Association (ADA) recommends that an RD, knowledgeable and skilled in implementing current principles and recommendations for diabetes, be the member of the diabetes care team who provides ongoing MNT as an integral part of overall diabetes care. It is, however, important for all members of the diabetes care and education team to communicate the basic principles of nutrition and lifestyle guidelines and support interventions for further training so the guidelines can be assimilated into the patient's life.

ACCESS TO MNT

Although referrals for diabetes self-management training (DSMT) are increasing, the sad fact remains that only ~30% of individuals with diabetes have had any education. Of those individuals, a smaller percentage has seen an RD for MNT. Studies of referral patterns indicate that the lack of referral by physicians and other health care professionals remains a major barrier. Lack of dissemination about the good news regarding improved reimbursement may be a factor. Table 16.11 provides information about how to access dietitians and diabetes education.

REIMBURSEMENT FOR DIABETES MNT AND DSMT

Although in the past lack of reimbursement has been a barrier for providers to refer patients, over the last decade reimbursement/coverage for diabetes MNT and DSMT have improved greatly. More health plans than ever before are covering MNT and DSMT. Providers should encourage people with diabetes to learn about their benefits and to be proactive in obtaining coverage for MNT and DSMT. For more information, Table 16.12 lists information resources about DSMT and MNT.

Table 16.10 Top Five Reasons to Refer to a Dietitian

Refer a patient to a dietitian when a patient:

1. is new to diabetes and doesn't know what to eat
2. has had diabetes awhile but needs to get back on track
3. wants help in deciding how to eat their favorite foods
4. has a schedule that makes it difficult to eat well
5. wants to feel better and improve their diabetes control
6. would like to improve food choices and/or lose weight

Table 16.11 Accessing Dietitians and Diabetes Education

- Find the ADA's Recognized Education Programs in your area (see Table 16.12).
- Locate a diabetes educator who is a dietitian by calling the American Association of Diabetes Educators (AADE) at 1-800-TEAMUP4 (800-832-6874) or go to AADE's website www.aadenet.org and go to "Find a Diabetes Educator" in the "General Public" section.
- Find a dietitian by calling The American Dietetic Association at 800-366-1655 or go to their website www.eatright.org.
- Ask colleagues about dietitians and diabetes education programs in your area.

State Laws

Forty-six states have passed laws that require health insurance companies and managed care plans to cover DSMT, which includes MNT. See Table 16.12 for help in finding out the law in your state. These laws have also typically required coverage of diabetes supplies, such as blood glucose meters and testing strips. Unfortunately, however, these state laws cover only ~30% of people with diabetes because they do not cover Medicaid or Medicare recipients or individuals employed by large businesses.

Medicare

Medicare now covers DSMT for people with diabetes who meet specific eligibility criteria and when it is provided by programs that have been reviewed and approved by the ADA Education Recognized Program or by the Indian Health Service. These programs must follow the National Standards for Diabetes Self-Management Education programs. There are 10 h of outpatient training available initially during the first 12 months of submitting for this service, and up to 2 h

---

Table 16.12 Information Resources about DSMT and MNT Reimbursement

State laws	www.diabetes.org/advocacy
	www.aadenet.org/ResourceCenter
List of recognized diabetes programs in each state	ADA Recognition Programs: call 1-800-DIABETES (800-342-2383)
	www.diabetes.org/education/eduprogram.asp
Medicare coverage for MNT and DSMT	www.diabetes.org
	www.aadenet.org
	www.eatright.org

---

annually thereafter, with provider referral. Medicare requires that the DSMT be provided in groups unless the provider has identified a specific barrier to group education.

In addition, Medicare coverage for MNT for Part B beneficiaries with type 1, type 2, and gestational diabetes and renal disease (exclusive of beneficiaries on dialysis and 6 months after renal transplant) went into effect January 2002. The beneficiary must be referred by the treating physician, and the service must be provided by a qualified nutrition professional (i.e., an RD) who has obtained a Unique Physician/Practitioner Identification Number (UPIN) from Medicare. The nutrition professional can then be directly reimbursed for MNT and DSMT or can assign reimbursement to his or her place of employment. The beneficiary is entitled to 3 h within a 12-month period for initial MNT and 2 h in the following years. Eligible beneficiaries are allowed to use both the MNT and DSMT benefit. The only restriction is that the services cannot be provided on the same day.

WHAT TO EXPECT

MNT is effective in lowering A1C, blood pressure, and lipid levels when used as monotherapy, and it improves the effectiveness of medication when needed (Table 16.2). At some point in the progression and management of these metabolic conditions, medications often are needed to support MNT. Continued support and reinforcement of behavioral goals needed to be successful are necessary and can now be reimbursed as part of recently established changes in federal and state laws governing health care. Establishing a referral network to dietitians will become easier as these reimbursement changes occur. Patients will ultimately benefit as they achieve their goals and decrease the risk of developing complications from diabetes, hypertension, or cardiovascular disease. This result is achieved through the implementation of individualized food plans that take into consideration the patient's lifestyle and metabolic needs.

BIBLIOGRAPHY

American Diabetes Association: Nutrition principles and recommendations in diabetes (Position Statement). *Diabetes Care* 27:S36-S46, 2004

American Diabetes Association and National Institute of Diabetes, Digestive and Kidney Diseases: The prevention or delay of type 2 diabetes (Position Statement). *Diabetes Care* 26:S62-S69, 2003

Cutler JA, Follmann D, Allender PS: Randomized trials of sodium restriction: an overview. *Am J Clin Nutr* 54 (Suppl. 1):643S-651S, 1997

Franz MJ, Monk A, Barry A, McClain K, Weaver T, Cooper N, Upham P, Gergenstal R, Mazze R: Effectiveness of medical nutrition therapy by dietitians in the management of non-insulin-dependent diabetes mellitus: a randomized, controlled clinical trial. *J Am Diet Assoc* 95:1009-1017, 1995

Franz M, Warshaw H, Pastors JG, Daly A, Arnold M: The evolution of diabetes medical nutrition therapy. *Postgrad Med J* 79:30–35, 2003

Kulkarni K, Castle G, Gregory R, Holmes A, Leontos C, Powers M, Snetselaar L, Splett P, Wylie-Rosett J: Nutrition practice guidelines for type 1 diabetes mellitus positively affect dietitian practices and patient outcomes. *J Am Diet Assoc* 98:62–70, 1998

Monk A, Barry B, McClain K, Weaver T, Cooper N, Franz M: Practice guidelines for medical nutrition therapy provided by dietitians for persons with non-insulin-dependent diabetes mellitus. *J Am Diet Assoc* 95:999–1006, 1995

National Institutes of Health (NIH) National Heart, Lung & Blood Institute (NHLBI): Clinical guidelines on the identification, evaluation and treatment of overweight and obesity in adults: the evidence report. *Obes Res* 6 (Suppl. 2):51S–209S, 1998

Pastors JG, Warshaw H, Daly A, Franz M, Kulkarni K: Evidence for effectiveness of medical nutrition therapy in diabetes management. *Diabetes Care* 25:608–613, 2002

Powers M: *American Dietetic Association Guide to Eating Right When You Have Diabetes.* Hoboken, NJ, John Wiley and Sons, 2003

Rickheim P, Weaver TW, Flader JL, Kendall DM: Assessment of group versus individual diabetes education. *Diabetes Care* 25:269–274, 2002

Rosett JW, Delahanty L: An integral role of the dietitian: implications of the Diabetes Prevention Program. *J Am Diet Assoc* 102:1065–1068, 2002

Sacks FM, Swetkey LP, Vollmer WM, Appel LJ, Bray GA, Harsha D, Obarzanek E, Conlin PR, Miller ER 3rd, Simons-Morton DG, Karanja N, Lin PH, DASH-Sodium Collaborative Research Group: Effects on blood pressure of reduced dietary sodium and the Dietary Approaches to Stop Hypertension (DASH) diet. *N Engl J Med* 344:3–10, 2001

United Kingdom Prospective Diabetes Study: Response of fasting plasma glucose to diet therapy in newly presenting type II patients with diabetes. *Metabolism* 39:905–912, 1990

Yu-Poth S, Zhao G, Etherton T, Naglak M, Jonnalagadda S, Kris-Etherton PM: Effects of the National Cholesterol Education Program's step I and step II dietary intervention programs on cardiovascular disease risk factors: a meta-analysis. *Am J Clin Nutr* 60:632–646, 1999

Ms. Daly is Director of Nutrition and Diabetes Education at the Springfield Diabetes and Endocrine Center, Springfield, IL. Ms. Powers is Manager of Health Programs at the International Diabetes Center, Park Nicollet Institute, Minneapolis, MN.

17. Pharmacological Treatment of Obesity

DONNA H. RYAN, MD, AND GEORGE A. BRAY, MD

Obesity has become a major focus of modern medicine, driven by the U.S. pandemic of overweight and obesity. The 1999–2000 National Health and Nutrition Examination Survey (NHANES) pegs obesity rates (BMI ≥30 kg/m²) at 30.5% of the U.S. population. The concern, of course, is the morbidities that accompany obesity. In particular, attention has recently focused on the metabolic syndrome—the constellation of lipid, vascular, and metabolic abnormalities associated largely with insulin resistance. A reanalysis of NHANES data shows that the metabolic syndrome affects 24% of the U.S. population. The 2001 National Cholesterol Education Program Adult Treatment Panel III (ATP III) guidelines target the metabolic syndrome as a focus for cardiovascular risk reduction. This shift from lipid management to "therapeutic lifestyle change" as a way to control metabolic syndrome stems from the knowledge that type 2 diabetes is a cardiovascular risk equivalent. By the time type 2 diabetes is diagnosed, cardiovascular disease is already entrenched, a concept bolstered by evidence that individuals with type 2 diabetes have the same risk for subsequent cardiovascular events as individuals without diabetes who have had a first cardiovascular event.

At the same time that there is alarm over the links between the obesity-diabetes-cardiovascular risk, there is an appreciation by our public health officials that even modest weight reduction can produce substantial health benefits. The U.S. Diabetes Prevention Program and the Finnish Diabetes Prevention Study both demonstrated significant reduction in risk for diabetes in individuals with impaired glucose tolerance who lost as little as 5–7% of baseline weight.

Physicians must develop effective office-based approaches to obesity management. Medicating for obesity is a tool unique to physicians, and if we are to stem the tide of obesity-related morbidities, physicians must be knowledgeable about the use of medications in at-risk patients. This chapter is a guide to current practices in evaluating and medicating for obesity management.

REALITIES OF TREATMENT

First, obesity is a chronic, relapsing, neurochemical disease that has many causes. Environmental, biological, and psychological factors all play a role in the current prevalence of obesity, which exceeds 30% of the U.S. population. In most patients presenting with obesity, a clear etiologic diagnosis is usually not possible. Because of its chronic nature and relative unknown cause, cure of obesity is rare, but palliation is a realistic clinical goal. Weight loss occurs with most treatments, and, except for surgery or very-low-calorie diets, it is usually slow (0.5–1.0 kg/week). Recidivism, or regain of body weight, is common after a weight loss program is terminated. In contrast to the relatively slow rate of weight loss, weight regain may be rapid. A regain in weight after termination of drug treatment is often ascribed to a failure of the drugs or other treatment. A more appropriate interpretation is that medications do not work if not taken. This is true of medications for the treatment of obesity, just as it is for medications used to treat hypertension, diabetes, heart disease, or asthma.

EVALUATION OF THE OBESE PATIENT

Classification and Risk Assessment of Obesity

The first step in assessing the obese patient is to consider potential causes of the condition. Table 17.1 outlines an etiologic classification of obesity. Whereas secondary causes of obesity are rare, endocrine and hypothalamic syndromes, such as hypothyroidism, Cushing's syndrome, Prader-Willi syndrome, and hypothalamic injury, must be considered. Although diet and a sedentary lifestyle are always contributory, physicians must remember that the amount of energy imbalance required to result in significant weight gain does not usually indicate sloth or gluttony. With a net excess energy intake of only 100 kcal/day, >10 lb will be gained in a year and 100 lb in 10 years. Whereas there are strong genetic influences on weight and body habitus, the cause of the obesity epidemic of the last 30 years is an environmental, rather than a genetic, shift.

Table 17.2 lists drugs that may be associated with weight gain. Many common medications promote weight gain, and physicians must be cognizant of the additional health risks imposed by such weight gain and seek alternative therapy for susceptible individuals. Another problem is the excessive gain and weight retention that can follow pregnancy or that is associated with menopause. Not all women are susceptible, but at least a subset report the onset of obesity with these life events.

Operationally, BMI is a useful way of communicating the degree of overweight. Table 17.3 shows BMI values for various heights and weights. Whereas BMI may be elevated in bodybuilders without a concomitant increase in body fat, a high BMI generally reflects an increased percentage of *total body fat*. BMI may overestimate health risks from obesity in African-American women and underestimate them in Asian and Indian individuals. The most reliable way to measure total body fat is with dual-energy X-ray absorptiometry, where body fat

Table 17.1 Etiologic Classification of Obesity

▪ Hypothalamic	▪ Dietary	▪ Genetic	▪ Idiopathic
▪ Endocrine	▪ Sedentary lifestyle	▪ Drug-induced	

Table 17.2 Drugs Associated with Weight Gain

Psychiatric/neurological
- Antipsychotics: olanzapine, clozapine, risperidone
- Antidepressants: tricyclic antidepressants, some selective serotonin-reuptake inhibitors
- Lithium
- Antiepileptics: valproate, gabapentin, carbamazepine

Diabetes treatment
- Insulin

- Sulfonylureas
- Thiazolidinediones

Others
- Hormonal contraceptives
- Corticosteroids
- Progestational agents
- Antihistamines
- β-Blockers,α-blockers

>25% for men and >33% for women can define obesity. On a practical level, clinical judgment usually suffices in interpreting BMI in relation to health risk. In particular, consideration of waist circumference, in addition to BMI, can aid in risk assessment and diagnosis of the metabolic syndrome.

Intra-abdominal fat increases with age and carries the highest risk for developing cardiovascular and other disease consequences. *Visceral fat distribution* can be estimated by several techniques. The ratio of the circumference of the waist to the circumference of the hips has been widely used in epidemiological studies, but this is no better than the waist circumference alone. Men with a waist circumference >102 cm (40 inches) and women with a waist circumference >88 cm (35 inches) are in the high-risk category. The top tertile in abdominal fat distribution nearly doubles the risk of mortality and morbidity from heart disease, diabetes, and hypertension. This extra risk is observed in men and women and rises sharply for the top 10th percentile of abdominal fat distribution. When the difference in fat distribution is corrected, the excess mortality observed between men and women is largely, if not completely, eliminated. The risk associated with excess central accumulation of fat probably reflects the increase in visceral fat. Abnormal glucose tolerance, hypertension, and hypertriglyceridemia and low HDL cholesterol are more closely associated with the amount of visceral fat than with total body fat. The sagittal diameter has been proposed as a way to estimate visceral fat, but currently the only reliable way to determine visceral fat is with a computed tomography or magnetic resonance imaging scan. The availability of newer, less expensive methods will be an important clinical advance.

METABOLIC SYNDROME

The National Cholesterol Education Program ATP III indicates the metabolic syndrome as a secondary target (in addition to lipid levels) for cardiovascular disease prevention. Table 17.4 lists the ATP III criteria for the metabolic syndrome. The levels chosen are less stringent than those generally used by physicians for categorizing disease states; for example, the blood pressure cut points are 130/85 mmHg, which are less than the 140/90 mmHg cut points usually indicating hypertension. The aim of using these criteria is to identify individuals

Table 17.3 BMI Using Either Pounds and Inches or Kilograms and Centimeters

Inches	19	20	21	22	23	24	25	26	27	28	29	30	31	32	33	34	35	36	37	38	39	40	Centimeters
58	*91*	*95*	*100*	*105*	*110*	*115*	*119*	*124*	*129*	*134*	*138*	*143*	*148*	*153*	*158*	*162*	*167*	*172*	*177*	*181*	*186*	*191*	
	41	**43**	**45**	**48**	**50**	**52**	**54**	**56**	**58**	**61**	**63**	**65**	**67**	**69**	**71**	**73**	**76**	**78**	**80**	**82**	**84**	**86**	147
59	*94*	*99*	*104*	*109*	*114*	*119*	*124*	*128*	*133*	*138*	*143*	*148*	*153*	*158*	*163*	*168*	*173*	*178*	*183*	*188*	*193*	*198*	
	43	**45**	**47**	**50**	**52**	**54**	**56**	**59**	**61**	**63**	**65**	**68**	**70**	**72**	**74**	**77**	**79**	**81**	**83**	**86**	**88**	**90**	150
60	*97*	*102*	*107*	*112*	*118*	*123*	*128*	*133*	*138*	*143*	*148*	*153*	*158*	*164*	*169*	*174*	*179*	*184*	*189*	*194*	*199*	*204*	
	44	**46**	**49**	**51**	**53**	**55**	**58**	**60**	**62**	**65**	**67**	**69**	**72**	**74**	**76**	**79**	**81**	**83**	**85**	**88**	**90**	**92**	152
61	*100*	*106*	*111*	*116*	*121*	*127*	*132*	*137*	*143*	*148*	*153*	*158*	*164*	*169*	*174*	*180*	*185*	*190*	*195*	*201*	*206*	*211*	
	46	**48**	**50**	**53**	**55**	**58**	**60**	**62**	**65**	**67**	**70**	**72**	**74**	**77**	**79**	**82**	**84**	**86**	**89**	**91**	**94**	**96**	155
62	*104*	*109*	*115*	*120*	*125*	*131*	*136*	*142*	*147*	*153*	*158*	*164*	*169*	*175*	*180*	*186*	*191*	*196*	*202*	*207*	*213*	*218*	
	47	**50**	**52**	**55**	**57**	**60**	**62**	**65**	**67**	**70**	**72**	**75**	**77**	**80**	**82**	**85**	**87**	**90**	**92**	**95**	**97**	**100**	158
63	*107*	*113*	*118*	*124*	*130*	*135*	*141*	*146*	*152*	*158*	*163*	*169*	*175*	*180*	*186*	*192*	*197*	*203*	*208*	*214*	*220*	*225*	
	49	**51**	**54**	**56**	**59**	**61**	**64**	**67**	**69**	**72**	**74**	**77**	**79**	**82**	**84**	**87**	**90**	**92**	**95**	**97**	**100**	**102**	160
64	*110*	*116*	*122*	*128*	*134*	*140*	*145*	*151*	*157*	*163*	*169*	*174*	*180*	*186*	*192*	*198*	*203*	*209*	*215*	*221*	*227*	*233*	
	50	**52**	**55**	**58**	**60**	**63**	**66**	**68**	**71**	**73**	**76**	**79**	**81**	**84**	**87**	**89**	**92**	**94**	**97**	**100**	**102**	**105**	162
65	*114*	*120*	*126*	*132*	*138*	*144*	*150*	*156*	*162*	*168*	*174*	*180*	*186*	*192*	*198*	*204*	*210*	*216*	*222*	*228*	*234*	*240*	
	52	**54**	**57**	**60**	**63**	**65**	**68**	**71**	**74**	**76**	**79**	**82**	**84**	**87**	**90**	**93**	**95**	**98**	**101**	**103**	**106**	**109**	165
66	*117*	*124*	*130*	*136*	*142*	*148*	*155*	*161*	*167*	*173*	*179*	*185*	*192*	*198*	*204*	*210*	*216*	*223*	*229*	*235*	*241*	*247*	
	54	**56**	**59**	**62**	**65**	**68**	**71**	**73**	**76**	**79**	**82**	**85**	**87**	**90**	**93**	**96**	**99**	**102**	**104**	**107**	**110**	**113**	168
67	*121*	*127*	*134*	*140*	*147*	*153*	*159*	*166*	*172*	*178*	*185*	*191*	*198*	*204*	*210*	*217*	*223*	*229*	*236*	*242*	*248*	*255*	
	55	**58**	**61**	**64**	**66**	**69**	**72**	**75**	**78**	**81**	**84**	**87**	**90**	**93**	**95**	**98**	**101**	**104**	**107**	**110**	**113**	**116**	170
68	*125*	*131*	*138*	*144*	*151*	*158*	*164*	*171*	*177*	*184*	*190*	*197*	*203*	*210*	*217*	*223*	*230*	*236*	*243*	*249*	*256*	*263*	
	57	**60**	**63**	**66**	**69**	**72**	**75**	**78**	**81**	**84**	**87**	**90**	**93**	**96**	**99**	**102**	**105**	**108**	**111**	**114**	**117**	**120**	173

BMI (kg/m²)

(continued)

Therapy for Diabetes Mellitus and Related Disorders

Table 17.3 BMI Using Either Pounds and Inches or Kilograms and Centimeters (*continued*)

BMI (kg/m^2)

Inches	19	20	21	22	23	24	25	26	27	28	29	30	31	32	33	34	35	36	37	38	39	40	Centimeters
69	*128*	*135*	*142*	*149*	*155*	*162*	*169*	*176*	*182*	*189*	*196*	*203*	*209*	*216*	*223*	*230*	*237*	*243*	*250*	*257*	*264*	*270*	
	58	**61**	**64**	**67**	**70**	**74**	**77**	**80**	**83**	**86**	**89**	**92**	**95**	**98**	**101**	**104**	**107**	**110**	**113**	**116**	**119**	**123**	**175**
70	*132*	*139*	*146*	*153*	*160*	*167*	*174*	*181*	*188*	*195*	*202*	*209*	*216*	*223*	*230*	*236*	*243*	*250*	*257*	*264*	*271*	*278*	
	60	**63**	**67**	**70**	**73**	**76**	**79**	**82**	**86**	**89**	**92**	**95**	**98**	**101**	**105**	**108**	**111**	**114**	**117**	**120**	**124**	**127**	**178**
71	*136*	*143*	*150*	*157*	*165*	*172*	*179*	*186*	*193*	*200*	*207*	*215*	*222*	*229*	*236*	*243*	*250*	*258*	*265*	*272*	*279*	*286*	
	62	**65**	**68**	**71**	**75**	**78**	**81**	**84**	**87**	**91**	**94**	**97**	**100**	**104**	**107**	**110**	**113**	**117**	**120**	**123**	**126**	**130**	**180**
72	*140*	*147*	*155*	*162*	*169*	*177*	*184*	*191*	*199*	*206*	*213*	*221*	*228*	*235*	*243*	*250*	*258*	*265*	*272*	*280*	*287*	*294*	
	64	**67**	**70**	**74**	**77**	**80**	**84**	**87**	**90**	**94**	**97**	**100**	**104**	**107**	**111**	**114**	**117**	**121**	**124**	**127**	**131**	**134**	**183**
73	*144*	*151*	*159*	*166*	*174*	*182*	*189*	*197*	*204*	*212*	*219*	*227*	*234*	*242*	*250*	*257*	*265*	*272*	*280*	*287*	*295*	*303*	
	65	**68**	**72**	**75**	**79**	**82**	**86**	**89**	**92**	**96**	**99**	**103**	**106**	**110**	**113**	**116**	**120**	**123**	**127**	**130**	**133**	**137**	**185**
74	*148*	*155*	*163*	*171*	*179*	*187*	*194*	*202*	*210*	*218*	*225*	*233*	*241*	*249*	*256*	*264*	*272*	*280*	*288*	*295*	*303*	*311*	
	67	**71**	**74**	**78**	**81**	**85**	**88**	**92**	**95**	**99**	**102**	**106**	**110**	**113**	**117**	**120**	**124**	**127**	**131**	**134**	**138**	**141**	**188**
75	*152*	*160*	*168*	*176*	*184*	*192*	*200*	*208*	*216*	*224*	*232*	*240*	*247*	*255*	*263*	*271*	*279*	*287*	*295*	*303*	*311*	*319*	
	69	**72**	**76**	**79**	**83**	**87**	**90**	**94**	**97**	**101**	**105**	**108**	**112**	**116**	**119**	**123**	**126**	**130**	**134**	**137**	**141**	**144**	**190**
76	*156*	*164*	*172*	*180*	*189*	*197*	*205*	*213*	*221*	*230*	*238*	*246*	*254*	*262*	*271*	*279*	*287*	*295*	*303*	*312*	*320*	*328*	
	71	**74**	**78**	**82**	**86**	**89**	**93**	**97**	**101**	**104**	**108**	**112**	**115**	**119**	**123**	**127**	**130**	**134**	**138**	**142**	**145**	**149**	**193**
BMI	19	20	21	22	23	24	25	26	27	28	29	30	31	32	33	34	35	36	37	38	39	40	BMI

BMI is shown as **bold underlined** numbers at the top and bottom.
To determine your BMI, select your height in either inches or centimeters and move across the row until you find your weight in pounds or inches. Your BMI can be read at the top or bottom.
Italic numbers are pounds and inches; **bold numbers are kilograms and centimeters.**
Copyright 1999 George A. Bray

Table 17.4 ATP III Metabolic Syndrome Criteria

Presence of three or more of the following risk factors:

Risk Factor	Defining Level
Abdominal obesity (waist circumference)	
Men	>40 inches (102 cm)
Women	>35 inches (88 cm)
Fasting glucose	≥110 mg/dl
Triglycerides	≥150 mg/dl
HDL cholesterol	
Men	<40 mg/dl
Women	<50 mg/dl
Blood pressure	≥130/≥85 mmHg

ATP III, National Cholesterol Education Program Adult Treatment Panel III.

with insulin resistance and the accompanying dyslipidemia (small, dense LDL particles; low levels of HDL cholesterol; and elevated triglycerides), vascular dysfunction (elevations in blood pressure), and increased risk for development of type 2 diabetes. Metabolic syndrome is best managed by weight reduction as evidenced by the results of the U.S. Diabetes Prevention Program and Finnish Diabetes Prevention Study. We believe that the presence of the metabolic syndrome is an indication for pharmacological interventions to aid weight loss because the health risks of the disorder justify that approach. We also provide a scheme to adjust risk using some of these risk factors, which we shall discuss later (Table 17.5).

EVALUATING RISK TO GUIDE TREATMENT

Because all treatments for obesity entail some risk, it is important to decide whether drug treatment is appropriate for the risks involved. This requires an assessment of the risk associated with total fat and fat distribution, as well as an assessment of metabolic status and complicating factors. In general, clinical judgment can be used to "adjust" BMI to assess risk. We propose here a scheme that relies on fat distribution assessed by waist circumference and evaluating other risk factors. Our scheme helps physicians codify the judgment decisions (adapted from Bray [2003]).

Body weights associated with a BMI of 19–25 kg/m² are good weights for most people. Body weights associated with BMI >30 kg/m² are almost invariably associated with increasing health risk. Risk assessment for a BMI between 25 and 30 kg/m² should include accounting for visceral fat and other comorbid factors that are affected by body weight, such as diabetes, hypertension, and dyslipidemia.

Table 17.5 illustrates our schema for the adjustment that can be made to reflect the increased risk imparted by the presence of comorbid risk factors, such as lipid levels, fasting glucose, blood pressure, sleep apnea, and

Table 17.5 BMI Adjustments for Metabolic Variables and Other Risk Factors

	Adjustment Scores			BMI Adjustment Score
	0	+1	+3	
Weight gain since age 18 (kg)	<5	5–15	>15	
Fasting glucose (mg/dl)	<110	≤110–125	≥125	
Triglyceride (mg/dl)	<150	≥150	≥200	
HDL cholesterol (mg/dl)				
Men	≥40	<40	<35	
Women	≥50	<50	<60	
Blood pressure (mmHg)	<130/<85	≥130/≥85	>140/≥90	
Sleep apnea	Absent		Present	
Osteoarthritis	Absent	Present		
Adjustment to BMI for central fat (Table 17.4)				
Calculated BMI				
Adjusted BMI				

osteoarthritis, and for degrees of weight gain since age 18 years. Once relative risk is evaluated, the appropriateness of various treatments can be determined from Figure 17.1. For adjusted BMI ≥30, pharmocotherapy is indicated. By adjusting the BMI for risk factors, one can identify patients who will benefit most from weight loss and in whom the risks associated with medications are justified.

INITIATING PHARMACOLOGICAL THERAPY

Practice guidelines, such as the National Institutes of Health, National Heart, Lung, and Blood Institute Clinical Guidelines on the Identification, Evaluation, and Treatment of Overweight and Obesity in Adults—the Evidence Report, recommend a trial of behavioral approaches before medications are initiated. We endorse this approach. In practice, however, most obese patients who are candidates for medications have had prior weight loss attempts without lasting success, and physicians need only document this history.

Before initiating drug therapy, a counseling session with patients is important. Because the amount of weight reduction is correlated with the degree of behavior change, assessing readiness to change is an important first step. The medications will, through biological measures, reinforce the intention to restrict food intake and modify eating behavior. However, patients can override their biological signals. If patients are to maximize the amount of weight lost during the active weight loss phase, they must be ready to change entrenched behavior patterns.

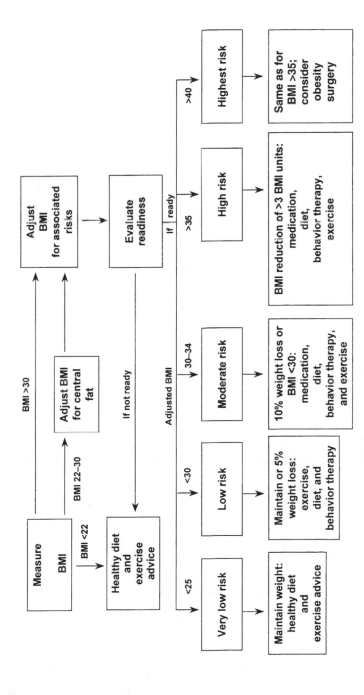

Figure 17.1 Algorithm for adjusting BMI for other comorbid risk factors and obtaining an overall assessment of risk, goal for weight loss, and rank order for potential treatments.

Patients must also have a realistic weight loss goal. It is unrealistic for very obese patients to expect to achieve the ideal BMI of 25 kg/m^2. However, loss of 5–10% initial body weight can translate into significant health benefits. A focus on a realistic weight loss goal of 10% and on health, rather than cosmetic benefits, is essential for the very obese. Once reached, the patient can then establish a new weight loss goal. One theory to the success of lifestyle change is setting small achievable goals to prevent failure.

A frank discussion of side effects must be preliminary to a patient's consent to undergo treatment. Sibutramine can cause blood pressure elevation, and patients must be prepared to return for monitoring. Orlistat causes fat malabsorption and anal leakage by blocking up to 30% of fat digestion, and occasional diarrheal steatorrhea must be anticipated. Another facet of the counseling interview is to describe the weight gain that is certain to occur if medications are stopped and there has not been permanent lifestyle adaptation to maintain weight loss.

MEDICATION AS ADJUNCTIVE TREATMENT

Medications for the treatment of obesity are considered adjuncts to the overall treatment plan. The other components of a standard treatment protocol include:

- use of meal replacements (e.g., shakes, nutrition bars, and frozen entrees) as means of portion and calorie control. These are important adjuncts in the active weight loss and weight loss maintenance phases.
- counseling on how to reduce fat and calorie intake
- an exercise program that will increase activity (by walking or other suitable means)
- the use of techniques for behavior modification that can help the patient monitor food intake, increase physical activity, and develop constructive cognitive strategies for dealing with the everyday demands to eat

STRATEGIES FOR RELAPSE PREVENTION AFTER WEIGHT LOSS

Physicians should develop a list of local resources for weight loss and lifestyle adaptation. Health clubs, hospital- or clinic-based programs, commercial programs (e.g., Weight Watchers, Jenny Craig, and Nutri/System), and support organizations (e.g., Overeaters Anonymous and TOPS Club, Inc.) can all play a role.

If the patient is an appropriate candidate, treatment options are discussed and medications are initiated with the behavioral program. Failure to lose >4 lb after 4–8 weeks of treatment is considered "treatment failure." Nonresponsive patients should not continue on medication. Evidence from clinical trials demonstrates that weight loss plateaus after 6 months or less. When patients discontinue the treatment, as they often do, they regain weight unless lifestyle changes have become a permanent part of daily life. Enrollees in our weight loss programs must commit to 1 year of treatment and then are given the option of either continued medication or an intensive lifestyle program that incorporates exercise (burning >2,000 kcal/week) and behavior modification techniques. We encourage them to resume medication whenever weight regain exceeds 5% and provide "refresher courses" of more intensive therapy.

The physician plays an important role in monitoring progress by providing positive reinforcement for success and devising constructive strategies for problem areas. Once weight has plateaued, the physician must shift emphasis to the lifelong goal of weight maintenance.

DRUGS APPROVED BY THE U.S. FOOD AND DRUG ADMINISTRATION FOR CLINICAL USE IN THE TREATMENT OF OBESITY

Drugs on the Market

There are only two drugs approved by the U.S. Food and Drug Administration (FDA) for long-term obesity management: orlistat (Xenical) and sibutramine (Meridia or Reductil). Phentermine is still widely prescribed but has approval only for short-term obesity management (usually interpreted to mean use up to 12 weeks). Phentermine is no longer patent-protected and is thus inexpensive. There are other noradrenergic drugs still available, although they are rarely used. Table 17.6 shows all drugs with an obesity indication currently listed in the *Physician's Desk Reference*.

Sibutramine. Sibutramine, marketed as Meridia in the U.S., entered the market in March 1998. It is a β-phenethylamine with a cyclobutyl group on the side chain. Sibutramine inhibits the reuptake of serotonin, norepinephrine, and, to a lesser extent, dopamine. Sibutramine produces weight loss by a dual mechanism of action. It promotes satiety and increases energy expenditure, blocking the reduction in metabolic rate that accompanies weight loss. One key to successful use of sibutramine is to prescribe an appropriate dietary approach. Because sibutramine promotes satiety (it does not produce anorexia), it works best in a program that enforces regular portion-controlled meals. One regimen for the active weight loss period is to use two meal replacements (breakfast and lunch) and a sensible dinner (~600–700 kcal or two frozen entrees) in addition to sibutramine.

There are three key factors to sibutramine's efficacy. First, weight loss is dose related. The usual starting dose is 10 mg, but the drug may be increased to 15 mg (or decreased to 5 mg if there are side effects). An advantage is sibutramine's once-a-day dosing. Second, the amount of initial weight loss is related to the intensity of the behavioral intervention. Highly structured, portion-controlled schemes produce the most weight loss. Third, sibutramine is very effective during weight loss maintenance. Placebo-controlled studies demonstrate successful weight loss maintenance with sibutramine for up to 2 years.

Table 17.6 Drugs Approved by the FDA for Treatment of Obesity

Drug	Trade Names	Dosage	DEA Schedule
Pancreatic Lipase Inhibitor Approved for Long-Term Use			
Orlistat	Xenical	120 mg t.i.d. before meals	—
Norepinephrine-Serotonin Reuptake Inhibitor Approved for Long-Term Use			
Sibutramine	Meridia Reductil	5–15 mg/day	IV
Noradrenergic Drugs Approved for Short-Term Use			
Diethylpropion	Tenuate Tenuate Dospan	25 mg t.i.d. 75 mg q. AM	IV
Phentermine	Adipex Ionamin Slow Release	15–37.5 mg/day 15–30 mg/day	IV
Benzphetamine	Didrex	25–50 mg t.i.d.	III
Phendimetrazine	Bontril Prelu-2	17.5–70 mg t.i.d. 105 mg q.d.	III

In general, clinical trials inform us that about three-quarters of patients treated with 15 mg/day sibutramine will achieve >5% weight loss, and 80% of those will maintain that loss for 2 years. About 5% of patients will not tolerate the drug because of adverse effects on blood pressure and pulse. Some patients (~20%) are nonresponders.

Sibutramine, like other sympathomimetic agents, produces a small increase in mean heart rate and mean blood pressure observed in clinical trials. However, the blood pressure response is variable. A subset (~5% of patients) appear to be sensitive to the blood pressure effects and cannot tolerate sibutramine. Some patients may need to discontinue sibutramine because of blood pressure elevations to a hypertensive range. Other side effects, including dry mouth, insomnia, and asthenia, are similar to those of other noradrenergic drugs. Sibutramine is not associated with valvular heart disease, primary pulmonary hypertension, or substance abuse.

Sibutramine should be used with caution in patients with cardiovascular disease and in individuals taking selective serotonin reuptake inhibitors. It should not be used within 2 weeks of taking monoamine oxidase inhibitors and should not be used with other noradrenergic agents.

Orlistat. Orlistat is marketed as Xenical. Fat digestion can be inhibited by blocking the enzymatic action of pancreatic lipase. In experimental studies, orlistat (tetrahydrolipstatin) has been shown to be a potent inhibitor of lipase activity that decreases intestinal triglyceride hydrolysis in a dose-dependent manner. In clinical trials, it also has a dose-dependent effect on fat absorption and weight loss. After a high-fat meal, steatorrheal diarrhea is expected, but gastrointestinal events in practice are mild to moderate, resolve spontaneously, and are usually limited to one or two episodes per patient. Deficiency of fat-soluble vitamins can occur, and vitamin supplementation should be used. In general, patients tolerate the drug very well, especially if it is combined with advance patient education.

Orlistat works best when given with a diet that has ~30% fat content, so patient counseling is important. If a high-fat meal or snack is consumed, gastrointestinal distress can result. For a very-low-fat meal, orlistat is not going to produce a caloric deficit, and patients on a low-fat diet will not lose weight on orlistat.

Orlistat is effective in producing and sustaining weight loss. It is given at a dose of 120 mg before meals three times daily. Data from clinical trials support that ~70% of patients will achieve >5% weight loss, and at 2 years, 70% of them will have maintained that loss. There are clinical trials documenting orlistat use for up to 4 years.

One advantage to orlistat's use is its beneficial effect on LDL cholesterol. Because orlistat blocks fat absorption, the LDL reduction is about twice that seen with weight loss alone.

Phentermine, diethylpropion, phendimetrazine, and benzphetamine. Phentermine and diethylpropion are classified by the U.S. Drug Enforcement Agency (DEA) as schedule IV drugs, and phendimetrazine and benzphetamine are classified as schedule III drugs. This regulatory classification indicates the government's belief that these drugs have the potential for abuse, although this potential appears to be very low. These drugs are only approved for a "few weeks" of use, which is usually interpreted as up to 12 weeks. Weight loss with phentermine and diethylpropion persists for the duration of treatment, suggesting that tolerance to these drugs does not develop. If tolerance developed, the drugs would lose their effectiveness or increased amounts of drugs would be required for patients to maintain weight loss. Of the agents in this group, phentermine is prescribed most frequently in the U.S., probably because it is no longer protected by patents and is therefore inexpensive. Phentermine is not available in Europe. A recent review in the *New England Journal of Medicine* (Yanovski and Yanovski [2002]) recommends obtaining written informed consent if phentermine is prescribed for longer than 12 weeks, because there are not sufficient published reports on the long-term use of phentermine.

The only published studies of these medications involve small numbers of patients treated for a short duration. Because of the lack of long-term studies and the lack of sufficient safety data, we do not recommend the use of these agents routinely. There is one 36-week study using phentermine that shows that intermittent (1 month on, 1 month off) use of phentermine is just as effective in producing weight loss as continuous therapy. This approach is occasionally useful.

The side effect profile for sympathomimetic drugs is similar. They produce insomnia, dry mouth, asthenia, and constipation. Sympathomimetic drugs can also increase blood pressure.

OFF-LABEL PRESCRIBING

Weight loss has been reported with bupropion (an approved antidepressant and aid to smoking cessation), venlafaxine (an antidepressant with structural similarity to sibutramine), and topiramate (an anticonvulsant). We discourage off-label prescribing for obesity. However, because many antidepressants produce weight gain, bupropion or venlafaxine are good choices for the depressed obese patient. Clinical trials of topiramate as an anti-obesity agent are underway. Because of the central nervous system effects (cognitive slowing) and other serious side effects (renal stones and acute blindness), physicians should not prescribe this medication for obesity management until adequate safety has been assessed.

SPECIAL ISSUES IN DIABETES

In regard to patients with diabetes, diabetic control improves with weight reduction, and hypoglycemia becomes a possibility for those patients on insulin or oral hypoglycemic medications. Some patients may develop increased hunger due to hypoglycemia, and weight loss may slow or stop. Physicians must remember to monitor glucose carefully and reduce or stop diabetic medications as weight loss occurs. In our clinics, we halve or discontinue insulin and sulfonylureas at the start of the weight loss program.

BIBLIOGRAPHY

Bray GA: *Contemporary Diagnosis and Management of Obesity.* 2nd ed. Newtown, PA, Handbooks in Health Care, 2003

Bray GA, Greenway FL: Current and potential drugs for treatment of obesity (Review). *Endocr Rev* 20:805–875, 1999

National Institutes of Health, National Heart, Lung, and Blood Institute: Clinical Guidelines on the Identification, Evaluation, and Treatment of Overweight and Obesity in Adults: the Evidence Report. *Obes Res* 6 (Suppl. 2):51S–210S, 1998

Yanovski SZ, Yanovski JA: Drug obesity. *N Engl J Med* 346:591–602, 2002

Dr. Ryan is Associate Executive Director for Clinical Research and Dr. Bray is Chief of the Division of Obesity and Metabolic Diseases at the Pennington Biomedical Research Center in Baton Rouge, LA.

18. Exercise

JEANNE H. STEPPEL, MD, AND EDWARD S. HORTON, MD

Regular physical exercise has been recommended as an important component of the treatment of all people with diabetes. However, exercise potentiates the action of insulin, resulting in lower insulin requirements and an increased risk of hypoglycemic reactions during and after exercise. Also, in patients with type 1 diabetes who are insulin deficient, exercise may cause a further rise in blood glucose and the rapid development of ketosis. Even in well-controlled patients, vigorous exercise may result in sustained hyperglycemia. Because of these problems with regulation of blood glucose and ketones during or after exercise, many patients with type 1 diabetes find it difficult to participate in sports or other recreational activities or to manage exercise as part of their daily lives. This result has led to the opinion that exercise should not be recommended for all patients with type 1 diabetes but that efforts should be focused on making it possible for those who want to exercise to be able to do so as safely as possible. The availability of self-monitoring of blood glucose and the increased use of multiple-dose insulin regimens have led to the development of strategies for the management of exercise in type 1 diabetes patients, making it possible for them to participate safely in a wide range of physical activities and thus to have a normal or near-normal lifestyle. In patients with type 2 diabetes, on the other hand, regular activity is an important component of treatment and should be prescribed along with appropriate diet and either oral hypoglycemic agents or insulin as part of a comprehensive treatment program. This requires a careful assessment of the expected benefits and associated risks of exercise in individual patients, the development of a well-planned exercise program, and appropriate monitoring to avoid complications.

BENEFITS

The benefits of exercise for patients with diabetes are listed in Table 18.1. Moderate sustained exercise in patients with either type 1 or type 2 diabetes may be used to help regulate glucose on a day-to-day basis and may be the mechanism by which regular physical exercise assists in achieving improved long-term metabolic control. Physical training results in lower fasting and postprandial insulin concentrations and increased insulin sensitivity. In patients with type 1 diabetes, increased insulin sensitivity results in lowered insulin requirements. In patients

Table 18.1 Benefits of Exercise for Patients with Diabetes

- Lower blood glucose concentrations during and after exercise
- Lower basal and postprandial insulin concentrations
- Improved insulin sensitivity
- Lower glycated hemoglobin levels
- Improved lipid profile
  - Decreased triglycerides
  - Slightly decreased LDL cholesterol
  - Increased HDL2 cholesterol
- Improvement in mild to moderate hypertension
- Increased energy expenditure
  - Adjunct to diet for weight reduction
  - Increased fat loss
  - Preservation of lean body mass
- Cardiovascular conditioning
- Increased strength and flexibility
- Improved sense of well-being and quality of life

with type 2 diabetes, the improvement in insulin sensitivity resulting from regular physical exercise may be of major importance in improving long-term glycemic control.

Another benefit of regular exercise is a reduction in cardiovascular risk factors through improvement of the lipid profile and reduction of hypertension in patients with diabetes. Physical training is associated with a significant decrease in serum triglycerides, particularly VLDLs, and an increase in HDL2 cholesterol. There is also usually a slight reduction in LDL cholesterol levels with exercise. This improvement in the lipid profile requires a fairly high intensity of physical training. It is observed with running ≥9–12 miles/week and increases progressively up to distances of ~40 miles/week. Lower levels of physical activity have little, if any, effect on serum lipids. The effect of physical training to improve mild to moderate hypertension is independent of weight loss or a change in body composition. Decreases in both systolic and diastolic blood pressures of 5–10 mmHg are common and are often correlated with decreases in serum insulin and triglyceride concentrations.

In addition to improvement in cardiovascular risk factors, physical exercise may be an effective adjunct to diet for weight reduction. This is usually seen when exercise is combined with moderate calorie restriction. When patients are treated with very-low-calorie diets (600–800 kcal/day), exercise may not have a significant effect on the amount or composition of weight loss beyond that of the diet alone.

Finally, exercise improves cardiovascular function (decreased resting heart rate, increased stroke volume, and decreased cardiac work), increases fitness and physical working capacity, and improves sense of well-being and quality of life.

RISKS

There are several risks associated with exercise for patients with diabetes (Table 18.2). In patients with type 1 diabetes, late-onset postexercise hypoglycemia can occur 6–15 h after completion of the exercise and may persist for up to 24 h after prolonged strenuous exercise. In contrast to hypoglycemia,

---

Table 18.2 Risks of Exercise for Patients with Diabetes

- Hypoglycemia, if treated with insulin or oral agents
  - Exercise-induced hypoglycemia
  - Late-onset postexercise hypoglycemia
- Hyperglycemia after very strenuous exercise
- Hyperglycemia and ketosis in insulin-deficient patients
- Precipitation or exacerbation of cardio-vascular disease
  - Angina pectoris
  - Myocardial infarction
  - Arrhythmias
  - Sudden death
- Worsening of long-term complications of diabetes
- Proliferative retinopathy
  - Vitreous hemorrhage
  - Retinal detachment
- Nephropathy
  - Increased proteinuria
- Peripheral neuropathy
  - Soft tissue and joint injuries
- Autonomic neuropathy
  - Decreased cardiovascular response to exercise
  - Decreased maximum aerobic capacity
  - Impaired response to dehydration
  - Postural hypotension

---

vigorous exercise may result in a rapid increase in blood glucose, which can persist for several hours after the exercise is discontinued. Even moderate-intensity exercise may result in hyperglycemia and the rapid development of ketosis or ketoacidosis in type 1 diabetes patients who are insulin deficient.

Careful screening for underlying cardiac disease is important for all patients with diabetes before starting an exercise program. In addition, degenerative joint disease is more common in obese individuals and may be exacerbated by weight-bearing exercises.

Several complications of diabetes may be aggravated by exercise, and all patients should be screened before they start an exercise program. The most important of these is proliferative retinopathy, in which exercise may result in retinal or vitreous hemorrhage. Exercises that increase blood pressure, e.g., heavy lifting or exercise associated with Valsalva-like maneuvers, are particularly dangerous and should be avoided by patients with proliferative retinopathy. Exercise resulting in jarring or rapid head motion may precipitate hemorrhage or retinal detachment. Physical exercise is also associated with increased proteinuria in patients with diabetic nephropathy, probably because of changes in renal hemodynamics. It has not been shown, however, that exercise leads to progression of renal disease, and the use of angiotensin-converting enzyme inhibitors does appear to decrease the amount of exercise-induced albuminuria.

Patients with peripheral neuropathy have an increased risk of soft tissue and joint injuries, and, if autonomic neuropathy is present, the capacity for high-intensity exercise is impaired because of a decrease in maximum heart rate and aerobic capacity. In addition, patients with autonomic neuropathy may have impaired responses to dehydration and develop postural hypotension after exercise. With proper selection of the type, intensity, and duration of exercise, most of these complications can be avoided.

GUIDELINES FOR EXERCISE

Screening

Before starting an exercise program, all patients should have a complete history and physical examination, with particular attention paid to identifying any long-term complications of diabetes. A cardiac stress test is recommended for all patients >35 years of age. This test will help identify silent ischemic heart disease and may identify patients who have an exaggerated hypertensive response to exercise and/or may develop postexercise orthostatic hypotension. A careful ophthalmologic examination to identify proliferative retinopathy, renal function tests (including screening for microalbuminuria), and a neurological examination to determine peripheral and/or autonomic neuropathy should be performed. If abnormalities are found, exercises should be selected that will not pose significant risks for worsening complications. In general, young active patients with diabetes of brief duration and no evidence of long-term complications do not require formal exercise prescriptions, although they need specific recommendations regarding strategies for managing exercise and avoiding injuries.

Selection of Types of Exercise

If there are no contraindications, the types of exercise a patient performs can be a matter of personal preference. In general, moderate-intensity aerobic exercises that can be sustained for ≥30 min are preferred, although intermittent high-intensity and -resistance exercises (e.g., weight lifting) can also be managed successfully.

Some types of exercise may be less desirable for people with diabetes. For example, high-resistance exercises (such as weight lifting) are less desirable because of the high incidence of orthopedic and vascular side effects. Exercises that traumatize the feet (e.g., running and jogging) should be limited in patients with peripheral neuropathy, and body-contact sports should be avoided by patients with proliferative retinopathy.

Exercise Sessions

Each exercise session should begin with a warm-up of low-intensity aerobic exercise and stretching for 5–10 min to prevent musculoskeletal injuries. The higher-intensity portion of the exercise session should last 20–45 min, except in highly trained individuals, in whom longer workouts are possible. Exercises should be of moderate intensity (50–75% of the individual's maximum aerobic capacity) if the complications of diabetes permit and blood pressure response is not excessive. In general, exercise intensity should be limited so that systolic blood pressure does not exceed 180 mmHg. The intensity of exercise can be estimated from the heart rate response (i.e., the resting pulse rate determined before arising in the morning and the maximum heart rate determined during exercise). Fifty percent of a subject's maximal effort can be estimated by the formula 0.5(maximum heart rate – resting heart rate) + resting heart rate. When the true maximal heart rate is unknown, it can be estimated by the formula 220 – patient's age. However, this is less accurate than a direct determination of the maximum heart rate under controlled conditions and may significantly overestimate the maximum heart rate in patients with autonomic neuropathy. Once the heart rate response to exercise is determined for an individual patient, exercise intensity can be conveniently monitored by teaching the patient to measure his or her own pulse periodically during exercise and recording the results. The end of each exercise session should consist of a cooldown for at least 5–10 min to reduce the risk of postexercise cardiac and musculoskeletal complications. This is best done at an intensity of ~30% of maximum aerobic capacity and should include activities such as walking, stretching, and slow rhythmic exercises.

Frequency of Exercise

Patients should exercise 3 5 days/week or on an every-other-day schedule to achieve cardiovascular conditioning and improved insulin sensitivity and glycemic control. If exercise is being used as an adjunct to diet for weight reduction, exercise should be done ≥5 days/week.

Special Precautions

Feet should be inspected daily and always after exercise for cuts, blisters, and infections. Exercise should be avoided in extreme hot or cold environments and during periods of poor metabolic control. Special guidelines for patients taking insulin are described below.

Compliance

Several things can be done to improve the patient's motivation and participation on a regular basis. These include choosing activities the patient enjoys, providing a variety in types and settings for exercise, performing exercise at a convenient time and location, encouraging participation in group activities, involving the patient's family and associates for reinforcement, and measuring progress to provide positive feedback. Most important is to start slowly, build up gradually, and not set excessive or unrealistic goals.

Instruction and Monitoring

For patients who have not participated regularly in exercise in the past or who have significant complications of diabetes or other impediments to exercise, supervised exercise programs may be beneficial. Often, cardiac rehabilitation programs will be of assistance in supervising exercise programs for people with diabetes, particularly if the patients are at high risk for cardiovascular disease. There are an increasing number of diabetes treatment centers that offer supervised exercise programs for patients with either type 1 or type 2 diabetes. Many patients, however, do not need formal supervision once an initial assessment has been completed and an appropriate exercise plan has been established.

MANAGEMENT IN PATIENTS WITH TYPE 1 DIABETES

Whereas changes in blood glucose are small in nondiabetic individuals during exercise, several factors may complicate glucose regulation during and after exercise in patients with type 1 diabetes. Plasma insulin concentrations do not decrease normally during exercise, thus upsetting the balance between peripheral glucose utilization and hepatic glucose production. With insulin treatment, plasma insulin concentrations stay the same or may even increase if exercise is undertaken within 1 h of an insulin injection. Enhanced insulin absorption during exercise is most likely to occur when the insulin injection is given immediately before or within a few minutes of the onset of exercise. The longer the interval between injection and onset of exercise, the less significant this effect will be and the less important it is to choose the site of injection to avoid an exercising area.

The sustained insulin levels during exercise increase peripheral glucose uptake and stimulate glucose oxidation by the exercising muscles. In addition, insulin inhibits hepatic glucose production. The hepatic glucose production rate cannot match the rate of peripheral glucose utilization, and blood glucose concentration falls. During mild to moderate exercise of short duration, this may be a beneficial effect of exercise, but during more prolonged exercise, hypoglycemia may result. On the other hand, if exercise is vigorous, sympathetic nervous stimulation of hepatic glucose production may result in a rapid and sustained rise in blood glucose concentrations. If there is also insulin deficiency, hepatic ketone production is stimulated, and ketosis or ketoacidosis may occur.

A checklist of factors to consider before the onset of exercise is provided in Table 18.3. Obviously, it is not possible to predict all situations, because exercise is often spontaneous or intermittent and varies greatly in intensity and duration.

By considering the exercise plan and making adjustments in insulin dosage and food intake, patients with type 1 diabetes can avoid severe hypoglycemia or hyperglycemia. If exercise is of moderate intensity and long duration, blood glucose levels will fall, whereas vigorous exercise of short duration will often cause blood glucose to rise. Attention should be paid to the amount, timing, and site of insulin administration. Food intake before, during, and after exercise should be considered. It is also important to measure blood glucose before starting exercise and, if necessary, during and after exercise. With this information, the strategies outlined in Table 18.4 can be used to avoid either hypoglycemia or hyperglycemia.

Usually, a snack containing 20–25 g carbohydrate every 30 min is sufficient to provide enough glucose to maintain normal blood levels during prolonged exercise. Carbohydrate requirements will depend on factors such as the intensity and duration of exercise, the level of physical conditioning, the antecedent diet, and the circulating insulin levels.

If the exercise is planned, the insulin dosage schedule may be altered to decrease the likelihood of hypoglycemia. Individuals who take a single dose of intermediate-acting insulin may decrease the dose by 30–35% on the morning before exercise or may change to a split-dose regimen, taking 65% of the usual dose in the morning and 35% before the evening meal. Those who are taking a combination of intermediate- and short-acting insulin may decrease the short-acting insulin by 50% or omit it altogether before exercise; they also may decrease

---

Table 18.3 Pre-exercise Checklist for Patients with Type 1 Diabetes

1. Consider the exercise plan.
   - What is the duration and intensity of the planned exercise?
   - Is the exercise habitual or unusual?
   - How does the exercise relate to the level of physical conditioning?
   - What is the estimated calorie expenditure?
2. Consider the insulin regimen.
   - What is the usual insulin dosage schedule? Should it be decreased?
   - What is the interval between injection of insulin and the onset of exercise?
   - Should the site of injection be changed to avoid exercising areas?
3. Consider the plan for food intake.
   - What is the interval between the last meal and the onset of exercise?
   - Should a pre-exercise snack be eaten?
   - Should carbohydrate feedings be taken during exercise?
   - Will extra food be required after exercise?
4. Check blood glucose.
   - If <100 mg/dl (<5.5 mmol/l), eat a pre-exercise snack.
   - If 100–250 mg/dl (5.5–14 mmol/l), it should be all right to exercise.*
   - If >250 mg/dl (>14 mmol/l), check urine ketones.
5. Check urine ketones (if glucose is >250 mg/dl [>14 mmol/l]).
   - If negative, it is all right to exercise.
   - If positive, take insulin; do not exercise until ketones are negative.

*See Table 18.4.

---

the intermediate-acting insulin before exercise and take supplemental doses of short-acting insulin later if needed. Many patients now are treated with once-daily long-acting glargine insulin with multiple daily doses of rapid-onset short-acting insulin (aspart or lispro). In these patients, the short-acting insulin dose before exercise may be decreased by 30–50%, and postexercise doses may be adjusted based on glucose monitoring and experience with postexercise hypoglycemia. If insulin infusion devices are used, the basal infusion rate may be decreased during exercise and premeal boluses decreased or omitted.

Table 18.4 Strategies for Avoiding Hypoglycemia and Hyperglycemia with Exercise

1. Eat a meal 1–3 h before exercise.
2. Take supplemental carbohydrate feedings at least every 30 min during exercise if exercise is vigorous and of long duration.
3. Increase food intake for up to 24 h after exercise, depending on intensity and duration of exercise.
4. Take insulin at least 1 h before exercise. If <1 h before exercise, inject in a nonexercising area.
5. Decrease insulin dose before exercise.
6. Alter daily insulin schedule.
7. Monitor blood glucose before, during, and after exercise.
8. Delay exercise if blood glucose is >250 mg/dl (>14 mmol/l) and ketones are present.
9. Learn individual glucose responses to different types of exercise.

EXERCISE PROGRAMS FOR TREATING TYPE 2 DIABETES

Exercise programs improve insulin sensitivity and lower average blood glucose concentrations. The increased energy expenditure associated with exercise, when combined with calorie restriction, may improve weight reduction. Thus, regular exercise is an important component of treating patients with type 2 diabetes.

On the other hand, type 2 diabetes patients are usually older, are frequently obese, and may have significant long-term complications, making the initiation of exercise programs difficult. In this group of patients, exercises with a decreased risk of injury that enhance motivation and participation should be selected. Increasing daily activities such as walking, climbing stairs, and other familiar activities is an excellent start.

Unlike patients with type 1 diabetes, problems in glucose regulation do not occur, with the exception of occasional problems with hypoglycemia in patients taking sulfonylureas, thiazolidinediones, or insulin. In patients treated with diet alone, supplemental feedings before, during, or after exercise are unnecessary, except when exercise is unusually vigorous and of long duration.

In patients being treated with low-calorie diets, physical exercise is generally well tolerated and does not pose any additional risks if the diet is adequately supplemented with vitamins and minerals and adequate hydration is maintained. In patients treated with very-low-calorie diets (600–800 kcal/day), the diet should contain at least 35% of calories as carbohydrate to maintain normal muscle glycogen stores, which are needed to maintain high-intensity exercise. On the other hand, very-low-calorie diets severely restricted in carbohydrate are compatible with moderate-intensity exercise after an adaptation period of ≥2 weeks. It is important to note that increasing activity while on a very-low-calorie diet in someone on a hypoglycemic agent will increase the risk of hypoglycemia.

An exercise program for obese patients with type 2 diabetes should start slowly, build up gradually, and include exercises that are familiar to the patient and least likely to cause injuries or worsening of long-term diabetes complications.

BIBLIOGRAPHY

American Diabetes Association: Physical activity/exercise and diabetes mellitus (Position Statement). *Diabetes Care* 26 (Suppl. 1):S73–S77, 2003

Steppel J, Horton E: Exercise for the patient with type 1 diabetes. In *Diabetes Mellitus: A Fundamental and Clinical Text*. LeRoith D, Olefsky J, Taylor S, Eds. Philadelphia, Lippincott-Raven, 2003, p. 671–681

Steppel J, Horton E: Exercise in patients with type 2 diabetes. In *Diabetes Mellitus: A Fundamental and Clinical Text*. LeRoith D, Olefsky J, Taylor S, Eds. Philadelphia, Lippincott-Raven, 2003, p. 1099–1105

Dr. Steppel is a Clinical Research Fellow at the Joslin Diabetes Center at Harvard Medical School, Boston, MA. Dr. Horton is Director of Clinical Research at the Joslin Diabetes Center and Professor of Medicine at Harvard Medical School, Boston, MA.

19. Prevention of Type 2 Diabetes Mellitus

JILL CRANDALL, MD, AND HARRY SHAMOON, MD

Treatment of established type 2 diabetes mellitus can prevent many, if not most, of its serious long-term complications; however, currently available therapies are rarely successful in achieving euglycemia and therefore cannot eliminate the risk of microvascular or macrovascular disease. Furthermore, treatment of diabetes is costly, in terms of financial resources and the time and effort expended by both the health care system and the affected individual. Type 2 diabetes is typically diagnosed relatively late in its course, at a time when many patients already have evidence of vascular complications. Fortunately, the risk factors for type 2 diabetes are well understood and include a number of modifiable factors, such as obesity and sedentary lifestyle. The natural history of type 2 diabetes is characterized by a prolonged period of milder pre-diabetic hyperglycemia (Fig. 19.1). Therefore, strategies to address modifiable risk factors in this pre-diabetic period offer enormous potential to prevent the serious health and economic consequences of the later stages of established diabetes.

IMPAIRED GLUCOSE TOLERANCE AND IMPAIRED FASTING GLUCOSE

There is abundant evidence from epidemiological studies that the natural history of type 2 diabetes includes a prolonged period of mild hyperglycemia that is usually not appreciated clinically, manifested as either impaired glucose tolerance (IGT) (fasting plasma glucose [FPG] <126 mg/dl and 2-h plasma glucose between 140 and 199 mg/dl on a 75-g oral glucose tolerance test [OGTT]) or impaired fasting glucose (IFG) (FPG 100–125 mg/dl) (Table 19.2). The presence of IGT increases the risk of developing diabetes 5- to 8-fold, with 1–9% per year progressing to diabetes, depending on the population studied. The risk of diabetes associated with IFG appears to be similar. In addition to preceding the development of overt diabetes, IGT is associated with increased cardiovascular risk and often occurs in conjunction with other components of the metabolic syndrome (hypertension, dyslipidemia, and insulin resistance). Primary prevention efforts initiated at the stage of IGT (or IFG) may be necessary to ultimately reduce the occurrence of the microvascular and macrovascular complications of diabetes.

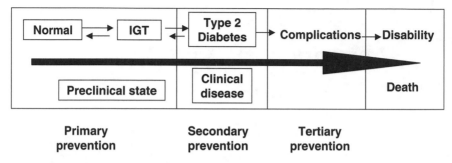

Figure 19.1 The natural history of type 2 diabetes.

IDENTIFICATION OF HIGH-RISK INDIVIDUALS

Although diabetes risk may be approximated by the presence of other variables, such as obesity and family history, testing for the presence of IGT/IFG is necessary to target intervention efforts to individuals most likely to benefit. Those most likely to have IGT/IFG are individuals who are overweight (BMI ≥25 kg/m²) and above age 45 years (Table 19.1). Younger individuals with additional risk factors, including prior gestational diabetes, family history of diabetes, and the presence of hypertension or dyslipidemia, should also be considered for screening. Members of ethnic and racial groups with a high prevalence of diabetes, such as African Americans, American Indians, Hispanic Americans, and Asian Americans, should also receive priority for screening efforts. Because the incidence of glucose intolerance and diabetes increases with age, at-risk patients should be retested periodically (typically every 2–3 years).

Screening may be accomplished by measurement of FPG or by an OGTT. An OGTT is necessary for the identification of IGT and may be the preferred test, because clinical trials thus far have been conducted in IGT populations and the benefits of intervention have been established for this group. Furthermore, an OGTT appears to be more sensitive and may identify a larger number of at-risk individuals than measurement of FPG. Concerns regarding use of the OGTT include inconvenience and lack of reproducibility, and the test must be performed carefully to obtain accurate results. As a practical matter, either

Table 19.1 Individuals to Be Screened for Pre-Diabetes

Highest risk Age ≥45 years and BMI ≥25 kg/m²	■ Prior gestational diabetes ■ First-degree relative with type 2 diabetes
Consider screening Age <45 years and BMI ≥25 kg/m², plus any of the following:	■ High-risk ethnicity ■ Hypertension ■ Dyslipidemia

Table 19.2 Categories of Glucose Tolerance Based on Fasting and 2-h Post-Challenge Glucose (75-g OGTT)

	Normal	IFG	IGT	Diabetes
Fasting	<100	100–125	≤125	≥126
2-h	<140		140–199	≥200

Data are given in milligrams per deciliter.

approach is reasonable when applied carefully to the appropriate population (see above), and clinicians should use whichever test is most feasible in their clinical setting. Screening for IGT/IFG has the added advantage of identifying cases of previously unrecognized diabetes, which can then be appropriately treated.

INTERVENTIONS TO PREVENT OR DELAY DIABETES

Lifestyle Modification

There is now convincing evidence from controlled clinical trials that lifestyle modification can prevent or delay the development of diabetes in high-risk individuals. The Diabetes Prevention Program (DPP) was a randomized controlled trial that enrolled 3,234 participants who were at high risk for diabetes on the basis of elevated fasting and postload glucose and a BMI >24 kg/m². Almost 50% of the cohort were members of high-risk racial or ethnic groups, and 20% were over the age of 60 years. DPP participants were randomized to one of three treatment arms (intensive lifestyle, metformin, or placebo) and were followed for an average of 2.8 years. The Finnish Diabetes Prevention Study (DPS) randomized 522 middle-aged European subjects to an intensive lifestyle program or an untreated control group. Both the Finnish DPS and the DPP reported a 58% reduction in the development of diabetes among subjects in the intensive lifestyle groups, compared with control subjects. In both studies, subjects in the intervention group received intensive individualized instruction on weight reduction, food intake, and exercise. The goals of the interventions were also similar and included weight loss of 5–7% of initial body weight, reduction of fat to <30% of calories, and physical activity of moderate intensity for at least 150 min/week. In the DPP, the majority of the subjects achieved the exercise goals and one-half lost 7% or more of body weight, although some weight regain occurred during the trial. It is important to note that although the lifestyle changes achieved in these studies were modest (mean weight loss was 7 kg, and typical exercise was equivalent to 30 min of brisk walking 5 days per week), the benefits in reducing diabetes were dramatic. In addition, lifestyle intervention was more effective than metformin or placebo in restoring normal fasting and post-challenge glucose. The benefits of lifestyle intervention in the DPP were consistent in both sexes, all age-groups, and among members of ethnic/racial groups who were highly represented in the DPP population.

Although the intensive and individualized lifestyle coaching provided in clinical trials is generally not feasible in routine medical practice, there is evidence that group-implemented weight loss and exercise programs are also effective. Community resources, such as schools, health clubs, exercise facilities, and even commercial weight loss programs, should be considered when prescribing lifestyle modification for individuals at risk for diabetes. Additional resources include information and patient education materials available from the National Diabetes Education Program at www.ndep.nih.gov. The DPP lifestyle program curriculum and manual are available to the public at www.bsc.gwu.edu/dpp/index.htmlvdoc. Currently, most health insurance programs do not cover medical nutrition therapy in the absence of a diagnosis of diabetes. However, the diagnosis of dysmetabolic syndrome (ICD9 277.7) will include most patients with IGT/IFG and may be used to bill insurance plans for medical visits. Continued support and reinforcement for patients who pursue lifestyle modification is critical to long-term success.

Medications

Metformin. Metformin, a drug that is used in the treatment of type 2 diabetes, may also be used to prevent diabetes. In the DPP, metformin at a dose of 850 mg b.i.d. reduced the incidence of diabetes by 31%, compared with placebo. Other than gastrointestinal side effects, metformin was well tolerated and medication adherence was high. Unlike lifestyle modification, which was effective in all groups, metformin was not effective in older (>60 years old) or leaner (BMI <30 kg/m^2) individuals. The benefit of metformin largely persisted following a 1- to 2-week withdrawal of the drug, suggesting there may be a mechanism beyond an acute pharmacological effect. Use of metformin requires appropriate monitoring of renal and hepatic function and standard precautions regarding the use of intravenous contrast and serious acute illness, when the risk of lactic acidosis is increased. In addition, patients must be informed that metformin should be discontinued during pregnancy. Women with oligoamenorrhea due to polycystic ovary disease should be advised that they may experience increased fertility when treated with metformin. Although not yet confirmed in a population with IGT, metformin treatment was associated with a reduction in cardiovascular risk among obese diabetic subjects in the United Kingdom Prospective Diabetes Study, suggesting that this treatment may have additional benefits beyond glucose lowering.

Acarbose. A modest amount of clinical trial data suggest that acarbose, an α-glucosidase inhibitor, may be useful in preventing type 2 diabetes. The STOP-NIDDM trial, which included individuals with IGT and a BMI between 25 and 40 kg/m^2, demonstrated that the α-glucosidase inhibitor acarbose reduced the risk of diabetes by 25% compared with placebo. Acarbose was initiated at a dose of 50 mg daily and gradually titrated up to 100 mg t.i.d. with meals to minimize gastrointestinal side effects. Despite this, almost 20% of individuals randomized to acarbose were unable to tolerate the drug and discontinued the study. The rate of conversion to diabetes during the 3.5-year study in both the placebo and acarbose groups was unusually high (42 vs. 32%, respectively). It was also reported that acarbose-treated subjects were somewhat more likely than placebo-treated patients to revert to normal glucose tolerance.

Thiazolidinediones. Studies in a small number of subjects suggest that insulin sensitizers of the thiazolidinedione (TZD) class may be effective in preventing type 2 diabetes. In a high-risk group of women with glucose intolerance and prior gestational diabetes, troglitazone reduced the risk of diabetes by 56%. Protection from diabetes was greatest in those women who had the best improvement in insulin sensitivity. The beneficial effect of troglitazone appeared to persist for up to 8 months after discontinuation of the drug, suggesting a true preventive effect and not merely treatment ("masking") of incident diabetes. A proposed mechanism for the beneficial effect of troglitazone is preservation of pancreatic β-cell function, through reduction of secretory demand on β-cells by reducing insulin resistance. It is not known whether currently available TZDs will share this effect. There is little information about the safety of long-term use of TZDs, and caution is necessary when considering their use as a preventive treatment, especially in a relatively young population. A number of clinical trials are currently underway with newer TZDs to test their ability to prevent diabetes.

Other drugs. A number of other agents may potentially prevent diabetes. Posthoc analysis of clinical trials designed to assess cardiovascular outcomes have suggested that both angiotensin-converting enzyme (ACE) inhibitors and HMG-CoA reductase inhibitors (statins) may reduce the risk of type 2 diabetes. In the Heart Outcomes Protection Evaluation (HOPE) trial, the relative risk of developing diabetes in the group treated with an ACE inhibitor was 0.66 when compared with the placebo group. Statin therapy was associated with a 30% reduction in diabetes incidence in the West of Scotland Coronary Prevention Study, which may be mediated by this drug's proposed anti-inflammatory effect. These observations remain to be confirmed by appropriately designed clinical trials.

RECOMMENDATIONS

1. Lifestyle modification, which is most effective, should be the initial approach for all patients who are at risk for type 2 diabetes (Table 19.3). Such interventions should ideally include input from professionals with nutritional and behavioral expertise. The goals should be weight loss of at least 7% of initial body weight and moderate physical activity for at least 30 min per day. Continued treatment, including education and support, is necessary to maintain weight loss.
2. Results of lifestyle modification should be evaluated after 6–12 months, and additional intervention should be considered for patients who have been unable to achieve weight loss goals. Metformin, at a dose of 850 mg b.i.d., can be used for such patients and for those who have other indications for its use, such as treatment of polycystic ovarian syndrome. Younger and more obese patients may be most likely to benefit from metformin. Decades of experience with metformin as an antidiabetic therapy and its excellent safety profile in carefully selected patients make this an appro-

Table 19.3 Recommendations for Lifestyle Modification

- Reduce caloric intake
- Smaller portion sizes
- Reduce total fat to <30% of calories
- Increase fresh fruits, vegetables, and dietary fiber
- Weight loss of 5–7% (minimum) of starting body weight
- Physical activity equivalent to brisk walking 30 min daily

priate agent to use for diabetes prevention. Other medications cannot be recommended for routine use until the results of preliminary studies are confirmed in larger populations and additional information is available about long-term safety.

3. Monitoring should include yearly measurement of FPG to determine if progression to diabetes has occurred. Periodic follow-up OGTTs are not likely to be helpful or cost-effective in routine clinical practice. Although there are insufficient data at this time to recommend use of glycated hemoglobin A1C in the diagnosis of diabetes, it may be useful as an adjunct to FPG in assessing response to intervention.

4. Patients with IGT or IFG should be screened for the presence of other cardiovascular risk factors, such as dyslipidemia and hypertension, and treated as indicated. Because of its presumed low frequency, screening for diabetes-specific microvascular disease is not indicated in this population.

CONCLUSION

Lifestyle modification is very effective in reducing the development of diabetes in individuals at high risk because of the presence of obesity and glucose intolerance. It is expected that prevention or delay of diabetes will ultimately result in reduction of long-term vascular complications, although this remains to be confirmed by additional studies. Current medical practice should include active efforts to identify and treat individuals at risk for diabetes. It is estimated that at least 10 million individuals in the U.S. share the high-risk characteristics of the DPP cohort and would therefore benefit from identification and intervention. Because of the size of the at-risk population and the lifelong need for lifestyle intervention, prevention of diabetes is a major public health issue and will require community-based and health care systems efforts to have a significant impact on the current epidemic of type 2 diabetes.

BIBLIOGRAPHY

Buchanan T, Xiang A, Peters R, Kjos S, Marroquin A, Goico J, Ochoa C, Tan S, Berkowitz K, Hodis H, Azen S: Preservation of pancreatic beta cell function and prevention of type 2 diabetes by pharmacological treatment of insulin resistance in high-risk Hispanic women. *Diabetes* 51:2796–2803, 2002

Chaisson J, Josse R, Gomis R, Hanefeld M, Karasik A, Laakso M, for the STOP-NIDDM Trial Research Group: Acarbose for prevention of type 2 diabetes mellitus: the STOP-NIDDM randomized trial. *Lancet* 359:2072–2077, 2002

Diabetes Prevention Program Research Group: Effects of withdrawal from metformin on the development of diabetes in the Diabetes Prevention Program. *Diabetes Care* 26:977–980, 2003

Diabetes Prevention Program Research Group: Reduction in the incidence of type 2 diabetes with lifestyle intervention or metformin. *N Engl J Med* 346:393–403, 2002

Eastman RC, Cowie CC, Harris MI: Undiagnosed diabetes or impaired glucose tolerance and cardiovascular risk. *Diabetes Care* 20:127–128, 1997

Edelstein SL, Knowler WC, Bain RP, Andres R, Barrett-Connor EL, Dowse GK, et al.: Predictors of progression from impaired glucose tolerance to NIDDM: an analysis of six prospective studies. *Diabetes* 46:701–710, 1997

Haffner SM: Do interventions to reduce coronary heart disease reduce the incidence of type 2 diabetes? *Circulation* 103:346–347, 2001

Pan XR, Li GW, Hu YH, Wang JX, Yang WY, An ZX, et al.: Effects of diet and exercise in preventing NIDDM in people with impaired glucose tolerance: the Da Qing IGT and Diabetes Study. *Diabetes Care* 20:537–544, 1997

Saydh S, Byrd-Holt D, Harris M: Projected impact of implementing the results of the Diabetes Prevention Program. *Diabetes Care* 25:1940–1945, 2002

Stern MP, Williams K, Haffner SM: Identification of persons at high risk of type 2 diabetes: do we need the oral glucose tolerance test? *Ann Intern Med* 136:575–581, 2002

Tuomilehto K, Lindstrom J, Eriksson J, Valle T, Hamalainen H, Ilanne-Parikka P, et al.: Prevention of type 2 diabetes mellitus by changes in lifestyle among subjects with impaired glucose tolerance. *N Engl J Med* 344:1343–1350, 2001

Walker EA: Preventing type 2 diabetes in adults. In *Practical Psychology for Diabetes Clinicians.* 2nd ed. Anderson BJ, Rubin RR, Eds. Alexandria, VA, American Diabetes Association, 2002, p. 181–190

Dr. Crandall is Assistant Professor and Dr. Shamoon is Professor and Associate Dean for Clinical Research in the Division of Endocrinology and Metabolism, Department of Medicine, and Diabetes Research Center, Albert Einstein College of Medicine, Bronx, NY. The authors were supported by the following grants from the National Institutes of Health: DK48349 (to J.P.C. and H.S.), DK62463 (to H.S.), and DK20541 (to H.S.)

20. Insulin Secretagogues: Sulfonylureas, Repaglinide, and Nateglinide

HAROLD E. LEBOVITZ, MD

Sulfonylurea drugs have been used in the management of hyperglycemia in patients with type 2 diabetes for >50 years. The mechanism of their antidiabetic action is complex. They act on the β-cell to increase both basal and meal-stimulated insulin secretion. Minor effects have been attributed in some studies to various extrapancreatic actions. Chronic improvement in glycemic control by sulfonylurea treatment decreases the metabolic effects of glucose toxicity in inhibiting insulin secretion and insulin action. As a consequence of their multiple actions, sulfonylureas cause improvement in several metabolic pathways in patients with type 2 diabetes. They decrease the exaggerated overproduction of glucose by the liver, partially reverse the postreceptor defect in insulin action at the level of muscle and adipose tissue, and increase the magnitude of meal-mediated insulin secretion.

The biochemical mechanism of sulfonylurea action has been defined recently. Insulin secretion is regulated by an ATP-dependent K^+ channel located in the plasma membrane of the β-cell. Under fasting conditions, most of the channels are open, and K^+ is actively extruded from the β-cell. When the plasma glucose rises, glucose is transported into the β-cell through a specific transport molecule (GLUT2 transporter), phosphorylated by glucokinase, and metabolized in the mitochondria, where ATP is generated from ADP. High intracellular ATP and low ADP concentrations cause the ATP-dependent K^+ channel to close. K^+ accumulates within the cell membrane, thereby causing it to depolarize. A voltage-dependent Ca^{2+} channel (also located in the plasma membrane) opens, and Ca^{2+} moves from the extracellular space into the β-cell cytosol. The rising cytosolic Ca^{2+} concentration causes the insulin granule to migrate to the cell surface, where its contents are released by exocytosis.

The ATP-dependent K^+ channel consists of two subunits: one (named SUR) contains a sulfonylurea binding site (receptor) and regulates whether the channel is open or closed. The other subunit (named Kir) comprises the channel itself. The ATP-dependent K^+ channel is functional only when its two subunits are united. The sulfonylurea receptor faces the extracellular space. When sulfonylureas bind to the ATP-dependent K^+ channel, it closes. This then causes insulin secretion. The potency of a sulfonylurea is a function of its binding affinity to the receptor. Sulfonylureas therefore potentiate glucose-mediated insulin secretion as well as stimulating basal insulin secretion.

Other tissues such as myocardium, vascular smooth muscle, and brain have ATP-dependent K^+ channels that contain sulfonylurea binding sites. In vascular smooth muscle and myocardial cells, the ATP-dependent K^+ channels are normally closed and open in response to ischemia to allow potassium to be released and calcium to enter. This causes vasodilation to occur and improves myocardial function. In experimental studies, sulfonylureas can prevent the ATP-dependent K^+ channel from opening and interfere with vasodilation and myocardial adaptation to ischemia. A second effect of preventing the channel from opening is a decrease in K^+ flux in the myocardium, which can protect against ventricular arrhythmias. If such effects were to occur in humans with ordinary pharmacological dosing of sulfonylureas, either a detrimental or beneficial effect on the cardiovascular system may occur during ischemia. The SUR subunits of the vascular smooth muscle and myocardial cells are different isoforms than those in the β-cell. In general, they have lower binding affinities for sulfonylureas than the β-cell isoform. The only sulfonylurea shown to significantly bind to those isoforms in cardiovascular ATP-dependent K^+ channels is glyburide. Glyburide has been shown in both normal and diabetic individuals to block cardiovascular ATP-dependent channels from opening during ischemic episodes, which prevents ischemic preconditioning of the myocardium. The role of ischemic preconditioning is to render the heart less susceptible to ischemic damage. Although these data are worrisome, it is important to note that several large long-term follow-up studies of diabetic patients taking glyburide have not shown an increase in adverse cardiovascular outcomes. The effect of sulfonylureas, if any, on brain cells is unknown.

Repaglinide, the only member of the meglitinide family approved for clinical use, is not a sulfonylurea. It binds to a different site on the SUR1 subunit of the β-cell ATP-dependent K^+ channel from sulfonylureas. Repaglinide binding leads to closure of the ATP-dependent K^+ channel with subsequent insulin release. Sulfonylureas and repaglinide seem to have similar but not identical modes of action in causing insulin release (Tables 20.1 and 20.2). Their effects are not additive.

Nateglinide is a derivative of phenylalanine and is a very rapid-acting insulin secretogogue. It binds to the sulfonylurea receptor on SUR1 but with different binding characteristics than sulfonylureas. Its rates of association and dissociation are much more rapid. It has very low binding affinity for cardiovascular ATP-dependent K^+ channels.

Several features are essential in understanding the proper use of drugs that stimulate insulin secretion. These drugs are ineffective in lowering blood glucose in patients who have a marked reduction or total loss of functioning β-cells. In contrast, hypoglycemia can be a serious consequence of their inappropriate use. For unknown reasons, not all type 2 diabetes patients respond to the antidiabetic action of sulfonylureas (primary failure), and many patients who respond very well initially may have a loss of effective antidiabetic response after several years of treatment (secondary failure). In the United Kingdom Prospective Diabetes Study (UKPDS), treatment with sulfonylureas (glyburide or chlorpropamide) achieved a glycated hemoglobin A1C (A1C) of <7% in 50% of patients at 3 years, 34% at 6 years, and only 24% at 9 years.

The 6- and 9-year data from the UKPDS show that this secondary failure is a characteristic of all antidiabetic treatments and not just sulfonylureas. Little is

Table 20.1 Characteristics of Specific Insulin Secretagogues

Drug	Dose Range (mg/dl)	Peak Level (h)	Half-Life (h)	Metabolites	Excretion
Sulfonylureas					
Tolbutamide	500–3,000	3–4	4.5–6.5	Inactive	Kidney
Chlorpropamide	100–500	2–4	36	Active or unchanged	Kidney
Tolazamide	100–1,000	3–4	7	Inactive	Kidney
Glipizide	2.5–40	1–3	2–4	Inactive	Kidney 80%, feces 20%
Glipizide GITS	5–20	Constant after several days of dosing		Inactive	Kidney 80%, feces 20%
Glyburide	1.25–20	~4	10	Inactive and weakly weakly	Kidney 50%, feces 50%
Glyburide, micronized formulation	1.5–12	2–3	~4	Inactive and weakly active	Kidney 50%, feces 50%
Glimeperide	1–8	2–3	9	Inactive and weakly active	Kidney 60%, feces 40%
Nonsulfonylurea Insulin Secretagogues					
Repaglinide	0.5–4 with each meal	1	1	Inactive	Feces
Nateglinide	60–120 with each meal	1.8	1.4	Weakly active	Kidney 80%, feces 10%

known about repaglinide's or nateglinide's antidiabetic effects beyond 1 or 2 years of treatment. Drugs that stimulate insulin secretion do not replace dietary management of type 2 diabetes; they complement it (i.e., they are unlikely to be effective if dietary management is ignored).

CHOOSING AN INSULIN SECRETAGOGUE

The clinical use of a particular insulin secretagogue is determined by the characteristics described in Table 20.3. Intrinsic antidiabetic activity varies considerably and is a function of the binding affinity to the sulfonylurea receptor or the other binding sites on the ATP-dependent K^+ channel. Repaglinide, glimeperide, and glyburide are the most potent, and tolbutamide is the least potent. The intrinsic potency of each drug is important in determining the effective dose of the drug

Table 20.2 Comparison Between Sulfonylureas and Nonsulfonylurea Insulin Secretagogues

Sulfonylureas	Nonsulfonylurea Insulin Secretagogues
Intermediate or long duration of action	Short duration of action
Administered once or twice daily	Must be given with each meal
Major effect is a decrease in FPG	Repaglinide has the same effect in decreasing FPG as sulfonylureas. Nateglinide causes an ~20 mg/dl decrease in FPG.
Little effect of early meal-mediated insulin secretion	Increases early meal-mediated insulin secretion
Little or no effect on postprandial glucose excursion	Significant reduction in meal-mediated glucose excursion
Clinically significant hypoglycemia occurs fasting and late postprandially	Hypoglycemia (particularly nocturnal) is uncommon.
Weight gain of 2–4 kg usually occurs with treatment	Weight gain is less of a problem.
Mean decrease in A1C is ~1.5%	Mean decrease in A1C with repaglinide is equivalent to that of sulfonylureas. Mean decrease in A1C with nateglinide is ~0.8%
Inexpensive	Relatively expensive

that is necessary. Clinical response in controlling hyperglycemia, however, is not significantly different among the various insulin secretagogues at their effective doses except for tolbutamide and nateglinide, which are less effective than the other drugs in controlling hyperglycemia in type 2 diabetes patients.

Type 2 diabetes is characterized by both a delay and a decrease in meal-stimulated insulin secretion. The delay in insulin secretion contributes to the excessive early postprandial rise in blood glucose levels. The more rapid the onset of action of an insulin secretagogue, the shorter the delay in the rise in postprandial insulin secretion. Repaglinide and nateglinide have a rapid onset of action

Table 20.3 Characteristics by Which to Select a Specific Insulin Secretagogue

- Intrinsic insulin secretory potency
- Rapidity of onset of action
- Duration of action
- Mode of metabolism and excretion
- Beneficial and detrimental side effects

and, when administered at the onset of the meal, effectively restore early post-prandial insulin secretion almost to normal. The interval between administration of the drug and the meal should be considered. With some sulfonylureas (glyburide and glipizide), better results are obtained if the drug is given 30 min before the meal. The ideal goal in administering an insulin secretogogue is to synchronize the peak insulin secretion with the peak postprandial glucose rise.

The duration of action of an insulin secretagogue is of considerable importance. A long-acting secretagogue is more likely to be associated with severe, prolonged, and sometimes fatal hypoglycemia in susceptible patients, i.e., those who are elderly (~70 years of age), have poor nutrition, are likely to miss meals, or have concomitant hepatic, renal, or cardiovascular disease. Shorter-acting insulin secretagogues are significantly safer in this population. The rapid-acting non-sulfonylurea secretogogues cause low rates of hypoglycemia because of their shorter duration of action.

The mode of metabolism and excretion are also important in determining the frequency and severity of hypoglycemic reactions. Insulin secretagogues that are metabolized to active metabolites are associated with more hypoglycemic reactions. Likewise, drugs or active metabolites primarily excreted by the kidney are more likely to cause hypoglycemia in patients with renal dysfunction than drugs excreted via the biliary tract.

Side effects occur that are independent of antidiabetic action. Some appear to be unique to chlorpropamide (e.g., water retention and hyponatremia). This may be the reason for the higher rate of development of hypertension and poorer risk reduction of diabetic retinopathy observed in the chlorpropamide-treated compared with the glyburide-treated patients in the UKPDS. Other side effects (e.g., alcohol-induced flushing) may occur with first-generation (low intrinsic potency) sulfonylureas such as chlorpropamide and tolbutamide but not with second-generation (high intrinsic potency) agents.

Characteristics of Specific Sulfonylurea Drugs

Table 20.1 lists the characteristics of the commonly used sulfonylurea drugs. The dose range is a function of the intrinsic potency, but the clinical effectiveness at the appropriate dose is the same for all sulfonylureas except tolbutamide. Onset and duration of action are determined by the unique pharmacokinetic properties of each agent and its specific formulation. Most sulfonylureas are metabolized in the liver to active or inactive metabolites, except chlorpropamide, which is excreted unchanged in significant quantities in the urine. Biliary excretion is significant with glyburide and glimeperide and to a lesser extent with glipizide. Major side effects other than hypoglycemia are most commonly seen with chlorpropamide.

Characteristics of Repaglinide

Repaglinide is a new nonsulfonylurea insulin secretagogue. Table 20.1 lists its characteristics and Table 20.2 compares them to sulfonylureas. Repaglinide is available in 0.5-, 1.0-, and 2.0-mg doses. Its oral absorption is rapid, with peak plasma levels occurring at 1 h. Its half-life in plasma is 1 h. Its metabolites are inactive, and it is excreted mainly by the liver. The duration of action of repaglinide is ~4 h. Because of its short duration of action, it must be taken 15 min before each meal, and the incidence of hypoglycemia is low. The usual dose is 0.5–2.0 mg at the start of each meal. Repaglinide reduces both fasting plasma glucose (FPG) and postprandial glucose excursions.

Characteristics of Nateglinide

Nateglinide is a phenylalanine derivative nonsulfonylurea insulin secretogogue. Tables 20.1 and 20.2 list its characteristics and compare them with the characteristics of sulfonylureas. Nateglinide is available as a 60- and 120-mg tablet. Its oral absorption is rapid (peak plasma level at 1.5–2.0 h). Its plasma half-life is 1.4 h. It has very rapid kinetics of both binding to and displacement from the β-cell ATP-dependent K^+ channel. It causes the most rapid release and shortest duration of release of insulin of any of the insulin secretogogues. Consequently, its effect is almost exclusively that of decreasing postprandial glucose excursions. The side effects of weight gain and hypoglycemia are less than with other insulin secretogogues. Nateglinide is administered as 120 mg before each meal. The dose may be reduced to 60 mg before each meal in individuals with minimal elevations in FPG.

HYPOGLYCEMIA

The most serious complication of insulin secretagogue therapy is hypoglycemia. This is best avoided or minimized by the following procedures:

1. Start insulin secretagogue therapy with the lowest possible dose and increase the dose incrementally every 4–7 days.
2. Patients susceptible to severe and prolonged hypoglycemia should be treated with shorter-acting insulin secretagogues.
3. Sulfonylureas should be used cautiously in patients with renal dysfunction. Sulfonylureas with short duration of action, inactive metabolites, and biliary excretion are preferred. The nonsulfonylurea insulin secretogogues are particularly useful in patients with renal dysfunction.
4. Encourage patients not to skip meals after taking insulin secretagogues. Patients who frequently miss or delay meals are ideal for treatment with repaglinide or nateglinide. Those medications are only taken at the start of the meal.
5. Be careful of drug interactions.

The treatment of mild hypoglycemia in insulin secretagogue–treated patients is managed by giving food, monitoring carefully, and reducing the dosage or changing the specific agent. The treatment of severe sulfonylurea-induced hypoglycemia requires vigorous and prolonged treatment. Patients who present with gluconeuropenic symptoms and plasma glucose levels <50 mg/dl (<2.8 mmol/l) should be given 50 ml of 50% glucose intravenously followed by continuous glucose (5 or 10%) and frequent monitoring of blood glucose. Occasionally, administration of 1 mg glucagon intramuscularly or slowly intravenously may be necessary. Patients with severe intractable hypoglycemia despite glucose administration have been successfully treated by the addition of 50 μg octreotide administered subcutaneously every 8 h for two or three doses.

Patients with insulin secretagogue–mediated severe hypoglycemia must be monitored and treated for at least 24 h. With long-acting sulfonylureas, patients should be monitored for 72 h, because recurrence of hypoglycemia is common. These patients cannot be given 50% glucose intravenously and sent home. The reason for the severe hypoglycemia must be sought and appropriate therapeutic changes made.

Repaglinide, because of its short duration of action, is associated with less frequent and less severe hypoglycemia. Nateglinide treatment is only rarely associated with significant hypoglycemia.

INDICATIONS FOR THERAPY WITH INSULIN SECRETAGOGUES

Ideal candidates for treatment with insulin secretagogues are type 2 diabetes patients who are significantly insulin deficient but still have enough β-cell function to respond to stimulation by the secretagogue. Patients likely to show good glycemic response to agents that stimulate insulin secretion

- had onset of hyperglycemia after age 30 years
- have had diagnosed hyperglycemia for <5 years
- are normal weight or obese
- are willing to follow a reasonable dietary program
- are not totally insulin deficient

Contraindications for insulin secretagogue therapy are given in Table 20.4.

PROPER USE OF INSULIN SECRETAGOGUES

Insulin secretagogues should be administered to type 2 diabetes patients who have been unable to adequately control their plasma glucose on a reasonable trial

Table 20.4 Contraindications for Insulin Secretagogue Therapy

■ Type 1 diabetes or pancreatic diabetes ■ Pregnancy ■ Major surgery ■ Severe infections, stress, or trauma ■ History of severe adverse reaction to sulfonylurea or similar compound (sulfa drug) (does not exclude repaglinide)	■ Predisposition to severe hypoglycemia, e.g., patients with significant liver or kidney disease

(4–6 weeks) of appropriate dietary therapy. When insulin secretagogue therapy is added, dietary management must continue. Patients who present with marked symptoms and random plasma glucose levels of ~300 mg/dl (16.7 mmol/l) should probably be started on dietary management and insulin secretagogue therapy together. Insulin secretagogue therapy alone is unlikely to have significant beneficial effects in an individual who has an FPG >275 mg/dl (>15.3 mmol/l) while on a reasonable dietary program.

Initiation of a newly diagnosed type 2 diabetes patient with random hyperglycemia >300 mg/dl (>16.7 mmol/l) on insulin secretagogue therapy is controversial. In general, most diabetologists are concerned that such patients are unlikely to achieve acceptable glycemic control initially because of the effects of glucose toxicity and the possibility of severe insulin deficiency. Such patients are best treated with insulin and placed on an appropriate diet. After adequate glycemic control is obtained (FPG <130 mg/dl [6.7 mmol/l]), insulin secretagogue therapy may replace insulin therapy. Peters and Davidson (1995) have disputed this approach and claim that most of their patients who present with marked symptoms and mean random plasma glucose levels of 456 mg/dl (25 mmol/l) can be well controlled by initiation of therapy with maximal doses of glyburide. Such an approach can be hazardous unless the initial evaluation shows no evidence of dehydration or acidosis and the patient is followed closely for lack of response and/or deterioration toward ketoacidosis or nonketotic hyperosmolar states. The combination of glyburide and metformin (Glucovance) has been shown to be effective in controlling initial hyperglycemia in a cohort of type 2 diabetes patients presenting with mean FPG of 283 mg/dl and mean A1C of 10.6%. A mean daily dose of 7.9 mg glyburide and 1,571 mg metformin reduced the mean FPG and A1C to 161 mg/dl and 7.1%, respectively, after 26 weeks of treatment.

Insulin secretagogue therapy should ordinarily be instituted with a low dose and increased at 4- to 7-day intervals until the maximal benefit is achieved. Many elderly or modestly symptomatic type 2 diabetes patients may be exquisitely sensitive to insulin secretagogues, and initial institution with moderate or high doses may precipitate severe hypoglycemia. The ideal goal of therapy is to maintain preprandial plasma blood glucose levels between 90 and 130 mg/dl (5.0 and 7.2 mmol/l) and an A1C of <7%. If such control is obtained and maintained, insulin secretagogue therapy might be tapered and discontinued to see whether dietary therapy alone will maintain near-normoglycemic control. There are, however, some data to suggest that long-term glycemic control is better achieved if low-dose insulin secretagogue therapy is maintained.

Chronic insulin secretagogue therapy should be continued only as long as it maintains glycemic control in the target range sought for that particular patient. Most patients will achieve the maximal benefit in improving glycemic control with one-half to two-thirds of the manufacturer's recommended maximal dose. With sulfonylurea drugs, use of the maximal recommended dose may actually be less effective than using more moderate doses. This may be the result of down-regulation or desensitization of the sulfonylurea receptor.

When target glycemic control is no longer achieved with insulin secretagogues, a change in therapy is indicated and should probably be the addition of other antihyperglycemic agents alone or in combination with insulin (see Chapter 26).

EFFECTS OF OTHER DRUGS ON INSULIN SECRETAGOGUE ACTIONS

Many commonly used drugs can potentiate insulin secretagogue effects and precipitate hypoglycemia or antagonize insulin secretagogue effects and worsen glycemic control. Table 20.5 lists some of the more important interactions. Alcohol and aspirin interactions may provide prolonged and severe hypoglycemia. β-Blockers interfere with both the recognition and counterregulatory responses to hypoglycemia. Anticoagulants are competitive inhibitors of sulfonylurea metabolism, and when both classes of drugs are used, the doses of both may have to be reduced appropriately.

Any concomitant drug treatment in a patient on or to be started on insulin secretagogue therapy must be evaluated for possible drug interactions. Because sulfonylureas with high intrinsic activity are given in smaller quantities and have somewhat different binding characteristics, they are likely to have fewer drug interactions than those with low intrinsic activity.

Repaglinide metabolism may be inhibited by antifungal agents such as ketoconazole and micronazole and antibacterial agents such as erythromycin. Drugs that increase cytochrome P_{450} enzyme system 3A4 may increase repaglinide metabolism in the liver. Such drugs include troglitazone and barbiturates. Repaglinide does not alter the metabolism of digoxin, warfarin, or theophylline. Its interactions with agents that increase hypoglycemia or worsen glycemic control are similar to those of the sulfonylureas (Table 20.5). Treating patients with repaglinide who are on other medications may require adjustments of its dose.

EXPECTED RESULTS

Initial treatment of patients with type 2 diabetes with either sulfonylureas or repaglinide is likely to result in a mean decrease in FPG of 60–70 mg/dl (3.3–3.8 mmol/l) and a drop in A1C of 1–2%. Nateglinide treatment primarily

Table 20.5 Drug Interactions with Sulfonylureas

Increase hypoglycemia

- Drugs that displace sulfonylurea from albumin-binding sites, e.g., aspirin, fibrates, trimethoprim
- Competitive inhibitors of sulfonylurea metabolism, e.g., alcohol, H^2 blockers, anticoagulants
- Inhibitors of urinary excretion of sulfonylureas, e.g., probenecid, allopurinol
- Concomitant use of drugs with hypoglycemic properties, e.g., alcohol, aspirin

- Antagonist of endogenous counterregulatory hormones, e.g., β-blockers, sympatholytic drugs

Worsen glycemic control

- Drugs that increase sulfonylurea metabolism, e.g., barbiturates, rifampin
- Agents that antagonize sulfonylurea action, e.g., β-blockers
- Inhibitors of insulin secretion or action, e.g., thiazides and loop diuretics, β-blockers, corticosteroids, estrogens, phenytoin

lowers postprandial hyperglycemia and therefore decreases mean A1C ~0.8%. As with all pharmacological treatments in patients with type 2 diabetes, the mean improvement in glycemic control with these agents is somewhat greater when the glycemic control is poor and somewhat less when the glycemic control is only moderately abnormal.

About one-third of newly diagnosed patients will achieve their target glycemic control on treatment with an insulin secretagogue and diet. Another third will achieve significant improvement in glycemic control but will require additional antihyperglycemic agents if the target goal is to be achieved. The other third will have a poor response and should be put on another therapeutic regimen.

With increasing duration of type 2 diabetes, the response to sulfonylureas and probably also to repaglinide and nateglinide (although data are not available) diminishes. This decreased effectiveness is ultimately due to decreasing endogenous β-cell insulin secretory function. It is unclear whether progressive β-cell functional loss is an intrinsic characteristic of type 2 diabetes or whether it is a consequence of chronic insulin resistance and/or chronic glucose and lipid toxicity from poor control. Chronic stimulation of insulin secretion by sulfonylureas does not appear to be a cause of β-cell exhaustion. The consequence of this diminishing effect of insulin secretogogues is that modifications in therapy will be necessary.

Table 20.6 is an extensive list of many of the factors that might contribute to diminished effectiveness of sulfonylurea therapy and probably repaglinide and nateglinide therapy. Before concluding that the diminished effectiveness is caused by decreasing β-cell function, the possibility that a correctable cause is the culprit should be excluded.

The major concerns regarding insulin secretagogue therapy are

- hypoglycemia
- weight gain
- cardiovascular disease risk

Hypoglycemia is a significant complication. The newer agents—glimeperide, repaglinide, and nateglinide—are claimed to have a significantly lower risk of hypoglycemia than the older agents. Glimeperide therapy is thought to be more

Table 20.6 Common Causes of Secondary Sulfonylurea Failure

Patient-related factors	Therapy-related factors
■ Overeating and weight gain ■ Poor patient compliance ■ Lack of physical activity ■ Stress ■ Intercurrent illnesses	■ Inadequate drug dosage ■ Desensitization to chronic sulfonylurea exposure ■ Impaired absorption of drug due to hyperglycemia ■ Concomitant therapy with diabetogenic drugs
Disease-related factors	
■ Decreasing β-cell function ■ Increasing insulin resistance	

effective with lower plasma insulin levels and to maintain physiological suppression of insulin secretion in response to low blood glucose levels. Repaglinide is a short-acting insulin secretagogue and is taken with each meal. Nateglinide is the shortest-acting insulin secretogogue and it too must be taken with each meal. Additional studies are needed to quantify the degree to which these agents are associated with less clinical hypoglycemia. Glyburide treatment is noteworthy in that many studies now indicate that hypoglycemia is more common and severe with it than with other insulin secretagogue therapies.

Weight gain is noted in almost all studies involving patients with type 2 diabetes on chronic sulfonylurea therapy. In the UKPDS, this amounted to ~12.5 lb or 7% of body weight. Weight gain is less when sulfonylureas are combined with other antihyperglycemic agents such as acarbose or metformin. There are some data to indicate that repaglinide and especially nateglinide treatments are associated with less weight gain than sulfonylurea treatment.

Cardiovascular disease risk associated with sulfonylurea therapy has been a concern since the University Group Diabetes Program results were published in 1970. That study suggested that tolbutamide therapy was associated with an increase in sudden death from cardiovascular disease. There has been no additional clinical validation for that study in the last 25 years. The UKPDS data settled this issue because there was no increase in macrovascular disease events in the large cohort treated with sulfonylureas for a mean of 11 years. The recent experimental studies of the myocardial and vascular smooth muscle effects of sulfonylureas, although interesting, have not been clinically validated. Glyburide has been shown to block ischemic preconditioning in the heart in individuals both with and without diabetes. However, there is no clinical evidence that glyburide increases cardiovascular morbidity or mortality in patients with diabetes. Nonetheless, studies with glimeperide, repaglinide, and nateglinide show that these agents have significantly less binding to myocardial and vascular smooth muscle ATP-dependent K^+ channels than glyburide. Glimeperide in contrast to glyburide does not block ischemic preconditioning. The effects of repaglinide and nateglinide on ischemic preconditioning have not been tested because their interactions with the SUR subunits in cardiovascular tissues are so weak.

BIBLIOGRAPHY

Groop LC, Pelkonen R, Koskimies S, Bottazzo GF, Doniach D: Secondary failure to treatment with oral antidiabetic agents in non-insulin-dependent diabetes. *Diabetes Care* 9:129–133, 1986

Lebovitz HE: Oral antidiabetic agents. In *Joslin's Diabetes Mellitus.* 14th ed. Kahn CR, Weir GC, Eds. Philadelphia, Lippincott, Williams & Wilkins. 2004

Lebovitz HE: Oral therapies for diabetic hyperglycemia. *Endocrinol Metab Clin North Am* 30:909–933, 2001

Lebovitz HE, Melander A: Sulfonylureas: basic aspects and clinical uses. In *International Textbook of Diabetes Mellitus.* 3rd ed. DeFronzo RA, Ferraninni E, Keen H, Zimmet P, Eds. Colchester, U.K., Wiley. 2004

Peters AL, Davidson MB: Maximal dose glyburide therapy in markedly sympto-matic patients with type 2 diabetes: a new use for an old friend. *J Clin Endocrinol Metab* 81:2423–2427, 1995

Riddle MC: Editorial: sulfonylureas differ in effects on ischemic pre-condition-ing: is it time to retire glyburide? *J Clin Endocrinol Metab* 88:528–530, 2003

Turner R, Cull C, Holman R: United Kingdom Prospective Diabetes Study 17: a 9-year update of a randomized, controlled trial on the effect of improved metabolic control on complications in non-insulin-dependent diabetes mel-litus. *Ann Intern Med* 124:136–145, 1996

UK Prospective Diabetes Study 33: Intensive blood glucose control with sul-fonylureas or insulin compared with conventional treatment and risk of complications in patients with type 2 diabetes. *Lancet* 352:837–853, 1998

Dr. Lebovitz is Professor of Medicine at the State University of New York Health Science Center at Brooklyn, Brooklyn, NY.

21. Metformin

Clifford J. Bailey, PhD

In 1995, metformin was introduced for the treatment of hyperglycemia in patients with type 2 diabetes in the U.S., having been used in Europe since the early 1960s. It acts to counter insulin resistance and has several potential benefits against risk factors for vascular disease that are independent of glycemic control. It may also be of use for other conditions associated with insulin resistance, such as polycystic ovarian syndrome (PCOS).

Metformin is a member the class of drugs known as biguanides, which are guanidine derivatives (Fig. 21.1). Guanidine is found in the plant *Galega officinalis* (goat's rue or French lilac), which was used in medieval Europe as a treatment for diabetes. Other biguanides, notably phenformin and buformin, were introduced for the treatment of type 2 diabetes but were withdrawn because of a significant incidence of associated lactic acidosis. Metformin does not have this risk if appropriately prescribed and is now used widely as a monotherapy and in combination with other antidiabetic agents.

MODE OF ACTION AND RATIONALE FOR USE

Key features of the therapeutic effect of metformin in patients with type 2 diabetes are as follows:

- Metformin counters insulin resistance; it does not stimulate insulin secretion.
- Metformin decreases mainly fasting (and also postprandial) hyperglycemia in type 2 diabetes patients.
- Monotherapy with metformin does not cause hypoglycemia.
- The antidiabetic action of metformin requires some circulating insulin.
- Metformin treatment does not cause weight gain and can assist modest weight loss in overweight type 2 diabetes patients.
- Metformin treatment often improves the lipid profile.
- Metformin treatment can improve other vascular risk factors (e.g., it can increase fibrinolysis).
- Metformin has been shown to reduce vascular mortality when used as initial antidiabetic therapy in overweight and obese patients with type 2 diabetes.

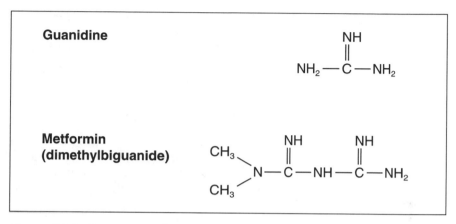

Figure 21.1. Structures of guanidine and metformin.

Blood Glucose Lowering

Metformin is an antihyperglycemic agent (rather than a hypoglycemic agent) because, when used as monotherapy, it lowers blood glucose concentrations in patients with type 2 diabetes without causing overt hypoglycemia. Also, it has little effect on blood glucose concentrations in nondiabetic individuals. Although the antihyperglycemic efficacy of metformin requires the presence of insulin, metformin does not stimulate insulin secretion. Some effects of metformin are mediated via increased insulin action (so-called insulin sensitizing effects), and some are not directly insulin dependent.

The main blood glucose–lowering effects of metformin are summarized in Table 21.1. Fasting hyperglycemia is reduced predominantly by decreased hepatic glucose production, principally due to reduced gluconeogenesis but also through reduced glycogenolysis. At therapeutic concentrations, metformin suppresses hepatic gluconeogenesis mostly by potentiating the effect of insulin. Metformin can also reduce hepatic extraction of lactate. The rate of glycogenolysis is decreased by reducing the effect of glucagon and impeding the activity of hepatic glucose-6-phosphatase.

Insulin-mediated glucose uptake and utilization by skeletal muscle is enhanced during treatment with metformin. Euglycemic-hyperinsulinemic clamp studies in

Table 21.1 Mechanisms for the Antihyperglycemic Effect of Metformin

▪ Suppression of hepatic glucose production	▪ Decreased fatty acid oxidation
▪ Increased insulin-mediated muscle glucose uptake	▪ Increased intestinal glucose utilization

patients with type 2 diabetes have typically noted an increase in glucose uptake by ~20%, although this is not a consistent finding and appears to be influenced by the severity of the diabetic state, extent of weight reduction, and duration of therapy. Metformin increases the translocation of insulin-sensitive glucose transporters into the cell membrane and promotes the insulin- and glucose-sensitive transport properties of glucose transporters. The increased cellular uptake of glucose is associated with increased glycogen synthase activity and glycogen deposition.

Other effects of metformin that contribute to a lowering of blood glucose include an insulin-independent suppression of fatty acid oxidation and a reduction of hypertriglyceridemia. Through these effects, metformin reduces the energy supply for gluconeogenesis and improves the glucose–fatty acid (Randle) cycle. Metformin also increases glucose turnover, particularly in the splanchnic bed, which may benefit both the blood glucose–lowering and weight-stabilizing effects of the drug.

Nonglycemic Effects

In addition to its antihyperglycemic actions, metformin has been reported to counter several features of the insulin resistance syndrome (metabolic syndrome), as summarized in Table 21.2. While reducing insulin resistance, metformin ther-

Table 21.2 Effects of Metformin to Counter the Insulin Resistance (Metabolic) Syndrome

Features of the Insulin Resistance Syndrome	Effects of Metformin to Counter the Insulin Resistance Syndrome
Insulin resistance	Counters insulin resistance (e.g., increases insulin action to suppress hepatic glucose production and enhance muscle glucose uptake)
Hyperinsulinemia	Reduces fasting hyperinsulinemia
Abdominal obesity	Usually stabilizes body weight; reduces weight gain and can facilitate weight loss
IGT or type 2 diabetes	Reduces progression of IGT to type 2 diabetes; improves glycemic control in type 2 diabetes
Dyslipidemia ($\uparrow$VLDL-TG, $\uparrow$LDL-C, $\uparrow$HDL-C)	Modest improvement of lipid profile often seen in dyslipidemic patients
Hypertension	No significant effect on blood pressure in most studies
Procoagulant state	Some antithrombotic activity (e.g., decreases in PAI-1, fibrinogen, and platelet aggregation)
Atherosclerosis	Evidence for anti-atherogenic activity from preclinical studies; no equivalent clinical studies

HDL-C, HDL cholesterol; IGT, impaired glucose tolerance; LDL-C, LDL cholesterol; VLDL-TG, very-low-density lipoprotein triglyceride; PAI-1, plasminogen activator inhibitor-1.

apy can lower fasting hyperinsulinemia, prevent weight gain, improve the lipid profile, and decrease certain thrombotic factors. Such actions could potentially reduce vascular risk.

Circulating concentrations of triglycerides and LDL cholesterol are usually reduced by metformin in individuals with raised levels, but there is little or no effect when these parameters are already within the normal range. HDL cholesterol concentrations are slightly raised in some individuals during metformin therapy.

Several actions of metformin oppose the procoagulant state of type 2 diabetes (e.g., fibrinolytic activity is increased, sensitivity to platelet aggregating agents is decreased, and plasminogen activator inhibitor-1 [PAI-1] levels are decreased). The United Kingdom Prospective Diabetes Study (UKPDS) found that use of metformin as initial antidiabetic therapy in overweight patients with type 2 diabetes reduced macrovascular complications and increased survival compared with equivalent glycemic control by other agents (sulfonylureas or insulin) during a mean follow-up of 10 years.

Despite occasional claims to the contrary, most studies and clinical experience have found no significant effect of metformin on blood pressure. However, there have been preliminary reports that metformin can reduce hepatic steatosis and reduce some pro-inflammatory markers associated with type 2 diabetes. Initial evidence suggests that metformin is helpful in the treatment of PCOS and can reinstate menstruation and fertility.

Thus, the rationale for use of metformin to treat patients with type 2 diabetes is its antihyperglycemic efficacy and its activity against insulin resistance, with reductions in several cardiovascular risk factors. Metformin may be preferred for obese patients because it does not cause weight gain, although it shows similar antihyperglycemic efficacy in nonobese patients.

TREATMENT

Metformin (proprietary name Glucophage) is available in two formulations: the standard (now called immediate-release [IR]) formulation and the extended-release (XR) formulation. The therapeutic effects of the two formulations are essentially the same, but the XR formulation is absorbed more slowly and can be given as once-daily dosing. Pharmacokinetic aspects of metformin are summarized in Table 21.3.

Indications

Metformin is indicated as monotherapy for the treatment of hyperglycemia in patients with type 2 diabetes who do not achieve appropriate target levels of glycemic control with nonpharmacological therapy such as diet, exercise, and health education (Table 21.4). It can also be used in combination with an insulin-releasing agent (sulfonylurea or meglitinide), α-glucosidase inhibitor (acarbose or miglitol), thiazolidinedione (rosiglitazone or pioglitazone), or insulin. Metformin is helpful in patients who require weight stabilization or weight loss or who are

Table 21.3 Pharmacokinetic Aspects of Metformin

Variable	Comment
Bioavailability	50–60%; absorbed mainly from the small intestine; estimated time to maximal plasma concentration 0.9–2.6 h for standard (IR) formulation, 4–8 h for XR formulation
Plasma concentration	Maximal 1–2 µg/ml (approximately 10^{-5} mol/l) 1–2 h after an oral dose of 500–1,000 mg for standard (IR) formulation; maximal concentration is ~20% lower (but area under the curve is similar) at same dose of XR formulation; negligible binding to plasma proteins
Plasma elimination half-life	~6 h
Metabolism	Not measurably metabolized
Elimination	About 90% of absorbed drug is eliminated in urine in 24 h; multiexponential pattern involving glomerular filtration and tubular secretion
Tissue distribution	Distributed in most tissues at concentrations similar to those in peripheral plasma; higher concentrations in liver and kidney; highest concentration in salivary glands and intestinal wall

vulnerable to hypoglycemia. Potential benefits against various atherogenic risk factors associated with insulin resistance (Table 21.2) are not specific indications but are usefully taken into account in the selection of metformin.

Elderly patients can be given metformin with appropriate adherence to the contraindications, especially renal function. Children can also receive metformin up to a maximum dose of 2,000 mg daily, although studies have not been conducted in subjects <10 years of age. Use in the elderly and in children warrants frequent monitoring.

Starting Metformin

Starting metformin therapy assumes attention to contraindications (detailed below) and appropriate monitoring of glycemic control, initially using fasting plasma glucose (FPG) and subsequently glycated hemoglobin A1C (A1C).

Standard (IR) metformin should be taken with meals, starting with one 500- or 850-mg tablet at breakfast or other main meal. The dose can then be increased one tablet at a time at 4- to 14-day intervals, leading to two or three divided doses with the main meals, until the desired level of blood glucose control is achieved or the maximum tolerated dose is reached. A total dose of three or four 500-mg tablets or two to three 850-mg tablets is often required, with the maximum dose being 2,550 mg daily.

Gastrointestinal side effects are not uncommon during initiation of therapy. These include abdominal discomfort, diarrhea, nausea, anorexia, and a metallic

Table 21.4 Clinical Use of Metformin

Indications	As monotherapy or in combination with other oral antidiabetic agents or insulin in type 2 diabetes patients inadequately controlled by diet, exercise, and health education
Usage	500-, 850-, and 1,000-mg standard (IR) tablets: take with meals; increase dose slowly; monitor glycemic control; maximal dose 2,550 mg/day (2,000 mg/day in children)
	500- and 700-mg XR tablet: take with evening meal; increase dose slowly; monitor glycemic control; maximal dose 2,000 mg/day
Contraindications and warnings	Renal and hepatic disease; cardiac or respiratory insufficiency; any hypoxic condition; severe infection; alcohol abuse; history of lactic acidosis; temporarily discontinue during use of intravenous radiographic contrast agents; pregnancy
Side effects	Gastrointestinal symptoms and metallic taste, which improve with dose reduction; may impair absorption of vitamin B12 and folic acid
Adverse reactions	Risk of lactic acidosis in patients with a contraindication; hypoglycemia can occur when taken in combination with another antidiabetic drug or during alcohol abuse
Precautions	Check for contraindications; check hemoglobin and plasma creatinine periodically; possible interaction with cimetidine therapy

taste. These symptoms are usually transient, remit with dose reduction, and are minimized by gradual dose escalation and administration with meals.

XR metformin is usually given once daily with the evening meal or occasionally twice daily with the breakfast and evening meals. The XR tablets (500 mg and 750 mg) should always be taken whole so that the inner and outer polymer compartments are undisturbed and continued slow release of metformin is provided for up to 24 h. Patients may experience lesser initial gastrointestinal side effects with the XR formulation.

Contraindications and Warnings

Metformin is contraindicated in patients with impaired renal function (e.g., a serum creatinine ≥ 1.5 mg/dl in men or ≥ 1.4 mg/dl in women). In older individuals, where serum creatinine is not a reliable measure of renal function, metformin is contraindicated if creatinine clearance is substantially impaired (e.g., <60 ml/min/1.73 m^2). Renal function should be checked at least yearly during metformin therapy. It is suggested that metformin be temporarily discontinued for about 48 h during/after use of an intravascular contrast medium until normal renal function is evidently reestablished.

Any hypoxic state should be regarded as a contraindication for metformin—notably chronic congestive heart failure, acute heart failure, severe respiratory insufficiency, septicemia, and other conditions with hypoperfusion or hypoxemia. Significant liver disease, history of lactic acidosis, alcohol abuse, or other disturbances of liver function likely to prevent normal hepatic lactate metabolism should be considered as contraindications for metformin.

Administration of metformin is not recommended during pregnancy or lactation because of insufficient clinical data. However, metformin is not teratogenic in animals, and no adverse effects on the fetus or nursing infant are apparent.

Metformin should be temporarily discontinued in favor of insulin administration during severe acute illnesses and major surgical procedures. Metformin is not effective as a primary treatment for type 1 diabetes.

Side Effects of Treatment

Lactic acidosis is a rare but serious adverse event associated with metformin therapy. Extensive worldwide experience indicates that the incidence is ~0.03 cases/1,000 patient-years of treatment, with a mortality of ~50%. Many of these cases have occurred when the drug was inappropriately prescribed, hence the importance of adequate renal function for the drug to be eliminated and the avoidance of hypoxemia and conditions that compromise lactate metabolism. Lactic acidosis can occur in diabetic patients unrelated to metformin therapy.

The most common side effects of metformin are the gastrointestinal disturbances described above. Although these often resolve with time, dose reduction, gradual titration, and administration with meals, ~5–10% of patients do not tolerate a full therapeutic dose of metformin (e.g., 2,000 mg/day).

Long-term therapy with metformin is associated with a small decrease in the absorption of vitamin B12 and occasionally folate; however, development of anemia from this cause is rare, can be associated with poor diet, and is usually reversed by vitamin B12 supplementation.

Severe hypoglycemia is unlikely with metformin unless administered with another antidiabetic agent. In general, the blood glucose–lowering effect of metformin is additive to that of other oral antidiabetic agents, while adequate β-cell function remains. Metformin usually increases the hypoglycemic effect of insulin. Use of metformin in combination with other antidiabetic agents requires appropriate adjustments of dosage based on glucose monitoring. Introduction of drugs that tend to increase blood glucose concentrations, such as corticosteroids, may also necessitate dosage adjustments.

Other clinically important drug interactions have not been identified with metformin. Metformin shows little binding to plasma proteins; it is not metabolized and is eliminated unchanged in the urine by glomerular filtration and tubular secretion. Increased metformin levels can occur with cimetidine, which shares the same transporter in the renal tubules, and other cationic drugs could theoretically compete with metformin elimination. Minor pharmacokinetic interactions occur with furosemide and nifedipine.

EXPECTED RESULTS

The reduction of hyperglycemia and improvement in glycemic control achieved with oral antihyperglycemic drugs is influenced by many factors, including the level of initial hyperglycemia, the pathophysiological status of β-cell function and insulin resistance, and the mechanism of drug action. The therapeutic action of metformin improves sensitivity to low or moderate concentrations of insulin and therefore requires adequate remaining β-cell function.

Typically, the antihyperglycemic effect of metformin is evident throughout the range of mild to moderately severe fasting hyperglycemia (110–275 mg/dl [6.1–15.5 mmol/l] or A1C 7–12%). In clinical trials involving a broad spectrum of patients with type 2 diabetes, metformin treatment produced an average lowering of FPG by 55 mg/dl (3.1 mmol/l) and A1C by 1.5%. The absolute drop in plasma glucose and A1C will be greater at higher starting levels of hyperglycemia (e.g., FPG of 275 mg/dl [15.5 mmol/l] and A1C of 12%) than at lower levels (e.g., FPG of 150 mg/dl [8.3 mmol/l] and A1C of 8%). However, it is likely that a smaller proportion of patients will achieve target levels of glycemic control (e.g., A1C of 6.5–7.5%) when the starting level of hyperglycemia is high.

The effect of metformin appears to be predominantly on fasting hyperglycemia, with a small effect on the meal-stimulated incremental rise in plasma glucose. A meta-analysis comparing metformin monotherapy with sulfonylurea monotherapy revealed that the two classes of drugs have comparable potency in reducing hyperglycemia and A1C.

Additional benefits ascribed to metformin therapy during trials with type 2 diabetes include a lack of weight gain or a small weight loss (mean reduction of 1–2 kg). Depending on the extent of initial dyslipidemia, there is often a small decrease in plasma LDL cholesterol and triglycerides (of ~5% in several trials) and a decrease in PAI-1. Severe episodes of hypoglycemia do not occur during metformin monotherapy, and fasting insulin concentrations are slightly reduced.

Because the cellular mechanism of action of metformin is different from that of other oral antidiabetic agents, its blood glucose–lowering efficacy is generally additive when combined with these agents, provided that adequate β-cell function remains. Single-tablet combinations of metformin with glyburide (Glucovance), metformin with glipizide (Metaglip), and metformin with rosiglitazone (Avandamet) are now available.

GLUCOVANCE

Glucovance is a single-tablet combination of metformin with the sulfonylurea glyburide. It was introduced in the U.S. in 2000. Glucovance can be used as initial antidiabetic drug therapy when substantial hyperglycemia persists after non-pharmacological interventions. Glucovance is convenient for patients transferring to a combination of metformin and glyburide because of inadequate glycemic control after monotherapy with one of these agents. Also, patients already receiving metformin and glyburide as separate tablets can be conveniently switched to Glucovance. Additionally, so-called "triple therapy" can be given using Glucovance plus a thiazolidinedione (rosiglitazone or pioglitazone).

Mode of Action and Rationale for Use

The two antidiabetic components of Glucovance, namely metformin and glyburide, act simultaneously to exert their individual blood glucose–lowering effects as described above and in Chapter 20. Provided there is adequate β-cell function, the blood glucose–lowering efficacy of the two components is approximately additive. This applies similarly whether metformin and glyburide are given as separate tablets or as Glucovance. However, there is preliminary evidence that the formulation of Glucovance may enhance the cumulative efficacy of metformin and glyburide, mainly to improve postprandial glycemic control.

Most patients with type 2 diabetes exhibit some degree of both insulin resistance and defective β-cell function. These two pathogenic facets of type 2 diabetes are addressed concurrently by Glucovance: metformin counters the insulin resistance and glyburide stimulates insulin secretion. While the single-tablet combination of Glucovance offers the additional therapeutic benefits attributed individually to metformin and glyburide, it also carries all of the contraindications of the two compounds. When used in combination, the effects of the two compounds are not mutually exclusive (e.g., the presence of metformin will reduce the extent of weight gain associated with glyburide, but the occurrence of hypoglycemia is likely to increase).

Thus, the rationale for use of Glucovance in the treatment of type 2 diabetes is the additive blood glucose–lowering efficacy of metformin and glyburide, which act by complementary mechanisms to address insulin resistance and defective function. Glucovance enables these agents to be given simultaneously in a convenient single-tablet formulation.

Treatment

Glucovance is available at three strengths of glyburide/metformin: 1.25 mg/ 250 mg, 2.5 mg/500 mg, and 5 mg/500 mg. Tablets should be swallowed whole. Pharmacokinetic features are generally the same as for the two agents given in separate tablets, except that the peak circulating concentration of the glyburide component is achieved earlier (~1–3 h compared with 4–8 h) depending on food consumption (for glyburide, see Chapter 20). This result reflects the distribution of glyburide particle size in the Glucovance formulation, which includes a high proportion of small particles.

As initial antidiabetic drug therapy, Glucovance can be started if glycemic control is inadequate with nonpharmacological measures. Contraindications for both metformin *and* glyburide must be respected, and monitoring of FPG is required for gradual dose escalation until the desired glycemic control is achieved. It is recommended that patients begin with the lowest-strength tablet (1.25 mg glyburide/250 mg metformin). If the starting A1C level is >9%, it is usually appropriate to begin with this strength tablet twice daily with the breakfast and evening meals. If the starting A1C level is between 8 and 9%, begin with this strength tablet once daily with breakfast. Titrate up to twice daily, then increase one tablet at a time to the next strength level, changing the morning tablet first. The suggested maximal daily dose is 10 mg glyburide/2,000 mg metformin in divided doses. Do *not* begin with the high-strength tablet (5 mg/500 mg) to reduce risk of hypoglycemia. Patients with a starting A1C level <8% may be more appropriately treated with a single oral antidiabetic agent.

As second-line therapy in patients inadequately controlled on a maximally effective amount of either glyburide or metformin, it is recommended to select a starting dose of Glucovance that contains a lower amount of glyburide or metformin than is already being taken. For example, a patient inadequately controlled on 2,000 mg metformin might start Glucovance at 2.5 mg/500 mg twice daily and then increase one tablet at a time. Although a maximal suggested daily dose is 10 mg/2,000 mg, a dose of 20 mg/2,000 mg is permitted when used as second-line therapy.

In patients already taking a combination of glyburide (or another sulfonylurea) and metformin as separate tablets, it is convenient to switch to a similar dosage regimen of Glucovance, but do not exceed the daily amounts of glyburide (or equivalent of another sulfonylurea) and metformin already being taken.

For patients inadequately controlled on Glucovance, a thiazolidinedione can be added (so-called triple therapy). This addition may assist patients to achieve the desired glycemic target while there is remaining β-cell function. Patients with severe and rapidly escalating hyperglycemia, often with unintentional weight loss, should be considered for insulin therapy.

Glucovance can be used in the elderly provided there is careful and frequent monitoring, avoiding the highest doses. Glucovance has not been studied in children and is not recommended during pregnancy and lactation. It is reemphasized that the contraindications and precautions associated with the use of metformin and glyburide separately must be observed with Glucovance. Likewise, the side effects of each drug should be borne in mind when using Glucovance, and gradual dose titration with monitoring is especially important to reduce the risk of hypoglycemia.

Expected Results

In type 2 diabetes, the blood glucose–lowering effect of oral antidiabetic agents is influenced by many features of the disease process (as noted above in the metformin section of this chapter), particularly the extent of starting hyperglycemia. Previous experience with the use of metformin and glyburide in combination as separate tablets has shown that the blood glucose–lowering effect of the two agents is approximately additive.

A 26-week trial conducted for registration purposes found that initial drug therapy with Glucovance in patients with type 2 diabetes who had a starting A1C of 7–11% and FPG up to 240 mg/dl reduced A1C by ~1.5% and FPG by ~40 mg/dl. The effect was generally greater among individuals with a starting hyperglycemia in the upper part of the range, and two-thirds of patients achieved a target A1C of <7%. A greater reduction in blood glucose was achieved in groups treated with Glucovance at a lower mean dose of each of the two active agents than in parallel groups treated with glyburide or metformin alone. Indeed, the Glucovance group treated with the 1.25 g/250 g strength tablets had a greater mean improvement in glycemic control than groups treated with glyburide or metformin as single therapies, and the average dosage of Glucovance contained about half of the dosage of glyburide or metformin as the single therapies. In particular, there was a greater improvement in the postprandial glucose excursion with Glucovance. This improvement may reflect the pharmacokinetic attribute of an initially rapid release of glyburide from the Glucovance tablet. The postprandial insulin response was greater than that with metformin alone but similar to that with glyburide alone: weight gain was greater compared with metformin alone, and there was little effect on the lipid profile. Fewer hypoglycemic symptoms were reported with the lowest strength of Glucovance than glyburide alone, but the higher strength of Glucovance was prone to more hypoglycemic symptoms, especially in patients with lower A1C levels (hence, the recommendation to initiate drug therapy with the 1.25 mg/250 mg strength of Glucovance).

An open-label study of patients with either a starting A1C >11% or FPG >240 mg/dl (>13.3 mmol/l) began with the 2.5 mg/500 mg strength Glucovance. After 26 weeks, there was a mean reduction of FPG from 283 to 161 mg/dl (15.7–8.9 mmol/l), with an average A1C of 7.1%, and this response was sustained to 52 weeks.

As second-line therapy, a 16-week study found that in patients inadequately controlled on a sulfonylurea, transfer to Glucovance and titration of the dosage enabled improvements in FPG, postprandial glucose, and A1C. For example, in patients with an A1C of ~9.5% on a maximal or near-maximal dose of glyburide, transfer to Glucovance reduced mean A1C by 1.7–1.9%, whereas continuation therapy with a sulfonylurea alone or switching to metformin alone was not effective.

Addition of the thiazolidinedione rosiglitazone to patients inadequately controlled with Glucovance (A1C ~8%) has been shown to produce an average decrease of A1C by 1% and FPG by 48 mg/dl after 24 weeks. Rosiglitazone was added at 4 mg/day and increased to 8 mg/day if target glycemic control was not achieved after 8 weeks.

METAGLIP

Metaglip is a single-tablet combination of metformin with the sulfonylurea glipizide. It was introduced in the U.S. in 2002 for use in the treatment of type 2 diabetes as initial antidiabetic drug therapy or for progression to a combination of metformin and glipizide if glycemic control is inadequate after monotherapy with metformin or glipizide (or another sulfonylurea) alone. Also, patients already taking a combination of metformin and glipizide as separate tablets can be switched to Metaglip for convenience.

Metaglip can be used in a similar manner to Glucovance (except the triple therapy indication) and provides an appropriate combination where glipizide is already used or is preferred as the sulfonylurea to give in combination with metformin.

Mode of Action and Rationale for Use

The mode of action and rationale for use of Metaglip follow the same principles as Glucovance. Thus, the single-tablet combination of metformin and glipizide (Metaglip) conveniently takes advantage of the additive blood glucose–lowering efficacy of metformin and a sulfonylurea, which act by complementary mechanisms to address insulin resistance and defective β-cell function. The shorter duration of action of glipizide may be preferred in older patients or individuals more prone to hypoglycemia, although there is no specific indication for these groups, and contraindications (especially declining renal function in the elderly) must be taken into account.

Treatment

Metaglip is available at three strengths of glipizide/metformin: 2.5 mg/250 mg, 2.5 mg/500 mg, and 5 mg/500 mg. Pharmacokinetic features are generally the same as the two agents given together in separate tablets, which are also almost identical to the agents given alone (for metformin, see above, and for glipizide, see Chapter 20).

The procedures for use of Metaglip (metformin/glipizide) are essentially the same as those of Glucovance (metformin/glyburide). Starting any oral antidiabetic drug treatment assumes that appropriate targets for glycemic control are not achieved with nonpharmacological therapy, and the nonpharmacological measures should continue to be reinforced throughout drug treatment. With Metaglip, the contraindications of both metformin *and* glipizide must be respected, and FPG monitoring is required for gradual dose escalation until the desired glycemic control is achieved. Gradual titration and taking the drug with meals should minimize the occurrence of gastrointestinal side effects and hypoglycemia.

As initial antidiabetic drug therapy, it is recommended to begin Metaglip with the lowest-strength tablet (2.5 mg glipizide/250 mg metformin) once daily with breakfast if the A1C level is <9% and twice daily with the breakfast and evening meals if the A1C level is >9%. Titrate up once daily to twice daily, then increase one tablet at a time to the next strength level, changing the morning tablet first. In patients with type 2 diabetes who present with severe hyperglycemia, consider starting with a higher-strength tablet (2.5 mg glipizide/500 mg metformin) twice daily. The suggested maximum daily dose is 10 mg glipizide/2,000 mg metformin in divided doses (maximum permitted daily dose is 20 mg glipizide/2,000 mg metformin). As with all oral antidiabetic drug therapies, provided there are no limiting adverse events or contraindications, continue dose titration until the desired glycemic control is achieved. If a titration step produces no further improvement in glycemic control, return to the previous dosage, which can be deemed the minimum dose with the maximum effect for that patient, and if the level of glycemic control is not acceptable, consider moving to the next stage of the treatment algorithm. Patients with a starting A1C <8% may be more appropriately treated with a single oral antidiabetic agent.

As second-line therapy in patients inadequately controlled on a maximally effective amount of either glipizide (or another sulfonylurea) or metformin alone, the starting dose of Metaglip should not exceed the daily dose of glipizide or metformin already being taken. This is likely to equate to Metaglip tablets of 2.5 mg/500 mg or 5 mg/500 mg strength. If glycemic control is close to target with monotherapy, it may be preferable to decrease a dosage level for the first dose of Metaglip.

In patients already taking a combination of glipizide (or another sulfonylurea) and metformin as separate tablets, a switch to Metaglip should use the nearest equivalent dosage regimen of Metaglip. Patients on a high dosage of Metaglip who are not adequately controlled and exhibit persistently severe and escalating hyperglycemia, often with unintentional weight loss, should be considered for insulin therapy.

Expected Results

Several studies in type 2 diabetes have confirmed that the blood glucose–lowering effects of metformin and a sulfonylurea are approximately additive, provided there is adequate β-cell function remaining.

Initial drug therapy with Metaglip (2.5 mg/250 mg and 2.5 mg/500 mg) has been studied in patients with type 2 diabetes during a 24-week trial for registration purposes. Patients had an average starting FPG of 203–210 mg/dl and A1C of ~9.1%, and Metaglip therapy produced mean decreases in FPG by 54–56 mg/dl and A1C by 2.1%. Thus, appropriate titration of the lower-strength tablets (2.5 mg/250 mg) gave similar results to the higher-strength tablets (2.5 mg/500 mg) in this study. These improvements in glycemic control were greater than those achieved with either glipizide alone (decreased A1C by 1.7%) or metformin alone (decreased A1C by 1.4%). Moreover, the amounts of glipizide and metformin given with the lower-strength Metaglip tablets were less than half of the amounts of these agents taken by the groups receiving each agent alone. The Metaglip groups also showed greater improvements in the postprandial glucose excursion than groups treated with either glipizide or metformin alone. Metaglip was associated with a small decrease in body weight (by 0.4–0.5 kg), which was less than the decrease in body weight with metformin alone (by 1.9 kg). No clinically significant effects of Metaglip or its separate component drugs were observed on lipid parameters in this study. More reports of hypoglycemic symptoms and fingerstick blood glucose values ≤50 mg/dl were made by patients taking Metaglip (7.6 and 9.3% of patients taking the lower- and higher-strength tablets, respectively) compared with metformin alone (0% of patients) and glipizide alone (2.9% of patients). Metaglip was discontinued by 2.6% of patients because of hypoglycemic symptoms. Gastrointestinal symptoms including diarrhea occurred more often in the group taking metformin alone, and 1.2% of patients on Metaglip discontinued because of gastrointestinal symptoms.

As second-line therapy, an 18-week study noted that patients inadequately controlled on either a sulfonylurea or metformin alone achieved an additional decrease in mean A1C by ~1% when taking Metaglip. Improvements in FPG and postprandial glucose were also noted with Metaglip, but body weight loss was trivial (–0.3 kg) compared with metformin alone (–2.7 kg), and there were no significant changes in lipids.

AVANDAMET

Avandamet is a single-tablet combination of metformin with the thiazolidinedione rosiglitazone. It was introduced in the U.S. in 2002 as a second-line oral antidiabetic drug therapy for patients with type 2 diabetes. Avandamet can be used in patients who are inadequately controlled by monotherapy with metformin or rosiglitazone; patients already receiving metformin and rosiglitazone as separate tablets can switch to the single-tablet formulation if more convenient.

Mode of Action and Rationale for Use

Metformin and rosiglitazone are used routinely in combination therapy as separate tablets, and their blood glucose–lowering effects are approximately additive, provided there is adequate β-cell function. They each improve insulin sensitivity, but they do so by different and complementary mechanisms that enable their effective use in combination. Rosiglitazone stimulates the nuclear receptor peroxisome proliferator-activated receptor-γ, and its mode of action is described in Chapter 23. The mode of action of metformin is described earlier in this chapter. The blood glucose–lowering effect of metformin predominantly involves a reduction in hepatic glucose production, whereas rosiglitazone mainly causes an increase in peripheral glucose uptake. Both agents act without stimulating insulin secretion: they are antihyperglycemic and rarely cause frank hypoglycemia when used alone. Hypoglycemia can occur when these agents are used in combination, but it is usually mild. Each agent has been reported to influence certain cardiovascular risk factors associated with the metabolic syndrome, at least in part by reducing insulin resistance. Introduction of antidiabetic therapy with metformin in the UKPDS has already been shown to improve long-term macrovascular outcomes. Long-term outcome trials with rosiglitazone are in progress.

The main rationale for use of Avandamet to treat type 2 diabetes is the convenience of single-tablet combination therapy with metformin and rosiglitazone to address insulin resistance by complementary actions with minimal risk of hypoglycemia.

Treatment

Avandamet is available at three strengths of rosiglitazone/metformin: 1 mg/500 mg, 2 mg/500 mg, and 4 mg/500 mg. Pharmacokinetic characteristics of each agent are unaltered by each other, and the single-tablet combination shows the same characteristics as the two components co-administered as separate tablets.

Use of Avandamet in type 2 diabetes assumes that monotherapy with metformin or rosiglitazone alone does not achieve adequate glycemic control. When starting Avandamet, it is important that the contraindications and cautions are respected for both metformin (described above) *and* rosiglitazone (see Chapter 23). In patients inadequately controlled on metformin monotherapy, start Avandamet at the same daily dose of metformin (up to 2,000 mg) plus 4 mg rosiglitazone daily, given in divided doses that correspond with the previous metformin regimen. For patients inadequately controlled on rosiglitazone monotherapy, start Avandamet with the same daily dose of rosiglitazone plus 1,000 mg metformin daily in divided doses, although it may be prudent to introduce metformin at 500 mg daily (with breakfast) for the first few days. Titrate the dosage gradually, bearing in mind that when initiating rosiglitazone there is a slow onset of the rosiglitazone component effect: monitor FPG and other parameters as required for each component drug.

To switch a patient from a combination of rosiglitazone and metformin as separate tablets, use the nearest equivalent daily dose of Avandamet. The maximum recommended daily dose of Avandamet is 8 mg rosiglitazone/2,000 mg metformin in divided doses.

Expected Results

Although there are no reported clinical trials with the single-tablet formulation of Avandamet, use of the two agents together as separate tablets has demonstrated the additive blood glucose–lowering effect of adding rosiglitazone to metformin. A 26-week trial in patients with type 2 diabetes inadequately controlled on metformin found that addition of rosiglitazone (8 mg daily) reduced A1C by 0.8% from baseline and by 1.2% compared with individuals continuing on metformin alone.

Introduction of Avandamet in patients who have not previously received rosiglitazone may cause a small increase in LDL and HDL cholesterol fractions, but the ratio of the two fractions is affected little. Circulating concentrations of free fatty acids are likely to fall by ~20% with Avandamet.

A small increase in body weight (e.g., 1–2 kg) can be expected in patients not previously receiving rosiglitazone. Prescribers are reminded that use of Avandamet carries the adverse events risks of both rosiglitazone (see Chapter 23) and metformin (described above).

BIBLIOGRAPHY

Bailey CJ, Campbell IW: United Kingdom Prospective Diabetes Study: implications for metformin. *Brit J Cardiol* 9:115–119, 2002

Bailey CJ, Turner RC: Drug therapy: metformin. *N Engl J Med* 334:574–579, 1996

Cusi K, DeFronzo RA: Metformin: a review of its metabolic effects. *Diabetes Rev* 6:89–130, 1998

DeFronzo RA, Goodman AM, Multicenter Metformin Study Group: Efficacy of metformin in patients with non-insulin-dependent diabetes mellitus. *N Engl J Med* 333:541–549, 1995

Fonseca V, Rosenstock J, Patwardhan R, Salzman A: Effect of metformin and rosiglitazone combination therapy in patients with type 2 diabetes mellitus. *JAMA* 283:1695–1702, 2000

Garber AJ, Larsen J, Schneider SH, Piper BA, Henry D: Simultaneous glyburide/metformin therapy is superior to component monotherapy as an initial pharmacological treatment for type 2 diabetes. *Diabetes Obes Metab* 4:201–208, 2002

Howlett HCS, Bailey CJ: A risk-benefit assessment of metformin in type 2 diabetes mellitus. *Drug Safety* 20:489–503, 1999

Misbin RI, Green L, Stadel BV, Gueriguian JL, Gubbi A, Fleming GA: Lactic acidosis in patients with diabetes treated with metformin. *N Engl J Med* 338:285–286, 1997

UK Prospective Study (UKPDS) Group: Effect of intensive blood-glucose control with metformin on complications in overweight patients with type 2 diabetes (UKPDS 34). *Lancet* 352:854–865, 1998

Wiernsperger NF, Bailey CJ: The antihyperglycaemic effect of metformin: therapeutic and cellular mechanisms. *Drugs* 58 (Suppl. 1):31–39, 1999

Dr. Bailey is Head of Diabetes Research at Aston University, Birmingham, U.K.

22. α-Glucosidase Inhibitors in the Treatment of Hyperglycemia

RÉMI RABASA-LHORET, MD, PhD, AND JEAN-LOUIS CHIASSON, MD

D ietary intervention remains the cornerstone of treatment strategies for patients with type 2 diabetes mellitus. Although the focus of dietary intervention is frequently on weight reduction, dietary intervention also has a direct effect on hyperglycemia. When diet and exercise fail, oral antidiabetic medications such as sulfonylureas, biguanides, or thiazolidinediones are added. These agents have been shown to decrease fasting plasma blood glucose, but in over 60% of patients, postprandial hyperglycemia persists and probably accounts for the sustained increase in glycated hemoglobin A1C (A1C). Such postprandial glycemic excursion contributes to the development of diabetes-specific complications (e.g., retinopathy and nephropathy) and could be involved in the development of macrovascular complications. Slowly absorbed carbohydrates and a high-fiber diet blunt the postprandial elevation of plasma glucose and insulin levels, but most patients find these regimens difficult to follow long term. Pharmacological agents (α-glucosidase inhibitors) have been developed to delay the digestion of complex carbohydrate. By their original mechanism of action, they significantly reduce postprandial glycemic and insulinemic excursion regardless of the current therapy in place and the type of diabetes (type 1 or type 2).

MECHANISM OF ACTION

α-Glucosidase inhibitors are competitive suppressants of small intestine brush border enzymes, which are needed to hydrolyze oligosaccharides and polysaccharides to monosaccharides. Normally, carbohydrates are primarily and rapidly absorbed in the first part of the small intestine. With α-glucosidase inhibitors, carbohydrate absorption and digestion are delayed and prolonged throughout the small intestine, resulting in a reduction of the postprandial plasma glucose elevation in both type 1 and type 2 diabetes mellitus. Acarbose, the principal medication of this class, is a pseudotetrasaccharide of microbial origin, structurally analogous to an oligosaccharide derived from starch digestion. It has a high affinity for the carbohydrate-binding site of various α-glucosidase enzymes, exceeding the affinity (10- to 100,000-fold) of regular oligosaccharides from nutritional carbohydrates. Because of its structure, acarbose cannot be cleaved and, therefore, enzymatic hydrolysis is blocked. Despite its high affinity for these enzymes, acarbose binding is reversible after 4–6 h. Owing to its specificity for α-glucosidases, β-glucosidases (e.g., lactases) are not inhibited by acarbose; therefore, the digestion and absorption of lactose are not affected by acarbose treatment. Oral glucose administration is also not affected by the drug. Acarbose is poorly absorbed, and <1–2% of the active compound appears in the plasma.

The delay of carbohydrate digestion and absorption in the small bowel increases the amount of fermentable carbohydrates reaching the colon. This results in gastrointestinal (GI) symptoms (flatulence and diarrhea) but does not interfere with use of the energy content of carbohydrates, which are metabolized by colonic microflora to short-chain fatty acids and then absorbed.

α-Glucosidase inhibitors also modify the secretion of GI peptides: gastric inhibitory peptide and glucagon-like peptide 1. When an α-glucosidase inhibitor is taken with a meal rich in carbohydrates, gastric inhibitory peptide secretion is decreased while glucagon-like peptide 1 is markedly increased, particularly in the late postprandial period. It is unclear whether such modifications in the secretion of these important GI hormones involved in glucose homeostasis play a role in the overall beneficial effect of α-glucosidase inhibitors.

CLINICAL USE

Three α-glucosidase inhibitors have been developed: acarbose, miglitol, and voglibose. Their pharmacological profiles are very similar, and acarbose is the most widely available and used.

Because of their mechanism of action, α-glucosidase inhibitors should be taken within the first 15 min of each of the three major meals. The mechanism of action also explains the necessity of initiating treatment at a low dose and increasing it slowly to minimize GI side effects. α-Glucosidases content in the small intestine is high in the upper jejunum and low in the distal jejunum and ileum. When initiating treatment at a low dose, the small amount of carbohydrates reaching the distal part of the small intestine will induce α-glucosidase synthesis, thus minimizing the carbohydrate load from reaching the large intestine, which is responsible for the side effects. It is recommended to start at a low dose (i.e., 25 or 50 mg o.d. for 1 week) and then increase slowly by 25–50 mg in each subsequent week based on GI tolerance and clinical efficacy. Some, though not all, studies suggest that the maximal benefit/side effect ratio is obtained at 50 mg t.i.d.

Titration should be based on 1-h postprandial plasma glucose. If GI side effects become significant during titration, the dose should be reduced for some time because these side effects decrease with time. Treatment efficacy is seen from the first week and is maintained over the long term. Maximal efficacy is obtained between 50 and 100 mg t.i.d.

INDICATIONS FOR α-GLUCOSIDASE INHIBITOR THERAPY

Prescription of α-glucosidase inhibitors should be considered in patients with diabetes in the following situations:

- **As primary therapy for**
  - □ patients with normal fasting blood glucose and postprandial hyperglycemia
  - □ type 2 diabetes patients with mild to moderate hyperglycemia (<180 mg/dl [10 mmol/l]) not controlled by diet and exercise
  - □ type 2 diabetes patients as an alternative when other oral hypoglycemic agents are contraindicated (existing or significant risk of hypoglycemia with sulfonylurea, risk of lactic acidosis with biguanides). Elderly patients with mild diabetes represent an important population for this indication.
- **As an adjunct therapy for**
  - □ patients with inadequate glycemic control under other oral agents
  - □ patients using insulin. Can be used with insulin to reduce insulin requirement, decrease postprandial glycemic excursion, and lessen hypoglycemia.

EFFICACY

Most published studies have shown a moderate but constant decline of A1C. This decrease is maintained long term and is mostly related to postprandial glycemic reduction because the fasting plasma glucose fall is generally not significant.

In Combination with Diet Therapy

In controlled trials compared with placebo, acarbose elicited a significant reduction of postprandial hyperglycemia (approximately –54 mg/dl) along with a mean 0.9% (0.5–1.4%) decrease of A1C (Table 22.1). Studies with miglitol gave comparable results.

In Comparison with Other Oral Hypoglycemic Agents

When compared in the same study with sulfonylurea and biguanides, α-glucosidase inhibitors showed a comparable reduction of A1C (~1%) in four of five trials. In the remaining study, miglitol was less efficient than glibenclamide.

In Association with Other Oral Hypoglycemic Agents

Because the mechanism of action of acarbose is different from that of other oral hypoglycemic agents, an additive benefit can be expected with coadministration. This additive effect has been confirmed in seven different trials. When acarbose is added to ongoing suboptimal treatment with sulfonylureas or biguanides, a mean 0.75% decrease of A1C can be expected (Table 22.1). Several small studies comparing the effect of adding either acarbose or metformin to existing sulfonylurea therapy have found the two drugs to be equivalent as adjunctive treatment. There is only one published comparison of thiazolidinediones and

Table 22.1 Mean Reduction of A1C and Fasting and Postprandial Plasma Glucose When Acarbose Is Added to Previous Antidiabetic Therapeutics

Treatment already in place (numbers of studies/ numbers of subjects)	A1C (%)	Plasma glucose mg/dl (mmol/l)	
		Fasting*†	Postprandial
Diet (14/1,136)	−0.89	−23.4 (−1.3)	−53.9 (−2.99)
Diet + sulfonylurea (6/342)	0.78	−10.2 (−0.57)	−54.4 (−3.02)
Diet + biguanides (2/148)	−0.72	−10.2 (−0.57)	−63.1 (−3.5)
Diet + insulin (4/338)	−0.59	−11.0 (−0.61)	−48.0 (−2.66)

*Mean of studies from which this information was available.
†In most studies, this reduction is not significant.

acarbose. In that small study, the addition of troglitazone to patients previously treated with acarbose produced significant glycemic improvement.

In Association with Insulin

In patients with type 2 diabetes, adding acarbose to insulin treatment evoked a mean 0.6% reduction of A1C in three different studies (Table 22.1). In patients with type 1 diabetes, a similar decrease of A1C was reported with no increase of hypoglycemic risk. Small studies have also suggested that acarbose could reduce the risk of nocturnal or exercise-induced hypoglycemia.

Long-Term Effect

Only two studies lasted ≥1 year. The results from these works support the hypothesis that the glucose-lowering effect of acarbose is maintained long term. In the United Kingdom Prospective Diabetes Study, a 3-year trial tested the addition of acarbose to other forms of antidiabetic treatment. Patients remaining on acarbose at the end of the trial benefited by a 0.5% reduction of A1C, but the dropout rate was extremely high. In a study by Chiasson et al., published in 1994, significant benefit was proven after 1 year of treatment regardless of the previous therapy in place.

For Type 2 Diabetes Prevention

In obese subjects with impaired glucose tolerance, lifestyle modification is highly effective in preventing or delaying the development of type 2 diabetes. In two important intervention trials, a 5–7% weight reduction and physical activity exceeding 150 min per week produced a reduction of nearly 60% of new cases of diabetes over 3 years. Pharmacological interventions have also been shown to be effective. Compared with placebo, acarbose resulted in a 35.6% risk reduction of new cases of diabetes. Although these new data offer potential new applications for α-glucosidase inhibitors, there is no current recommendation for pharmacological interventions in patients with impaired glucose tolerance.

TOLERABILITY

As monotherapy, α-glucosidase inhibitors are safe agents that do not induce hypoglycemia and have a neutral effect on weight. However, they may potentiate the hypoglycemic action of sulfonylureas and insulin. A reduction in the dosage of concomitant hypoglycemic agents may be necessary when α-glucosidase inhibitor treatment is introduced. If a patient given acarbose experiences hypoglycemia, it should be treated with glucose because the absorption of sucrose and complex carbohydrates is delayed by the drug. Patients should be well educated on this potential occurrence.

The main side effects of α-glucosidase inhibitors are GI symptoms consisting of abdominal distention, flatulence, diarrhea, and borborygmus in ~50% of patients. Safety studies have shown no deleterious effects on digestive tract morphology. The side effects are related to intra-colonic fermentation and consequent gas production of carbohydrates not absorbed in the small bowel. The symptoms are dose dependent and tend to decrease with continued treatment. The best strategy to minimize the GI side effects is to "start low and go slow." It is estimated that ~5% of patients are unable to tolerate acarbose, a rate comparable to biguanides. Despite these frequent GI symptoms, the quality of life of patients on acarbose has been shown to be as good as with sulfonylurea or insulin therapy.

An elevation of liver enzymes has been reported on rare occasions in patients on high doses of acarbose (300 mg t.i.d.); it was moderate and always returned to normal after cessation of the drug. There are a few reports of ileus associated with acarbose treatment in Japanese patients.

Concurrent administration of antacids, bile acid resins, intestinal absorbents, or digestive enzyme preparations may reduce the effect of α-glucosidase inhibitors. Rare interaction with digoxin has also been reported, resulting in decreased drug absorption with acarbose.

Formal contraindications to α-glucosidase inhibitor therapy are intestinal malabsorption syndromes, inflammatory bowel disease, intestinal obstruction, and hepatic disease. However, small studies have suggested that acarbose is safe for patients with severe hepatic impairment. It is also contraindicated in cases of severe renal impairment (creatinine clearance <25 ml/min), in pregnant or lactating women, and in children <12 years of age because of a lack of data in these patient groups.

CONCLUSION

α-Glucosidase inhibitors significantly decrease postprandial plasma glucose and insulin, resulting in a reduction of A1C regardless of the therapeutic regimen already in place. This decline of A1C is sufficient to be associated with a long-term fall in microvascular complications. Recent data indicate that α-glucosidase inhibitors could be an option in the treatment of impaired glucose tolerance to prevent the development of diabetes. Although α-glucosidase inhibitors are safe agents, frequency of GI side effects may limit their use. It is thus recommended to initiate treatment with a low dose and to titrate upward slowly. These agents also have potential implications in the prevention of atherosclerosis.

BIBLIOGRAPHY

Chiasson J-L, Josse RG, Gomis R, Hanefeld M, Karasik A, Laakso M: Acarbose for prevention of type 2 diabetes mellitus: the STOP-NIDDM randomised trial. *Lancet* 359:2072–2077, 2002

Chiasson J-L, Josse RG, Hunt JA, Palmason C, Rodger NW, Ross SA, et al.: The efficacy of acarbose in the treatment of patients with non-insulin-dependent diabetes mellitus. *Ann Intern Med* 121:928–935, 1994

Holman RR, Cull C, Turner RC, UKPDS Study Group: A randomized double-blind trial of acarbose in type 2 diabetes shows improved glycemic control over 3 years (UKPDS 44). *Diabetes Care* 22:960–964, 1999

Lebovitz H: Alpha-glucosidase inhibitors as agents in the treatment of diabetes. *Diabetes Reviews* 6:132–145, 1998

Tattersall R: Alpha-glucosidase inhibition as an adjunct to the treatment of type 1 diabetes. *Diabet Med* 10:688–693, 1993

Dr. Rabasa-Lhoret is Assistant Professor of Medicine, Department of Medicine, Université de Montréal. Dr. Chiasson is Professor of Medicine, Department of Medicine, Université de Montréal. Both authors are from the Research Group on Diabetes and Metabolic Regulation, Université de Montréal, Montréal, Canada.

23. Thiazolidinediones

Harold E. Lebovitz, MD

The thiazolidinediones are a new class of antihyperglycemic agents whose primary action is to decrease peripheral insulin resistance. Clinical and laboratory studies have revealed that they also have dramatic actions in ameliorating many of the components of the metabolic (insulin resistance) syndrome. The first drug of this class, ciglitazone, was shown in 1982 to markedly improve hyperglycemia in rodent models of insulin-resistant diabetes. It was not developed as a treatment for human diabetes because of toxic side effects. Several analogs have been developed that are considerably more potent and have a better safety profile. Troglitazone was the first member of the thiazolidinedione family to be approved in 1997 for the treatment of type 2 diabetes. It was very effective in improving insulin resistance and glycemic control; however, a rare complication of hepatic toxicity leading to hepatic failure and death caused its removal from the market in March 2000. Several other thiazolidinediones (e.g., pioglitazone and rosiglitazone) have been approved for clinical use since 1999. Extensive clinical trials and clinical use in several millions of patients with type 2 diabetes have shown these drugs to be highly effective in the management of patients with type 2 diabetes and not to have significant hepatotoxicity.

MECHANISM OF ACTION

Thiazolidinediones exert their primary effects through activation of specific nuclear receptors named peroxisome proliferator-activated receptors (PPARs). There are three subtypes of these receptors: PPAR-α, PPAR-γ, and PPAR-δ. Most data suggest that the antidiabetic effects of thiazolidinediones are closely related to their ability to bind to and activate the PPAR-γ subtype. PPARs, when activated, increase transcription of genes that have recognition sites for the specific PPAR subtype that was activated. Some of the gene products that are activated by PPAR-γ are important regulators of adipocyte differentiation, lipid homeostasis, and insulin action. GLUT1 and GLUT4 glucose transporter gene expression is among the activities stimulated by thiazolidinediones.

The in vivo effects of thiazolidinediones in humans (Table 23.1) have been studied extensively and can be divided into effects that directly regulate insulin action on glucose metabolism and effects that affect the other nonglycemic components of the metabolic syndrome. In general, the reported effects of pioglita-

---

Table 23.1 Clinically Relevant Metabolic Effects of Thiazolidinediones

Glycemic effects

- Increase insulin-mediated glucose uptake and utilization
- Decrease hyperglycemia in insulin-resistant type 2 diabetes patients

Nonglycemic effects

- Lipids
  - Convert small, dense LDL particles to large, buoyant LDL particles
  - Increase plasma HDL cholesterol
  - Decrease plasma triglycerides if they are elevated (>200 mg/dl)
  - Increase adipogenesis
  - Decrease plasma free fatty acids
- Vascular
  - Improve endothelial dysfunction
  - Reduce vascular peripheral resistance with 4-mmHg decreases in 24-h mean systolic and diastolic blood pressure
  - Improve procoagulant state by decreasing plasma fibrinogen and PAI-1
  - Decrease non-infective inflammation as measured by decreases in markers such as CRP
  - Decrease carotid artery intimal and medial thickness
  - Decrease neo-intimal proliferation after coronary stent implantation
  - Reduce microalbuminuria
- Pancreatic β-cells
  - Slows the rate of loss of β-cell insulin secretory function

---

zone and rosiglitazone are very similar, and because there are no valid blinded, randomized studies comparing the two, the subsequent discussion about effects will apply equally to both unless otherwise stated.

Effects on Insulin Action and Glucose Metabolism

The effects of thiazolidinediones on glucose metabolism in type 2 diabetes patients have been discovered using isotopic techniques that measure hepatic glucose production, insulin-mediated peripheral glucose uptake, and lipid metabolism as well as the standard parameters of glycemic control and lipoprotein homeostasis. Because thiazolidinediones act largely through activating gene transcription, their metabolic effects are not maximal until 3–6 weeks after initiating treatment.

The effect of thiazolidinediones in decreasing hepatic glucose production in type 2 diabetes patients appears moderate, because they reduce fasting hyperglycemia by a mean of 50–70 mg/dl. As noted later, the mechanism by which thiazolidinediones improve fasting hyperglycemia differs from that of metformin, and their effects in suppressing hepatic glucose production and fasting hyperglycemia are additive to those of metformin.

Both pioglitazone and rosiglitazone dramatically improve insulin sensitivity in patients with type 2 diabetes and insulin resistance. The magnitude of improvement depends on the baseline state and can vary from 25% to 70%. The improvement in insulin sensitivity has been demonstrated using the euglycemic-hyperinsulinemic clamp, the frequently sampled intravenous glucose tolerance test (analyzed by Bergman's minimal model), and the homeostasis model assessment for insulin resistance (HOMA-IR) model of Matthews.

The improvement in postprandial hyperglycemia is in large part the consequence of an increase in muscle responsiveness to insulin. The thiazolidinedione improvement in insulin action is thought to be secondary to the effects on adipose tissue. Insulin resistance in the ordinary type 2 diabetes patient is thought to be the result of an excess release of plasma free fatty acids, certain cytokines such as tumor necrosis factor (TNF)-α, and deficient release of the adipocyte hormone adiponectin. These changes cause alterations in the intracellular insulin action cascade in muscle and diminish transmission of the insulin signal. The thiazolidinediones partially correct these adipose abnormalities, improving the intracellular transmission of the insulin signal.

Nonglycemic Actions of Thiazolidinediones

Thiazolidinediones are PPAR-γ agonists. PPAR-γ nuclear receptors are present in many tissues, including adipose tissue, endothelial cells, macrophages, vascular smooth muscle cells, and skeletal muscle. Treatment with thiazolidinediones improves many of the components of the metabolic syndrome.

- Insulin resistance dyslipidemia
  The dyslipidemia of insulin resistance is characterized by an increase in plasma free fatty acids and triglycerides, a decrease in plasma HDL cholesterol, and a shift in the LDL cholesterol particle pattern from predominately large, buoyant particles to predominately small, dense particles. Treatment with thiazolidinediones decreases plasma free fatty acids; increases plasma HDL cholesterol levels between 10% and 20%; converts LDL cholesterol particles from small, dense to large, buoyant particles; and modestly reduces plasma triglycerides if they are >200 mg/dl.
- Endothelial dysfunction
  Normal endothelium maintains the balance between vasoconstriction and vasodilation, prevents platelets and inflammatory cells from attaching, prevents vascular smooth muscle cell and fibroblast proliferation, and impedes lipid deposits. Insulin resistance shifts the pattern of endothelial function from the anti-atherosclerotic profile above to a pro-atherosclerotic one. Treatment with thiazolidinediones restores arterial vasodilation with mean decreases in 24-h ambulatory systolic and diastolic blood pressures of 4 mmHg. These PPAR-γ agonists decrease the production of adhesion molecules and growth factors and decrease vascular smooth muscle cell and fibroblast proliferation.
- Procoagulant state
  Insulin resistance leads to increases in serum fibrinogen and an increase in plasminogen activator inhibitor type 1 (PAI-1) production by adipose tissue and endothelial cells. PAI-1 is a known risk factor for clinical cardiovascular events. Treatment of insulin resistance with thiazolidinediones decreases the elevated levels of PAI-1.

- Inflammation
  Insulin resistance is associated with a non-infective inflammatory state. Various cytokines such as TNF-α, interleukin (IL)-1, and IL-6 and markers of inflammation such as C-reactive protein (CRP), serum amyloid A, and fibrinogen are increased in insulin resistance. Inflammatory markers have been shown to be risk factors for myocardial infarction. Thiazolidinedione treatment of insulin-resistant patients decreases these markers (TNF-α and CRP), suggesting that the inflammatory process is being reduced.

CLINICAL USE

The primary beneficial effect of thiazolidinedione treatment in type 2 diabetes patients is improving insulin-mediated effects on glucose metabolism in insulin-resistant individuals (Table 23.2). This result improves glycemic control and reduces insulin requirements. Secondary benefits are a reduction in plasma free fatty acids, an improvement in lipid profile, a return of endothelial function toward normal, a decrease in blood pressure, a lessening of the procoagulant state, and a reduction in the inflammatory response. These secondary benefits, which are reductions in cardiovascular risk factors, have been demonstrated with all thiazolidinediones and suggest that therapy with thiazolidinediones has the potential to decrease clinical cardiovascular events. Another likely secondary benefit that

Table 23.2 Reported Results of Rosiglitazone and Pioglitazone Treatment on Glycemic Control in Type 2 Diabetes Patients

	A1C (%)		Fasting Plasma Glucose (mg/dl)	
	Baseline	Decrease	Baseline	Decrease
Monotherapy				
Pioglitazone	10.3	1.6	276	65
Rosiglitazone	8.8	1.5	220	76
Combination with metformin				
Pioglitazone	9.9	0.8	252	38
Rosiglitazone	8.9	1.2	219	53
Combination with insulin secretogogues				
Pioglitazone	9.9	1.3	239	58
Rosiglitazone	9.2	1.0	205	44
Combination with insulin				
Pioglitazone	9.8	1.0	229	49
Rosiglitazone	9.0	1.3	209	47

Pioglitazone dose was 45 mg/day in monotherapy and 30 mg/day when added to metformin, sulfonylureas, and insulin. Rosiglitazone dose was 8 mg/day in monotherapy and when added to metformin and insulin and 4 mg/day when added to sulfonylureas.

has been shown for troglitazone, and is probably a class effect, is a preservation of pancreatic β-cell function, which leads to a decrease in the rate of progression of type 2 diabetes to more severe hyperglycemia. For thiazolidinediones to be effective in improving glycemia, insulin resistance must exist and adequate amounts of circulating endogenous or exogenous insulin must be present.

Pioglitazone should be taken once daily without regard to meals. The usual dose for monotherapy is 15–45 mg/day; however, in combination with metformin, sulfonylureas, or insulin, the maximum approved dose is 30 mg daily.

Rosiglitazone should be started at 4 mg once a day or 2 mg twice a day without regard to meals. In monotherapy or in combination with metformin, the dose can be increased to 8 mg daily as a single dose or divided in two daily doses. The maximum approved daily dose of rosiglitazone when combined with insulin is 4 mg. It is recommended that the maximal daily dose when combined with sulfonylureas also be limited to 4 mg daily.

Monotherapy with thiazolidinediones is indicated in type 2 diabetes patients who are not adequately controlled with diet and increased physical activity. The glycemic responses to pioglitazone and rosiglitazone are listed in Table 23.2. As monotherapy, thiazolidinediones should not replace sulfonylurea or metformin treatment, because they have not been shown to be more effective than the other agents. The glycemic response to thiazolidinediones as measured by blood glucose levels develops slowly over a period of 6–8 weeks. The maximal decrease in glycated hemoglobin A1C (A1C) occurs after 12–14 weeks.

A more effective glycemic response to thiazolidinediones is seen when they are combined with either insulin secretogogues or insulin treatment in patients with type 2 diabetes. These combinations make more insulin available to be sensitized by the thiazolidinediones. Combination therapy of thiazolidinediones with metformin also has increased effectiveness in improving glycemic control, since the two classes of sensitizers have different mechanisms of action and their insulin-sensitizing effects are additive.

Table 23.2 lists the effects of treatment of type 2 diabetes patients with thiazolidinediones on the parameters of glycemic control. Because it is known that the absolute magnitude of the glycemic response to oral antidiabetic agents is a function of the baseline level of glycemia, it is difficult to compare the therapy-mediated decrease in A1C in type 2 diabetes patients whose baseline A1C levels are different. In monotherapy, both pioglitazone and rosiglitazone decrease mean A1C 1.5% in type 2 diabetes patients whose mean baseline A1C is ~9.0%. With rosiglitazone, 30% of that cohort achieved an A1C ≤7.0%. The addition of thiazolidinediones to patients inadequately controlled with metformin, sulfonylureas, or insulin results in further decreases in A1C of 0.8–1.3% (Table 23.2). Combination therapy of thiazolidinediones with metformin generally carries very little risk of hypoglycemia. However, when thiazolidinediones are added to sulfonylurea or insulin therapy, blood glucose must be closely monitored because the dose of the insulin-providing drug frequently needs to be decreased to avoid significant hypoglycemia.

Rosiglitazone (Avandia) is available in 2-, 4-, and 8-mg tablets. The combination of rosiglitazone plus metformin is being widely prescribed, and a combination tablet (Avandamet) is available as 1 mg rosiglitazone/500 mg metformin, 2 mg/500 mg, 4 mg/500 mg, 2 mg/1,000 mg, and 4 mg/1,000 mg. Pioglitazone (Actos) is available in 15-, 30-, and 45-mg tablets.

Rosiglitazone has not been reported to have significant drug interactions. Pioglitazone may potentially interact with oral contraceptives through their common metabolism by cytochrome CYP 3A4. Ketoconazole may affect the metabolism of pioglitazone, and their combined use requires careful monitoring of pioglitazone's effects.

SIDE EFFECTS

Troglitazone, the first thiazolidinedione to be approved and marketed, was associated with a rare idiosyncratic hepatotoxicity that led to liver failure and death. This condition led to the removal of troglitazone from the market in March 2000. There was an initial concern that liver toxicity might be a class effect of all thiazolidinediones. During its clinical trials, troglitazone treatment caused a threefold increase in the number of patients developing significant elevations of alanine aminotransferase (ALT) levels compared with placebo treatment, and two patients developed jaundice. During the clinical trials with pioglitazone and rosiglitazone, there was no increase in the number of patients developing significantly elevated ALT levels compared with placebo treatment, and no cases of drug-related jaundice occurred. In the 3 years that pioglitazone and rosiglitazone have been on the market, there has been no indication of significant drug-related hepatotoxicity. Despite this, it is still recommended that pioglitazone and rosiglitazone not be given to individuals with baseline ALT levels >2.5 times the upper limit of the normal range. Patients on thiazolidinediones should have liver function tests at baseline, every 2 months for the first year, and periodically thereafter. In the event that liver enzymes rise to more than three times the upper limit of the normal range, the thiazolidinedione should be discontinued.

A recent study showed that 48 weeks of rosiglitazone therapy actually improves the clinical and pathological features of patients with nonalcoholic steatohepatitis.

Weight gain has been a constant feature of therapy with all of the thiazolidinediones. The weight gain is due to both an increase in body fat and fluid retention. PPAR-γ agonists play a key role in the differentiation of precursor cells into fat cells. During treatment of type 2 diabetes patients, thiazolidinediones increase subcutaneous adiposity but have no effect on visceral adiposity. The increase in total body fat averages ~1.5 kg at low doses and 3.5 kg at the maximal doses. The weight gain is somewhat greater when thiazolidinediones are combined with sulfonylureas and greatest with combination therapy with insulin (~4–5.4 kg). The increase occurs only in subcutaneous fat because visceral fat mass is generally unchanged or slightly reduced. A rare individual will gain 5–20 kg. It is unclear as to what is different about these rare individuals.

Fluid retention is also seen during treatment with all thiazolidinediones. Hemoglobin and hematocrit are decreased on average ≤1 g/dl and ≤3.3%, respectively. These changes occur during the first 12 weeks of therapy and reflect increases in plasma volume because red blood cell mass is unchanged. Mild to moderate peripheral edema is observed in 4–5% of patients on thiazolidinedione monotherapy. This increases to 6–8% on thiazolidinedione and sulfonylurea combination therapy and 15% on thiazolidinedione and insulin combination treatment. The mechanism of the fluid retention is poorly understood but appears to be kidney mediated and is unresponsive to loop diuretics and angiotensin-converting enzyme inhibitors. The magnitude of fluid retention is ordinarily modest, although a rare patient may experience >5 kg of fluid retention. Discontinuation of the thiazolidinedione in such patients results in excretion of the retained fluid.

There have been case reports of the development of heart failure in type 2 diabetes patients treated with thiazolidinediones. This is likely a manifestation of excess fluid retention in individuals who have an increased susceptibility to develop heart failure. Most reported cases were in individuals given the maximum dose of the thiazolidinedione. Risk factors included combination therapy with insulin, female sex, and predisposing conditions such as chronic renal failure or prior cardiovascular disease. The incidence of thiazolidinedione-precipitated heart failure is difficult to determine because heart failure in type 2 diabetes patients is relatively common. Heart failure that can be attributed to thiazolidinedione therapy occurs within the first several months of treatment. In patients at risk, therapy with thiazolidinediones should be initiated with the lowest dose (15 mg pioglitazone daily or 2 mg rosiglitazone daily) and gradually titrated up with careful observation of weight gain and evidence of fluid retention. The maximal dose of the thiazolidinedione is to be avoided if possible, particularly when combined with insulin.

CONTRAINDICATIONS

Thiazolidinediones are not effective in the treatment of patients with type 1 diabetes (Table 23.3). Its effects on fetal development are unknown, and it should not be used during pregnancy. As noted above, thiazolidinediones are not recommended for treatment of diabetes in individuals with active liver disease.

Table 23.3 Thiazolidinedione Therapy

Indications/FDA-approved

- Treatment of hyperglycemia in insulin-resistant type 2 diabetes patients
  - Monotherapy
  - Combination with sulfonylureas, metformin, or insulin

Pending further study and approval

- Treatment of androgen excess and anovulation in polycystic ovarian syndrome
- Prevention of progression of impaired glucose tolerance to type 2 diabetes

Contraindications

- Type 1 diabetes
- Patients with clinical liver abnormalities
- Pregnant patients

EXPECTED RESULTS

Thiazolidinedione treatment decreases insulin resistance and improves insulin sensitivity to physiological levels of insulin by 35–70%. These improvements can be measured by sophisticated techniques such as the euglycemic-hyperinsulinemic clamp or the frequently sampled intravenous glucose tolerance test or by simpler and more clinically available procedures such as the HOMA-IR.

In the average type 2 diabetes patient with a mean A1C of 8.5–9.0%, monotherapy with a thiazolidinedione will achieve a target A1C of ≤7.0% in ~30% of patients. Early use of combination rosiglitazone plus glipizide was able to achieve an A1C ≤7.0% in 56% of patients and an A1C ≤6.5% in 34% of patients in a recent study in which glipizide alone was able to achieve an A1C ≤7% in only 22% of the recently diagnosed type 2 diabetes patients. Early use of a combination of rosiglitazone and metformin achieved target goals of ≤7.0% and ≤6.5% in 55% and 35%, respectively, of recently diagnosed type 2 diabetes patients. The data indicate that early use of thiazolidinediones plus either metformin or an insulin secretogogue is highly effective in improving glycemic control. As noted in Table 23.2, addition of a thiazolidinedione to patients not achieving adequate glycemic control on metformin, insulin secretogogues, or insulin is highly effective in improving glycemic control at the appropriate stage of type 2 diabetes. Several nonglycemic effects of thiazolidinedione therapy are to be expected. These include improvement of the dyslipidemia of insulin resistance and other aspects of the metabolic syndrome, as described in Table 23.1. Although clinical outcome data are not yet available, there are circumstantial data to suggest that therapy with thiazolidinediones will have beneficial effects on cardiovascular events and in the progression from impaired glucose tolerance through the various stages of type 2 diabetes by virtue of their ability to stabilize and preserve pancreatic β-cell function. These aspects of thiazolidinedione actions are being assessed in ongoing long-term studies such as DREAM (Diabetes REduction Assessment with ramipril and rosiglitazone Medication), BARI-2 (Bypass Angioplasty Revascularization Investigation), and PRO-ACTIVE (Prospective Pioglitazone Clinical Trial in Macrovascular Events).

There are no studies directly comparing the effects of rosiglitazone and pioglitazone. The only area where questions have been raised of differences in their actions has been that of lipid metabolism. Several open-label clinical studies in which patients were switched from troglitazone to either rosiglitazone or pioglitazone have reported that pioglitazone significantly decreases plasma triglycerides while rosiglitazone does not. These data need to be substantiated by double-blind randomized controlled comparative studies for the conclusions to be validated. On the other hand, investigative studies show that both increase HDL cholesterol and increase LDL particle size.

Thiazolidinediones decrease hyperinsulinemia in women with polycystic ovarian disease. This results in reduction in androgen secretion and, in some anovulatory women, restoration of ovulation. Such diabetes patients may be at risk of becoming pregnant during thiazolidinedione treatment. Thiazolidinediones should not be administered during pregnancy because of the potential increase in fetal mortality and growth retardation that have been demonstrated during midgestation and late gestation in laboratory animals.

BIBLIOGRAPHY

Aronoff S, Rosenblatt S, Braithwaite S, Egan JW, Mathisen AL, Schneider RL: Pioglitazone hydrochloride monotherapy improves glycemic control in the treatment of patients with type 2 diabetes. *Diabetes Care* 23:1605–1611, 2000

Fonseca VA, Rosenstock J, Patwardhan R, Salzman A: Effect of metformin and rosiglitazone combination therapy in patients with type 2 diabetes mellitus. *JAMA* 283:1695–1702, 2000

Lebovitz HE: *Clinician's Manual on Insulin Resistance.* London, Science Press, 2002

Lebovitz HE, Banerji MA: Insulin resistance and its treatment by thiazolidine-diones. *Recent Prog Horm Res* 56:265–294, 2001

Lebovitz HE, Dole JF, Patwardhan R, Rappaport EB, Freed MI: Rosiglitazone monotherapy is effective in patients with type 2 diabetes. *J Clin Endocrinol Metab* 86:280–288, 2001

Lebovitz HE, Kreider M, Freed MI: Evaluation of liver function in type 2 diabetic patients during clinical trials: evidence that rosiglitazone does not cause hepatic dysfunction. *Diabetes Care* 25:815–821, 2002

Mudaliar S, Chang AR, Henry RR: Thiazolidinediones, peripheral edema, and type 2 diabetes: incidence, pathophysiology, and clinical implications. *Endocr Pract* 9:406–416, 2003

Parulkar AA, Pendergrass ML, Granda-Ayala R, Lee TR, Fonseca VA: Non-hypoglycemic effects of thiazolidinediones. *Ann Intern Med* 134:61–71, 2001

Raskin P, Rendell M, Riddle MC, Dole JF, Freed MI, Rosenstock J: A randomized trial of rosiglitazone therapy in patients with inadequately controlled insulin-treated type 2 diabetes. *Diabetes Care* 24:1226–1232, 2001

Dr. Lebovitz is Professor of Medicine at the State University of New York Health Science Center at Brooklyn, Brooklyn, NY.

24. Insulin Treatment

JAY S. SKYLER, MD

Insulin was isolated and became available for clinical use in the early 1920s. It revolutionized the treatment of diabetes mellitus. Today, essentially all patients with type 1 diabetes and many patients with type 2 diabetes require insulin therapy. Although insulin has been available for >80 years, major advances have been made over the past 2 decades in the way insulin therapy is used in clinical practice. Much of the progress is a consequence of three factors:

1. The introduction of self-monitoring of blood glucose (SMBG) into routine practice
2. A change in philosophy of diabetes management, such that patient self-management and flexibility in lifestyle have come to drive contemporary treatment approaches
3. The development of insulin analogs that have time-action profiles aligned with physiological insulin secretion—both meal-related insulin secretion and basal insulin secretion

This chapter emphasizes these changing practices. Because of major differences in both pathophysiology and treatment strategy, type 1 and type 2 diabetes are considered separately.

GENERAL CONSIDERATIONS

Types of Insulin

There are four major characteristics of insulin preparations:

1. Time course of action
2. Degree of purity
3. Concentration
4. Species of origin

The time course of action falls into four general categories:

1. Rapid-acting, including the genetically engineered insulin analogs insulin lispro, insulin aspart, and insulin glulisine
2. Short-acting, specifically regular insulin (also known as soluble insulin)

3. Intermediate-acting, including NPH insulin (also known as isophane insulin) and lente insulin (also known as insulin zinc suspension)
4. Long-acting, including ultralente insulin (also known as extended insulin zinc suspension) and the insulin analogs insulin glargine and insulin detemir

There are preparations of mixtures of regular and NPH insulins, including a human insulin mixture containing 70% NPH and 30% regular insulin (called "70/30") and a human insulin mixture containing 50% NPH and 50% regular insulin (called "50/50"). There are also preparations of mixtures of insulins based on insulin lispro (containing 75% intermediate-acting and 25% rapid-acting insulin, called "lispro 75/25") and insulin aspart (containing 70% intermediate-acting and 30% rapid-acting insulin, called "aspart 70/30"). The action profiles of the various insulin preparations available in the U.S. are summarized in Table 24.1.

Purity of insulin preparations generally is reflected by the amount of noninsulin proteins in the preparation. Insulins are defined as purified when they contain <10 ppm of noninsulin proteins and highly purified when they contain <1 ppm of noninsulin proteins. All insulin preparations sold in the U.S. are highly purified, and this is becoming the case for most Western countries.

Table 24.1 Time Course of Action of Human Insulin Preparations

Insulin Preparation	Onset of Action	Peak Action	Effective Duration of Action
Rapid-acting insulin analogs			
Insulin lispro	5–15 min	30–90 min	3–5 h
Insulin aspart	5–15 min	30–90 min	3–5 h
Insulin glulisine*	5–15 min	30–90 min	3–5 h
Short-acting insulin			
Regular	30–60 min	2–3 h	5–8 h
Intermediate-acting insulins			
NPH	2–4 h	4–10 h	10–16 h
Lente	3–4 h	4–12 h	12–18 h
Long-acting insulins			
Ultralente	6–10 h	10–16 h	18–24 h
Insulin glargine	2–4 h	Peakless	20–24 h
Insulin detemir*	2–4 h	6–14 h	16–20 h
Insulin mixtures			
70/30 human mix (70% NPH, 30% regular)	30–60 min	Dual	10–16 h
75/25 lispro analog mix (75% intermediate, 25% lispro)	5–15 min	Dual	10–16 h
70/30 aspart analog mix (70% intermediate, 30% aspart)	5–15 min	Dual	10–16 h
50/50 human mix (50% NPH, 50% regular)	30–60 min	Dual	10–16 h

* FDA approval pending.

Insulin potency is measured in units. Originally, units were based on biological activity, but more recently, 1 mg insulin was defined to have 27.5 units of activity. In the U.S. (and many other countries), insulin preparations contain 100 units/ml and are known as U-100 insulin. For special circumstances, highly concentrated U-500 short-acting (regular) insulin (500 units/ml) is available. In some parts of the world, insulin preparations contain 40 units/ml and are known as U-40 insulin.

For many years, insulin was derived by extraction from bovine and porcine pancreas (mostly either mixtures of beef and pork insulin or only of pork origin). Today, most insulin is commercially produced by recombinant DNA technology. Preparations may be of the same amino acid sequence as native human insulin and thus are called "human insulin." The amino acid sequence may be intentionally altered to produce insulin analogs with altered pharmacological profiles—both rapid-acting analogs (insulin lispro, insulin aspart, and insulin glulisine) and long-acting basal analogs (insulin glargine and insulin detemir). Recombinant insulin preparations (both insulin and analogs) are less immunogenic than animal extracts.

Adverse Effects of Insulin Therapy

The major potential problem with insulin therapy is the risk of hypoglycemia. Other problems are cutaneous reactions to insulin and immunological reactions to insulin, leading to insulin allergy and insulin resistance (see Chapter 31).

THERAPY FOR TYPE 1 DIABETES

Insulin Secretion

There are two types of physiological insulin secretion:

1. Continuous basal insulin secretion
2. Incremental prandial insulin secretion, controlling meal-related glucose excursions

This is schematically depicted in Fig. 24.1. Basal insulin secretion restrains hepatic glucose production, keeping it in equilibrium with basal glucose utilization

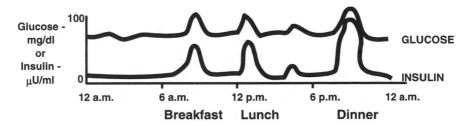

Figure 24.1 Twenty-four-hour plasma glucose and insulin profiles in a hypothetical nondiabetic individual.

by brain and other tissues that are obligate glucose consumers. After meals, meal-related prandial insulin secretion stimulates glucose utilization and storage while inhibiting hepatic glucose output. Patients with type 1 diabetes lack both basal and meal-related prandial insulin secretion.

Flexible Insulin Programs

Contemporary insulin regimens for type 1 diabetes have multiple components that attempt to mimic the two normal types of endogenous physiological insulin secretion:

1. By providing components that give meal-related prandial insulin every time the person eats
2. By providing a separate insulin component to provide basal insulinemia overnight and between meals

Meal-related prandial insulin therapy. Prandial incremental insulin secretion is best duplicated by giving preprandial injections of a rapid-onset insulin analog (insulin lispro, insulin aspart, or insulin glulisine) before each meal by syringe or pen. Each preprandial insulin dose is adjusted individually to provide meal insulinemia appropriate to the size of the meal. Thus, the size of the premeal insulin dose parallels the size of the meal, ideally by relating the dose of insulin to the composition of the meal, particularly the carbohydrate content. In addition, the timing of meals need not be fixed, and meals may be omitted along with the accompanying preprandial insulin dose. The use of preprandial insulin doses permits total flexibility in meal timing. Patients may consume any number of meals per day—one, two, three, or more—taking meal-related prandial insulin with each meal, the dose determined by the meal content.

Rapid-onset insulin analogs (insulin lispro, insulin aspart, and insulin glulisine) may be given immediately before eating a meal. In contrast, short-acting regular insulin administered subcutaneously has an onset of action that is not immediate, and prandial injections of regular insulin are best given at least 20–40 min before eating a given meal in an attempt to have prandial insulinemia parallel meal-related glycemic excursions. Moreover, its profile is less optimal than that of the rapid-onset analogs in that it has sustained action for a number of hours and thus may lead to postprandial hypoglycemia.

Basal insulin therapy. Basal insulinemia is best duplicated by giving one or two daily injections of long-acting insulin (insulin glargine, insulin detemir, or ultralente insulin). The long-acting insulin analogs (insulin glargine and insulin detemir) are peakless and provide optimal basal insulinemia. Insulin glargine has action up to 24 h and often may be given once daily, although occasionally may be divided into two doses. Insulin detemir almost always needs to be given twice daily to provide adequate duration of action. Although human ultralente insulin is relatively peakless in most patients after steady state has been attained, it does have a broad peak (~12–16 h after injection) and a less predictable time course of action than the analogs. As a consequence of the waning insulin effect at ~24 h with insulin glargine and with human ultralente insulin, it may be desirable to divide these long-acting insulins into two doses, particularly in patients who do not have any endogenous insulin. In fact, by dividing these basal insulins into two doses—half on awakening and half on retiring—there may be greater flexibility in lifestyle, facilitating such things as varying times of going to bed and sleeping late some days.

Basal insulin replacement may be attempted with intermediate-acting insulins (NPH insulin or lente insulin) at bedtime and in a small morning dose, but this is far less optimal because these insulins do not have flat insulin profiles, but rather clear peaks of activity. The intermediate-acting insulins have their onset of action ~2 h after injection and produce peak insulin levels ~8–10 h after injection, and their action often is not sustained beyond 12 or 14 h. When used, bedtime intermediate-acting insulin is given to provide overnight basal insulinemia, with peak serum insulin levels before breakfast, the time of relative insulin resistance known as the dawn phenomenon. Bedtime administration of intermediate-acting insulin also eliminates nocturnal peaks of insulin action, reducing the risk of nocturnal hypoglycemia. A small morning dose of intermediate-acting insulin provides basal insulinemia during the day. It is essential to include a morning dose of intermediate-acting insulin in patients using rapid-acting insulin analogs to ensure adequate basal insulinemia during the day, but may be obviated if regular insulin is used for meals, because of the prolonged "tail" of insulin action with regular insulin. Indeed, some patients may need a little intermediate-acting insulin with the predinner injection of a rapid-acting insulin analog if there is a long interval until bedtime and bedtime hyperglycemia occurs as a consequence of the waning effect of predinner rapid-acting insulin. In fact, a group in Perugia, Italy, used multiple small doses (four to six per day) of intermediate-acting insulin to replicate basal insulinemia by allowing curves to run together and creating flat insulinemia at steady state.

Blood glucose targets. Blood glucose targets must be individualized for each patient. Targets must be explicitly defined if they are to be achieved. For healthy young patients, who readily recognize hypoglycemic symptoms and spontaneously recover from hypoglycemia, such targets may nearly approximate the levels of glycemia seen in nondiabetic individuals (Table 24.2). Targets are lower during pregnancy and should be raised in subjects who have difficulty perceiving hypoglycemic symptoms, who do not spontaneously recover from hypoglycemia, or in whom hypoglycemia might be particularly dangerous (e.g., patients with angina pec-

Table 24.2 Representative Plasma Blood Glucose Levels Suitable for Young, Otherwise Healthy Patients with Type 1 Diabetes

	mg/dl	mmol/l
Preprandial	70–130	3.9–7.2
1-h postprandial	100–180	5.6–10.0
2-h postprandial	80–150	4.4–8.3
2:00 to 4:00 a.m.	100–140	5.6–7.8

toris or transient ischemic attacks). In motivated patients, realistic targets are achievable 70–80% of the time.

    Insulin programs. Basal/meal-related insulin programs are schematically depicted in Fig. 24.2. The multiple-dose premeal insulin plus basal insulin regimen has become increasingly popular in recent years for various reasons. It offers flexibility in meal size and timing. It is straightforward and easy to both understand and implement. Moreover, the introduction of insulin pens has stimulated its popularity. As a consequence, this regimen has become widely used.

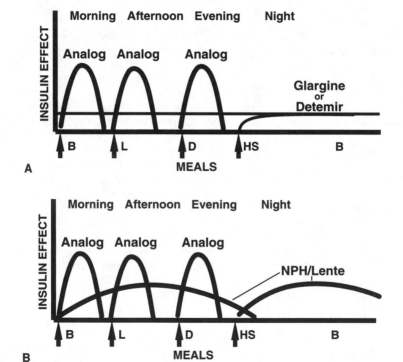

Figure 24.2 Idealized insulin effect provided by flexible multiple-dose regimens separately providing basal insulin and prandial insulin. *A:* Prandial injections of a rapid-acting insulin analog (insulin lispro, insulin aspart, or insulin glulisine) and basal insulin as a bedtime injection of insulin glargine. *B:* Prandial injections of a rapid-acting insulin analog (insulin lispro, insulin aspart, or insulin glulisine) and basal insulin as an intermediate-acting insulin (NPH or lente) at bedtime and before breakfast.

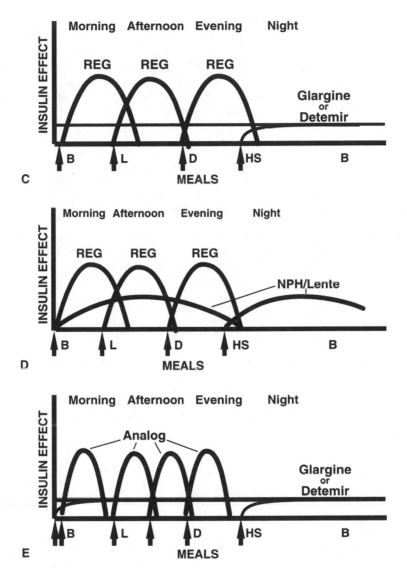

Figure 24.2 (Continued) *C:* Prandial injections of short-acting regular insulin and basal insulin as a bedtime injection of insulin glargine or detemir. *D:* Prandial injections of short-acting regular insulin and basal insulin as intermediate-acting insulin (NPH or lente) at bedtime and before breakfast. *E:* Example of insulin program involving four prandial injections of a rapid-acting insulin analog before meals and before an afternoon snack and basal insulin in which insulin glargine or detemir is administered one-half of the daily dose on arising and one-half of the daily dose on retiring, giving greater flexibility in sleeping hours. B, breakfast; D, dinner; HS, bedtime snack; L, lunch; REG, regular insulin. Arrows indicate the time of insulin injection.

Initial insulin doses and distribution. The insulin dosage required for meticulous glycemic control in typical patients with type 1 diabetes within 20% of their ideal body weight, in the absence of intercurrent infections or other periods of instability, is ~0.5–1.0 units/kg body weight/day. During the relative remission (honeymoon period) early in the course of the disease, insulin requirements generally are less. During intercurrent illness, dosage requirements may increase markedly. Dosage also increases during the adolescent growth spurt, and some adolescents may have a sustained increased dose requirement.

About 50% of the total daily insulin dose is used to provide basal insulinemia. The remainder is divided among the meals either empirically, proportionate to the carbohydrate content of the meals, or by giving ~1.0–1.5 units insulin/10 g carbohydrate consumed.

Dose alteration. Patients are provided with an action plan to alter their therapy to achieve individual defined blood glucose targets. These actions are guided by SMBG determinations and daily records. For prandial doses, the action taken may depend on the answers to several questions the patient needs to ask before any premeal insulin injection:

- What is my blood glucose level now?
- What do I plan to eat now (i.e., usual-size meal, large meal, or small meal; how much carbohydrate)?
- What do I plan to do after eating (i.e., usual activity, increased activity, decreased activity)?
- What has happened under these circumstances previously?

The answers dictate treatment response. The intervention actions may include altering

- food intake (size or content of food)
- activity
- insulin dosage
- timing of insulin injections in relation to meals

An example of an action plan for dose alteration is given in Table 24.3. The plan assumes that the preprandial and bedtime blood glucose targets are 70–130 mg/dl (3.9–7.2 mmol/l). The plan should also call for separate action in response to a pattern of glycemia over several days. Such actions presuppose that the patient has a relatively stable pattern of meals and activities, has no intercurrent illness, and is free from unusual stress.

Considerable patient education is required to implement the management plan. Moreover, the patient needs continued access to and interaction with an expert multidisciplinary diabetes management team if successful management is to be achieved.

Other Insulin Programs

Considering prandial and basal insulin needs separately permits flexibility in eating and activity. Yet such an approach requires a motivated, educated patient who carefully monitors blood glucose several (usually four or more) times daily.

Table 24.3 Sample Plan for Premeal Rapid-Acting Insulin Dosing

Once insulin dosage is stable, use the following scheme for premeal alteration of dosage of rapid-acting insulin (insulin lispro, insulin aspart, or insulin glulisine):

BG <50 mg/dl (<2.8 mmol/l)
– Reduce premeal dose by 2–3 units.
– Delay injection until 10–15 min after starting to eat.
– Include at least 10 g rapidly available carbohydrate in the meal.

BG 50–70 mg/dl (2.8–3.9 mmol/l)
– Reduce premeal dose by 1–2 units.
– Delay injection until after starting to eat.

BG 70–130 mg/dl (3.9–7.2 mmol/l)
– Take prescribed premeal dose.

BG 130–150 mg/dl (7.2–8.3 mmol/l)
– Increase premeal dose by 1 unit.

BG 150–200 mg/dl (8.3–11.1 mmol/l)
– Increase premeal dose by 2 units.

BG 200–250 mg/dl (11.1–13.9 mmol/l)
– Increase premeal dose by 3 units.

BG 250–300 mg/dl (13.9–16.7 mmol/l)
– Increase premeal dose by 4 units.
– Consider delaying meal to 10–20 min after injection.

BG 300–350 mg/dl (16.7–19.4 mmol/l)
– Increase premeal dose by 5 units.
– Delay meal to 15–20 min after injection.
– Check urine ketones. If moderate to high, increase fluid intake and consider extra insulin (1–2 units). Recheck BG and urine ketones in 2–3 h.

BG 350–400 mg/dl (19.4–22.2 mmol/l)
– Increase premeal dose by 6 units.
– Delay meal to 20–30 min after injection.
– Check urine ketones. If moderate to high, increase fluid intake and consider extra insulin (1–2 units). Recheck BG and urine ketones in 2–3 h.

BG >400 mg/dl (>22.2 mmol/l)
– Increase premeal dose by 7 units.
– Delay meal to ~30 min after injection.
– Check urine ketones. If moderate to high, increase fluid intake and consider extra insulin (1–2 units). Recheck BG and urine ketones in 2–3 h.

Planned meal is larger than usual
– Increase dose by 1–2 units.

Planned meal is smaller than usual
– Decrease dose by 1–2 units.

Plan to be unusually active after eating
– Eat extra carbohydrate and/or decrease dose by 1–2 units.

Plan to be unusually sedentary after eating
– Consider increasing dose by 1–2 units.

Plan assumes target goals in Table 24.2 and should be individualized for each patient. BG, blood glucose.

In the absence of motivation, education, or frequent blood glucose monitoring, an alternative approach is to maintain day-to-day consistency both of activity and of timing and quantity of food intake and thus permit prescription of a relatively constant insulin dose. This permits use of either *1*) twice-daily administration of mixtures of short- or rapid-acting insulin plus intermediate-acting insulin (NPH or lente), the so-called "split-mixed" insulin regimen, or *2*) morning administration of a mixture of short- or rapid-acting insulin plus intermediate-acting insulin, with predinner short- or rapid-acting insulin and bedtime intermediate-acting insulin—an approach used to minimize nocturnal hypoglycemia and to counteract the dawn phenomenon. These insulin programs are schematically depicted in Fig. 24.3.

Generally, it is not possible to adequately control glycemia in type 1 diabetes using one or two injections of intermediate-acting insulin alone. The exception may be early in the course of the disease when some endogenous insulin secretion remains.

THERAPY FOR TYPE 2 DIABETES

Pathophysiological Defects

Patients with type 2 diabetes have defects in both insulin secretion and insulin action. The impairments in insulin secretion are manifest in at least three ways:

1. Blunted or absent first-phase insulin response to glucose, so that insulin secretion is delayed and fails to restore prandial glycemic excursions in a timely manner
2. Decreased sensitivity of insulin response to glucose, such that hyperglycemia may fail to trigger an appropriate insulin response
3. Decreased overall insulin secretory capacity, progressive in nature with more prolonged and therefore more severe type 2 diabetes

This impairment in insulin secretory response is not static but dynamic, such that chronic hyperglycemia may itself aggravate the impairment in insulin secretion, a phenomenon known as glucose toxicity. Thus, with decompensation of glycemic control in type 2 diabetes, there is concomitant deterioration in insulin secretory response. Moreover, and most important, when there is correction of hyperglycemia, there is some reversal of the impairment in endogenous insulin response to a meal challenge (i.e., a demonstrable improvement in insulin secretion). Thus, attainment of glucose control facilitates maintenance of glucose control.

Patients with type 2 diabetes also have impaired insulin action (insulin resistance) at target cells. This increases the overall insulin requirement. Like the defect in insulin secretion, this impairment in insulin action is not static but dynamic. Chronic hyperglycemia may aggravate the impairment of insulin action, another manifestation of glucose toxicity. Thus, with decompensation of glycemic

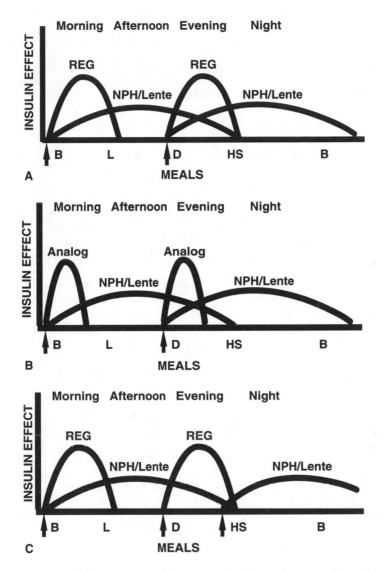

Figure 24.3 Idealized insulin effect provided by split-mixed insulin regimens. *A:* Two daily injections of short-acting regular insulin and intermediate-acting insulin (NPH or lente) before breakfast and before dinner. *B:* Two daily injections of a rapid-acting insulin analog (insulin lispro, insulin aspart, or insulin glulisine) and intermediate-acting insulin before breakfast and before dinner. *C:* Regimen consisting of a morning injection of short-acting regular insulin and intermediate-acting insulin (NPH or lente), a predinner injection of short-acting regular insulin, and a bedtime injection of intermediate-acting insulin. B, breakfast; D, dinner; HS, bedtime snack; L, lunch; REG, regular. Arrows indicate the time of insulin injection.

control, insulin action is diminished. Moreover, when hyperglycemia is corrected, some reversal in the impairment of insulin action occurs.

Insulin Programs for Type 2 Diabetes

Recommended blood glucose targets for patients with type 2 diabetes are summarized in Table 24.4. When patients have been placed on a stable diet and activity program, they can be divided by degree of severity into four groups—mild, moderate, severe, and very severe—based on their level of fasting glycemia and their ability to restore postprandial glycemia to basal levels (as a measure of intactness of prandial insulin secretion).

Mild type 2 diabetes. Insulin therapy is rarely used for patients with mild type 2 diabetes, i.e., individuals with fasting plasma glucose <126 mg/dl (<7.0 mmol/l).

Moderate type 2 diabetes. For patients with moderate type 2 diabetes, i.e., individuals with fasting plasma glucose 126–200 mg/dl (7.0–11.1 mmol/l), if insulin therapy is used, basal insulin therapy alone is often sufficient, with endogenous insulin secretion (perhaps facilitated by oral agents) being adequate to control meal-related prandial glucose excursions. Basal insulinemia may be initiated by long-acting (or intermediate-acting) insulin at bedtime. These insulin programs are schematically depicted in Fig. 24.4. Required doses are generally in the range of 0.3–0.4 units/kg/day, but may be initiated by 10 units at bedtime and increasing the dose every week based on prevailing fasting glucose, as outlined in Table 24.5. Basal insulin therapy serves to supplement the patient's basal insulin secretion and provides sufficient insulin to overcome the prevailing insulin resistance.

Severe type 2 diabetes. For patients with severe type 2 diabetes, i.e., individuals with fasting plasma glucose >200 mg/dl (>11.1 mmol/l), around-the-clock insulinization is necessary (bedtime intermediate-acting insulin cannot be used). Most patients in this category require the addition of short-acting insulin to attain adequate glucose control. Doses required are generally in the range of 0.5–1.2 units/kg/day. However, large doses, even >1.5 units/kg/day, may be required at least

Table 24.4 Representative Plasma Blood Glucose Levels Suitable for Patients with Type 2 Diabetes

	Goal	
	mg/dl	mmol/l
Fasting, preprandial	70–100	3.9–5.6
Postprandial	100–180	5.6–10.0
Bedtime	100–140	5.6–7.8

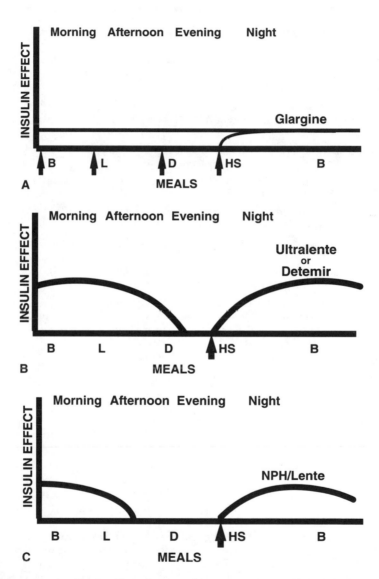

Figure 24.4 Idealized basal insulin effect provided by a bedtime injection. *A:* Bedtime injection of long-acting insulin glargine. *B:* Bedtime injection of long-acting ultralente insulin or insulin detemir. *C:* Bedtime injection of intermediate-acting insulin (NPH or lente). B, breakfast; D, dinner; HS, bedtime snack; L, lunch; REG, regular. Arrows indicate the time of insulin injection.

Table 24.5 Sample Plan for Bedtime Basal Insulin Dosing in Type 2 Diabetes

This action plan assumes that the FBG target is 70–100 mg/dl (3.9–5.6 mmol/l). Plans should be individualized for each patient.

Start with 10 units at bedtime of basal insulin (insulin glargine, insulin detemir, NPH insulin, or ultralente insulin). Adjust the dose weekly based on the following guidelines:

If mean FBG during the previous 4 days is >180 mg/dl (>10.0 mmol/l)
- Increase bedtime basal insulin dose by 8 units.

If mean FBG during the previous 4 days is 140–180 mg/dl (7.8–10.0 mmol/l)
- Increase bedtime basal insulin dose by 6 units.

If mean FBG during the previous 4 days is 120–140 mg/dl (6.7–7.8 mmol/l)
- Increase bedtime basal insulin dose by 4 units.

If mean FBG during the previous 4 days is 100–120 mg/dl (5.6–6.7 mmol/l)
- Increase bedtime basal insulin dose by 2 units.

If mean FBG during the previous 4 days is 70–100 mg/dl (3.9–5.6 mmol/l)
- Maintain current bedtime basal insulin dose.

If any FBG during the previous week is <70 mg/dl (<3.9 mmol/l)
- Return to previous bedtime basal insulin dose

If any FBG during the previous week is <56 mg/dl (<3.1 mmol/l) or if there is any episode of severe hypoglycemia
- Reduce the bedtime basal insulin dose by 2–4 units.

FBG, fasting blood glucose.

initially to overcome prevailing insulin resistance. Such high-dose therapy may be necessary only to attain control, with subsequent control maintained on lower doses, on a basal insulin program, or even with oral hypoglycemic agents. Often, insulin therapy is continued at doses in the range of 0.3–1.0 units/kg/day. Premixed insulin may be used.

Very severe type 2 diabetes. The last category is patients with very severe type 2 diabetes, i.e., individuals with nonintact endogenous insulin response to meals, such that postprandial glycemia is not restored to basal levels within 5 h of meal consumption. In such individuals, fasting plasma glucose is usually quite elevated as well, i.e., >250–300 mg/dl (>13.9–16.7 mmol/l), but this category may include individuals with lesser degrees of fasting hyperglycemia. The insulin deficiency is so profound that, initially, these patients may be difficult to distinguish from patients with type 1 diabetes, although they generally do not manifest ketosis. Indeed, because of their similarity to type 1 diabetes patients, they are best treated like type 1 diabetes patients initially.

In all patients with type 2 diabetes, pathophysiological defects improve as glycemic control is attained and maintained. This facilitates control and may permit patients initially treated with insulin to be maintained with oral hypoglycemic agents or even on a diet and activity program alone.

Most patients with type 2 diabetes can be controlled with insulin if adequate doses are given and if the patient follows an appropriate meal and exercise program. The latter facilitates insulin action. Failure to follow a diet may countermand the effects of insulin and lead to a vicious cycle of progressively increasing insulin doses with failure to control glycemia.

TEMPORARY INSULIN THERAPY

One important use of insulin is as temporary therapy

- to initially attain glycemic control in patients with severe type 2 diabetes
- to overcome glucose toxicity
- to re-regulate decompensated patients

Indeed, type 2 diabetes may be considered a disease of periodic decompensation with the need for re-regulation, usually with insulin. For this reason, all patients with type 2 diabetes should learn insulin administration techniques and be prepared to initiate insulin therapy in the face of expected periodic decompensation, which occurs both spontaneously and with intercurrent illness or stress. Unfortunately, however, the temporary use of insulin is one of the more neglected principles of management of type 2 diabetes.

The hypothesis that short-term insulin therapy may induce long-lasting metabolic improvements in patients with type 2 diabetes has been tested. The degree of success varies depending on the stage of the disease. This approach works extraordinarily well early in the disease to initially attain glycemic control and to re-regulate decompensated patients with intercurrent illness or stress. When used in long-standing patients in whom other therapy has failed to achieve adequate glycemic control, results with temporary insulin therapy are variable. These patients probably have progressive pancreatic β-cell failure.

When using insulin to initially attain glycemic control, vigorous insulin therapy is needed to overcome insulin resistance and glucose toxicity. The plan here is a program of "sequential therapy" in which insulin is used initially to attain glycemic control, with subsequent control maintained by oral agents, diet and exercise, or basal insulin therapy.

When using insulin to re-regulate decompensated patients with intercurrent illness, it is often possible to merely add the insulin to existing oral therapy. As such, insulin may be used for a few days to a few weeks. Dosage may be either as supplemental insulin based on the prevailing level of preprandial glycemia (e.g., 1–2 units rapid-acting or short-acting insulin for every 50 mg/dl [2.7 mmol/l] above the preprandial glucose target) or as a relatively small total dose (e.g., 0.2–0.3 units/kg/day) added to the existing therapy, either as basal insulin or a combination of prandial and basal insulin.

INSULIN PROGRAMS FOR ELDERLY PATIENTS

Insulin therapy is often used in the elderly as a last resort—after failure of dietary management and maximum doses of oral hypoglycemic agents. The aim of therapy in the elderly is to relieve symptoms and prevent both hypoglycemia and acute complications of uncontrolled diabetes (e.g., hyperosmolar states). Schedules for the injection of insulin should be kept as simple as possible, because self-administration may be difficult and dosage errors are not uncommon. Either long-acting basal insulin or premixed insulin may be used.

BIBLIOGRAPHY

DeWitt DE, Dugdale DC: Using new insulin strategies in the outpatient treatment of diabetes mellitus: clinical applications. *JAMA* 289:2265–2269, 2003

DeWitt DE, Hirsch IB: Outpatient insulin treatment in type 1 and type 2 diabetes mellitus: scientific review. *JAMA* 289:2254–2264, 2003

Gerich JE: Novel insulins: expanding options in diabetes management. *Am J Med* 113:308–316, 2002

Hirsch IB, Farkas-Hirsch R, Skyler JS: Intensive insulin therapy for treatment of type 1 diabetes. *Diabetes Care* 13:1265–1283, 1990

Porcellati F, Rossetti P, Pampanelli S, Fanelli CG, Torlone E, Scionti L, Perriello G, Bolli GB: Better long-term glycemic control with the basal insulin glargine as compared to nph in patients with type 1 diabetes mellitus given mealtime lispro insulin. *Diabet Med* In press

Riddle MC, Rosenstock J, Gerich J, on behalf of the Insulin Glargine 4002 Study Investigators: The Treat-to-Target Trial: Randomized addition of glargine or human NPH insulin to oral therapy of type 2 diabetic patients. *Diabetes Care* 26:3080–3086, 2003

Schade DS, Santiago JV, Skyler JS, Rizza R: *Intensive Insulin Therapy*. Princeton, NJ, Excerpta Med, 1983

Skyler JS: Insulin pharmacology. *Med Clin North Am* 72:1337–1354, 1988

Skyler JS: Insulin therapy in type II diabetes: who needs it, how much of it, and for how long? *Postgrad Med* 101:85–90, 92–94, 96, 1997

Skyler JS: Insulin therapy in type 1 diabetes mellitus. In *Current Therapy of Diabetes Mellitus*. DeFronzo RA, Ed. St. Louis, MO, Mosby, 1998, p. 36–49

Skyler JS: Insulin therapy in type 2 diabetes mellitus. In *Current Therapy of Diabetes Mellitus*. DeFronzo RA, Ed. St. Louis, MO, Mosby, 1998, p. 108–116

Zinman B: The physiologic replacement of insulin. *N Engl J Med* 321:363–370, 1989

Dr. Skyler is Professor of Medicine, Pediatrics and Psychology, and Director of the Division of Endocrinology, Diabetes, and Metabolism at the University of Miami, Miami, FL.

25. Insulin Pump Therapy

BRUCE BODE, MD

Both insulin pump therapy, also known as continuous subcutaneous insulin infusion (CSII), and multiple daily injection (MDI) therapy are effective means of implementing intensive diabetes management with the goal of achieving near-normal blood glucose levels. These methods of basal/bolus therapy require the patient and health care team to be adept at all aspects of intensive diabetes management, including self-monitoring of blood glucose (SMBG), insulin dose adjustment, correction of blood glucose levels that are out of range, record keeping, medical nutrition therapy with the use of carbohydrate counting, troubleshooting high and low blood glucose values to prevent both hypoglycemia and hyperglycemia, and appropriate insulin injection technique and site care.

ADVANTAGES OF CSII

The advantages of CSII over MDI therapy are primarily from the result of better insulin pharmacokinetics. Only short- or rapid-acting insulin is used, with all food intake being covered by insulin boluses. Normal blood glucose levels are maintained at other times by continuous delivery of short-acting basal insulin. The modified insulins (NPH, lente, and ultralente, as well as the long-acting basal analog glargine) have been shown to vary in absorption anywhere from 20 to 52% in the same individual, resulting in unpredictable glucose excursions. In contrast, the soluble short-acting insulins that are used in CSII vary in absorption by <3% on a daily basis. As a result, there is decreased variability in insulin absorption and glucose values. Additionally, with CSII, there is a decreased risk of nocturnal hypoglycemia and an improved control of the "dawn phenomenon" through the use of variable basal rates, a decreased risk of hypoglycemia at other times during the day because of better timing of meal boluses and basal rates, and a greater freedom in the timing of meals and snacks. As a result, CSII has often resulted in better glycemic control, less risk of major hypoglycemia, and improvement in lifestyle flexibility and quality of life.

CSII EVOLUTION

Use of insulin pumps for patients with type 1 diabetes was first reported in the late 1970s and demonstrated the ability to achieve strict glucose control in a select group of individuals. Since then, pumps have become dramatically smaller, more durable, and easier to use. Current pumps have electronic memory, multiple basal rates, different bolus options, safety alarms with child-block features, and remote controls on certain models. New software changes have recently been implemented to aid the patient in determining the correction bolus for an out-of-range glucose level and how much insulin to give for a certain amount of carbohydrate. Other alert features are being added to insulin pumps to help remind the patient to change his or her infusion set, to give a meal bolus, and to check glucose values. Modern-day infusion sets now have soft cannulas with quick-release options and better adhesive properties.

CSII EXPERIENCE

In the Diabetes Control and Complications Trial (DCCT), 42% of the experimental group used insulin pump therapy during the last full year of study. DCCT investigators observed a 0.2–0.4% decrease in glycated hemoglobin A1C (A1C) using CSII, as well as an improvement in lifestyle flexibility. Since the DCCT, CSII use has increased from 15,000 patients in 1993 to over 200,000 patients in the U.S. in 2003.

Glycemic control during pump therapy has been shown to improve in adults, as well as in adolescents and children, with type 1 diabetes. In large nonrandomized and randomized studies, the average A1C has decreased from 0.2% to >1%, with the average being between 0.4 and 0.6%. Several factors have been identified as keys to successful treatment, with the most important being frequency of blood glucose monitoring. Patients who monitor three or more times a day have an average A1C of 7.2%, with patients monitoring two or less times a day having an average A1C of 8.0%. Each additional glucose test often results in a significant drop in A1C of up to 0.2 points, with the majority of patients monitoring five or more times a day achieving an average A1C of <7.0%. Other significant factors affecting glycemic control are *1*) recording of insulin doses and blood glucose values on a log sheet, *2*) counting carbohydrates and taking appropriate amounts of insulin, and *3*) use of rapid-acting insulin such as insulin lispro or aspart.

Experience with CSII in patients with type 2 diabetes is limited but encouraging. Glycemic control has been shown to be as good as or better than multiple daily injections, with better fasting and postbreakfast glucose values and a marked improvement in the quality of life.

Other advantages of insulin pump therapy include a reduction in the occurrence of severe hypoglycemia. On average, people on MDI therapy have rates of severe hypoglycemia ranging anywhere from 60 to 170 episodes per 100 patient-years. In contrast, people on CSII have rates of hypoglycemia ranging from 20 to 30 per 100 patient-years (Fig. 25.1). This reduction in severe hypoglycemia appears to be the result of the better pharmacokinetic delivery of insulin provided when only short- or rapid-acting insulin is used for both basal and bolus components, as well as a 15–20% reduction in long-term insulin requirements as compared with MDI.

Reduced insulin requirements and flexibility in food intake minimize the weight gain that often occurs in insulin pump therapy patients. However, as a result of the greater flexibility in taking insulin to cover any type of food, patients must be cautioned that any excess calorie intake, with improving glycemic control, can result in weight gain.

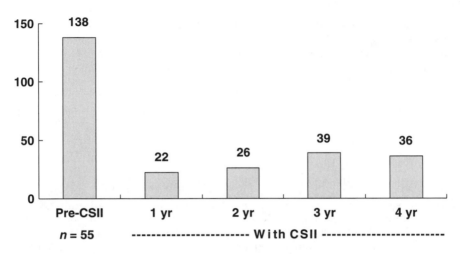

Figure 25.1 Reduction in severe hypoglycemia during CSII.

Patients using CSII are at greater risk of developing diabetic ketoacidosis (DKA) and hyperglycemic crisis than individuals using MDI therapy because of the absence of a depot of long-acting insulin. However, with appropriate training and troubleshooting of high blood glucose values, the CSII rates of DKA have only been slightly higher than the MDI rates. Teaching patients to treat high blood glucose levels (by giving manual injections of subcutaneous insulin when ketones are positive or glucose values are >250 mg/dl on two consecutive readings, followed by a change of their infusion set) has resulted in minimizing the risk of DKA. Alternatively, adolescents who are prone to ketoacidosis because they miss their insulin injections often have a reduction in DKA and hospitalizations with CSII as a result of the continual delivery of basal insulin.

Another important advantage of CSII over MDI therapy is that it allows patients to lead more normal lives and simplifies irregular meal schedules and other unplanned activities. Patients can eat, snack, work, exercise, and sleep based on their own personal schedules and needs rather than on the peaks of insulin given many hours earlier. This explains why more than 60% of the members of the American Diabetes Association and the American Association of Diabetes Educators who are health care providers with insulin-dependent diabetes are currently on insulin pump therapy. Because of these benefits, long-term continuation rates for CSII are now >95%.

IMPLEMENTING PUMP THERAPY

The best candidates for CSII are patients who are currently practicing diabetes self-management, including frequent blood glucose monitoring, maintaining records of blood glucose values and insulin doses on a flow sheet, visiting a medical team on a regular basis, and counting carbohydrates. However, some patients exhibiting poor self-management on MDI therapy may be very successful with CSII. These are often patients who have become frustrated and discouraged on MDI therapy as a result of inadequate success in achieving their goals because of the limitations of MDI therapy. These patients are often able to achieve their goals on CSII and thus become much more active in their daily self-management, including all aspects of intensive long-term diabetes management. It is important for the health care provider to offer realistic expectations when discussing pump therapy with a prospective pump user, CSII is not a cure, but a tool to aid in successful management of diabetes. The indications for CSII are listed in Table 25.1.

Starting Insulin Dose on CSII

There are two methods for calculating the initial starting insulin dose on CSII: one method is based on the prior total daily insulin dose while on MDI therapy, and the other is based on weight. The most common method is to reduce the total daily insulin dose on MDI therapy by 25–30%, using one half as a basal dose and the other half as the total bolus doses given for meals and snacks (Fig. 25.2). The starting total daily dose on CSII is 0.45 times the patient's weight in kilograms, with the average total daily dose in well-controlled patients on CSII being higher at 0.53 times the weight in kilograms. The type of insulin used in CSII is either regular or rapid-acting insulin analogs, with insulin aspart being the only FDA approved insulin analog.

The basal dose is initially divided by 24 to get the units per hour, given often as a single basal rate. The bolus doses are divided according to the carbohydrate content of the meal. Basal and bolus doses are adjusted based on monitoring of the patient's blood glucose before meals, 2 h after eating, and at bedtime, midnight, and 3:00 a.m. The basal rate is increased or decreased by 0.1 unit/h to keep the premeal and overnight blood glucose levels within a 30 mg/dl glucose excursion from baseline glucose levels. If the glucose rises >30 mg/dl from 3:00 a.m. to prebreakfast, a second basal rate is implemented, usually starting 2–3 h before the patient awakens from sleep. The basal rate is adjusted during the day only if there are significant glucose excursions occurring >4 h after a meal bolus is given. To guide daytime basal rate adjustments, the patient should delay or skip a meal and monitor blood glucose levels every 2 h in the fasting state. This should be done periodically (at least once a year) to ascertain that basal rates are not set too high

---

Table 25.1 Indications for CSII

1. Inadequate glycemic control, defined as:
   - A1C above target (>7%)
   - Dawn phenomenon with glucose levels >140–160 mg/dl (>8–9 mmol/l) in the morning
   - Marked variability in glucose on a day-to-day basis
2. History of hypoglycemia unawareness or of hypoglycemic events requiring assistance
3. Need for flexibility in lifestyle (e.g., shift worker, business traveler, or worker in a safety-sensitive job)

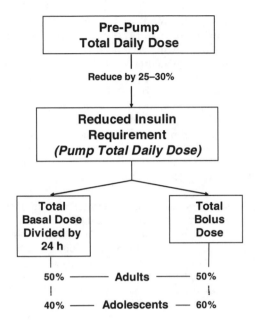

Figure 25.2 Establishing initial basal and bolus doses.

or too low. At each visit to the health care provider, the total basal rate and the total daily dose should be obtained from the insulin pump memory. The ratio of basal rate to total daily insulin dose should be between 40 and 50% (optimal basal rates are ~48% of total daily dose). It is important to note that children and young adolescents on CSII may have different basal rate requirements than adults. It is often shown that children need more basal insulin given in the evening hours and early morning hours (between 9:00 p.m. and 3:00 a.m.), which is in marked contrast to adults, who often need more basal insulin in the early dawn hours between 3:00 a.m. and breakfast. Such changes can easily be made by frequent monitoring of bedtime and nocturnal glucose readings.

Bolus doses are often 50–60% of the total daily insulin requirement on CSII. Bolus doses are adjusted based on 2-h postmeal blood glucose levels. The patient is provided specific guidelines to adjust insulin boluses or the carbohydrate-to-insulin ratio to keep blood glucose levels within a reasonable glucose excursion (<160 mg/dl [<8.9 mmol/l] at 2 h postmeal). Once the individual has fine-tuned boluses to a stable meal plan, a carbohydrate-to-insulin ratio can be calculated for the patient's ongoing use in modifying bolus doses based on carbohydrate content of meals. The ratio rate varies from 1 unit per 5 g carbohydrate to 1 unit per 25 g carbohydrate, with the average being 1 unit per 10–15 g carbohydrate. An estimate for the appropriate carbohydrate-to-insulin ratio can be obtained by using mathematical formulas. Two mathematical formulas exist. The first method includes taking the total daily dose of insulin and dividing it into 450. The second, more recent, formula supports taking 2.8 times the body weight in pounds divided by total daily insulin. Both of these methods will give an estimate of how many grams of carbohydrate are covered by 1 unit of insulin. The carbohydrate-to-insulin ratio can then be adjusted accordingly, based on 2-h postmeal glucose monitoring.

In addition to bolus doses, all patients on intensive insulin therapy should be provided with correction bolus or supplemental bolus guidelines to correct out-of-range glucose values. These are best initially estimated by using another mathematical formula, initially known as the 1500 rule and now known as the 1700 rule. The total daily dose of insulin is divided into 1700, which gives an estimate of how much reduction in milligrams per deciliter of glucose 1 unit of insulin provides. With an appropriate insulin sensitivity factor or glucose correction factor, out-of-range glucose values can be corrected by taking the glucose value obtained before the meal, subtracting it from the ideal glucose, and dividing by the glucose correction factor. Patients should use this correction bolus algorithm before each meal, in addition to troubleshooting any high glucose values. By monitoring the response to using this correction bolus, adjustments can be made to obtain an appropriate response for returning glucose back to within goal range.

Guidelines for prevention of hypoglycemia and hyperglycemic crisis must be provided accordingly. Patients are encouraged to treat all low blood glucose values with a set amount of carbohydrate (specifically rapid-acting glucose in the form of glucose tablets or glucose gel). Patients are taught to adjust both their bolus and basal doses to avoid hypoglycemia, defined as any glucose below the individual target range for that patient.

Hyperglycemia troubleshooting and prevention, as well as sick-day management, is taught upon initiation of pump therapy and reviewed at each follow-up visit. Patients must be able to understand that they are only using short-acting insulin with no long-acting insulin depot. If they experience hyperglycemia >250 mg/dl (>13.9 mmol/l), they should troubleshoot this accordingly by taking a correction bolus dose. If they are nauseated or feel sick in any way, patients should check urine ketones. If positive, they should give their correction bolus by manual insulin injection, change their insulin infusion set line, and repeat delivery of correction bolus doses by injection until glucose levels are back within normal range. Patients are taught to troubleshoot hyperglycemia by not only inspecting the infusion site area, but also inspecting the infusion site line, luerlock, and basal/bolus doses set in the pump memory. Such meticulous attention to troubleshooting hyperglycemia should prevent DKA; however, hyperglycemic crisis can still occur because of crimping of the soft-set cannula, leakage of insulin from the insulin syringe or luerlock, air in the insulin tubing, dislodgement of the soft cannula from underneath the skin, as well as other potential problems including not giving the insulin dose, no insulin in the syringe, no basal delivery, and so forth.

The patients should wear the pump continuously but they are able to disconnect for periods of up to 2 to 4 hours without any adverse consequences. If one is off their pump longer than 4 hours, supplemental insulin should be given to cover the basal rate along with bolus insulin to cover food intake. If they desire a pump holiday or they must return to MDI for a period of greater than 24 hours, they should take insulin glargine at a dose equal to their CSII basal rate daily along with bolus injections until they return to CSII.

INSULIN PUMP THERAPY FOLLOW-UP

Clinical follow-up of patients on insulin pump therapy is similar to follow-up of individuals on other forms of intensive diabetes management with MDI therapy. Patients are encouraged to continue monitoring their glucose four to six times a day, initially faxing or e-mailing their blood glucose values and insulin log sheets to the health care provider's office once or twice a week until normalized. Follow-up with a registered dietitian is often scheduled within 2–4 weeks and as needed thereafter, with definite follow-up on a yearly basis to review carbohydrate counting practices, guidelines for normal nutrition, and weight management. Follow-up with the physician and other health care providers is often done initially 2–4 weeks after starting pump therapy. Once glucose levels are stabilized, visits are done on a quarterly basis. At each visit, hypoglycemia, hyperglycemia, DKA prevention and troubleshooting, and sick-day management should be reviewed. Adjustment of the basal rate, bolus doses, carbohydrate-to-insulin ratio, and correction boluses should be done to obtain the glycemic targets set for that individual patient.

When the patient's A1C is above goal, it is important to note the frequency of SMBG, along with the individual's record-keeping habits. Diet and knowledge of food intake should be examined, as should bolusing practices with food and snacks. The memory features on blood glucose meters and on insulin pumps are helpful in verifying the patient's record of glucose monitoring and bolus frequency. Infusion site areas should be examined for atrophy, hypertrophy, and inflammation. Appropriate rotation of sites should be encouraged. If evidence of infection exists, appropriate use of anti-staphylococcal soap should be used before insertion of the infusion set, along with eradication of the staph-carrier state by using mupirocin calcium cream 2% (Bactroban) or another anti-staphylococcal ointment in the nares of the nose. Other factors affecting glycemic control, such as marked fear of hypoglycemia or overtreatment of low blood glucose values, need to be explored if glycemic targets are not met.

If the A1C goal is still not met, the patient should then be placed on a continuous glucose monitoring system to determine the reasons for suboptimal glycemic control, with appropriate changes made in both the basal and bolus doses, as well as treatment of high and low blood glucose values.

FUTURE OF PUMP THERAPY

The future of pump therapy is promising. Newer pumps are being developed with enhanced software features. These features will not only aid in calculating the bolus dose for a set amount of carbohydrate, but will also aid in calculating the correction bolus for an out-of-range glucose value. Features will include setting reminders for when to change the infusion set and when to check glucose both before and after a meal, as well as other safety alerts. Once continuous glucose monitoring is available in real time, the effectiveness of pump therapy in achieving near-normal glycemia will be enhanced. Patients can then correct any out-of-range glucose values and are warned before any significant out-of-range glucose level occurs, thus avoiding a hypoglycemic or hyperglycemic crisis. Eventually, closed-loop systems will be developed, in the form of either an external or implantable sensor feeding back to an external or implantable pump, resulting in near-normal glycemia without hypoglycemia.

BIBLIOGRAPHY

Bode BW, Hirsch I, Hu P, Santiago O: Type 1 diabetes patients can temporarily switch from continuous subcutaneous insulin therapy with insulin aspart to basal bolus therapy with insulin aspart and insulin glargine. *Diabetes* 52 (Suppl. 1):438, 2003

Bode BW, Schleusener DS, Strange P: Switch to multiple daily injections (MDI) with insulin glargine (lantus) and insulin lispro (humalog) from continuous subcutaneous insulin infusion (CSII) with insulin lispro–a randomized, open-label, study using continuous glucose monitoring system (CGMS). *Diabetes* 52 (Suppl. 1):439, 2003

Bode BW, Steed RD, Davidson PC: Reduction in severe hypoglycemia with long-term continuous subcutaneous insulin infusion in type I diabetes. *Diabetes Care* 19:324–327, 1996

Bode BW, Tamborlane WV, Davidson PC: Insulin pump therapy in the 21st century: strategies for successful use in adults, adolescents, and children with diabetes. *Postgrad Med* 111:69–77, 2002

Boland E, Weinzimer S, Ahern JA, Steffan A, Tamborlane W: Randomized, prospective trial of CSII vs MDI with glargine in children: a preliminary report. *Diabetes* 52 (Suppl. 1):192, 2003

Davidson PC, Hebblewhite HR, Bode BW, Steed RD, Welch NS, Greenlee MC, Richardson PL, Johnson J: Statistically based CSII parameters: correction factor, CF (1700 Rule), carbohydrate-to-insulin ratio, CIR (2.8 Rule), and basal-to-total ratio. *Diabetes Techno & Ther* 5:237, 2003

Diabetes Control and Complications Trial Research Group: The effect of intensive treatment of diabetes on the development and progression of long-term complications in insulin-dependent diabetes mellitus. *N Engl J Med* 329:977–986, 1993

Pickup JC, Keen H: Continuous subcutaneous insulin infusion in type 1 diabetes is beneficial in selected patients and should be more widely available. *BMJ* 322:1262–1263, 2001

Raskin P, Bode B, Marks J, Hirsch I, Weinstein R, McGill J, Peterson G, Mudaliar S, Huang WC, Reinhardt R: Continuous subcutaneous insulin infusion and multiple daily injection therapy are equally effective in type 2 diabetes: a randomized, parallel-group, 24 week study. *Diabetes Care.* 26:2598–2603, 2003

Dr. Bode is Medical Director at the Diabetes Resource Center of Atlanta, Atlanta Diabetes Associates, Atlanta, GA.

26. Combination Therapy for Hyperglycemia

HAROLD E. LEBOVITZ, MD

Conclusive data showing that appropriate glycemic control can reduce both microvascular and macrovascular complications provide compelling arguments that we should strive for glycemic control that achieves glycated hemoglobin A1C (A1C) levels of ≤7%. It is clear from the results of numerous recent large clinical trials that the treatment of type 2 diabetes patients with lifestyle intervention and a single pharmacological agent is unlikely to achieve such glycemic control. The question then arises as to the strategies that should be used to achieve such goals when they are unmet by monotherapy with an oral agent. The possibilities are to combine oral agents that have different mechanisms of action, to switch to an insulin treatment regimen, or to use a combination of insulin and an oral agent. This chapter focuses on the rationale and use of combination therapy for hyperglycemia in patients with type 2 diabetes.

RATIONALE FOR COMBINATION THERAPY

Factors influencing glucose metabolism are as follows:

- rate of gastrointestinal absorption of carbohydrate
- insulin secretory rate
- glucose balance (production versus uptake) across the liver
- peripheral (muscle) glucose uptake and utilization

Most of these regulatory sites are abnormal in type 2 diabetes, and all are amenable to modification by the antidiabetic agents now available. Table 26.1 highlights the primary pharmacological actions of currently available agents. Judicious use of combinations of oral antidiabetic agents or combinations of insulin with oral antidiabetic agents takes advantage of these different modes of action. Additive and potentiated effects in reducing glycemia are possible. Equally important, the nonglycemic effects of these combinations can improve other aspects of the metabolic derangements seen with type 2 diabetes.

Table 26.1 Currently Available Classes of Antidiabetic Agents

Class/drug	Primary Mode of Action				Primary Effect on Glycemia	
	Delay Carbohydrate Absorption	Increased Insulin Secretion	Decreased Hepatic Glucose Production	Increased Peripheral Glucose Uptake	Decreased FPG	Decreased Postprandial Plasma Glucose
α-Glucosidase inhibitor (acarbose, miglitol)	+++	0	+	0	+	+++
Sulfonylurea (glipizide, glyburide, glimepiride)	0	+++	+++	+++	+++	+
Repaglinide	0	+++	++	+++	++	+++
Nateglinide	0	+++	++	+++	+	+++
Metformin	±	0	+++	+	+++	+
Thiazolidinediones (pioglitazone, rosiglitazone)	0	0	++	+++	++	++
Rapid- and short-acting insulin	0	—	+	+++	+	+++
NPH, lente, or glargine insulin at 10:00 p.m.	0	—	+++	+	+++	+

0, no effect; +, small effect; ++, moderate effect; +++, marked effect ±, variable effect.

COMBINATIONS OF ORAL ANTIDIABETIC AGENTS

Combinations of oral antidiabetic agents that have been used to treat patients with type 2 diabetes are listed in Table 26.2. Combinations of agents that increase insulin secretion, e.g., sulfonylureas, repaglinide, or nateglinide, with agents that decrease insulin requirements, e.g., metformin, acarbose, and thiazolidinediones (pioglitazone and rosiglitazone), have been sufficiently well studied and their effects have been validated; hence, they are approved by the U.S. Food and Drug Administration (FDA). The effects expected are the mean data reported from the largest and most rigorous clinical trials reported. The combinations of α-glucosidase inhibitors such as acarbose with insulin secretagogues or insulin sensitizers are useful when additional effects in specifically lowering postprandial hyperglycemia are desired. The thiazolidinediones and metformin improve insulin sensitivity by different mechanisms and seem to preferentially affect different organs (metformin

Table 26.2 Combinations of Oral Agents Used to Treat Type 2 Diabetes

	Expected Decrease from Addition of Second Agent		
	FPG (mg/dl)	A1C (%)	Weight Change (lb)
Approved for use by FDA			
Sulfonylureas + metformin	64 (3.5)	1.7	0.9
Sulfonylureas + acarbose	25 (1.4)	0.9	NS
Sulfonylureas + rosiglitazone or pioglitazone	38–56 (2.1–3.1)	1.3–1.4	6–13
Repaglinide + metformin	31 (1.7)	1.0	
Nateglinide + metformin	31.8 (1.8)	1.1	0.7
Rosiglitazone + metformin	53 (3.0)	1.2	6.8
Pioglitazone + metformin	38 (2.1)	0.8	
Supported by peer-reviewed publications			
Acarbose + metformin	10 (0.5)	0.8	NS

Values in parentheses are SI units in mmol/l.

affects the liver and thiazolidinediones the skeletal muscle). Recent studies indicate that combination therapy with these two classes of insulin sensitizers has added benefits in improving insulin sensitivity and achieving glycemic control.

All of the combinations discussed above are effective only if endogenous insulin secretion is adequate to support their effects. As endogenous insulin secretion continues to decrease, as occurs with increasing duration of type 2 diabetes, combinations of oral antidiabetic agents will become increasingly less effective.

COMBINATIONS OF ORAL ANTIDIABETIC AGENTS WITH INSULIN

At the later stages of type 2 diabetes when deficient insulin secretion has limited the effectiveness of oral antidiabetic agents, effectiveness can be restored by combining the administration of oral agents with insulin. Several mechanisms account for this. Metformin and thiazolidinediones act by increasing tissue sensitivity to insulin. α-Glucosidase inhibitors lower postprandial glycemic rise and therefore decrease insulin requirements. Thus, insulin is needed for the action of metformin, thiazolidinediones, and acarbose, but all three also lower the amount of insulin required for effective action. Oral agents that release endogenous insulin can provide a physiological insulin response when combined with exogenous insulin.

Table 26.3 lists combinations of oral antidiabetic agents and insulin for which there are sufficient data to evaluate their effects. Pioglitazone or rosiglitazone

Table 26.3 Combinations of Insulin and Oral Agents Used to Treat Type 2 Diabetes

	Expected Decrease from Addition of Insulin		
	FPG (mg/dl)	A1C (%)	Weight Change (lb)
Approved for use by FDA			
Pioglitazone or rosiglitazone + insulin	49–54 (2.7–3.0)	1.0–1.3	8.0–12.0
Glimepiride + insulin*			
Supported by peer-reviewed publications			
Metformin + bedtime insulin	60–80 (3.3–4.4)	1.7–2.5	2
Sulfonylureas + bedtime insulin	60–80 (3.3–4.4)	0.5–1.8	9
Acarbose + insulin	0–16 (0–0.8)	0.4–0.5	NS

Values in parentheses are SI units in mmol/l. *Treatment FPG and A1C levels were no different between placebo + insulin and glimiperide + insulin, but less insulin was required (49 units/day compared with 78 units/day).

added to insulin therapy has been shown to significantly improve glycemic control in insulin-resistant type 2 diabetes patients who are inadequately controlled despite taking an average of ~70 units/day of insulin. The improvement in glycemic control is accompanied by a decrease in mean insulin requirements of 15–20%. Care must be exercised when adding thiazolidinediones to the regimen for insulin-treated patients. The combination causes significant increases in fluid retention, and ~15% of patients develop mild to moderate edema. A few case reports in the literature suggest that in a rare type 2 diabetes patient, the addition of a thiazolidinedione may precipitate heart failure. This is thought to be due to plasma volume expansion in a patient with unrecognized borderline cardiac compensation. Therefore, it is recommended that patients at risk for heart failure be started on low doses of thiazolidinediones, be observed carefully, and have their dose titrated upward slowly.

Several recent studies have evaluated the effect of combining insulin treatment with metformin. These studies show a mean decrease in A1C of 1.7–2.5%. Insulin requirements are reported in some studies to decrease but in others to stay the same. One particularly useful way of combining insulin and metformin is to administer NPH or glargine insulin at bedtime and metformin during the day. This combination has been reported to decrease A1C as well as or better than multiple injections of insulin but without clinically significant weight gain. Combining insulin and acarbose can smooth out postprandial glycemic oscillations and modestly improve glycemic control as well as reduce episodes of hypoglycemia.

Considerable controversy exists concerning combination of sulfonylureas with insulin. The combination will improve glycemic control. Hypoglycemia, however, is a problem, and improvement in glycemic control is less consistent than with other insulin and oral antidiabetic combinations.

The addition of a basal insulin regimen at night to oral medications during the day achieves improved glycemic control because overnight hepatic glucose production is reduced, and the target is to administer sufficient insulin to achieve a fasting plasma glucose (FPG) level between 90 and 110 mg/dl (5 and 6.1 mmol/l). Table 26.4 provides the titration scheme that was used in a recent treat-to-target study that added either NPH or glargine insulin at bedtime to the regimen of type 2 diabetes patients who were not well controlled on combinations of oral antidiabetic agents.

WHEN AND HOW TO INSTITUTE COMBINATION THERAPY

Figure 26.1 is a general guide that can be used to determine when and how combination therapy is instituted. Individuals with predominantly postprandial hyperglycemia (FPG ≤150 mg/dl [≤8.3 mmol/l]) can be well controlled with diet and increased physical activity. Most, however, will require the addition of monotherapy with acarbose, metformin, or a thiazolidinedione to achieve an A1C between 6.0 and 7.0%. Severely hyperglycemic and symptomatic patients are best treated initially with an insulin regimen. Most type 2 diabetes patients (FPG 151–270 mg/dl [8.4–15 mmol/l]) should be started on diet, increased physical activity, and monotherapy with an oral antidiabetic agent. Those who are predominantly insulin resistant (central and/or generalized obesity) might best be treated with an agent that decreases insulin resistance (metformin or a thiazolidinedione). Those who are predominantly insulin deficient (nonobese with FPG >200 mg/dl [<11.1 mmol/l]) might be better candidates for an agent that increases insulin secretion (sulfonylureas, repaglinide, or nateglinide).

Most patients will not achieve their target glycemic control on monotherapy either initially or after several years of treatment. These individuals require combination therapy. Several combinations of oral antidiabetic drugs are effective in

Table 26.4 Scheme for Adding Basal or Intermediate-Acting Insulin to Oral Agents

Start with 10 units of basal (glargine) or intermediate-acting (NPH) insulin at bedtime (~10:00 p.m.). Adjust insulin dose weekly according to the following guidelines.

Self-monitored FPG (mg/dl)	Increase in insulin dose (units/day)
≥180	8
≥140 but <180	6
≥120 but <140	4
≥100 but <120	2
Treat-to-target FPG ≤100 mg/dl	

Do not increase insulin dose if FPG is <72 mg/dl on 2 days. Decrease insulin dose 2–4 units/day if FPG is <56 mg/dl or clinically significant hypoglycemia occurs.

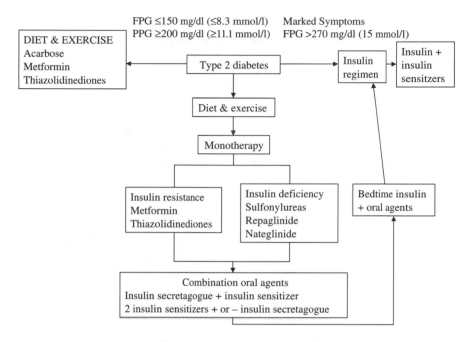

Figure 26.1 An approach to the management of hyperglycemia in patients with type 2 diabetes. Details are described in the text. PPG, postprandial plasma glucose. Insulin secretagogue: sulfonylurea, repaglinide, or nateglinide; insulin sensitizer: metformin or thiazolidinedione; acarbose could be added to various combinations if additional PPG lowering is desired.

controlling glycemia as described in Fig. 26.1 and Table 26.1. The doses to be used are given in Table 26.5.

Combination oral agent therapy will lose its effectiveness when endogenous insulin secretion becomes markedly deficient. At that stage, the β-cell is so depleted after the three meals that overnight insulin secretion is virtually nil. The consequence of insufficient overnight insulin secretion is unrestrained hepatic glucose production, which causes marked increases in fasting hyperglycemia. This can be ameliorated by administering an intermediate-acting or a basal insulin at bedtime (10:00 p.m.) and giving oral agents during the day. This treatment option has been shown to be as effective as multiple injections of insulin in most type 2 diabetes patients and is without the extensive weight gain or hypoglycemia seen with multiple injections of insulin.

If insulin secretion declines even further so that little or no insulin secretion occurs with meals, then oral antidiabetic agents become ineffective and a multiple-insulin injection regimen becomes necessary. This can usually be intermediate- and short-acting insulin before breakfast, short-acting insulin before the evening

Table 26.5 Recommended Doses for Combination Therapy*

Sulfonylureas	
Glipizide	20 mg/day
Glyburide	10 mg/day
Glipizide-GITS	5 mg/day
Glimiperide	4–8 mg/day
Repaglinide	1–2 mg/meal
Nateglinide	60–120 mg/meal
Metformin	1.5–2.0 g/day
Pioglitazone	15–30 mg/day
Rosiglitazone	4–8 mg/day
Acarbose	50–100 mg/meal
Bedtime NPH, lente, or glargine insulin	Start with 5–10 units; increase by 2–3 units every 3 days until FPG is between 110 and 120 mg/dl (6.1–6.6 mmol/l); an alternative scheme is given in Table 26.4.
Multiple insulin doses	Insulin dose is very variable and needs to be individualized.

*Combinations that include insulin or insulin secretagogues drugs will need reduced doses if hypoglycemia occurs. GITS, gastrointestinal therapeutic system.

meal, and intermediate-acting insulin at 10:00 or 11:00 p.m. An alternative is to give a basal insulin such as glargine insulin once a day and precede each meal with a rapid-acting insulin analog such as lispro or aspart insulin. Because many type 2 diabetes patients are severely insulin resistant, it may be necessary to treat them with very large doses of insulin (>100 units/day), and in this instance, better glycemic control at lower doses of insulin can often be achieved by adding pioglitazone, rosiglitazone, or metformin to the insulin regimen.

USEFUL HINTS FOR COMBINATION THERAPY IN TYPE 2 DIABETES PATIENTS

The following are useful guidelines when contemplating combination therapy in patients with type 2 diabetes:

1. About 5–10% of adults who have phenotypic type 2 diabetes are in reality slowly evolving type 1 diabetes patients (latent autoimmune diabetes in adults [LADA]). These individuals tend to be younger and leaner than the classic patients with type 2 diabetes. This occurs primarily in white and some Asian populations. They will probably require insulin therapy within the first 6 years after diagnosis.
2. Measurement of plasma C-peptide, fasting and after a meal challenge, can be used to identify insulin resistance. This is usually not necessary because insulin resistance can be suspected on the basis of clinical features of the

insulin resistance syndrome (central obesity, acanthosis nigricans, hypertension, elevated plasma triglycerides, decreased plasma HDL cholesterol).
3. Most oral antidiabetic agents achieve their effects at two-thirds of the maximal dose recommended by the manufacturer. Giving maximal doses of single agents before adding a second agent is usually not cost-effective and frequently increases side effects.
4. The use of three different oral antidiabetic agents, although appealing on an intellectual basis, has few clinical data to validate it and may not be cost-effective. The data that are available indicate that adding the third oral agent rarely lowers the A1C to ≤7% if the A1C before adding the third agent is much above 8%.
5. If one oral antidiabetic agent does not lower glycemia to the target range, changing to a different oral agent rarely achieves better glycemic control. However, combining two oral agents with different modes of action will result in improved glycemic control.
6. Bedtime insulin and oral agents during the day are frequently as effective in achieving glycemic control as multiple injections of insulin in patients with type 2 diabetes.

BIBLIOGRAPHY

Aviles-Santa L, Sinding J, Raskin P: Effects of metformin in patients with poorly controlled, insulin-treated type 2 diabetes mellitus: a randomized, double-blind, placebo-controlled trial. *Ann Intern Med* 131:182–188, 1999

DeFronzo RA, Goodman AM: Efficacy of metformin in patients with non-insulin-dependent diabetes mellitus: the Multicenter Metformin Study Group. *N Engl J Med* 333:541–549, 1995

Fonseca V, Rosenstock J, Patwardhan R, Salzman A: Effect of metformin and rosiglitazone combination therapy in patients with type 2 diabetes mellitus: a randomized controlled trial. *JAMA* 283:1695–1702, 2000

Inzucchi SE, Maggs DG, Spollett GR, Page SL, Rife FS, Walton V, Shulman GI: Efficacy and metabolic effects of metformin and troglitazone in type 2 diabetes mellitus. *N Engl J Med* 338:867–872, 1998

Lebovitz HE: Alpha-glucosidase inhibitors as agents in the treatment of diabetes. *Diabetes Rev* 6:132–145, 1998

Lebovitz HE: Oral therapies for diabetic hyperglycemia. *Endocrinol Metab Clin North Am* 30:909–933, 2001

Lebovitz HE: Treating hyperglycemia in type 2 diabetes: new goals and strategies. *Cleve Clin J Med* 69:809–820, 2002

Raskin P, Rendell M, Riddle MC, Dole JF, Freed MI, Rosenstock J, for the Rosiglitazone Clinical Trials Study Group: A randomized trial of rosiglitazone therapy in patients with inadequately controlled insulin-treated type 2 diabetes. *Diabetes Care* 24:1226–1232, 2001

United Kingdom Prospective Diabetes Study Group: United Kingdom Prospective Diabetes Study 24: a 6-year, randomized, controlled trial comparing sulfonylurea, insulin and metformin therapy in patients with newly diagnosed type 2 diabetes that could not be controlled with diet therapy. *Ann Intern Med* 128:165–175, 1998

Yki-Jarvinen H, Dressler A, Zieman M, Study Group HOE 901/3002: Less nocturnal hypoglycemia and better post dinner glucose control with bedtime insulin glargine compared with bedtime NPH insulin during combination therapy in type 2 diabetes. *Diabetes Care* 23:1130–1136, 2001

Yki-Jarvinen H, Ryysy L, Kauppila M, Kujansuu E, Lahti J, Marjanen T, Niskanen L, Rajala S, Salo S, Seppala P, Tulokas T, Vükari J, Taskinen MR: Effect of obesity on the response to insulin therapy in non-insulin-dependent diabetes mellitus. *J Clin Endocrinol Metab* 82:4037–4043, 1997

Yki-Jarvinen H, Ryysy L, Nikkila K, Tulokas T, Vanamo R, Heikkila M: Comparison of bedtime insulin regimens in patients with type 2 diabetes mellitus: a randomized, controlled trial. *Ann Intern Med* 130:389–396, 1999

Dr. Lebovitz is Professor of Medicine at the State University of New York Health Science Center at Brooklyn, Brooklyn, NY.

27. Glycemic Control and Chronic Diabetes Complications

HAROLD E. LEBOVITZ, MD

O ur understanding of the relationship between glycemic control and the chronic complications of diabetes has been greatly enhanced by the results of several recent seminal intervention studies. Those studies demonstrated that microvascular complications are highly correlated with mean glycemic control, as measured by glycated hemoglobin A1C (A1C), and that improvement in glycemic control results in reduction in all microvascular complications. In contrast, they failed to show a significant reduction in macrovascular complications with improved glycemic control, suggesting that macrovascular complications are the result of multiple metabolic abnormalities. An unexpected result of the studies and their extensions is the remarkable finding that vascular tissues have a long memory of their previous glycemic control and that this influences the rate of development of complications for many future years. Table 27.1 lists some of the more noteworthy studies.

INTERVENTION STUDIES

The Diabetes Control and Complications Trial (DCCT) was both a primary and secondary intervention trial in patients with type 1 diabetes that tested the effects of intensive glycemic control versus ordinary glycemic control on the development or progression of microvascular and neuropathic complications. For the study, 1,441 patients were recruited and treated for an average of 6.5 years. Intensive treatment involved insulin injections three or four times per day or insulin pump therapy. Ordinary treatment was insulin injections one or two times per day. The glycemic control for the ordinary-treatment group over the 6.5 years of the study was a mean A1C of 9.1% and a daily average plasma glucose of 231 mg/dl (12.8 mmol/l) (nondiabetic values: A1C ≤6%, plasma glucose 110 mg/dl [6.1 mmol/l]). The intensively treated group maintained an A1C of 7.2% and a daily average plasma glucose of 155 mg/dl (8.6 mmol/l). The results of both the primary and secondary intervention arms showed that this degree of difference in glycemic control resulted in risk reductions of 63% for retinopathy, 60% for neuropathy, and 54% for nephropathy. Specific details of the results of this remarkable study are given in Tables 27.2 and 27.3. Intensive glycemic control was associated with a greater than threefold increase in severe hypoglycemia (62 vs. 19 episodes/100 patient-years) and a remarkable increase in body weight.

Table 27.1 Studies Demonstrating the Relationship Between Glycemic Control and Chronic Complications

	Diabetes Patients (*n*)	Data Reported
Intervention studies		
DCCT	1,441 type 1	1993
EDIC (follow-up of the DCCT)	1,229 type 1	Ongoing reports
Kumamoto study	110 Japanese type 2	1995
UKPDS	5,102 newly diagnosed type 2	1998
Epidemiologic studies		
Wisconsin	1,516	1994
Steno type 2 diabetes	328	1995
Finnish elderly study	229	1994

The Kumamoto study, a much smaller study carried out in 110 thin Japanese type 2 diabetes patients, with essentially the same protocol as the DCCT, showed similar results. Their ordinary-treatment group maintained an A1C of 9.4% and a fasting plasma glucose (FPG) of 164 mg/dl (9.1 mmol/l), and their intensively treated patients had a mean A1C of 7.1% and a mean FPG of 126 mg/dl (7 mmol/l). Their intensive-treatment patients had a risk reduction of 69% for retinopathy and 70% for nephropathy compared with their ordinary-treatment group.

The United Kingdom Prospective Diabetes Study (UKPDS) was designed primarily to assess the chronic effects of intensive glycemic control on the development of clinical microvascular and macrovascular complications in newly diagnosed type 2 diabetes patients. A secondary goal was to compare the outcomes of treatment with a first-generation sulfonylurea (chlorpropamide), a second-generation sulfonylurea (glyburide), and insulin to that of conventional (diet and exercise) treatment in non-overweight patients and the same treatments and metformin

Table 27.2 Results of Primary Prevention Study (DCCT)

Complication	Conventional Therapy (rate/100 patient-yr)	Intensive Therapy (rate/100 patient-yr)	Risk Reduction (%)
≥3-step sustained retinopathy	4.7	1.2	76
Urinary albumin excretion ≥40 mg/24 h	3.4	2.3	34
Clinical neuropathy at 5 yr	9.8	3.1	69

Table 27.3 Results of Secondary Intervention Study (DCCT)

Complication	Conventional Therapy (rate/100 patient-yr)	Intensive Therapy (rate/100 patient-yr)	Risk Reduction (%)
Laser treatment	2.3	0.9	56
Urinary albumin excretion ≥300 mg/24 h	1.4	0.6	56
Clinical neuropathy at 5 yr	16.1	7.0	57

treatment in overweight patients. A total of 5,102 newly diagnosed type 2 diabetes patients were recruited and initially treated for 3 months with a diet and an increased physical activity program. The 4,209 patients who were symptom free and had an FPG between 108 mg/dl (6.0 mmol/l) and 270 mg/dl (15 mmol/l) after the 3-month run-in were randomized to the various treatments. The mean duration of treatment was 11 years. The target glycemic goal was an FPG of 108 mg/dl (6.0 mmol/l). However, to evaluate both the individual treatments as well as intensive glycemic control, the researchers did not add additional therapies to the treatment regimens of the individual patients until the patients became symptomatic or the FPG exceeded 270 mg/dl (15 mmol/l). This conflict frequently interfered with the principle of obtaining early intensive glycemic management. Despite this shortcoming, the intensively treated patients (insulin and sulfonylurea treatments) had a median A1C during the study of 7.0% and the conventionally treated group had a median A1C of 7.9%. The 0.9% difference in the intensively treated patients resulted in a significant reduction in microvascular complications (Table 27.4).

Thus, it can be extrapolated from the intervention studies in both type 1 and type 2 diabetes patients that a 1% decrease in A1C reduces the risk of microvascular complications by ~30%.

Neither the DCCT nor the Kumamoto study had enough macrovascular events to determine the effects of glycemic control on the development or

Table 27.4 Results of Intensive Glycemic Control in the UKPDS

Complication	Risk Reduction	Statistical Significance (P)
Any diabetes-related endpoint	↓ 12%	0.029
Myocardial infarction	↓ 16%	0.052
Microvascular endpoints	↓ 25%	0.0099
Retinal photocoagulation	↓ 29%	0.0031
Cataract extraction	↓ 24%	0.046
Microalbuminuria at 12 yr	↓ 33%	<0.001

progression of macrovascular disease. Whereas the UKPDS had a 16% reduction in the risk of myocardial infarctions in the intensively treated group, this failed to achieve statistical significance. Therefore, both studies failed to demonstrate a clear benefit of intensive glycemic control in reducing macrovascular complications.

EPIDEMIOLOGIC STUDIES

Several epidemiologic studies suggest that glycemic control does influence both the number and severity of macrovascular events. For 10 years, the Wisconsin epidemiology study followed 682 individuals who had developed diabetes before the age of 30 years and 834 who developed diabetes after age 30 years.

The data showed that there was a progressive increase in mortality, development of ischemic heart disease, development of proteinuria, and progression of retinopathy in both groups of diabetes patients as the patients' HbA_1 values went from the lowest fourth (5.4–8.5%) to the highest fourth (11.6–20.8%) of the population. In 328 white type 2 diabetes patients followed for 5 years at Steno hospital in Denmark, cardiovascular mortality was two- to threefold greater in individuals who maintained an A1C >7.8% compared with those who maintained an A1C <7.8%. Similarly, in the Finnish elderly study reported by Kuusisto et al. (1994), cardiovascular events and mortality during a 3.5-year follow-up were five- to eightfold greater in type 2 diabetes patients who had an A1C >7% compared with those with an A1C <7%.

An analysis of the epidemiologic data from the UKPDS indicated that each 1% decrease in mean A1C of the entire study population was associated with a statistically significant 14% decrease in myocardial infarctions.

From currently available data, it is reasonable to conclude that microvascular and probably macrovascular complications in both type 1 and type 2 diabetes patients will increase as glycemic control worsens. Complications can be minimized at an A1C level of ≤7%. Our current criteria for the goals of glycemic control are based on the results of studies such as those discussed.

ADDITIONAL KEY FINDINGS FROM THE INTERVENTION STUDIES

Metformin Reduces Macrovascular Disease

An additional important finding in the UKPDS in the overweight cohort was that treatment with metformin significantly reduced myocardial infarctions and diabetes-related deaths (Table 27.5). These effects were not observed with insulin or sulfonylurea treatments, which gave the same reduction in A1C, compared with conventional treatment (0.6%), as metformin. These observations suggest that it is the effects of metformin on the metabolic syndrome that account for its benefits on macrovascular disease.

Table 27.5 Effects of Metformin Treatment in United Kingdom Prospective Diabetes Study Overweight Type 2 Diabetes Cohort

Complication	Risk Reduction	Statistical Significance (*P*)
Any diabetes-related endpoint	↓ 32%	0.0023
Diabetes-related deaths	↓ 42%	0.017
All-cause mortality	↓ 36%	0.011
Myocardial infarction	↓ 39%	0.01

Vascular Tissues Have a Memory for Previous Glycemic Control that Influences Complication Rates

In both the DCCT and the UKPDS, there was a long lag time between the establishment of intensive glycemic control and the observed decrease in microvascular complications. This time lag was 3–3.5 years in the DCCT and almost 9 years in the UKPDS. The corollary of the concept that the effects of poor glycemic control persist even after good control is established is that early intensive glycemic control protects the microvascular system against poor glycemic control for many years, and this was demonstrated in the Epidemiology of Diabetes Interventions and Complications (EDIC) study. The EDIC study is the long-term follow-up of DCCT cohort subjects after they return to community health providers. Within a year or two of returning to the community-based health care system, the glycemic control of the previously intensively treated cohort worsened from a mean A1C of 7.3% to 7.9%. The previous control group improved their A1C from 9.1% to 8.3%. For the next 5 years of follow-up, the two cohorts maintained equal glycemic control, with mean A1C levels of ~8.1%. Despite the same A1C, the previously

Table 27.6 Renal Disease at the Fifth and Sixth Yr of Follow-up in 1,298 Subjects in Epidemiology of Diabetes Interventions and Complications Study

	Conventional Therapy	Intensive Therapy
Development of microalbuminuria		
4 yr	11%	5%
5–6 yr	12.3%	4.5%
Development of albuminuria		
4 yr	5%	1%
	Risk reduction = 86%	
5–6 yr	Risk reduction = 84%	
Aggregate endpoint	17 (2.7%)	6 (0.9%)
Serum creatinine ≥2 mg/dl		
Chronic dialysis Rx		
Renal transplantation		

intensively treated cohort developed retinopathy and nephropathy at statistically significantly lower rates than the previous control cohort (Table 27.6), indicating that the protective effect of early intensive glycemic control lasts for many years. These observations emphasize that aggressive early treatment of glycemia in patients with diabetes provides the maximal protection against chronic microvascular complications.

BIBLIOGRAPHY

DCCT Research Group: The effect of intensive treatment of diabetes on the development and progression of long-term complications in IDDM. *N Engl J Med* 329:977–986, 1993

DCCT Research Group: Effect of intensive therapy on the microvascular complications of type 1 diabetes mellitus. *JAMA* 287:2563–2567, 2002

Gall MA, Borch-Johnsen K, Hougaard R, Nielsen FS, Parving HH: Albuminuria and poor glycemic control predict mortality in NIDDM. *Diabetes* 44:1303–1309, 1995

Klein R: Hyperglycemia and microvascular and macrovascular disease in diabetes: Kelly West Lecture 1994. *Diabetes Care* 18:258–268, 1995

Kuusisto J, Mykkanen L, Pyorala K, Laakso M: NIDDM and its metabolic control predict coronary heart disease in elderly subjects. *Diabetes* 43:960–967, 1994

Ohkubo Y, Kishikawa H, Araki E, Mirata T, Isami S, Motoyoshi S, Kojima Y, Furuyoshi N, Shichiri M: Intensive insulin therapy prevents the progression of diabetic microvascular complications in Japanese patients with non-insulin-dependent diabetes mellitus: a randomized prospective 6-year study. *Diabetes Res Clin Pract* 28:103–117, 1995

Turner R, Cull C, Holman R: United Kingdom Prospective Diabetes Study 17: a 9-year update of a randomized, controlled trial on the effect of improved metabolic control on complications in non-insulin-dependent diabetes mellitus. *Ann Intern Med* 124:136–145, 1996

UK Prospective Diabetes Study Group: Intensive blood-glucose control with sulphonylureas or insulin compared with conventional treatment and risk of complications in patients with type 2 diabetes (UKPDS 33). *Lancet* 352:837–853, 1998

UK Prospective Diabetes Study Group: Effect of intensive blood glucose control with metformin on complications in overweight patients with type 2 diabetes (UKPDS 34). *Lancet* 352:854–865, 1998

Dr. Lebovitz is Professor of Medicine at the State University of New York Health Science Center at Brooklyn, Brooklyn, NY.

28. Surgery and Anesthesia

LARISSA AVILÉS-SANTA, MD, AND PHILIP RASKIN, MD

Approximately 50% of all patients with diabetes will undergo surgery at least once in their lifetime. The types of surgery performed are usually influenced by the presence of long-term diabetes complications, including amputations, ulcer debridement, and renal transplantation. However, patients with diabetes are also subject to the same types of surgery performed on patients without diabetes, such as cardiothoracic, peripheral vascular, and ophthalmologic procedures. Approximately 17% of all diabetes patients who undergo surgery will have some type of complication, the most common being postsurgical infections and cardiovascular complications (Table 28.1). Therefore, a thorough assessment of the patient's actual metabolic status and glycemic control, the cardiovascular status, and the presence of underlying complications related to diabetes (e.g., neuropathy and nephropathy) in the preoperative period is necessary to predict or prevent certain adverse events.

PATHOPHYSIOLOGY

Several factors that predispose diabetes patients to metabolic decompensation include the patient's insulin reserve, endocrine response to surgical stress, volume status (particularly dehydration), and the need to be fasting.

During anesthesia and surgery, there is an increase in the plasma concentration of counterregulatory hormones (Table 28.2). An elevation in the levels of glucagon, catecholamines, cortisol, and growth hormone is observed in individuals with and without diabetes. Increased secretion of these hormones leads to a marked increase in hepatic glucose production (due to both glycogenolysis and gluconeogenesis), a decrease in insulin-mediated glucose uptake, increased lipolysis with elevated levels of nonesterified fatty acids, and decreased insulin secretion. In nondiabetic individuals, major surgery is frequently associated with elevations in blood glucose into the range of 150–200 mg/dl (8.3–11.1 mmol/l). In individuals with diabetes, insulin secretion is impaired; thus, in the presence of a major surgical stress, severe hyperglycemia with or without ketosis can occur unless adequate insulin replacement is provided. The severity of the metabolic abnormality is proportional to the extent and duration of the surgical procedure and the impairment of insulin secretion. Because surgical patients are always fasting, administration of insulin will cause hypoglycemia if an adequate and constant source of carbohydrate is not available.

Table 28.1 Complications of Diabetes During Surgery, Anesthesia, and Postoperative Periods

Metabolic
  Diabetic ketoacidosis
  Nonketotic hyperosmolar states
  Hypoglycemia
  Hyperkalemia
  Hypokalemia

Cardiovascular
  Hypotension (related to autonomic diabetic neuropathy)

Arrhythmia
  Postoperative myocardial infarction
  Other thrombotic phenomena

Renal
  Acute kidney failure
  Volume overload

Infections

Other perioperative complications often faced by diabetes patients include myocardial ischemia and infarction, cerebrovascular accidents, fluid and electrolytic abnormalities, hemodynamic abnormalities during anesthesia, and impaired healing and infection of surgical wounds.

Depending on the surgical procedure and its duration, life-support measures and instrumentation, and the type of anesthesia and anesthetic agent used, cardiac output and peripheral vascular resistance will temporarily change. This can lead to

Table 28.2 Endocrine and Metabolic Response to Surgery in Patients with Diabetes

Endocrine
  Increased secretion of counterregulatory hormones
  Decreased insulin secretion
  Decreased insulin action

Metabolic
  Hyperglycemia
  Ketosis or ketone body formation
  General increase in metabolic rate and catabolism

Others
  Dehydration: intravascular and extravascular volume depletion
  Electrolytic imbalance
  Impaired wound healing and decreased resistance to infection secondary to
    hyperglycemia

blood pressure and heart rate changes, which could precipitate or aggravate underlying myocardial and coronary disease, sometimes occult or asymptomatic in some individuals with diabetes. The risks of postoperative cardiovascular complications become more evident in individuals with known coronary or peripheral arterial disease and cardiomyopathy. Autonomic neuropathy can cause severe hypotension during the induction of anesthesia, and its presence should be evaluated before any procedure involving general and/or spinal anesthesia. The anesthesiologist must be informed about the findings of the autonomic nervous system evaluation.

Intravascular and extravascular fluid status will influence the sudden shifts in volume status and electrolytic changes experienced during acute stress associated with surgery. Hyperglycemia, whether chronic or acute, is almost always associated with intravascular fluid depletion, which in turn can alter cardiac output and peripheral vascular resistance. If not corrected, volume depletion can contribute to increased morbidity during the perioperative period. Diabetic nephropathy, with or without proteinuria, makes fluid and electrolyte management difficult, and the use of intravenous fluids, vasopressors, vasodilators, and diuretics must be carefully planned.

Chronic hyperglycemia has been associated with delayed wound healing as a consequence of inadequate collagen repair and remodeling. In addition, because of impaired leukocyte chemotaxis and defective immune defense mechanisms, infections at surgical sites are common. This picture becomes more complicated by underlying poor nutrition, which many poorly controlled diabetic individuals suffer, therefore impairing healing even further.

EVALUATION OF DIABETES PATIENTS BEFORE SURGERY

Metabolic Control

The degree of metabolic control should be evaluated before surgery, and attempts should be made to improve poor control on an outpatient basis before elective procedures. Chronically hyperglycemic patients are frequently dehydrated. Dehydration can be accompanied by electrolytic abnormalities, particularly sodium and potassium loss, and by intravascular volume depletion, with subsequent hemodynamic imbalance. Admission to the hospital to optimize metabolic control 12–16 h before elective procedures is recommended for all patients with type 1 diabetes and those with type 2 diabetes who have inadequate metabolic control. A stabilization period of 12–16 h is also recommended for semi-urgent procedures if severe hyperglycemia is present, although, given the current problems with third-party carriers and reimbursement, this may be difficult. In patients with severe metabolic derangements (diabetic ketoacidosis or hyperosmolar nonketotic states) who need urgent surgical intervention, 6–8 h of intensive treatment usually improves the general condition of the patient. This period also allows clarification of the diagnosis in cases of acute abdominal pain that could be the consequence of diabetic ketoacidosis rather than a surgical abdomen.

Correction of chronic hyperglycemia and assessment of nutritional status before surgery or immediately after surgery will supplement benefits from increased protein and caloric intake to improve collagen formation and healing. In addition, depending on other coexistent medical conditions (e.g., obstructive pulmonary disease or chronic renal insufficiency), specific nutritional needs may need to be addressed.

Cardiovascular Status

Atherosclerotic heart disease is highly prevalent in the diabetes population, especially in individuals with type 2 diabetes. Most of the time, long-standing diabetes is accompanied by arterial hypertension and dyslipidemia, increasing the risk of ischemia, myocardial infarction, and cerebrovascular accidents during the perioperative period. A preoperative assessment and evaluation of risk factors for coronary artery disease is crucial, with special attention to the patient without symptoms, because the risk of silent ischemia is present.

The risk of cardiovascular complications should be stratified depending on the urgency (elective versus emergent) and type of procedure (cardiac versus noncardiac) to determine the need for preoperative testing. Recent cardiovascular history, physical examination, and electrocardiographic findings generally provide sufficient information to determine risks. Further tests to estimate functional capacity and rule out (and treat) coronary disease may be needed in individuals with a positive cardiovascular review of systems and unstable coronary syndromes.

Well-controlled hypertension does not pose a major risk to surgery, but patients receiving β-blockers may develop hypoglycemia without warning symptoms and should be monitored accordingly. Type 1 diabetes patients receiving β-blockers are also at a greater risk for prolonged episodes of insulin-induced hypoglycemia. Diabetes patients have increased thrombotic risk. Antithrombotic therapy (including unfractionated or low-weight heparin, anti-embolic graduated pressure stockings, and ambulation) should be considered unless specifically contraindicated during the period the patient is confined to bed.

The use of vasopressors for the treatment of severe hypotension associated with sepsis or extreme intravascular volume loss has been associated with remarkable peripheral vasoconstriction. Patients with poor peripheral pulses and who require high doses of vasopressors during the course of a critical illness are at risk of gangrene of the digits. Vasopressors, however, should not be restricted or halted if their benefits outweigh the risk of amputation.

Neurological Status

Disordered gastrointestinal motility may increase the risk of aspiration and may delay the resumption of enteral feeding. In addition, general anesthesia may cause nausea and vomiting. Bladder dysfunction may lead to urinary retention and subsequent obstructive uropathy and fluid overload. Urinary retention due to decreased bladder contractility has been observed with the use of narcotics for pain management. Therefore, if a patient has evidence of either gastrointestinal dysmotility or bladder dysfunction, with the use of anti-emetic and/or narcotic analgesic agents, careful monitoring of fluid intake and urinary output should be addressed before and after surgery. As mentioned before, the anesthesiologist should be alerted to the presence of orthostatic blood pressure changes associated with advanced neuropathy to predict possible hemodynamic changes during anesthesia induction.

Renal Function

Measurement of blood urea nitrogen, serum creatinine, electrolytes, and proteinuria should be performed before surgery. Azotemic patients may have problems with fluid management, and monitoring of central venous or pulmonary artery wedge pressure may be necessary. Hyperkalemia with or without hyponatremia is often seen in patients with mild to moderate renal insufficiency, and hyperkalemia can precipitate an acute cardiac arrhythmia. This metabolic finding often results from diabetic autonomic neuropathy and hyporeninemic hypoaldosteronism. Hypokalemia may be present, and insulin and glucose infusion therapy may aggravate this condition. Proteinuria, with resulting hypoalbuminemia, can cause extravasation of fluid to the interstitial space, therefore potentiating problems with intravascular volume, cardiac output, and alveolar oxygen exchange. Depending on the severity of proteinuria, the combination of diuretics, fluid restriction, hemodialysis, or ultrafiltration will be necessary for stabilization of intravascular volume status.

METABOLIC MANAGEMENT AND MONITORING

Insulin and Glucose Administration During Surgery

The use of an insulin and glucose infusion is recommended for all type 1 diabetes patients, insulin-treated type 2 diabetes patients, and poorly controlled drug- or diet-treated type 2 diabetes patients who are undergoing general anesthesia, regardless of the planned duration of the surgical procedure. Several methods of insulin administration during the perioperative period are recommended. Most of the protocols include the intravenous administration of short-acting insulin and 5–10% glucose solution. Subcutaneous administration of insulin is associated with unpredictable absorption and variable plasma insulin levels and is not recommended for surgical patients except for those undergoing minor procedures. In some of the protocols with intravenous insulin, the glucose and insulin are contained in the same infusion mixture. The theoretical advantage of this approach is that, if the glucose infusion is accidentally disconnected or obstructed, so is the insulin infusion, avoiding the risk of hypoglycemia. The disadvantage of this method is that no flexibility is allowed for changes in the delivery rate of either insulin or glucose infusion.

Another approach is to administer insulin and glucose in separate bags but through the same vein, i.e., to piggyback the insulin infusion onto the glucose infusion. This allows independent adjustments to each infusion according to the levels of hourly capillary blood glucose measurements. An example of such a protocol is shown in Table 28.3. With this protocol, a blood glucose level in the range of 100–125 mg/dl (5.6–6.9 mmol/l) is easily maintained during the entire perioperative period. As with every therapeutic protocol, clinical judgment must be used. Depending on the individual patient, increases or decreases in the rate of insulin or glucose infusion for a given capillary blood glucose range may be necessary. Electrolyte solutions are administered as needed into the glucose infusion or with a separate infusion as needed. In patients with azotemia or other problems with fluid

Table 28.3 Representative Protocol for Insulin-Glucose Infusion for Perioperative Periods

1. Discontinue all subcutaneous insulin after initiation of glucose-insulin infusion.
2. Measure capillary blood glucose levels at 1-h intervals.
3. Infuse 5% dextrose (D_5W) intravenously via infusion pump.
4. Make insulin solution with 0.5 units/ml short-acting insulin (i.e., 250 units regular insulin in 500 ml normal saline). Give piggyback via infusion pump into D_5W infusion.
5. Based on hourly blood glucose determination, adjust each infusion according to the following schedule:

Blood Glucose		Insulin Infusion		
mg/dl	mmol/l	ml/h	units/h	D_5W Infusion (ml/h)
≤70*	<3.9	1.0	0.5	150
71–100	3.9–5.6	2.0	1.0	125
101–150	5.6–8.3	3.0	1.5	100
151–200	8.3–11.1	4.0	2.0	75
201–250	11.1–13.9	6.0	3.0	50
251–300	13.9–16.7	8.0	4.0	0
≥300	≥16.7	12.0	6.0	0

Modified from Rosenstock and Raskin.
*Give 10 ml $D_{50}W$ intravenously and repeat blood glucose measurement 15 min later.

management or those receiving large amounts of other solutions, 10% dextrose ($D_{10}W$) can be substituted for the 5% dextrose (D_5W) solution. If $D_{10}W$ is not available, it can be made easily by adding 100 g 50% dextrose ($D_{50}W$) to 1,000 ml D_5W.

Patients with severe fluid management problems, e.g., those with congestive heart failure or end-stage renal disease, may not tolerate the amounts of fluids administered with either a D_5W or $D_{10}W$ infusion. Thus, to provide an adequate carbohydrate supply, $D_{50}W$ must be administered through a central venous line. Table 28.4 shows a protocol for diabetes patients who are at high risk for fluid overload. Again, clinical judgment dictates individual changes in the protocol as necessary.

Patients undergoing coronary artery bypass graft surgery and/or cardiopulmonary bypass often require higher doses of insulin to achieve glycemic control during the perioperative period. Intensive glycemic control using intravenous insulin and dextrose solution during the perioperative period and during the subacute phase of myocardial infarction has been shown to improve cardiovascular morbidity and mortality as well as general postoperative outcome in diabetes patients. Therefore, its use should be encouraged both during and after surgery, and treatment goals should approach blood glucose levels of 100–125 mg/dl (5.6–6.9 mmol/l).

The blood glucose level must be monitored at hourly intervals. Capillary blood glucose measurements taken in the operating and recovery rooms with bedside glucose monitoring devices are adequate for perioperative management. Hourly measurements are necessary to keep the blood glucose level between 100

Table 28.4 Protocol for Insulin-Glucose Infusion for Perioperative Patients at Risk of Volume Overload

1. Discontinue all subcutaneous insulin after initiation of glucose-insulin infusion.
2. Measure capillary blood glucose levels at 1-h intervals.
3. Infuse 50% dextrose ($D_{50}W$) intravenously into central venous line via infusion pump.
4. Make insulin solution with 0.5 units/ml short-acting insulin (i.e., 250 units regular insulin in 500 ml normal saline). Give piggyback via infusion pump into $D_{50}W$ infusion.
5. Based on hourly blood glucose determination, adjust each infusion according to following schedule:

Blood Glucose		Insulin Infusion		
mg/dl	mmol/l	ml/h	units/h	$D_{50}W$ Infusion (ml/h)
≤70*	<3.9	1.0	0.5	25
71–100	3.9–5.6	2.0	1.0	22
101–150	5.6–8.3	4.0	2.0	20
151–200	8.3–11.1	6.0	3.0	17
201–250	11.1–13.9	8.0	4.0	12
251–300	13.9–16.7	10.0	5.0	0
≥300	>16.7	12.0	6.0	0

*Give 10 ml $D_{50}W$ intravenously and repeat blood glucose measurement 15 min later.

and 125 mg/dl (5.6 and 6.9 mmol/l) and to ensure safety should the glucose infusion inadvertently be discontinued.

The management of stable diabetes patients undergoing minor procedures (e.g., endoscopic techniques or surgery performed under local anesthesia) involves withholding the morning dose of insulin or oral agent if the patient is going to be fasting and measuring capillary blood glucose every 2–4 h. Type 1 diabetes patients should not have insulin withheld. Depending on the individual, taking either one-third or one-half of the intermediate-acting insulin usually taken in the morning is a potential alternative. Also, supplemental subcutaneous short-acting insulin can be administered following a variable insulin schedule, and the patient's usual insulin dosage or oral agent can be resumed after surgery when the patient can eat (Table 28.5). However, if the period of time that the patient must wait to go to surgery is unknown, then it would be prudent to use the insulin-glucose infusion instead. In critically ill patients or those who have undergone emergency surgery, insulin therapy can be continued after surgery for better stabilization of glucose levels.

Postoperative Metabolic Management

The glucose and insulin infusion should be continued until the metabolic condition is stable and the patient is able to tolerate oral feeding. The insulin and glucose infusions should not be stopped until 1–2 h after the administration of

Table 28.5 Diabetes Management During Minor Surgical Procedures

Day of procedure (if patient NPO)
1. Withhold morning dose of insulin or oral agent.
2. Measure capillary blood glucose level before procedure and every 2–4 h.
3. Give short- or fast-acting insulin subcutaneously every 2–4 h as follows:

Blood Glucose		
mg/dl	mmol/l	Short- or Fast-Acting Insulin (units)
≤150	≤5.6	0
151–200	5.6–11.1	2
201–250	11.1–13.9	3
251–300	13.9–16.7	5
≥300	≥16.7	6

4. Give usual afternoon insulin or oral agent dose.

Day of procedure (if breakfast allowed)
1. Give normal morning dose of insulin or oral agent.
2. Measure blood glucose levels before and after procedure.
3. Give supplemental 4 units of short- or fast-acting insulin subcutaneously if blood glucose >250 mg/dl.
4. Give usual afternoon insulin or oral agent dose.

Modified from Rosenstock and Raskin.

subcutaneous insulin. After major surgery, the glucose and insulin infusions should be continued until the patient is able to eat solid food without difficulty. In these patients, the use of multiple subcutaneous injections of short-acting insulin before meals and intermediate- or long-acting insulin at bedtime is recommended during the first 24–48 h after the insulin and glucose infusions are stopped and before the patient's usual insulin regimen is resumed. Table 28.6 shows an example of such an insulin injection schedule. If a patient had been taking a long-acting insulin (such as insulin glargine) before surgery, we recommend stopping the insulin-glucose infusion 1–2 h after resuming the long-acting insulin to avoid hyperglycemia due to a lack of basal insulin.

Depending on the type of procedure, some patients will require continuous enteral nutrition. In these cases, we recommend multiple short-acting insulin injections, for example, every 6 h. Because the patient is receiving food continuously, the risk of hypoglycemia is low. Intermediate- or long-acting insulin should be used with caution, because hypoglycemia may take place in the case of sudden or inadvertent removal of the enteral tube.

The use of total parenteral nutrition (TPN) is frequently required in the postoperative period. Diabetes patients can develop serious metabolic derangements with TPN. A variable insulin infusion schedule (similar to that shown in Table 28.3) with hourly determinations of blood glucose is also recommended under these circumstances, but additional glucose infusion is not required because it is contained within the TPN solution. Initially, the insulin should be given as a separate continuous infusion from the TPN solution. Once a stable dose of insulin

Table 28.6 Postoperative Diabetes Management When Patient Tolerates Solid Food

1. Do not discontinue intravenous insulin-glucose infusion until after first subcutaneous insulin is administered.
2. Measure capillary blood glucose before meals, at 10:00 p.m., and at 3:00 a.m.*
3. Provide three meals and three snacks (20–30 kcal/kg/day).
4. Administer preprandial short- or fast-acting insulin subcutaneously according to the following variable insulin dosage schedule:

Blood Glucose		Short- or Fast-Acting Insulin (units)			
(mg/dl)	mmol/l	Breakfast	Lunch	Dinner	10:00 p.m.
≤70	<3.9	3	2	2	0
71–100	3.9–5.6	4	3	3	0
101–150	5.6–8.3	6	4	4	0
151–200	8.3–11.1	8	6	6	0
201–250	11.1–13.9	10	8	8	1
251–300	13.9–16.7	12	10	10	2
≥300	≥16.7	14	12	12	3

5. Administer intermediate- or long-acting insulin 10–20 units subcutaneously at 10:00 p.m.

Modified from Rosenstock and Raskin. *If hypoglycemia is present at 3:00 a.m., reduce the 10:00 p.m. insulin dose.

is ascertained (often within 12–24 h), the total amount of insulin required over 24 h can be added to the TPN bag, and the frequency of the capillary blood glucose measurements can be reduced to every 2–4 h. The doses of insulin needed during TPN can be high and are often >100 units in 24 h, depending on the patient's metabolic status and insulin sensitivity.

Postoperative Cardiovascular Evaluation

Serial postoperative electrocardiograms are recommended for older diabetes patients, patients with long-standing type 1 diabetes, and patients with known heart disease. Postoperative myocardial infarction may be silent and has a high mortality. Intravascular fluid and wedge pressure monitoring after surgery might be necessary in some patients with cardiomyopathy depending on the procedure performed. When ambulation of the patient begins, attention must be paid to the possibility of orthostatic hypotension. Evaluation and reevaluation of the mental and neurological status will help to assess changes associated with possible embolism of unstable carotid or aortic plaques after instrumentation during heart surgery.

Early ambulation should be encouraged, depending on the type of surgical procedure. If ambulation is not allowed or is not possible, antithrombotic measures should be instituted soon after surgery.

Postoperative Renal Evaluation

Careful monitoring of blood urea nitrogen and serum creatinine levels will help to detect acute kidney failure that may occur, especially after procedures with iodinated contrast material. If contrast material is to be used, the patient should be well hydrated before and after the procedure. Patients on metformin should be advised to withhold this medication 2 days before receiving intravenous contrast and resume metformin 3 days after the test is performed.

Postoperative Infection

Wound infections are common among diabetes patients with poor metabolic control. Fever may not always be present, so warning signs can be subtle, followed by a precipitous course. Impaired granulocyte function due to hyperglycemia may predispose the patient to bacterial infections. Poor circulation due to macroangiopathy or microangiopathy can also contribute to postoperative infection. Tight metabolic control during the perioperative period can decrease the risk of postoperative infection and improve the postoperative outcome.

Wound infections in individuals with diabetes are usually caused by mixed flora, and antibiotic coverage must include coverage for anaerobic bacteria, gram-negative enteric bacteria, and *Staphylococcus aureus*. If surgical debridement and drainage is needed, it should be performed early. Cultures should be obtained during drainage procedures and before antibiotic therapy is started. In patients with severe infections that are not responding to antibiotic therapy, *Candida* species or other fungal species should be suspected.

In addition to surgical wounds, other sources of infection during the postoperative period include intravenous catheter insertion sites, pressure and decubitus ulcers, nasopharynx (due to nasotracheal or orotracheal tubes for ventilatory support or nasotracheal tubes for feeding purposes), and urinary catheterization. Blood and urine cultures, chest radiography, removal or replacement of intravenous catheters, and cultures of the catheter tips should be performed if the infection focus cannot be easily identified. Guidelines for prevention of decubitus ulcers and replacement of intravenous lines should be followed to prevent infections in those sites.

The elderly and poorly nourished patients of all ages are at a higher risk of developing pressure ulcers after just a few hours of bed confinement. Prevention of pressure ulcers and maintenance of skin integrity should be established as soon as possible.

SUMMARY

Cardiovascular complications and infections are the most common complications patients with diabetes experience after surgery. A thorough history and physical evaluation will help to determine the presence of potential long-term diabetes complications that could influence the postoperative outcome. Glycemic, metabolic, and nutritional status and cardiovascular, neurological, and renal function should be evaluated and optimized, if possible, before surgery. Cardiovascular, hemodynamic, and intravascular volume status should be carefully monitored during and after surgery, and normoglycemia should be achieved and maintained during surgery and recovery. Depending on the procedure and coexistent physical conditions, further guidelines for prevention of infections and other postoperative complications should be addressed.

BIBLIOGRAPHY

Babineau TJ, Bothe A: General surgery considerations in the diabetic patient. *Infect Dis Clin North Am* 9:183–193, 1995

Burgos LG, Ebert TJ, Asiddas C, Turner LA, Pattison CZ, Wang-Cheng R, Kamysine JP: Increased intraoperative cardiovascular morbidity in diabetics with autonomic neuropathy. *Anesthesiology* 70:591–597, 1989

Caruso M, Orszulak TA, Miles JM: Lactic acidosis and insulin resistance associated with epinephrine administration in a patient with non insulin-dependent diabetes mellitus. *Arch Intern Med* 147:1422–1424, 1987

Dean D, Burchard KW: Fungal infections in surgical patients. *Am J Surg* 171:374–382, 1996

Furnary AP, Zerr KJ, Grunkemeier GL, Starr A: Continuous intravenous insulin infusion reduces the incidence of deep sternal wound infection in diabetic patients after cardiac surgical procedures. *Ann Thorac Surg* 67:352–362, 1999

Gavin LA: Perioperative management of the diabetic patient. *Endocrinol Metab Clin North Am* 21:457–475, 1992

Hirsch IB, McGill JB: Role of insulin in management of surgical patients with diabetes mellitus. *Diabetes Care* 13:980–991, 1990

Hollenberg SM: Preoperative cardiac risk assessment. *Chest* 115:51S–57S, 1999

Jeejeebhoy KN: Total parenteral nutrition: potion or poison? *Am J Clin Nutr* 74:160–163, 2001

John R, Choudhri AF, Weinberg AD, Ting W, Rose EA, Smith CR, Oz MC: Multicenter review of preoperative risk factors for stroke after coronary artery bypass grafting. *Ann Thorac Surg* 69:30–36, 2000

Lazar HL, Fitzgerald C, Gross C, Heeren T, Aldea GS, Shemin RJ: Determinants of length of stay after coronary artery bypass graft surgery. *Circulation* 92 (Suppl. 9):II20–II24, 1995

Leppo JA: Preoperative cardiac risk assessment of noncardiac surgery. *Am J Cardiol* 75:42D–51D, 1995

Malmberg K: Prospective randomized study of intensive insulin treatment on long term survival after acute myocardial infarction in patients with diabetes mellitus. *Br Med J* 314:1512–1515, 1997

Malmberg K, Norhammar A, Wedel H, Rydén L: Glycometabolic state at admission: important risk marker of mortality in conventionally treated patients with diabetes mellitus and acute myocardial infarction: long term results from the Diabetes and Insulin-Glucose Infusion in Acute Myocardial Infarction (DIGAMI) Study. *Circulation* 99:2626–2632, 1999

Malmberg K, Rydén L, Efendic S, Herlitz, Nicol P, Waldenstrom A, Wedel H, Welin L: Randomized trial of insulin-glucose infusion followed by subcutaneous insulin treatment in diabetic patients with acute myocardial infarction (DIGAMI Study): effects on mortality at 1 year. *J Am Coll Cardiol* 26:57–65, 1999

Malmberg K, Rydén L, Hamsten A, Herlitz J, Waldenstrom A, Wedel H: Mortality prediction in diabetic patients with myocardial infarction: experiences from the DIGAMI Study. *Cardiovasc Res* 34:248–253, 1997

Rosenberg CS: Wound healing in the patient with diabetes mellitus. *Nurs Clin North Am* 25:247–261, 1990

Rosenstock J, Raskin P: Surgery! Practical guidelines for diabetes management. *Clinical Diabetes* 5:49–61, 1987

Schade DS: Surgery and diabetes. *Med Clin North Am* 72:1531–1543, 1988

van den Berghe G, Wouters P, Weekers F, Verwaest C, Bruyninckx F, Schetz M, Vlasselaers D, Ferdinande P, Lauwers P, Bouillon R: Intensive insulin therapy in critically ill patients. *N Engl J Med* 345:1359–1367, 2001

Zerr KJ, Furnary AP, Grunkemeier GL, Bookin S, Kanhere V, Starr A: Glucose control lowers the risk of wound infection in diabetics after open heart operations. *Ann Thorac Surg* 63:356–361, 1997

Dr. Avilés-Santa is Assistant Professor of Internal Medicine and Dr. Raskin is Professor of Internal Medicine at the University of Texas Southwestern Medical Center at Dallas, Dallas, TX.

29. Geriatric Patients

JEFFREY B. HALTER, MD

D iabetes mellitus is an important health problem among the elderly population. The dramatic age-related increase in the prevalence rate of diabetes
mellitus is demonstrated in Fig. 29.1, indicating that >10% of people in
the U.S. >60 years of age have been diagnosed with diabetes. An equal number of
elderly people meet current American Diabetes Association criteria for diabetes
but are not aware that they have diabetes. Thus, the total prevalence rate of diabetes in elderly adults is ~25%. The rapid growth of the U.S. aging population
suggests that there will be continued growth in the number of elderly people
with diabetes mellitus. Hyperglycemia in elderly people is not a benign condition because it is associated with risk for long-term diabetes complications. Thus,
the management of hyperglycemia in an elderly patient with diabetes mellitus
should be considered seriously.

PATHOPHYSIOLOGY AND RATIONALE FOR TREATMENT

Most elderly people with diabetes mellitus have type 2 diabetes mellitus. The
pathogenesis of type 2 diabetes in this group is similar to that in other age-groups.
Many factors may contribute to the high rate of development of type 2 diabetes
in elderly patients (Fig. 29.2). Age-related impairments of both pancreatic β-cell
function and insulin action appear to be important factors in the pathophysiology of hyperglycemia in elderly people with diabetes mellitus. An age-related
increase in body adiposity and a decrease in physical activity both contribute to the
insulin resistance during aging. In addition, the prevalence of coexisting illnesses
and use of various drugs may contribute to the development of hyperglycemia.

The short-term risks of poor diabetes control for elderly patients merit intervention. Marked hyperglycemia associated with glucosuria and weight loss is a
catabolic state that predisposes the patient with diabetes to various acute illnesses,
particularly infections. The most extreme example of poor diabetes control among
elderly patients is the syndrome of hyperosmolar coma, which is associated with
a high mortality rate and requires aggressive intervention (see Chapter 26).

Elderly patients are also at risk for many long-term complications. This risk may
not be simply a function of known duration of diabetes, because the patient is likely
to have had asymptomatic undetected hyperglycemia for years before the initial
diagnosis was made. Older patients with diabetes mellitus have an approximately

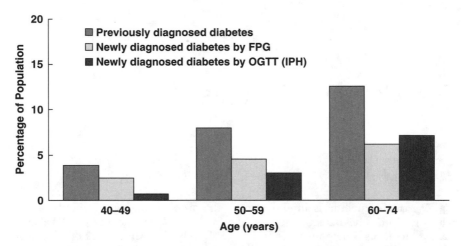

Figure 29.1 Prevalence of type 2 diabetes among elderly people according to age and American Diabetes Association diagnostic criteria (the Third National Health and Nutrition Examination Survey). FPG, fasting plasma glucose; IPH, isolated postchallenge hyperglycemia; OGTT, oral glucose tolerance test. Adapted from Harris et al. 1998 and Resnick et al. 2000.

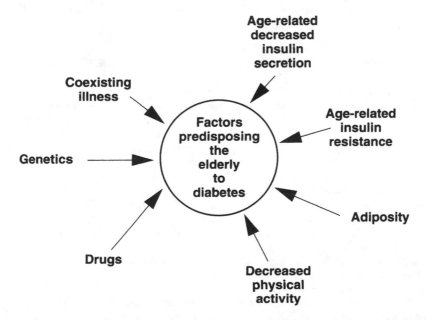

Figure 29.2 Factors predisposing elderly people to the development of diabetes mellitus. From Halter 1990.

twofold increased risk for myocardial infarction, stroke, and renal insufficiency than patients of the same age without diabetes. The risk for amputation in an elderly patient with diabetes is increased almost 10-fold.

THERAPY

General Approach to Management

The overall treatment goals of a basic diabetes care plan for an elderly patient are to prevent metabolic decompensation and to control other factors that may contribute to the high risk of cardiovascular complications in such a patient. This chapter focuses on control of hyperglycemia, a goal that should be part of an overall strategy of risk reduction. Such a strategy must also include intensive effort at identifying and controlling hypertension, lipid disorders, and cigarette smoking (see Chapters 33 and 34). Thus, a complex, multifaceted treatment program may be needed for many elderly patients with diabetes.

Severe symptomatic hyperglycemia must be treated to control excessive fatty acid mobilization and oxidation, excessive protein catabolism and muscle wasting, excessive glucose production, and urinary loss of calories in the form of glucose. Development of a rational long-term treatment plan for hyperglycemia in an elderly (>65 years old) diabetic patient must take into consideration *1*) remaining life expectancy, *2*) presence of diabetes complications, *3*) presence of coexisting medical or neuropsychiatric disorders, and *4*) the patient's ability and willingness to comply with the proposed diabetes treatment program (Table 29.1). In a healthy 70-year-old individual without associated medical problems or diabetes complications in whom a reasonable life expectancy (10–20 years or more) is anticipated, the physician should strive for the best possible glycemic control without predisposing the individual to the unnecessary risks of hypoglycemia. One approach is to strive for a fasting glucose level of 100–120 mg/dl (5.6–6.7 mmol/l), a postprandial glucose level of 160 mg/dl (9 mmol/l), and a glycated hemoglobin value within 1% of the upper limit of normal. Unfortunately, such targets are not often achieved in elderly patients.

Table 29.1 Important Factors to Consider for Diabetes Management in Elderly Patients

- The patient's remaining life expectancy
- Patient commitment
- Availability of support services
- Economic issues
- Coexisting health problems
  - □ Psychiatric or cognitive disorder
  - □ Other medical problems
  - □ Diabetes complications
  - □ Major limitation of diabetes functional status
- Complexity of medical regimen

In elderly diabetic patients with advanced microvascular complications (especially diabetic nephropathy and retinopathy), the likelihood of ameliorating their progression may be less. Therefore, more conservative therapeutic targets (e.g., fasting glucose <140 mg/dl [<7.8 mmol/l] and a postprandial glucose of 200–240 mg/dl [11.1–13.3 mmol/l]) may be more prudent. Elderly diabetes patients with serious associated medical problems, especially cardiovascular or cerebrovascular, should be treated in a manner similar to patients with advanced diabetes complications. A less aggressive approach is also advocated in patients with a major cognitive disorder, neuropsychiatric disorders, or a demonstrated inability to comply with the proposed therapeutic regimen.

Once a therapeutic goal for glycemic control has been established, an orderly approach to treatment, including diet, exercise, oral agents, and insulin, should be developed as described in Chapters 16, 18, 20, and 24.

Nutrition Therapy

Dietary intervention as a primary mode of diabetes management should be considered first for an overweight elderly person because of the potential effectiveness of weight reduction and its relative safety (see Chapter 16). Even a modest amount of weight reduction in an obese elderly patient can lead to a marked improvement in the degree of hyperglycemia, presumably by reducing resistance to insulin.

Substantial barriers may limit the effectiveness of a weight-reducing diet in an elderly patient. Lifelong dietary habits, often based on long-standing cultural traditions, may be particularly challenging to modify. Many elderly patients have changes in taste, vision, or smell that may lead to difficulties with food preparation. Arthritis or other neurological or muscular disorders may also limit the patient's access to the most appropriate kinds of foods, and financial factors may also be important. Because of these complexities, the skills of an experienced dietitian and the help of family may be of considerable importance in instituting and maintaining an appropriate dietary regimen.

Exercise

A carefully developed exercise program can benefit elderly patients with diabetes. The same principles that guide the choice of exercise program in younger patients with diabetes apply to elderly patients. It is important to recognize that the intensity of physical training must be commensurate with the patient's degree of physical fitness. Because of the high incidence of clinically silent coronary artery disease among elderly people with diabetes, any physical training program should be based on an appropriate exercise tolerance test and carried out with careful supervision. A foot injury resulting from an exercise program could have devastating effects in an elderly patient who is at a high risk for infection and amputation. Therefore, choice of appropriate footwear is critical. As with any exercise program, the risk of hypoglycemia should be minimized (see Chapter 18).

Oral Agents

If the defined treatment goal is not achieved with a program of diet and exercise, it is appropriate to consider the use of one or more oral agents. The dosage, mechanism of action, efficacy, and specific side effects of available oral agents are discussed in other chapters. Although no major differences in the clinical pharmacology of these agents in elderly adults have been defined, a prudent approach to the use of these agents in this population is to start with a relatively small dose and increase slowly while observing the patient's response. Use of a combination of two or more oral agents with different mechanisms of action may be attractive for a given patient, although there is limited information on the use of such combinations in elderly patients. The main concern is the potential for polypharmacy and drug interactions in an elderly patient who is also being treated for multiple coexisting medical problems.

Oral agents can cause hypoglycemia in elderly patients. Because of the importance of the kidneys and liver for drug elimination and the importance of the liver for glucose counterregulation, both renal and hepatic insufficiency are substantial risk factors for the development of severe hypoglycemia during sulfonylurea therapy. An age-related decline in renal function would contribute to this susceptibility. Despite the potential for hypoglycemia with use of sulfonylurea drugs, the risk appears to be small in elderly patients who have good nutrition status and who do not have major problems with renal or hepatic insufficiency. When hypoglycemia does occur, patients need to be carefully observed for a considerable period, particularly with some of the longer-acting agents. Chlorpropamide should be avoided in elderly people because of the concern for prolonged hypoglycemia.

Metformin should be avoided in elderly adults with renal or hepatic insufficiency, during heart failure, or during any severe acute illness because of the potential risk for these coexisting conditions to predispose a patient to the development of lactic acidosis. The gastrointestinal side effects associated with use of α-glucosidase inhibitors may limit their utility in elderly patients who have an underlying gastrointestinal disorder or for whom adequate calorie intake and maintenance of body weight is a coexisting health problem. Thiazolidinediones should not be used in elderly patients with heart failure.

Insulin

When the treatment goal for a patient has not been met by use of a weight reduction diet, exercise, and use of oral agents, insulin therapy should be considered. Institution of insulin therapy and subsequent adjustment of the insulin regimen should be carried out as discussed in Chapter 24.

Insulin does not have any major drug interactions, and there are virtually no contraindications to its use. It is important to emphasize, however, that the use of insulin requires that the patient or care provider be trained in self-monitoring of blood glucose (SMBG). Skills required for independence in insulin administration and SMBG that must be evaluated in elderly individuals with diabetes include the following:

- sufficient cognitive function to manage a complex regimen
- adequate vision to read labels, syringes, and glucose monitoring equipment
- fine motor control to draw up and use insulin

Limitations in some of these areas can be overcome. Family members and home health aides can help with administering insulin. The developing technology of SMBG can make up for limitations in vision and some of the fine motor skills.

Table 29.2 Potential Risk Factors for Hypoglycemia in Elderly Diabetes Patients

- Impaired autonomic nervous system function
- Impaired counterregulatory responses
- Poor or irregular nutrition
- Cognitive disorder
- Use of alcohol or other sedating agent
- Polypharmacy
- Kidney or liver failure

The major risk associated with insulin administration in elderly people is the development of hypoglycemia. Treatment of this complication is discussed in Chapter 24. Risk factors that may increase the likelihood of a hypoglycemic reaction in elderly patients are described in Table 29.2. Whereas age-related changes in hypoglycemia counterregulatory mechanisms have been described, the changes are subtle in otherwise healthy elderly people and are unlikely to result in greater risk of hypoglycemia during insulin therapy.

BIBLIOGRAPHY

Blaum CS, Velez L, Hiss RG, Halter JB: Characteristics related to poor glycemic control in NIDDM patients in community practice. *Diabetes Care* 20:7–11, 1997

California Health Foundation/American Geriatrics Society Panel on Improving Care for Elders with Diabetes: Guidelines for improving the care of the older person with diabetes mellitus. *J Am Geriatr Soc* 51:S265–S280, 2003

Caruso LB, Silliman RA, Demissie S, Greenfield S, Wagner EH: What can we do to improve physical function in older persons with type 2 diabetes? *J Gerontol Med Sci* 55A:M372–M377, 2000

Funnell MM: Role of the diabetes educator for older adults. *Diabetes Care* 13 (Suppl. 2):60–65, 1990

Funnell MM, Herman WH: Diabetes care policies and practices in Michigan nursing homes, 1991. *Diabetes Care* 18:862–866, 1995

Halter JB: Aging and carbohydrate metabolism. In *Handbook of Physiology, Volume on Aging.* Masoro EJ, Ed. New York, Oxford University Press, 1995, p. 119–145

Halter JB: *Diabetes Update: Elderly Patients With Non-Insulin-Dependent Diabetes Mellitus.* Kalamazoo, MI, Upjohn, 1990

Harris MI, Flegal KM, Cowie CC, Eberhardt MS, Goldstein DE, Little RR, et al.: Prevalence of diabetes, impaired fasting glucose, and impaired glucose tolerance in U.S. adults. *Diabetes Care* 21:518–524, 1998

Resnick HE, Harris MI, Brock DB, Harris TB: American Diabetes Association diabetes diagnostic criteria, advancing age, and cardiovascular disease risk profiles: results from the Third National Health and Nutrition Examination Survey. *Diabetes Care* 23:176–180, 2000

Shorr RI, Franse LV, Resnick HE, Di Bari M, Johnson KC, Pahor M: Glycemic control of older adults with type 2 diabetes: findings from the Third National Health and Nutrition Examination Survey, 1988–1994. *J Am Geriatr Soc* 48:264–267, 2000

Shorr RI, Ray WA, Daugherty JR, Griffin MR: Incidence and risk factors for serious hypoglycemia in older persons using insulin or sulfonylureas. *Arch Intern Med* 157:1681–1686, 1997

Sinclair AJ, Robert IE, Croxson SC: Mortality in older people with diabetes mellitus. *Diabet Med* 14:639–647, 1997

Dr. Halter is Professor of Internal Medicine, Chief of the Division of Geriatric Medicine, and Director of the Geriatrics Center, University of Michigan, Ann Arbor, MI.

30. Hypoglycemia in Patients with Type 1 Diabetes

ALICIA SCHIFFRIN, MD

Hypoglycemia occurs with varying degrees and frequency in every person with type 1 diabetes. Very few people affected with diabetes are free of the fear of hypoglycemia and its physical and psychological sequelae. The clinical experience of hypoglycemic symptoms can be so disabling to many that, on a day-to-day basis, it can cause as much anxiety as the fear of developing long-term complications. Hypoglycemia is mostly iatrogenic. Insulin regimens are unphysiological and lead to peripheral hyperinsulinemia. This is thought to result in defective counterregulation and various syndromes of absent to delayed warning symptoms in response to hypoglycemia. Hypoglycemia is one of the main limiting factors in achieving the glycemic goals required to prevent long-term diabetes complications. The Diabetes Control and Complications Trial (DCCT) demonstrated that the maintenance of near-normal glucose and glycated hemoglobin A1C (A1C) levels results in a 40–60% reduction of microvascular complications in patients with type 1 diabetes. Thus, the gold standard of diabetes care has become to achieve A1C levels similar to those reached in the DCCT. The study also showed that the intensively treated group had a threefold increase in the incidence of severe hypoglycemic reactions. A total of 65% of patients in the intensive group versus 35% of patients in the conventional group had at least one episode of severe hypoglycemia by the end of the study. The overall rates of severe hypoglycemia were 61.2 per 100 patient-years versus 18.7 per 100 patient-years in the intensive and conventional groups, respectively, with a relative risk of 3.28. There was a quadratic relationship between the A1C concentration and the risk of severe hypoglycemia, with the frequency of hypoglycemia increasing as A1C levels decreased. The A1C concentration achieved did not account for all of the estimated difference of severe hypoglycemia risk because the intensively controlled group still had an excess risk of severe hypoglycemia after adjustment for A1C concentration. However, an interesting finding was that the incidence of severe hypoglycemia was not higher in clinics with patients who had the lowest A1C levels than in clinics with patients who had the highest A1C levels. This finding suggests that quality of care may influence the incidence of hypoglycemia independently of A1C level. These findings are supported by other studies as well.

Every patient treated with insulin is at risk of hypoglycemia and should be instructed to take measures to prevent and treat its occurrence. Self-monitoring of blood glucose should be done often. Instruction should allow patients to become comfortable adjusting their insulin dosage according to glucose level, food intake, and physical activity.

DEFINITIONS

Hypoglycemia can be defined biochemically as a blood glucose level <50 mg/dl (<3.1 mmol/l). However, people with diabetes experience symptoms at varying degrees of blood glucose concentration, and, thus, many people accept Whipple's triad as confirmation of hypoglycemia. This triad consists of symptoms compatible with hypoglycemia, a low blood glucose level, and relief of symptoms after blood glucose is raised. The exact level of blood glucose that defines hypoglycemia remains a matter of debate.

When blood glucose levels decrease to ~3.1 mmol/l, secretion of counterregulatory hormones occurs in a majority of individuals. Glucagon and epinephrine are the most rapid-acting counterregulatory hormones, with effects measurable in minutes, whereas cortisol and growth hormone effects are slower and become apparent a few hours after the hypoglycemic episode. α-Adrenergic stimulation results in insulin suppression, and β stimulation results in glucagon secretion with inhibition of glucose utilization and increased glucose production. The clinical responses to hypoglycemia result in neurogenic (autonomic) and neuroglycopenic symptoms. The neurogenic symptoms involve the discharge of the sympathoadrenal and parasympathetic system, which release epinephrine, norepinephrine, and other peptides such as acetylcholine. Symptoms include hunger, sweating, tachycardia, palpitations, trembling, anxiety, and tingling. In mild hypoglycemia, the patient is able to self-treat. In a moderate episode, the patient will have neuroglycopenic symptoms but will be able to either self-treat or seek help for self-treatment. Moderate hypoglycemia can occur with or without previous warning symptoms. When the central nervous system is deprived of glucose, patients experience neuroglycopenic symptoms such as marked impairment of motor function, difficulty speaking, blurred vision, changes in body temperature, decreased ability to concentrate, drowsiness, confusion, or abnormal behavior. Any episode requiring complete assistance to treat from a third party should be considered a severe hypoglycemic episode. Usually, these episodes involve severe confusion, difficulty awakening, loss of consciousness, coma, seizures, and even death. Some patients with long-standing diabetes appear to have hypoglycemia unawareness (i.e., the presence of hypoglycemia without warning symptoms). The threshold for warning symptoms is lower than the threshold for neuroglycopenia, so that the first signs to appear will be confusion or loss of consciousness. Hypoglycemia unawareness is more frequent in patients with diabetes of longer duration and in intensively managed patients with shorter duration of diabetes. It is due to defective counterregulation. Asymptomatic hypoglycemia may occur as biochemical hypoglycemia without any clinical symptoms.

CAUSES AND PREVENTION OF HYPOGLYCEMIA

Conventional wisdom suggests that hypoglycemia results from absolute or relative excess of insulin due to the inability of most insulin regimens to mimic physiological insulin secretion. To correct this problem, patients are instructed to constantly match the intake of nutrients, in particular carbohydrates, to the expected timing of insulin peaks. Conditions of relative or absolute insulin excess can occur when:

- the insulin dosage is excessive or improperly timed
- access to exogenous glucose is decreased during an overnight fast
- a meal is delayed or missed, or the meal has insufficient carbohydrates
- gastric emptying is delayed because of high fat content of the meal or the presence of gastroparesis in autonomic neuropathy or episodes of gastroenteritis
- glucose utilization is increased during exercise
- insulin sensitivity is increased during the night or after prolonged exercise and during regular physical training, weight loss, recovery from infections, postpartum, lactation, and menopause
- hepatic glucose production is decreased because of inhibited gluconeogenesis caused by excessive alcohol intake
- insulin clearance is decreased as in renal failure

Other causes of insulin excess can be related to daily variations in insulin absorption from the subcutaneous sites. On any given day, there may be a 20–30% variation in the rate of absorption depending on body or ambient temperature, blood flow, anatomical site, or depth of injection among other factors.

Relative or Absolute Insulin Excess

Absolute insulin excess is usually more common before noon and in the evening before dinner, coinciding with the insulin peak after the morning injection. Many patients experience frequent prelunch hypoglycemia. This situation can be avoided by reducing the morning short-acting insulin dose and delaying the morning meal by 30–45 min if the patient's lifestyle permits it, or by administering rapid-acting analogs. Sometimes these maneuvers also fail, but usually hypoglycemia can be avoided by dividing the breakfast meal into two smaller meals.

Insulin excess is also frequent during the early morning hours, when less insulin is required to maintain normoglycemia and there is in addition a peak insulin effect from the evening predinner short-acting insulin dose. Close to 50% of severe hypoglycemic reactions occur during sleep, when the individual cannot perceive symptoms or is not alert enough to respond to the symptoms. Furthermore, it has been shown (in individuals both with and without diabetes) that deep sleep diminishes epinephrine response to hypoglycemia, which may explain the absence of adrenergic symptoms alerting the individual to respond. Nighttime asymptomatic hypoglycemia is very frequent. The availability of a continuous glucose monitoring system that provides data after completion of a 3-day recording has revealed a greater incidence of nocturnal hypoglycemia than previously thought. In one study, nocturnal hypoglycemia was present in 44% of nights in 97% of the subjects studied, regardless of the method of insulin delivery. However, bedtime snacks reduced the frequency by ~36%. Thus, it appears that providing a bedtime snack adjusted to blood glucose level is a good strategy to decrease hypoglycemia at night.

Exercise

In nondiabetic individuals who exercise, there is a reduction in insulin secretion in the portal circulation and an increase in hepatic glucose release such that normoglycemia is maintained. In contrast, individuals with type 1 diabetes are particularly predisposed to hypoglycemia either during or after exercise because of the inability to suppress exogenous insulin concentrations. Glucose utilization in peripheral tissues is increased, and there is simultaneous absorption from up to two to three previously injected sites (subcutaneous insulin pockets from which a few units of insulin can be absorbed at once in a delayed fashion). This results in decreased blood glucose levels during or after exercise. The risk of hypoglycemia is enhanced if the patient has not adequately increased caloric intake in anticipation of exercise, the insulin dose was not reduced accordingly, or if the patient takes a hot shower after exercising.

In addition, young children and lean individuals with type 1 diabetes who exercise for long periods are at greater risk of late hypoglycemia if their glucose stores are not adequately replenished, because hepatic glycogen stores can be depleted during prolonged exercise. In these people, gluconeogenic substrates may be insufficient to adequately maintain blood glucose levels during fasting, and hypoglycemia may occur several hours later. If severe hypoglycemia occurs, subcutaneous glucagon may be ineffective in the face of depletion of glycogen stores, and intravenous glucose will be required for treatment. In addition, patients who exercise regularly should be taught that insulin sensitivity may increase and total daily insulin requirements decrease, in addition to the pre-exercise adjustments required to avoid hypoglycemia.

Alcohol

Alcohol predisposes patients to hypoglycemia because it interferes with hepatic glucose production, the main source of blood glucose during the fasting state. When large amounts of ethanol are oxidized, there is an accumulation of NADH that is removed by conversion of pyruvate to lactate, resulting in decreased substrate for gluconeogenesis. In addition, alcohol can interfere with the ability to perceive hypoglycemic symptoms, resulting in delayed treatment. Individuals with diabetes should be aware of their potential inability to perceive the symptoms of hypoglycemia triggered by alcohol and should therefore be instructed to drink alcohol with moderation. In the case of adolescents who may not follow these recommendations, rigorous realistic instructions should be given to consume adequate amounts of carbohydrates if they intend to drink at parties. They should check their blood glucose repeatedly during the party, particularly during the early morning hours, and alert one or two nondrinking friends of the potential occurrence of severe hypoglycemia and what action should be taken.

Nocturnal Hypoglycemia

Close to 50% of episodes of severe hypoglycemia occur between bedtime and breakfast. Patients with type 1 diabetes are more vulnerable during these hours because, during sleep, they are less able to perceive the warning symptoms of hypoglycemia before neuroglycopenia ensues, and by then, it is too late for them to ask for help. In addition, insulin requirements are lower during the early morning hours and higher around awakening. Moreover, during the night, the patient's decreased insulin requirements may not be met by matching glucose output because the subject is fasting. With conventional insulin injections, it is not possible to accommodate these decreased insulin requirements unless the individual uses programmable insulin infusion pumps. However, even with infusion pumps, there is the risk of nocturnal hypoglycemia.

The risk of hypoglycemia during this period is so great that every person with type 1 diabetes should be encouraged to determine his or her nocturnal glycemic pattern from time to time and each time that insulin doses are changed. In the real world, blood glucose monitoring at bedtime and between 2:00 and 4:00 a.m. and between 6:00 and 7:00 a.m. for three consecutive nights every few months should suffice. Ideally, the blood glucose nadir should not drop below 80 mg/dl (4 mmol/l), even at the expense of mild fasting hyperglycemia. Monitoring blood glucose levels during the night should also be done after days of intense physical activity, after changes in work shifts, when staying up unusually late, when changing time zones, etc. Adolescents during their most rebellious periods of refusal to do blood glucose testing should be encouraged to test their blood glucose at least at bedtime to minimize the occurrence of severe hypoglycemia. Patients, relatives, and roommates should be taught that unusual or aggressive behavior, nightmares, excessive sweating, tremor, morning headaches, seizures, and difficulty awakening are all signs of hypoglycemia. These instances should always be monitored with frequent blood glucose levels, and preventive measures should be taken as soon as possible. These measures include not only an immediate decrease of the next day's evening insulin dose, but also a careful review of the treatment plan.

Practical recommendations to minimize the occurrence of nocturnal hypoglycemia in young children and sedentary people (who retire around 9:00 p.m.) is to adjust the carbohydrate and protein content of the bedtime snack following a prescribed algorithm according to the blood glucose level obtained at that time. However, nonobese patients who remain active after dinner and go to bed much later can consume a small standard snack at 9:00 p.m. Later on, at bedtime, an extra snack following a pre-fixed algorithm should be consumed if the blood glucose level is <140 mg/dl (<7.0 mmol/l). This strategy provides an extra measure of safety and helps prevent hypoglycemia in very active patients. The size of that snack is determined on a trial-and-error basis according to fasting blood glucose readings. It appears that bedtime snacks with complex carbohydrates and no less than 12–15 g of protein can be effective in minimizing the risk of hypoglycemia. Protein is converted into glucose and also stimulates glucagon release. Orally, it has a delayed effect on blood glucose rise; therefore, it may be ideal in people who tend to have hypoglycemia in the early morning hours.

Many individuals with type 1 diabetes do not take a bedtime snack. The lack of symptoms during the night and the presence of normal to high blood glucose levels upon rising may give a false sense of security. Recently, the availability of ambulatory, continuous blood glucose monitoring has made it evident that asymptomatic nocturnal hypoglycemia is much more common than previously thought, and consuming a bedtime snack substantially minimizes the risk of nocturnal hypoglycemia. The need for a bedtime snack appears to be less if the patient is on lispro or aspart insulin at dinner and the blood glucose level at bedtime is >180 mg/dl (>10 mmol/l).

Rapid-Acting Insulin Analogs

Rapid-acting insulin seems to have some benefits with regard to reducing the incidence of hypoglycemia (during the night in particular). A meta-analysis looked at pooled data from all studies in more than 4,000 subjects. There was a reduced frequency of severe hypoglycemia in the patients taking lispro versus regular insulin

(3.1 vs. 4.4%), despite similar levels of A1C. Patients with a history of severe hypoglycemia were not included; therefore, the actual rates of severe hypoglycemia may have been underestimated. However, these data suggest that people experiencing severe nocturnal hypoglycemia may derive some benefit from dinnertime rapid-acting insulin, because it may not have the delayed nighttime effect of regular insulin.

Long-Acting Insulin Analogs

A long-acting insulin analog, insulin glargine (Lantus, Aventis) may last up to 24 h or more in some patients. It has the advantage of not having a significant peak effect and not requiring resuspension before administration. In addition, it has recently been shown that in comparison with NPH, the incidence of nocturnal hypoglycemia is reduced when this analog is used in the morning. Another long-acting analog, insulin detemir (Novo Nordisk), can also provide basal insulin with an attenuated peak effect but, it is not clear yet if it will last 24 h. As with glargine, a lower incidence of nocturnal hypoglycemia has been reported with insulin detemir in comparison with NPH.

RISK FACTORS FOR HYPOGLYCEMIA

Statistical evidence from the DCCT supports that the most important risk factors for severe hypoglycemia include history of a previous severe hypoglycemic episode, longer duration of diabetes, lower recent A1C, higher baseline insulin dose, hypoglycemia unawareness, and lower residual β-cell secretory response. Autonomic neuropathy is a moderate risk factor for severe hypoglycemia and is not required for the presence of hypoglycemia unawareness. However, in addition to the relatively easier-to-ascertain risk factors mentioned above, there are other important factors that play crucial roles in the triggering of severe hypoglycemia. These risk factors are modifiable, and their impact can be reduced by appropriate intervention, as described below.

Inadequate Education

Important but difficult-to-measure risk factors for hypoglycemia include lack of adherence to a regular treatment plan and inappropriate insulin adjustment. Infrequent blood glucose monitoring, insufficient carbohydrates, or lack of adjustment of the insulin dose in anticipation of exercise are frequent causes of hypoglycemia during the day. Forgetting to monitor blood glucose levels and to take a snack at bedtime are frequent causes of hypoglycemia at night. Patients who are poorly trained (for whatever reason) can have more problems with hypoglycemia. It is therefore necessary to simplify the treatment regimen as much as possible. Other common errors include switching the morning dose with the evening dose, mistakes in measuring insulin, taking excessive doses of insulin with the evening meal, skipping meals, and failure to compensate for increased activity.

Degree of Glycemic Control

Data from studies comparing intensive insulin therapy and conventional therapy suggest that it is the glycemic goal and not the mode of therapy that determines the risk for hypoglycemia. Intensive insulin therapy lowers the glycemic thresholds at which symptoms are perceived and at which counterregulation is elicited. Studies in individuals with type 1 diabetes and in nondiabetic individuals demonstrate that a greater hypoglycemic stimulus is required to initiate a hormonal and symptom response after prior exposure to an episode of hypoglycemia. Thus, it appears that unrealistic goals to achieve normoglycemia or normal A1C values may lead to frequent episodes of severe hypoglycemia and suggest that glycemic goals need to be reviewed on a regular basis.

Acquired Hypoglycemia Syndrome

Defective counterregulation. Children tend to respond to hypoglycemia with symptoms and epinephrine responses at higher blood glucose levels (~68 mg/dl [3.8 mmol/l] compared with 56 mg/dl [3.8 mmol/l] in adults).

Conventional risk factors for hypoglycemia resulting from relative or absolute insulin excess do not always explain unexpected hypoglycemic episodes. An explanation for this is the interaction between hyperinsulinemia and the development of abnormal counterregulation. People with diabetes of longer duration may experience more hypoglycemia because they require larger doses of insulin. Insulin is passively absorbed from the subcutaneous injection sites, and plasma insulin levels do not fall as plasma glucose levels fall. After 2–5 years of diabetes, the ability to secrete glucagon in response to hypoglycemia is lost, although glucagon responses to other stimuli such as exercise are maintained. However, the responses to hypoglycemia are still normal because release of epinephrine partially compensates for the defective glucagon secretion. Later on in the course of type 1 diabetes (~10–12 years after diagnosis), the epinephrine response to hypoglycemia (in contrast with the glucagon that is glucose specific) exhibits a threshold effect. This means that an epinephrine response can still be elicited by hypoglycemia, but at a lower blood glucose level. When hypoglycemia develops in individuals who have this combined deficiency, the risk of severe hypoglycemia is increased 25-fold. The glucose recovery may be seriously impaired, and, consequently, if these patients are treated with intensive insulin therapy this should be done with extreme caution. This diminished epinephrine response is not the result of diabetic neuropathy.

Hypoglycemia unawareness. Hypoglycemia unawareness is the loss of warning neurogenic symptoms (irrespective of duration of diabetes), which makes the patient unable to react and prevent progression to neuroglycopenia. These symptoms may not be readily recognized, and patients may lapse into coma or develop seizures without any warning. As in patients with defective counterregulation, patients with this syndrome require lower glycemic thresholds to elicit symptomatic responses to hypoglycemia. Patients with this syndrome do not necessarily have autonomic neuropathy.

Altered glycemic thresholds. Altered glycemic thresholds may be iatrogenically induced by exposure to repeated episodes of hypoglycemia. A single hypoglycemic episode of 2 h duration can change the epinephrine and symptomatic response to subsequent hypoglycemia in both nondiabetic and diabetic individuals. This probably explains the altered thresholds observed in individuals with type 1 diabetes treated with intensive therapy. People with altered thresholds have a sixfold increase in the prevalence of severe hypoglycemia compared with individuals who retain normal glycemic awareness.

The syndromes of defective counterregulation, hypoglycemia unawareness, and altered glycemic threshold are associated with a high frequency of iatrogenic hypoglycemia; they tend to coexist in the same individuals; and they share some similar features, such as the much lower glycemic thresholds for symptoms of autonomic and symptomatic responses to hypoglycemia, suggesting that they have hypoglycemia as a common pathogenic cause. Accordingly, these conditions have been named "hypoglycemia-associated autonomic failure." However, these different mechanisms do not explain the defective glucagon response, which is the key defect and first to appear in abnormal glucose counterregulation. Antecedent hypoglycemia elevates the threshold for autonomic and symptomatic responses to subsequent hypoglycemia. The overall hypothesis is that antecedent hypoglycemia causes hypoglycemia-associated autonomic failure by reducing epinephrine responses (in addition to the already-reduced glucagon response) and symptoms of hypoglycemia (reduced awareness), resulting in repeated severe hypoglycemia, which thus perpetuates the cycle. In many cases, increasing blood glucose monitoring and meticulously avoiding hypoglycemia (maintaining blood glucose levels within a target of 80–180 mg/dl [4.4–10.0 mmol/l]) can reverse hypoglycemia unawareness, improve glucose counterregulation, or both. The potential for disappearance of warning symptoms should be used to motivate patients to monitor blood glucose levels more frequently, particularly at times when hypoglycemia is more likely to occur. Usually, the ability to perceive warning symptoms can be recovered after 2–3 weeks of careful avoidance of hypoglycemia. There is some recent evidence that patients with hypoglycemia-associated autonomic failure may have reduced β-adrenergic sensitivity compared with patients with normal counterregulation. This abnormal sensitivity could be recovered if hypoglycemia is avoided for several months, despite persistent blunted epinephrine responses. In some studies, beverages containing caffeine were shown to increase the threshold for hypoglycemic symptoms. In contrast, β-blockers inhibit the perception of neurogenic symptoms, and people on these medications should test their blood glucose often because they are at increased risk for severe hypoglycemia.

Blood glucose awareness training allows patients with hypoglycemia unawareness to improve their ability to detect a larger number of hypoglycemic episodes. Instruction involves interpretation of symptoms, performance cues, and moods, and careful planning of insulin dosing and its relation to expected blood glucose results.

In a not too distant future, subcutaneous glucose sensors for continuous glucose monitoring with sophisticated software may make it possible to trigger an alarm when hypoglycemia risk is detected. Such a system is being tested successfully in experimental animals.

COMPLICATIONS OF SEVERE HYPOGLYCEMIA

Hypoglycemia causes physical and psychosocial morbidity and may cause death. Physical morbidity ranges from unpleasant symptoms to errors in judgment, accidents, decreased performance, and behavioral changes leading to episodes that can be mistaken for alcohol intoxication or illegal drug use. More extreme cases may lead to severe neurological manifestations such as hemiplegia, focal or generalized seizures, or coma. The depth of impairment is related to the duration of symptoms and the blood glucose levels reached. It is very difficult to ascertain the mortality rate, but one retrospective study estimated death due to hypoglycemia at 4%.

Over the long term, repeated episodes may lead to decreased cognitive function and decreased memory in children and perhaps in adults as well. Prospective data in young children suggest that severe hypoglycemia is associated with lower IQ and speed in processing information, as well as reduced motor speed tasks. Adult studies do not definitively answer the question of whether severe hypoglycemia impairs cognitive function. The problem with prospective studies is that they use many different tests for evaluation and it is not possible to make useful comparisons. Furthermore, to evaluate the impact of hypoglycemia, it would be necessary to start evaluation at the time of diagnosis of diabetes, with careful ascertainment of severe hypoglycemic episodes over the long term and repeat neuropsychological testing over many years to assess if any changes have occurred.

TREATMENT

Every person taking insulin should be taught how to recognize warning symptoms of hypoglycemia and how to treat promptly, even if symptoms are subtle, to prevent progression to neuroglycopenia. Verification of blood glucose level immediately after treatment of suspected hypoglycemia is an excellent teaching tool because it helps the patient recognize unusual or unexpected symptoms in subsequent episodes. All hypoglycemic episodes, even in the absence of symptoms, require treatment. The goal of treatment is to increase the blood glucose to a safe level to prevent sequelae, using an intervention that works fast and relieves symptoms quickly while avoiding rebound hyperglycemia.

Relatives, friends, teachers, and coworkers should be taught how to recognize symptoms of hypoglycemia and, in general, should be suspicious of any unusual behavior on the part of the person with diabetes. In case of doubt, they should be taught to treat immediately as if the person had hypoglycemia, and only after treatment is administered should they verify the blood glucose level. Education for these people includes the administration of adequate amounts of glucose-containing solutions and/or subcutaneous glucagon in case of loss of consciousness or seizures. The amounts of glucose to be given will depend on the size of the person, the blood glucose level, and the time of day.

Mild to moderate hypoglycemia is usually treated with food, oral glucose tablets, or sucrose solutions. A good rule of thumb is to administer 15–20 g glucose as glucose tablets (3–5 g/10 kg body weight) to raise the blood glucose by ~65 mg/dl (3 mmol/l). Sports drinks containing pure glucose will be sufficient as well. Fruit juice is absorbed more slowly than glucose (because it contains half glucose and half sucrose) and is not as effective in raising the blood glucose level as glucose tablets or liquid glucose. Likewise, honey (1 tsp = 5 g glucose) is less efficient than glucose because it contains only 40–50% glucose and the same amount of fructose. However, for children older than 2 years of age and adults, it is very convenient to carry around in small packets and can also be used in case of severe hypoglycemia as the initial treatment because it can be administered by an unskilled third party without any risk. Sucrose solution as granulated sugar in orange juice or milk does not provide a quick rise in blood glucose levels for rapid symptomatic relief and may require the administration of larger volumes. The absorption of glucose gels is poor, and their administration is generally not advisable because the absorption is quite slow.

After the administration of the first 15–20 g glucose, patients should wait 15 min for symptoms to subside. Administration of glucose can be repeated after that time if the symptoms persist or the blood glucose level falls again. Moderate hypoglycemia may require twice that amount of glucose over a longer period of time. Some patients make the mistake of deferring treatment, particularly if the meal is half an hour away. This may lead to severe hypoglycemia. Ideally, for hypoglycemia occurring shortly before meals, patients should be taught to take the carbohydrate portion of that meal to raise their blood glucose and complete the rest of the meal at the usual time, thus preventing both further hypoglycemia and hyperglycemia. In cases of hypoglycemia occurring at night, 10–15 g of glucose may suffice. However, if there has been an error with the insulin dose or a missed meal, the glucose requirements may be four to five times higher.

In cases of loss of consciousness, the treatment is 10–25 g (20–50 ml) of 50% glucose injected intravenously over 1–3 min despite the risk of extravasation or phlebitis. Glucagon is ideal to use at home, and the standard dose is 1 mg given subcutaneously (for children <5 years old, 0.5 mg will suffice). The maximal blood glucose response occurs after 15 min, with a peak at 20 min to 1 h. However, if severe hypoglycemia occurs after strenuous exercise, decreased food intake (as in illness), prolonged fasting, alcohol ingestion, high doses of insulin, or antecedent hypoglycemia, glucagon injection may not be effective because glycogen stores may be depleted. When glucagon is used, it is important to remember that post-glucagon nausea and vomiting are common and that careful monitoring of blood glucose levels should be continued until the patient is able to eat normally.

BIBLIOGRAPHY

Boyle PJ, Kempers SF, O'Connor AM, Nagy RJ: Brain glucose uptake and unawareness of hypoglycemia in patients with insulin-dependent diabetes mellitus. *N Engl J Med* 333:1726–1731, 1995

Brunelle BL, Llewelyn J, Anderson JH Jr, Gale EA, Koivisto VA, et al.: Meta-analysis of the effect of insulin lispro on severe hypoglycemia in patients with type 1 diabetes. *Diabetes Care* 21:1726–1731, 1998

Chase HP, Lockspeiser T, Peery B, Shepherd M, MacKenzie T, Anderson J, et al.: The impact of the Diabetes Control and Complications Trial and humalog insulin on glycohemoglobin and severe hypoglycemia in type 1 diabetes. *Diabetes Care* 24:430–434, 2001

Cox DJ, Gonder-Frederick L, Polonsky W, Schlundt D, Kovatchev B, Clarke W: Blood glucose awareness training (BGAT-2): long-term benefits. *Diabetes Care* 24:637–642, 2001

Cryer PE: Banting lecture: Hypoglycemia: the limiting factor in the management of IDDM. *Diabetes* 43:1378–1389, 1994

Cryer PE: Iatrogenic hypoglycemia as a cause of hypoglycemia-associated autonomic failure in IDDM. *Diabetes* 41:255–260, 1992

DCCT Research Group: Adverse events and their association with treatment regimens in the Diabetes Control and Complications Trial. *Diabetes Care* 18:1415–1427, 1995

DCCT Research Group: Hypoglycemia in the Diabetes Control and Complications Trial. *Diabetes* 46:271–286, 1997

Dagogo-Jack S, Fanelli CG, Cryer PE: Durable reversal of hypoglycemia unawareness in type 1 diabetes. *Diabetes Care* 22:866–867, 1999

Davis SN, Tate D: Effects of morning hypoglycemia on neuroendocrine and metabolic responses to subsequent afternoon hypoglycemia in normal man. *J Clin Endocrinol Metab* 86:2043–2050, 2001

Diedrich L, Sandoval D, Davis S: Hypoglycemia associated autonomic failure. *Diabetologia* 12:358–365, 2002

Fanelli C, Pampanelli S, Lalli C, Del Sindaco P, Ciofetta M, Lepore M, et al.: Long-term intensive therapy of IDDM patients with clinically overt autonomic neuropathy: effects on hypoglycemia unawareness and counterregulation. *Diabetes* 46:1172–1181, 1997

Fritsche A, Stefan N, Haring H, Gerich J, Stumvoll M: Avoidance of hypoglycemia restores hypoglycemia unawareness by increasing beta-adrenergic sensitivity in patients with type 1 diabetes. *Ann Intern Med* 134:729–736, 2001

Gold AE, MacLeod KM, Frier BM: Frequency of severe hypoglycemia in patients with type 1 diabetes with impaired awareness of hypoglycemia. *Diabetes Care* 17:697–703, 1994

Hamman A, Matthaei S, Rosak C, Sivestre L: A randomized clinical trial comparing breakfast, dinner or bedtime administration of insulin glargine in patients with type 1 diabetes. *Diabetes Care* 26:1738–1744, 2003

Hershey T, Bhargava N, Sadler M, White NH, Craft S: Conventional versus intensive diabetes therapy in children with type 1 diabetes: effects on memory and motor speed. *Diabetes Care* 22:1318–1324, 1999

Jones TW, Porter P, Sherwin RS, Davis EA, O'Leary P, Frazer F, et al.: Decreased epinephrine responses to hypoglycemia during sleep. *N Engl J Med* 338:1657–1662, 1998

Slama G, Traynard PY, Desplanque N, Pudar H, Dhunputh I, Letanoux M, et al.: The search for an optimized treatment of hypoglycemia: carbohydrates in tablets, solution, or gel for the correction of insulin reactions. *Arch Intern Med* 150:589–593, 1990

Vague P, Selam JL, Skeie S: Insulin detemir is associated with more predictable glycemic control and reduced risk of hypoglycemia than NPH insulin in patients with type 1 diabetes on a basal-bolus regimen with pre-meal aspart. *Diabetes Care* 26:590–596, 2003

Dr. Schiffrin is Director of the Metabolic Day Center, Division of Endocrinology, Sir Mortimer B. Davis Jewish General Hospital, and Professor of Medicine and Pediatrics, McGill University, Montreal, Québec, Canada.

31. Insulin Allergy and Insulin Resistance

JOHN H. HOLCOMBE, MD, AND S. EDWIN FINEBERG, MD

T he use of human insulins has dramatically reduced the immunological complications of insulin therapy. However, insulin allergy continues to occur, albeit at a much lower frequency than when the use of insulins from animal sources predominated. Antibodies induced by the insulin molecule itself are the most likely cause of immunological complications. The presence of such antibodies may increase insulin dosage requirements or alter insulin absorption profiles. Occasionally, antibody-mediated insulin resistance has been associated with diabetic ketoacidosis. This chapter focuses on allergic responses to human insulin and to the newer insulin analogs.

Three insulin analogs are now commercially available: insulin lispro, insulin aspart, and insulin glargine. Insulin lispro and aspart are similar in their rapid onset of action after subcutaneous injection. Insulin glargine, which at physiological pH precipitates in the subcutaneous space, has a prolonged duration of action with no pronounced peak. These insulin analogs are relatively weak immunogens.

Other potential antigens may be found in pharmaceutical insulins. Circulating antibodies to protamine have been detected in ~40% of individuals treated with NPH insulins. These antibodies are rarely the cause of insulin-associated allergic phenomena but have been associated with anaphylaxis during the reversal of intraoperative heparin anticoagulation. However, the presence of antibodies to protamine does not predict protamine-related anaphylaxis. In patients previously treated with NPH insulins, heparin anticoagulation should be allowed to reverse spontaneously; if protamine reversal is necessary, it should be carried out with precautions against anaphylaxis.

Insulin dimers and oxidative products form during the storage of pharmaceutical insulins, especially at high temperatures; only the former incite specific antibodies. There are few cases of zinc-related insulin allergy despite the common demonstration of skin test reactions to zinc acetate or zinc sulfate. Rarely, patients may react to plasticizers, preservatives, or latex contaminants. Human insulin of recombinant DNA origin is made by insertion of insulin genes into the DNA of bacteria (*E. coli*) or yeast, yet we are not aware of any patients who have developed antibodies to yeast or bacterial peptides.

Local insulin allergic phenomena are encountered in 2–3% of patients treated with human insulins. Systemic allergy has rarely been reported to be associated with human insulins when individuals were begun and continued only on that type of insulin. However, in cases of systemic allergy, a desensitization procedure using human insulin or an insulin analog is often successful. Desensitization is the process of introducing low but increasing doses of an allergen, insulin in this case, to decrease the allergic response to that allergen. Insulin antibody–mediated insulin resistance resulting in insulin requirements of >1.5 units/kg/day (>10 nmol/l/kg/day) in adults and >2.5 units/kg/day (>16.7 nmol/l/kg/day) in children is an extremely rare complication of therapy and has been associated with few individuals begun on human insulin therapy.

All three human insulin analogs (insulin lispro, insulin aspart, and insulin glargine) have proven useful in treating insulin allergic reactions.

PATHOPHYSIOLOGY OF INSULIN ALLERGY

1. Insulin allergy is usually local and occurs within the first 2 weeks of therapy (Table 31.1). About 90% of individuals with local allergy have spontaneous remissions within 2 months while on the same therapy, and an additional 5% will improve within 6–12 months.
2. Isolated wheal-and-flare and biphasic reactions are mediated by reaginic antibodies (IgE). The late phase of a biphasic reaction is characterized by pain and erythema.
3. Arthus reactions (inflammatory response to the deposition of antigen-antibody complexes) are uncommon and are characterized by localized small-vessel injury and neutrophilic infiltrates.
4. Delayed reactions are indurated and often pruritic and painful with well-defined borders. Histologically, these lesions are associated with perivascular "cuffing" with mononuclear cells.
5. Systemic allergic reactions are seen most commonly in individuals with histories of atopy and/or intermittent insulin therapy. Anti-insulin IgG and

Table 31.1 Allergic Reactions to Insulin

Type	Description
Local Isolated wheal-and-flare reaction	Occurs within 30 min, resolves within 1 h; wheal-and-flare reaction followed by a late-biphasic phase reaction peaking in 4–6 h and persisting for 24 h
Arthus reaction	Develops over 4–6 h, peaks at 12 h
Delayed (tuberculin-like)	Develops nodule or "deep hive" over 8–12 h, peaks in 24 h
Systemic Urticaria to anaphylaxis	Immediate reaction

Modified from DeShazo et al.

IgE levels are not predictive of types of local reactions but are significantly elevated in individuals with systemic insulin allergy.

THERAPY FOR INSULIN ALLERGY

1. In individuals with severe persistent local allergy and individuals with systemic allergy, further therapy is indicated and is summarized in Tables 31.2–31.4.
2. Therapy of systemic allergy is based on intradermal testing to ascertain the least reactive insulin (i.e., insulin evoking the least hypersensitivity in the patient), desensitization, and, less frequently, the use of glucocorticoids and/or antihistamines.
3. With systemic or severe insulin allergy, insulin therapy must be continued to avoid future anamnestic reactions. Both human and insulin analogs have been used successfully for desensitization. More than 94% of individuals with systemic allergy can be desensitized as described above. Glucocorticoids and/or antihistamines may rarely be required to modify persisting insulin allergic symptoms.

Table 31.2 Therapy for Persistent Severe Local Allergy to Human Insulin (Present for 14–30 Days)

Rule out improper injection technique (also infection and contaminated alcohol).

Skin test to select least reactive insulin, 0.02-ml intradermal injections of 1:1 dilution of U-100 human regular insulin, insulin lispro, or insulin aspart diluted in phenol-saline; 700 µg/ml (4.3 mmol/l) zinc sulfate, ~0.1 mg/ml (0.48 mmol/l) histamine phosphate (positive control); and phenol-saline (negative control). Observe for reactions at 20 min, 6 h, and ~24 h. A positive wheal-and-flare reaction is 5 mm > phenol-saline 20 min after injection, surrounded by erythema. Significant induration is >1 cm.

Treat with least reactive insulin.

If the severe local allergy persists:

Divide dosage and deliver into multiple sites; use soluble insulin delivered by continuous subcutaneous insulin infusion; add dexamethasone to each unit of insulin delivered (1 or 2 mg dexamethasone/1,000-unit vial); systemic antihistamines; two relatively untested approaches have been suggested: cimetidine 300 mg t.i.d. or oral insulin plus aspirin in individuals unresponsive to dermal desensitization.

If reactive to zinc sulfate, consider using low-zinc insulin, such as NPH. If reactive to NPH insulins, avoid protamine. Protamine insulins are typically low in zinc. Modified from DeShazo et al. and Galloway and DeShazo.

Table 31.3 Therapy for Systemic Insulin Allergy

Is insulin necessary? ──No──► Diet and exercise, with or without oral antidiabetic agents

Yes ↓

Skin test for least reactive insulin: at 20-min intervals, 0.02 ml by intradermal injections of 0.001, 0.01, and 0.1 units (0.007, 0.07, and 0.7 nmol/l, respectively) of human insulin diluted in sterile phenol-saline or neutral insulin-dilution fluid. If wheal-and-flare reaction is 5 mm > phenol-saline control 20 min after injection of any dilution, proceed to insulin lispro or insulin aspart. A positive test results in a wheal-and-flare reaction 5 mm greater than negative control. If initial testing is negative, then proceed to test with 1 unit of insulin and, if negative, proceed to treat the patient with this insulin. If skin testing is positive, proceed to formal desensitization. Use saline and/or insulin-diluting fluid as negative-control solutions. If negative (<5 mm larger than control), test with 1 unit (6.7 nmol/l).

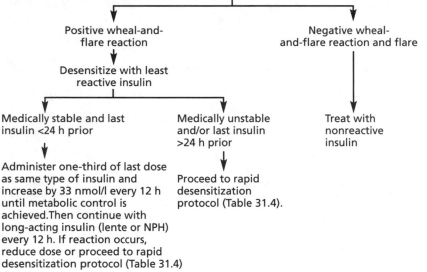

Positive wheal-and-flare reaction

↓

Desensitize with least reactive insulin

Medically stable and last insulin <24 h prior

↓

Administer one-third of last dose as same type of insulin and increase by 33 nmol/l every 12 h until metabolic control is achieved. Then continue with long-acting insulin (lente or NPH) every 12 h. If reaction occurs, reduce dose or proceed to rapid desensitization protocol (Table 31.4)

Medically unstable and/or last insulin >24 h prior

↓

Proceed to rapid desensitization protocol (Table 31.4).

Negative wheal-and-flare reaction and flare

↓

Treat with nonreactive insulin

Neutral insulin-diluting fluid and empty insulin mixing vials are available from Lilly. Modified from Galloway and DeShazo.

ANTI-INSULIN ANTIBODY–MEDIATED INSULIN RESISTANCE

1. Individuals with this complication of therapy commonly have histories of intermittent insulin therapy or atopy. Historically, therapy with beef-containing insulin often preceded the antibody-mediated insulin resistance.
2. To demonstrate that antibodies are the primary cause of insulin resistance, other etiologies, including intercurrent illness and neoplasia, must be elim-

Table 31.4 Rapid Desensitization Protocol

Prepare serial 1:10 dilutions of least reactive insulin (after an initial 1:1 dilution of U-100 insulin, then serial 1:10 dilutions of the least reactive insulin in neutral insulin-diluting fluid of 50, 5, 0.5, 0.05, and 0.005 units/ml).

| | Step (every 20–30 min) | | | | | | | | | | | |
| | Intradermal | | | | | | | | | Subcutaneous | | |
	1	2	3	4	5	6	7	8	9	10	11	12
Volume (ml)	0.02	0.04	0.08	0.02	0.04	0.08	0.02	0.04	0.08	0.02	0.04	0.08
Units/ml	0.05	0.05	0.05	0.5	0.5	0.5	5	5	5	50	50	50
Units	0.001	0.002	0.004	0.004	0.02	0.04	0.1	0.2	0.4	1	2	4

Instructions
1. Precede with skin testing as described in Table 31.3.
2. Carry out in the hospital under medical supervision. If reactions have been severe, carry out procedure in intensive care unit.
3. Avoid concomitant use of antihistamines or steroids. Have a syringe filled with 1 ml of 1:1,000 epinephrine, life-support equipment, and an allergy consultant available.
4. If patient reacts to initial dosage, begin with 0.005 units/ml.
5. If patient has more than a wheal-and-flare reaction or induration >1 cm, reduce by two dilution steps and then proceed again.
6. After step 12, double dose subcutaneously every 4 h until metabolic stability is established. Then long-acting insulin may be administered (lente or NPH as described in Table 31.3).

Insulin: 1 pmol/l = 0.139 mU/ml.

inated. Possible factitious resistance (e.g., resistance absent when insulin is administered by an MD or RN) must also be eliminated.

3. Occasionally, insulin antibody–mediated insulin resistance may be an early manifestation of the insulin autoimmune syndrome or the manifestation of a lymphoma. Identification and treatment of such insulin resistance is described in Table 31.5.

4. The use of a newer insulin analog may be advantageous. Occasionally, the use of U-500 regular human insulin may be of benefit, in lieu of a course of steroid therapy or if such therapy fails to decrease insulin volume requirements. Because of its concentration, U-500 insulin acts as a repository insulin due to its delayed time action.

5. In general, immunological resistance spontaneously remits in <1 year, but durations up to 5 years have been reported.

Table 31.5 Identification and Treatment of Antibody-Mediated Insulin Resistance

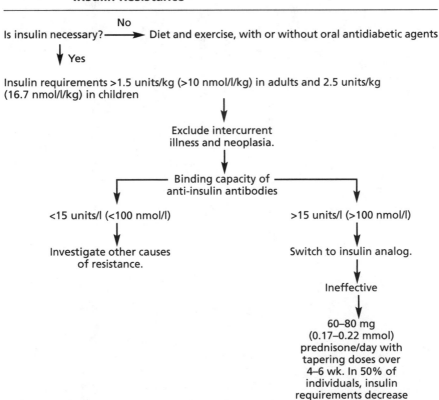

6. Approximately 50% of patients will benefit from a course of high-dose glucocorticoid (initially 40–80 mg prednisone daily) that is tapered over 2–4 weeks. Occasionally, dramatic decreases in insulin dosage requirements are seen within days after the institution of such therapy, and thus hypoglycemia must be avoided.

BIBLIOGRAPHY

Abraham M, Al-Sharif BA, Saavedra GA, Khardori R: Lispro in the treatment of insulin allergy. *Diabetes Care* 22:1916–1917, 1999

Airaghi L, Lorini M, Tedeschi A: The insulin analog aspart: a safe alternative in insulin allergy (Letter). *Diabetes Care* 24:2000, 2001

Chideckel EW, Mullin CJ, Michael BE: Cimetidine in insulin allergy. *Diabetes Care* 4:503–504, 1981

DeShazo RD, Mather P, Grant W, Carrington D, Frentz JM, Lueg M, et al.: Evaluation of patients with local reactions to insulin with skin tests and in vitro techniques. *Diabetes Care* 10:330–336, 1987

Dozio N, Beretta A, Castiglioni M, Rosa S, Scavini M, Belloni C, et al.: Insulin antibodies do not preclude optimization of metabolic control in women with IDDM during pregnancy. *Diabetes Care* 19:979–982, 1996

Fineberg NS, Fineberg SE, Anderson JH, Birkett M, Gibson RG, Hufferd S: Effects of insulin lispro [Lys (B28), Pro (B29) human insulin] in IDDM and NIDDM previously treated with insulin. *Diabetes* 45:1750–1754, 1996

Fineberg SE: Insulin allergy and insulin resistance. In *Therapy for Diabetes Mellitus and Related Diseases*. Leibovitz HE, Ed. Alexandria, VA, American Diabetes Association, 1995, p. 178–184

Galloway J, DeShazo R: Insulin chemistry and pharmacology: insulin allergy, resistance, and lipodystrophy. In *Ellenberg and Rifkin's Diabetes Mellitus: Theory and Practice*. 4th ed. Rifkin H, Porte D, Eds. New York, Elsevier, 1990, p. 504–508

Holdaway IM, Wilson JD: Cutaneous allergy responsive to oral desensitization and aspirin. *Br Med J (Clin Res Ed)* 289:1565–1566, 1984

Lassmann-Vague V, Belicar P, Alessis C, Raccah D, Vialettes B, Vague P: Insulin kinetics in type I diabetic patients treated by continuous intraperitoneal insulin infusion: influence of anti-insulin antibodies. *Diabet Med* 13:1051–1055, 1996

Lahtela JT, Knip M, Paul R, Antonen J, Salmi J: Severe antibody-mediated human insulin resistance: successful treatment with the insulin analog lispro. *Diabetes Care* 20:71–73, 1997

Lindholm A, Jensen LB, Home P, Raskin P, Boehn BO, Rastam J: Immune responses to insulin aspart and biphasic insulin aspart in people with type 1 and type 2 diabetes. *Diabetes Care* 25:876–882, 2002

Moriyama H, Nagata M, Fujihira K, Yamada K, Chowdhury SA, Chakrabarty S, et al.: Treatment with human analog (GlyA21, ArgB31, ArgB32) insulin glargine (HOE901) resolves a generalized allergy to human insulin in type 1 diabetes. *Diabetes Care* 24:411–412, 2001

Ottesen JL, Nilsson P, Jami J, Weilguny D, Duhrkop M, Bucchini D, et al.: The potential immunogenicity of human insulin and insulin analogues evaluated in a transgenic mouse model. *Diabetologia* 37:1178–1185, 1994

Peters A, Klose O, Hefty R, Keck F, Kerner W: The influence of insulin antibodies on the pharmacokinetics of NPH insulin in patients with type 1 diabetes treated with human insulin. *Diabet Med* 12:925–930, 1995

Weiler JM, Gellhaus MA, Carter JG, Meng RL, Benson PM, Hottel RA, et al.: A prospective study of the risk of an immediate adverse reaction to protamine sulfate during cardiopulmonary bypass surgery. *J Allergy Clin Immunol* 85:713–719, 1990

Yki-Jarvinen H, Dressler A, Ziemen M: Less nocturnal hypoglycemia and better post diner glucose control with bedtime insulin glargine compared with bedtime NPH insulin during combination therapy in type 2 diabetes. *Diabetes Care* 23:1130–1136, 2000

Dr. Holcombe is Clinical Associate Professor of Pediatrics at the Indiana University School of Medicine and Medical Advisor at Eli Lilly and Company, Indianapolis, IN. Dr. Fineberg is Emeritus Professor of Medicine at the Indiana University School of Medicine, Indianapolis, IN.

32. Drugs and Hormones That Increase Blood Glucose Levels

STEPHANIE ANN MORAN, MD, AND DEREK LEROITH, MD, PHD

A lthough certain medications may be associated with the development of hyperglycemia, none are contraindicated for use in diabetic patients because of this reason alone. As hormonal therapy becomes more common, it is important to be aware of the effect these natural substances may have on glucose metabolism.

MEDICATIONS

Many prescription and nonprescription drugs have been associated with hyperglycemia (Table 32.1). They cause elevated blood glucose levels by several different mechanisms, and in many cases the mechanism is unknown.

Antihypertensive Agents

Thiazide diuretics are associated with an increased risk of diabetes. The exact mechanism by which this class of drugs causes hyperglycemia is unknown. Associated potassium depletion and its effect on β-cell insulin secretion may be involved. β-Adrenergic stimulation promotes insulin secretion from the pancreatic β-cell in response to glucagon or glucose; therefore, blockade of this signal may result in hyperglycemia and insulinopenia. This effect is seen more commonly with the nonselective β-blocker propranolol; however, hyperglycemia has also been observed in patients treated with metoprolol and atenolol. Interestingly, the mixed α- and β-adrenergic antagonist, carvediolol, improves insulin sensitivity through its anti–α-adrenergic effects. Calcium-channel blockers cause decreased insulin secretion from the β-cell. Several case reports link these medications to the induction of hyperglycemia. Indapamide and acetazolamide have also been observed to be associated with hyperglycemia in a few patients. In general, hyperglycemia may be more commonly seen in hypertensive patients because of an increased prevalence of the metabolic syndrome in the population. Clinical judgment should therefore be exercised in evaluating patients with hyperglycemia who are also on antihypertensive medication, so that a more serious disease process is not overlooked.

Table 32.1 Medications Associated with Development of Hyperglycemia

Antihypertensive agents

Diuretics
  Chlorthalidone
  Ethacrynic acid
  Thiazide
  Indapamide
  Acetazolamide
β-Adrenergic blockers
  Propranolol
  Metoprolol and atenolol
Calcium-channel blockers
  Nifedipine, verapamil, diltiazem,
    nicardipine
α-Adrenergic agonists
  Clonidine

Anti-inflammatory agents

Glucocorticoids
  Prednisone
  Megestrol
Indomethacin
Glucosamine sulfate

Sympathomimetic and neuromodulatory agents

Catecholamines
α-Adrenergic agonists
β-Adrenergic agonists (terbutaline)
Caffeine
Nicotine
Anticholinesterase poisoning
Rodenticide, vacor (Pyriminil)
Chlorinated hydrocarbon pesticide
  (Endosulfan)

Psychiatric medication

Chlorpromazine
Mianserin
Clozapine
Olanzapine (Zyprexa)
Seroquel
Risperidone
Quetiapine
Paroxitine

Antibiotics

Pentamidine
Streptozocin

Immunomodulatory agents

L-Asparaginase
Cyclosporin
Tacrolimus (FK506)
Cytokine therapy: TNF-α, IL-1, IL-6
Protease inhibitors
Nucleoside analog therapy (Didanosine)

Others

Alcohol
Nicotinic acid
Cimetidine
Diazoxide
Diphenylhydantoin/phenytoin
Oral contraceptives: estrogen and
  progesterone
TPN

These medications cause elevations in blood glucose levels, as documented in the medical literature.

Anti-Inflammatory Agents

Glucocorticoids (GCs) cause hyperglycemia by increasing hepatic glucose output and by creating insulin resistance. GCs also result in increased synthesis and release of catecholamines. The hyperglycemia that they cause may be reversible in normal patients or may progress to frank diabetes in those patients who may already have underlying glucose intolerance. Glucosamine therapy for arthritis and indomethacin therapy for psoriatric arthritis have been observationally associated with hyperglycemia.

Sympathomimetic and Neuromodulatory Agents

The response of the sympathetic nervous system is to protect against hypoglycemia. Drugs that mimic this response result in hyperglycemia mediated through increased hepatic glucose production from glycogenolysis and gluconeogenesis. They also cause decreased tissue insulin sensitivity and inhibit insulin secretion. A concomitant increase in growth hormone (GH) after use of a sympathomimetic agent further contributes to insulin resistance. These effects are seen after treatment with α-adrenergic agonists such as catecholamines, caffeine, and nicotine. β-Adrenergic stimulation may also result in hyperglycemia by impairing insulin secretion. Opiates also cause hyperglycemia via this mechanism. Agents such as terbutaline, used in the treatment of premature labor, are associated with an increased risk of gestational diabetes, especially when this therapy is combined with corticosteroid therapy. Hyperglycemia has not been associated with inhaled β-adrenergic agonists. The rodenticide vacor acts as a nicotinimide antagonist and causes severe β-cell toxicity that may not be reversible and can cause ketoacidosis and diabetes. Organophosphate insecticides that cause anticholinesterase poisoning result in hyperglycemia in some cases, although hypoglycemia has also been observed. Endosulfan, a chlorinated hydrocarbon insecticide similar to DDT, acts as a central nervous system stimulant and has also been observed to cause hyperglycemia after an acute ingestion.

Anti-Psychotic Agents

Several new anti-psychotic medications have been associated with hyperglycemia that resolves after discontinuation of the drug. More recent studies question the causative nature of these medications and the resultant hyperglycemia, because the prediction of diabetes in this population was only found to be significantly associated with patients' BMI and psychiatric diagnosis but not their medication history. Chlorpromazine has been observed to cause hyperglycemia and glycosuria, but reports of hypoglycemia have also been noted. In a single psychiatric patient, hyperglycemia developed after treatment with paroxitine (Paxil).

Antibiotics

Infection creates an insulin-resistant state, so there is an expected coincidence of hyperglycemia; however, most antibiotics are not known to cause increased blood glucose levels. Pentamidine is β-cell toxic and causes injury to the pancreas in a dose- and time-dependent manner. Streptozocin is also β-cell toxic and has been used extensively to produce an experimental mouse model of type 1 diabetes.

Immunosuppressive Agents

A reversible hyperglycemia has been seen with L-asparaginase treatment, which coincides with decreased insulin levels. Cyclosporin and tacrolimus (FK506) treatment in transplant patients has been associated with the development of diabetes. These medications may inhibit islet cell function or may contribute to insulin resistance. Often these medications are used in conjunction with steroids, which adds to the risk of hyperglycemia. Cytokine therapy is becoming more commonly used in medical practice. The infusion of tumor necrosis factor (TNF)-α or interleukin (IL)-1 has been observed to cause an increase in catecholamines, which may result in hyperglycemia. Subcutaneous injection of IL-6 is associated with increased levels of plasma glucagon and higher glucose levels in normal healthy male volunteers. Cases of hyperglycemia have not yet been documented but are a plausible result of cytokine therapy and may be seen as more patients are treated with this immunomodulatory therapy. Didanosine, a nucleoside analog, appears to cause hyperglycemia via two mechanisms: a direct injury to β-cells and the suppression of insulin release by associated hypokalemia. The mechanism by which protease inhibitors cause hyperglycemia is largely unknown, but this treatment has been associated with the development of hypertriglyceridemia and centripetal obesity, both of which are associated with an increased risk of diabetes.

Others

The mechanism by which many medications cause hyperglycemia is unknown; however, their use has been linked to the development of elevated glucose levels or diabetes. In some cases, the mechanism has been better studied and may be known. The effect of alcohol consumption on carbohydrate metabolism is complex and differs between acute and chronic ingestion. Both hypoglycemia and hyperglycemia have been observed. The hyperglycemia induced by alcohol is usually seen in the setting of chronic ingestion and may be caused by an increased insulin resistance that occurs at the cellular level, resulting in decreased insulin-stimulated glucose disposal, and in the liver, with dysregulation of hepatic glucose metabolism, as seen in patients with alcoholic steatohepatitis. Nicotinic acid used in the treatment of hypertriglyceridemia may contribute to an insulin-resistant state. This medication causes a decreased availability of free fatty acids and then results in less substrate available for gluconeogenesis. However, the short-acting preparations may cause a rebound effect on the liver, which then results in increased free fatty acids and then an augmentation of glucose output. Cimetidine has been observed to cause elevated glucose levels that are thought to be due to decreased secretion of insulin. Diazoxide and diphenylhydantoin/phenytoin inhibit insulin secretion and cause reversible hyperglycemia that usually resolves after the medication is stopped. Total parenteral nutrition (TPN) and hyperglycemia frequently occur simultaneously. Most patients receiving TPN are often critically ill and therefore in a stressed state distinguished by catecholamine excess. In this situation, the patient receives an infusion of glucose that then may not be cleared because of their insulin resistance, resulting in hyperglycemia.

HORMONES

Blood glucose levels are hormonally mediated. Therefore, treatment with hormones and certain disease states of hormone excess are associated with hyperglycemia (Table 32.2).

Table 32.2 Hormones That Cause Hyperglycemia

Hormone	Associated Disease
Growth hormone	Acromegaly
Glucagon	Glucagonoma
Thyroid hormone	Thyrotoxicosis
Cortisol	Cushing's syndrome
Catecholamines Norepinephrine and epinephrine	Pheochromocytoma Stress response
Somatostatin	Somatostatinoma
Testosterone	Androgen excess, polycystic ovarian syndrome
Estrogen/progesterone	Pregnancy or hormone replacement therapy
Human somatomammotropin (human placental lactogen)	Pregnancy

Growth Hormone

GH, when acutely administered, causes an increase in insulin-like effects, but this effect only lasts a short time. Chronic administration or pathological states of GH excess are characterized by inducing insulin resistance with elevated hepatic glucose output.

Glucagon

Glucagon promotes hepatic gluconeogenesis and glycogenolysis, therefore contributing to hyperglycemia. Also, this hormone promotes release of epinephrine, which inhibits insulin secretion from the pancreas. Hyperglucagonemia may be caused by a glucagon-secreting tumor, but elevations in this hormone are more commonly seen in ketoacidosis, hyperosmolar syndrome, renal failure, and acute pancreatitis. The most common clinical situation of elevated glucagon may occur after the administration of this hormone for profound hypoglycemia. In this setting, remember that the glucagon injection may only temporarily raise the blood glucose level, after which the patient may again become hypoglycemic, as would occur in a long-acting sulfonylurea ingestion, if the original cause of the low blood glucose has not been treated.

Thyroid Hormone

Thyroid hormones, when in excess, may inhibit the secretion of insulin from the β-cell and cause increased gluconeogenesis. Thyrotoxicosis is a hypermetabolic stressed state that affects glucose metabolism in a similar fashion to catecholamine excess. Hyperglycemia does not occur in conjunction with exogenous administration of thyroid hormone as long as serum levels are maintained within a normal physiological range.

Cortisol

Glucocorticoids (GC) such as cortisol or exogenous steroids in excess promote hyperglycemia and impaired glucose tolerance. They cause the release of amino acids and free fatty acids and they upregulate the key enzyme in gluconeogenesis (phosphoenolpyruvate carboxykinase). Both of these effects promote the production and release of glucose into the blood. The clearance of glucose is inhibited by GCs, which decrease cellular uptake and processing of glucose and reduce the amount of insulin secretion from the β-cell. GC-induced hyperglycemia is common and has been well documented because these hormones are widely used in the treatment of inflammatory conditions.

Catecholamines

Norepinephrine and epinephrine release antagonizes the actions of insulin and promotes the release of glucagon. As expected, this process results in an increase in blood glucose by the stimulation of gluconeogenesis and glycogenolysis and fat lipolysis. These compounds cause β- and α-adrenergic stimulation. Glucagon release is promoted by both types of adrenergic stimulation. Insulin secretion from the pancreatic β-cell is promoted by β-adrenergic stimulation; however, in states of catecholamine excess, the α-adrenergic stimulation often exerts the dominant action, causing an inhibition of insulin release.

Somatostatin

Somatostatin inhibits the secretion of neuropeptides such as insulin and glucagon. Hyperglycemia and diabetes may occur in patients with somatostatin-producing tumors. However, pharmacological use of somatostatin analogs for the treatment of other neuroendocrine tumors has not resulted in diabetes. However, these synthetic compounds may result in impaired glucose tolerance, especially after a meal. The difference in the effect between endogenous somatostatin and the synthetic form on carbohydrate metabolism may be due to a variable stimulation of the subtypes of the somatostatin receptor.

Human Somatomammotropin (Human Placental Lactogen)

Human somatomammotropin, which increases throughout the first 3 months of pregnancy and then plateaus at an elevated level, antagonizes the action of insulin and promotes free fatty acid release, which then stimulates gluconeogenesis. Excess of this hormone promotes an abundance of nutrients available to the developing fetus and may chiefly contribute to the development of gestational diabetes in predisposed individuals.

Testosterone/Estrogen/Progesterone

Elevated androgens, whether administered exogenously in males or occurring in conjunction with polycystic ovarian syndrome in females, have been associated with insulin resistance and hyperglycemia. Estrogen and progesterone decrease insulin sensitivity. Higher-dose formulations of oral contraceptives were shown to cause hyperglycemia, but this relationship has not been supported by studies using modern low-dose or triphasic preparations.

TREATMENT OF DRUG-INDUCED HYPERGLYCEMIA

When a medication or hormone therapy is suspected of causing hyperglycemia, the agent should be discontinued if possible and the patient should be reevaluated. In many cases, this intervention will return the patient to a euglycemic state. If the medication suspected of causing hyperglycemia cannot be discontinued, then the patient should be treated to control his or her blood glucose levels.

Before starting therapy with either a drug or hormone that may cause hyperglycemia, evaluate the patient for his or her risk of developing hyperglycemia. A family history or the presence of disease that is associated with the metabolic syndrome (such as obesity, hypertension, and dyslipidemia) indicate a greater risk for hyperglycemia. A fasting blood glucose or a glucose level after a glycemic challenge may also be helpful. Throughout the therapy, monitor the patient closely for the development of hyperglycemia, which may be done by asking about the presence of any symptoms of hyperglycemia (polyuria or polydypsia) and obtaining periodic laboratory evaluation. Patients at high risk for developing hyperglycemia or who already have known diabetes should monitor their own blood glucose and then be treated accordingly.

Traditionally, short-term treatment of drug/hormone-induced hyperglycemia has been achieved by using insulin therapy. A classic example of this is in the treatment of gestational diabetes. Similarly, if the patient has type 1 diabetes, the insulin requirement may just be adjusted to treat a newly developed hyperglycemia.

In type 2 diabetes patients or those patients with impaired glucose tolerance who then develop hyperglycemia after beginning treatment with a drug, the choice of agent used to treat the hyperglycemia is less apparent. A trial of diet and exercise may improve their insulin sensitivity and resolve their hyperglycemia. Although effective, this intervention may not be realistic in a patient who is requiring treatment for another medical condition. Insulin therapy may be quite effective in these patients when they develop hyperglycemia due to a medication. Because of its fast action and effect, insulin may be the treatment of choice for a patient who only requires treatment with the agent causing the hyperglycemia for a short period of time. The initiation of insulin therapy may be cumbersome because this is an injectable therapy and compliance may be difficult. Oral agents may be more effective and easier for the patient. Sulfonylureas may be used but may not be terribly efficacious, and when adding additional medications, the side effect profile must be considered. With the introduction of shorter-acting agents in this class of medication, such as repaglinide or nateglinide, this may be a convenient preliminary therapy. This patient group, which is characterized by the presence of insulin resistance instead of deficiency, may not respond to therapy that causes an increase in circulating insulin levels. Therefore, use of an insulin sensitizer such as a thiazolidinedione or metformin may be a better choice; however, there have been few clinical trials that have studied the effectiveness of these agents in this setting of drug-induced hyperglycemia.

In summary, the most important approach is to follow the patient carefully and to reevaluate both the presence of hyperglycemia and the effectiveness of the treatment for this condition. Long-term hyperglycemia is still associated with the development of diabetes complications regardless of the cause. Some patients may require treatment with these drugs or hormones that cause hyperglycemia for several years; therefore, an aggressive approach to the treatment of their high blood glucose levels is indicated.

SUGGESTED READINGS

Becker KL, Bilezikian JP, Bremner WJ, Hung W, Kahn CR, Loriaux DL, NylTn ES, Rebar RW, Robertson GL, Snider, Jr. RH, Wartofsky L: *Principles and Practice of Endocrinology and Metabolism.* 3rd ed. Philadelphia, Lippincott, 2001

Chan NN, Osaki R, Chow CC, Chan JC, Cockram CS: Drug-related hyperglycemia. *JAMA* 287:714–715, 2002

Knowler WC, Barrett-Connor E, Fowler SE, Hamman RF, Lachin JM, Walker EA, Nathan DM, Diabetes Prevention Program Research Group: Reduction in the incidence of type 2 diabetes with lifestyle intervention or metformin. *N Engl J Med* 346:393–403, 2002

LeRoith D, Taylor SI, Olefsky JM: *Diabetes Mellitus: A Fundamental and Clinical Text.* 2nd ed. Philadelphia, Lippincott, 2000

Luna B, Feinglos MN: Drug-induced hyperglycemia. *JAMA* 286:1945–1948, 2001

Thomson Micromedex website: http://www.micromedex.com

Dr. Moran is a Clinical Endocrinology Fellow and Dr. LeRoith is Chief of the Diabetes Branch at the National Institute of Diabetes and Digestive and Kidney Diseases, National Institutes of Health, Bethesda, MD.

33. Diabetic Dyslipidemia

HENRY N. GINSBERG, MD

Numerous prospective cohort studies have indicated that diabetes mellitus is associated with a three- to fourfold increase in risk for coronary heart disease (CHD). The increase in risk is particularly evident in younger age-groups and in women: females with type 2 diabetes appear to lose a great deal of the protection that characterizes nondiabetic females. Furthermore, patients with diabetes have a 50% greater in-hospital mortality and a twofold increased rate of death within 2 years of surviving a myocardial infarction. Overall, CHD is the leading cause of death in individuals with diabetes who are over the age of 35 years.

Although a significant portion of this increased risk is associated with the presence of well-characterized risk factors for CHD, a significant proportion remains unexplained. Patients with diabetes, particularly those with type 2 diabetes, have abnormalities of plasma lipids and lipoprotein concentrations that are less commonly present in nondiabetic individuals. Patients with poorly controlled type 1 diabetes can also have a dyslipidemic pattern, although this is much less common and probably occurs on a background of insulin resistance or the metabolic syndrome.

In recent years, several large clinical trials have shown that reducing levels of LDL cholesterol and plasma triglycerides and/or raising levels of HDL cholesterol is associated with reduced rates of CHD events. There is now strong evidence that health care professionals caring for patients with diabetes should treat lipid abnormalities aggressively. This review will provide a brief pathophysiological basis for the dyslipidemia commonly present in patients with diabetes and then review treatment approaches. Because of the much greater prevalence of lipid abnormalities in type 2 diabetes, most of the emphasis in this review will focus on that group of patients.

LIPOPROTEIN METABOLISM IN DIABETES

Lipoproteins are spherical, macromolecular complexes carrying various lipids and proteins in plasma. The hydrophobic triglyceride and cholesteryl ester molecules comprise the core of the lipoproteins, and this core is covered by amphipathic (both hydrophobic and hydrophilic) phospholipids and proteins. Hundreds to thousands of triglyceride and cholesteryl ester molecules are carried in the core of different lipoproteins. Apolipoproteins are the proteins on the surface of the lipoproteins. They not only help to solubilize the core lipids but also play a critical role in the regulation of plasma lipid and lipoprotein transport. Apolipoprotein (apo) B100 is required for the secretion of hepatic-derived VLDLs, intermediate-density lipoproteins (IDLs), and LDLs. Apo B48 is a truncated form of apo B100 that is required for secretion of chylomicrons from the small intestine. Apo A-I is the major structural protein in HDLs. Other apolipoproteins will be discussed in the context of their roles in lipoprotein metabolism.

ABNORMAL CHYLOMICRON METABOLISM IN DIABETES

After ingestion of a meal, dietary fat (triglyceride) and cholesterol are absorbed into the cells of the small intestine and are incorporated into the core of nascent chylomicrons, which traverse the lymphatic system and enter the circulation via the superior vena cava. In the capillary beds of adipose tissue and muscle, chylomicrons interact with the enzyme lipoprotein lipase (LpL), the chylomicron core triglyceride is hydrolyzed, and the generated free fatty acids are taken up by fat cells and made back into triglyceride, or by muscle cells where they can be used for energy. Chylomicron remnants, products of this lipolytic process that have lost ~75% of the triglyceride, interact with several receptor pathways on hepatocytes and are removed rapidly from the circulation by the liver. Hepatic triglyceride lipase (HL), which hydrolyzes chylomicron remnant triglycerides, also plays a role in remnant removal. Defective metabolism of chylomicrons and chylomicron remnants has been observed commonly in type 2 diabetes, where LpL may be modestly reduced. Recent studies in animal models suggest that chylomicron formation in intestinal cells may also be increased in insulin-resistant states such as type 2 diabetes. Patients with well-controlled type 1 diabetes usually have normal fasting and postprandial triglyceride levels. The role of HL in the defective chylomicron metabolism in diabetes is unclear. In uncontrolled type 1 diabetes, however, LpL can be significantly reduced and marked postprandial lipemia has been observed. In most of those cases, however, a partial genetic defect in LpL production or function probably plays a key role along with insulin deficiency.

ABNORMAL VLDL METABOLISM IN DIABETES

VLDLs are assembled in the liver. The core of the VLDL comprises triglycerides and cholesteryl esters. Apo B100 and phospholipids form its surface. Recent studies indicate that an increased flow of fatty acids to the liver from adipose tissue (Fig. 33.1), along with the possibility for increased fatty acid synthesis in the liver, can drive the assembly and secretion of VLDL that is central to the dyslipidemia present in patients with type 2 diabetes (Fig. 33.2). Abnormalities of cholesterol metabolism, with excess hepatic cholesterol, may also contribute to the overproduction of VLDL. Such abnormalities have not been well defined in patients with diabetes.

Once in the plasma, VLDL triglyceride is hydrolyzed by LpL, generating smaller and more dense VLDL, and then IDL. IDLs are similar to chylomicron

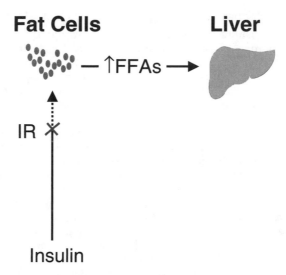

Figure 33.1 Insulin resistance (IR) at the level of the fat cells leads to increased release of free fatty acids (FFAs) into the circulation. The fatty acids are mainly cleared from the circulation by the liver.

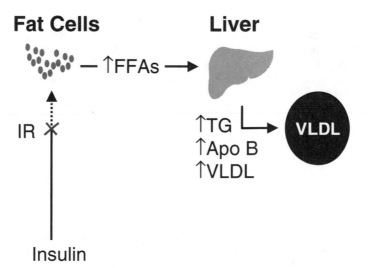

Figure 33.2 Increased fatty acids entering the liver will stimulate triglyceride (TG) synthesis, and this will stimulate the assembly and secretion of increased numbers of VLDL particles.

remnants, except that IDLs, in addition to removal by the liver, can undergo further plasma catabolism to become LDLs. Some LpL activity appears necessary for normal functioning of the metabolic cascade from VLDL to IDL to LDL. It also appears that HL, apo E (another surface apolipoprotein), and LDL receptors also play important roles in this process. Apo B100, the sole protein on the surface of LDL, is a ligand for the LDL receptor, and the concentration of LDL in plasma is determined by both the production of LDL and the availability of LDL receptors.

Plasma levels of VLDL triglyceride are commonly elevated in patients with type 2 diabetes. In population studies, levels of triglyceride greater than the 90th percentile for nondiabetic individuals are two to three times more common in individuals with diabetes. Overproduction of VLDL, with increased secretion of both triglyceride and apo B100, seems to be the common etiology of the increased plasma VLDL levels. Individuals with type 1 diabetes who have good glycemic control usually have average or better than average plasma triglyceride levels. This may be due in part to the ability of insulin to inhibit apo B100 secretion from the liver. As noted above, decreased LpL-mediated hydrolysis of VLDL triglycerides may contribute significantly to elevated triglyceride levels, particularly in patients with either type 1 or 2 diabetes who have poor glycemic control. Obesity and insulin resistance are important contributors to the hypertriglyceridemia of type 2 diabetes. Regulation of plasma levels of LDL cholesterol in type 2 diabetes is complex. In the presence of hypertriglyceridemia, small, dense, cholesterol-depleted, triglyceride-enriched LDLs are present (Fig. 33.3). This means that there will be more LDL particles for any LDL cholesterol level compared with people without diabetes who have LDLs of normal size and composition. Removal of LDL, mainly via LDL receptor pathways, can be increased, normal, or reduced in type 2 diabetes (it is important to remember that lipoprotein particles enter the artery wall). Glycosylated and/or oxidatively modified lipoproteins, which can be present in increased amounts in the blood of patients with either type 1 or type 2 diabetes, interact less efficiently with the LDL receptor and have the potential to increase plasma LDL levels. On the other hand, modified LDLs can be removed from plasma by alternative metabolic pathways, including retention in the arterial wall. Insulin also plays a role in stimulating the expression of the gene for LDL receptors; severe insulin deficiency in poorly controlled type 1 or type 2 diabetes may be associated with reduced LDL receptor function and increased LDL cholesterol levels.

ABNORMAL HDL METABOLISM IN DIABETES

HDL may be the most complex of all the lipoprotein classes. The majority of HDLs are formed by the coalescence of individual apolipoproteins, including apo A-I, A-II, and A-VI, with phospholipids. The resulting nascent disc-like HDLs, also called pre-beta HDLs, function as acceptors of cellular-free cholesterol and are the initial HDL particles involved in reverse cholesterol transport (the movement of cholesterol from peripheral tissues to the liver for excretion from the body). The movement of cellular free cholesterol to apo A-I is mediated via a recently discovered protein, ABCA1. Conversion of cholesterol to

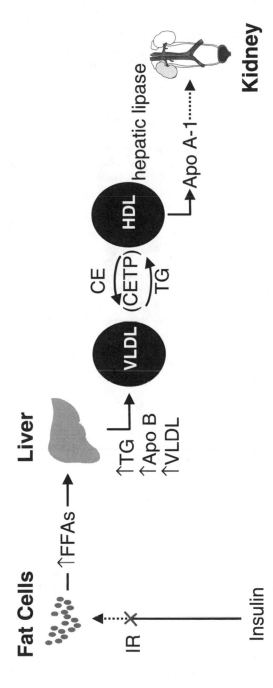

Figure 33.3 Increased VLDL in the circulation, in the presence of CETP, will stimulate increased exchange of HDL cholesterol for VLDL triglycerides (TG). This will deplete HDL of cholesterol. Additionally, hepatic lipase in the capillary bed of the liver will hydrolyze the TG in HDL, the HDL will become smaller, and apo A-I will dissociate. Free apo A-I will be cleared much faster than normal from the circulation, leading to fewer HDLs in the blood.

cholesteryl ester, by the addition of a fatty acid in a reaction catalyzed by lecithin cholesterol acyl transferase (LCAT), produces HDL_3. HDL_3 continues to accumulate cholesteryl ester and becomes HDL_2, which can deliver cholesteryl ester to the liver via a process called selective uptake. The selective uptake of cholesteryl esters from HDL to several organs, including the liver (without entry of the entire HDL particle), was demonstrated to be the result of the HDL interaction with a receptor called scavenger receptor B-1 (SRB-1). Whole HDL particle uptake into cells can occur by undefined pathways. Finally, plasma HDL cholesteryl esters can move from the HDL particle into VLDL and chylomicron particles in the presence of the cholesteryl ester transfer protein (CETP). LpL activity can modulate HDL levels by influencing plasma levels of triglyceride in VLDL or chylomicrons. HL can affect HDL levels by breaking down phospholipids on the surface of the particles; this leads to dissolution of the HDL and loss of apo A-I from the circulation.

Low levels of plasma HDL cholesterol are almost universally present in patients with type 2 diabetes. An important underlying mechanism for this is the CETP-mediated transfer of cholesteryl ester from HDL into VLDL and chylomicrons, both of which are increased in most patients with type 2 diabetes (Fig. 33.4). Low HDL levels in type 2 diabetes can also be present in the absence of fasting hypertriglyceridemia, and the mechanism for this is undefined, although it may reflect high postprandial triglyceride levels or some direct effect of insulin resistance. HDL levels are normal or even increased in patients with well-controlled type 1 diabetes, and this seems to be related to effects of insulin treatment, possibly through suppression of HL.

THERAPEUTIC APPROACHES TO DIABETIC DYSLIPIDEMIA

Dietary Therapy

The centerpiece of therapy for the treatment of diabetes is always diet, irrespective of the absence or presence of dyslipidemia. However, the presence of dyslipidemia increases the rationale for intensive diet intervention. It is important to remember that improvements in plasma triglyceride and total cholesterol levels during dietary intervention can be observed even in the absence of weight loss. Thus, reductions in dietary fat and saturated fat intake, along with reduced cholesterol consumption, can improve the lipid profile even if caloric intake is unchanged.

There is, however, a longstanding and continuing controversy concerning the composition of the "optimal diet" for patients with diabetes. Clearly, reducing dietary saturated fat and cholesterol intake is central to lipid lowering. Such changes will lower LDL ~10%; this may not seem like much, but this degree of reduction is equivalent to almost two doublings of an HMG-CoA reductase inhibitor (see below) once the starting dose has been initiated. The optimal replacement for saturated fat is the focus of the controversy. The issue of whether poly- or monounsaturated fats, rather than carbohydrates, should replace saturated fats has become much larger than it deserves based on the data. Certainly, high-fiber (not just "complex") carbohydrates should be consumed, and even then,

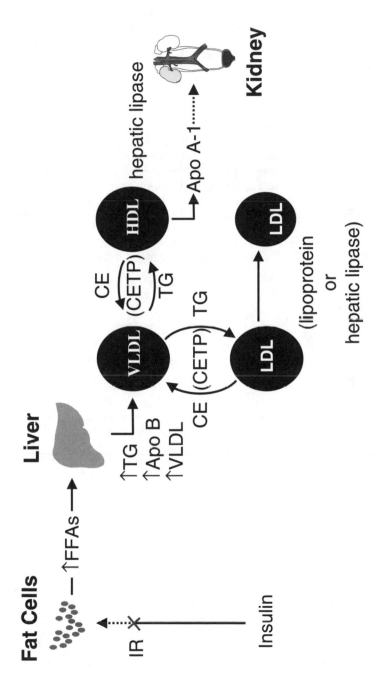

Figure 33.4 Increased VLDL in the circulation, in the presence of CETP, will stimulate an increased exchange of LDL cholesterol for VLDL triglycerides (TG). This will deplete LDL of cholesterol. Additionally, hepatic lipase and/or lipoprotein lipase will hydrolyze the TG in LDL, producing small, dense LDL.

high-fiber carbohydrates are not a panacea. A diet that is varied in poultry and fish, with many vegetables and legumes and with skim or 1% dairy products, should be recommended for patients with diabetes needing plasma lipid modification. Most importantly, because almost all individuals with type 2 diabetes would benefit from weight loss, removing saturated fat from the diet without replacing it is the optimal approach, at least initially.

Weight Loss

Weight reduction is an essential part of dietary therapy in individuals with type 2 diabetes; it is usually not an issue in patients with type 1 diabetes. Weight loss has been shown not only to improve glycemic control and reduce insulin resistance, but to positively affect lipoprotein patterns as well. Several groups have shown that when weight reduction is achieved and maintained in type 2 diabetes patients, there is a sustained decrease in triglyceride levels. Most, but not all, studies show an increase in HDL cholesterol as well with weight loss. The optimal weight loss diet in individuals with diabetes is controversial. Most physicians would agree that a lower-fat diet, with high-fiber foods replacing high-fat foods, is a reasonable approach.

Glycemic Control

Therapy of type 2 diabetes with either insulin or oral agents only partly corrects lipid abnormalities in the majority of patients. This is almost certainly because dyslipidemia is closely related to insulin resistance. Therapeutic approaches to type 2 diabetes that affect insulin sensitivity, such as metformin and thiazolidinediones, should theoretically lower VLDL secretion from the liver by improving insulin sensitivity. Improved LpL function may also result from such therapies. However, clinical trials indicate that metformin only lowers plasma triglyceride concentrations ~10%, whereas pioglitazone treatment is associated with ~15% reductions in plasma triglyceride levels. Unexpectedly, rosiglitazone does not affect triglyceride concentrations in plasma. The effects of the two thiazolidinediones on plasma LDL cholesterol have been variable, although rosiglitazone seems to increase LDL 5–10%, whereas pioglitazone is neutral in its effects. Metformin has been observed to reduce LDL 5–10%. Insulin treatment tends to lower LDL, whereas sulfonylurea therapy has little or no effect. Intensive insulin treatment in patients with type 1 diabetes lowers triglyceride and LDL cholesterol levels significantly.

Control of hyperglycemia does not correlate well with HDL cholesterol levels in patients with type 2 diabetes. Therapy with sulfonylureas does not seem to increase HDL cholesterol concentrations. On the other hand, modest increases in HDL levels, concomitant with modest decreases in triglyceride concentrations, have been observed with metformin therapy. More recently, the thiazolidinediones have been shown to raise HDL cholesterol levels in patients with type 2 diabetes. Of interest, although rosiglitazone and pioglitazone appear to differ in their effects on plasma triglyceride levels, they raise HDL cholesterol concentrations similarly.

Overall, some improvement should be expected in plasma lipid levels, with better glycemic control. In individuals with type 2 diabetes, however, lipid-altering therapy will almost always be necessary. In patients with type 1 diabetes, tight glycemic control with intensive insulin treatment may be adequate, depending on the individual's CHD risk profile.

Lipid-Lowering Drugs

If therapeutic goals have not been achieved after an adequate trial of diabetic control, diet, weight loss, and exercise, drug therapy should be initiated for the treatment of dyslipidemia. The length of time devoted to lifestyle changes should depend on the initial presentation of the patient, the severity of the dyslipidemia, and the presence of other risk factors for CHD or CHD itself. Patients with many correctable lifestyle habits and/or poorly controlled glycemia require more time devoted to those problems before initiation of specific hypolipidemic drug treatment. It is clear that lipid-lowering agents will be less efficacious, or actually ineffective, if these related factors are not approached first. In contrast, when patients are severely dyslipidemic, and/or have very high risk for development of CHD, earlier progression to pharmacotherapy may be prudent. If the patient already has clinically significant CHD or other vascular disease, then drug treatment can be initiated concomitant with lifestyle interventions. The severity of the dyslipidemia, independent of glycemic control, is an indicator of the presence of other genetic causes of lipid abnormalities, and this can also be taken into account when considering initiation of specific lipid-lowering therapy. Clearly, physicians cannot "wait forever" to control plasma glucose or achieve significant weight loss before moving on to specific lipid-altering treatment.

The American Diabetes Association recommends initiation of therapy to lower LDL cholesterol if it is >130 mg/dl in patients without existing clinical cardiovascular disease or >100 mg/dl if there is preexisting cardiovascular disease. The latter is a more aggressive approach than the one taken by the National Cholesterol Education Program (NCEP) Adult Treatment Panel III guidelines. In both guidelines, however, the goal of treatment, once initiated, is an LDL cholesterol level <100 mg/dl. Goals for triglycerides and HDL cholesterol are less well defined, but it is reasonable to try to reach a triglyceride level <150 mg/dl and an HDL cholesterol concentration >45 mg/dl. Women should attempt to get an HDL cholesterol level >50 mg/dl.

HMG-CoA Reductase Inhibitors

During the past decade, the treatment of hypercholesterolemia has undergone a revolution with the availability of potent, safe HMG-CoA reductase inhibitors, also known as statins. Lovastatin, pravastatin, fluvastatin, simvastatin, and atorvastatin are available drugs in this category in the U.S. These drugs work to competitively inhibit HMG-CoA reductase, the rate-limiting enzyme in cholesterol synthesis, and this results in both decreased hepatic production of apo B100–containing lipoproteins and upregulation of LDL receptors. The overall effect is a dramatic lowering of plasma levels of LDL cholesterol. VLDL triglyceride concentrations are also reduced in many subjects with moderate hypertriglyceridemia, including patients with type 2 diabetes. The reduction of triglycerides is directly related to the reduction of LDL cholesterol achieved. At their starting doses, which now range between 10 and 40 mg/day, statins lower LDL cholesterol by 25–40%. The most potent statins (simvastatin and atorvastatin), at the highest doses, can lower LDL cholesterol by up to 45–55% and decrease triglycerides 20–45%. The reduction in triglycerides achieved at these high levels of LDL cholesterol reduction will also depend on the starting triglyceride level; higher baseline triglycerides can be lowered more. Reductase inhibitors can raise HDL cholesterol by up to 5–10% but should not be considered as first-line HDL-raising drugs.

The main side effect associated with statin therapy is a myositis, characterized by diffuse severe muscle tenderness and weakness and elevated levels of creative phosphokinese (usually >1,000 units). In severe cases, rhabdomyolysis and concomitant myoglobinemia can place patients at risk for renal failure due to myoglobinuria. This is a risk particularly in patients with diabetes who have preexisting proteinuria. However, the incidence of myositis when statins are used as monotherapy is ~1 in 1,000 patients, and careful patient instruction about the signs and symptoms, with advice to stop the medication and consume large volumes of liquids if symptoms occur, should obviate more serious outcomes. Statins can also cause non–clinically significant elevations in liver function tests in 1–2% of patients, but only at the higher doses of each agent. It is important for physicians and patients to realize that, despite the package insert warnings and the need for liver function tests at initiation of treatment, the statins are not hepatotoxic drugs; clinically significant hepatotoxicity is extremely rare. The statins do not appear to affect diabetic control. Importantly, we now have results from several clinical trials demonstrating reductions in CHD events and deaths in patients with type 2 diabetes receiving statins. Based on those studies, statins are the first-line approach to diabetes patients with isolated high levels of LDL cholesterol, with combined hyperlipidemia, or with moderate hypertriglyceridemia and an LDL cholesterol level above the NCEP goal. Thus, despite the fact that the most common lipid abnormality in diabetes is a dyslipidemia characterized by high triglycerides and low HDL cholesterol levels, with average or slightly elevated LDL cholesterol concentrations, statins should be considered as the first agents to be used.

Although the use of statins is widespread, these outstanding agents are still underused. More importantly, the proportion of patients reaching LDL goals is well below optimal, particularly when the goal is an LDL cholesterol <100 mg/dl, as it is for patients with diabetes. Titrating the statin is an important priority if trying to reach goal LDL levels, and physicians must realize that statins are extremely safe drugs with proven benefits. In the recent Heart Protection Study conducted in England, several thousand patients with diabetes, with and without prior cardiovascular diseases, benefited significantly from therapy with 40 mg simvastatin daily. The benefit was observed at all levels of baseline LDL, including LDL cholesterol levels <100 mg/dl at baseline. As in all of the clinical trials, the subjects with diabetes had very high absolute rates of cardiovascular events.

Bile Acid–Binding Resins

Cholestyramine, colestipol, and colesevelam are resins that bind bile acids in the intestine, thus interrupting the enterohepatic recirculation of those molecules.

A fall in bile acids returning to the liver results in increased conversion of hepatic cholesterol to bile acids, which results in a diminution of a regulatory pool of hepatic cholesterol and upregulation of the gene for hepatic LDL receptors. All of these changes lead to decreased plasma LDL concentrations. Usual doses are 8–24 g/day for cholestyramine, 10–30 g/day for colestipol (both as granular powders), and 6.5 g/day for colesevelam (as tablets). Cholestyramine is mixed with sucrose, but there is a "light" form that is made with NutraSweet. Colestipol is also available in 1-g tablets. Colesevelam is available in tablets—six tablets per day is the standard dose. At full doses, cholestyramine and colestipol can reduce LDL levels ~25%; however, compliance is usually low and, in most patients, only mid-level doses are achieved. At six tablets per day, colesevelam lowers LDL cholesterol by 15–20% and compliance is significantly better. Bile acid–binding resins are not absorbed and therefore have no systemic toxicities. A drawback to the use of bile acid–binding resin in patients with diabetes is an increase in hepatic VLDL triglyceride production and plasma triglyceride levels commonly associated with their use. An additional major side effect of these agents is bloating and constipation, which may pose a significant problem in the diabetes patient with gastroparesis. The resins can also interfere with the absorption of other oral medications, although this problem has been significantly reduced with colesevelam. With the availability of HMG-CoA reductase inhibitors, however, the need for resins has been markedly reduced. However, they can add greatly to LDL lowering when added to statins.

Fibric Acid Derivatives

Fibric acid derivatives are peroxisome proliferator-activated receptor-α agonists that have potent lipid-altering effects and are very useful in patients with diabetes. In general, fibrate use in patients with type 2 diabetes results in lowering of triglycerides from 35% to 45% and increases in HDL cholesterol from 10% to 20%. Fenofibrate and gemfibrozil are the agents presently available in the U.S. (clofibrate is still available, but its use has been restricted by the U.S. Food and Drug Administration). Several other agents are available in Europe and Canada. Although their mechanism of action is unclear, these agents appear to work by both decreasing hepatic VLDL production and increasing the activity of LpL. Unfortunately, fibrates have modest and variable effects on LDL cholesterol in most patients with diabetes. That is because fibrates can have some LDL-lowering effect, no effect, or even an LDL-raising effect in patients with hypertriglyceridemia. The basis for these variable outcomes is complex and has to do with the efficiency with which VLDL is converted to LDL, how efficiently LDL is removed from plasma, and the cholesterol content of LDL. In the latter instance, fibrate treatment, with concomitant triglyceride lowering, usually converts small, dense, cholesterol-depleted LDL into more normal cholesterol-enriched LDL. The usual dose is 600 mg gemfibrozil twice daily and 160 mg once daily for micronized fenofibrate. These agents are contraindicated in patients with gallstones, and because they are tightly bound to plasma proteins, levels of other drugs (e.g., Coumadin) should be monitored carefully. Fibrates do not significantly affect glycemic control.

The rise in LDL cholesterol concentration that can accompany reduced triglyceride levels during fibrate therapy must be viewed in the context of clinical trials of fibrate therapy that included patients with diabetes. In the Helsinki Heart Study, the two groups with hypertriglyceridemia (with and without concomitant elevations in LDL cholesterol) had increases or no changes in LDL cholesterol levels during gemfibrozil therapy and yet achieved the same reduction in CHD events as the group with isolated LDL elevations, in which LDL cholesterol levels fell 10–12% with treatment. The two groups in which LDL changed little or not at all included the majority of participants with diabetes (a small number overall). A more recent study, the Veterans Administration HDL Intervention Trial, showed that gemfibrozil was efficacious in a group of men who had CHD and a mean LDL cholesterol that was low (111 mg/dl) at baseline and did not change during the trial. The treated group did show a 7% increase in HDL cholesterol and a 25% reduction in triglycerides; these changes were associated with a 22% reduction in CHD events. In the 25% of the subjects in this trial who had diabetes (almost certainly type 2 diabetes in most), relative benefit was equal to that seen in the nondiabetic cohort. The subjects with diabetes had, as expected, higher absolute rates of events in both the placebo and the treatment group.

When statins have been compared with fibrates in patients with type 2 diabetes, the expected results were observed. The statins produced much greater LDL lowering, while the fibrates lowered triglycerides and raised HDL cholesterol more than the statins. Importantly, several recent studies of combination treatment of patients with type 2 diabetes have shown the powerful, positive effects on the entire dyslipidemic pattern with this approach. Of note, however, is that the risk of myositis increases to ~1% when statins are combined with fibrates. On the other hand, myositis (a CPK level more than ten times ULN and muscle pain) should never progress to rhabdomyolysis if the patient and the doctor pay attention to the symptoms and if the patient stops the drugs and drinks large volumes of fluids if symptoms occur.

Nicotinic Acid (Niacin)

As noted above, the most common lipid abnormalities present in patients with diabetes are elevated triglycerides and low HDL cholesterol levels. Niacin, when used in pharmacological doses (1–3 g/day), has the ability to potently lower triglycerides (25–40%) and raise HDL cholesterol (10–25%). Niacin also lowers LDL cholesterol (15–20%), and this adds to its potential efficacy in a high-risk population. The mechanism of action is generally thought to be through lowering hepatic VLDL apo B100 production and increasing the synthesis of apo A-I. Unfortunately, niacin has several side effects that often limit its utility in nondiabetic individuals: niacin produces a prostaglandin-mediated flush that occurs ~30 min after ingestion and can last as long as 1 h; patients turn red and feel hot. Niacin can cause gastric irritation and can exacerbate peptic ulcer disease, has been associated with dry skin, causes hyperuricemia and can precipitate gouty attacks, and is associated with elevations of hepatic transaminases in ~3–5% of patients. Rarely, regular short-acting niacin can also cause a clinically significant hepatitis. All of these side effects can occur in anyone using niacin, but in patients with type 2 diabetes, hyperuricemia is already more common. Most importantly, some studies have demonstrated that niacin therapy worsens diabetic control, likely by inducing insulin resistance. This finding is interesting at a theoretical level because niacin's ability to inhibit lipolysis and lower plasma free fatty acid levels after a single dose might be expected to improve insulin sensitivity. Two recent studies, one using regular short-acting niacin and the other an intermediate-release formulation of niacin (Niaspan), demonstrated that niacin was efficacious in terms of lipid-altering activity with modest but manageable effects on glycemic control. If a physician is faced with persistent low HDL and/or significant hyper-triglyceridemia after statin treatment, or even statin plus fibrate therapy, addition of niacin in either of the available forms can be considered. Of note, "long-acting, no flush" niacin preparations can cause severe hepatotoxicity and should not be used. Niaspan appears to have the same safety profile as short-acting niacin. There are some "no-flush" short-acting niacin preparations available (i.e., niacin inositol), but their efficacy is not well documented.

Omega-3 Fatty Acid Supplements

Fatty fish from the northern oceans are enriched in ω-3 (omega-3) fatty acids, docosahexanoic acid, and eicosapentanoic acid. Their use has, in epidemiologic studies, been associated with lower rates of cardiovascular disease. Diets rich in plant sources of the ω-3 fatty acid, α-linolenic acid, have also been associated with reduced cardiovascular events. ω-3 fatty acids provided as supplements, in doses of 3–6 g/day, are potent triglyceride-lowering agents and can be very useful in rare diabetes patients who have triglyceride levels >600 mg/dl, especially those not responsive to other drug therapies. The question of whether low doses of ω-3 fatty acids, as supplements, should be given to patients with type 2 diabetes remains incompletely answered. In the GISSI Prevention Trial, 1 g of an ω-3 fatty acid supplement significantly reduced fatal and nonfatal myocardial infarction and stroke in both nondiabetic individuals and subjects with diabetes. A prevailing theory is that these fatty acids reduce arrhythmic sudden death. The use of 1 g per day of ω-3 fatty acids is not associated with alterations of glycemic control, but their use with aspirin therapy could increase the risk of bleeding.

Hormone Replacement Therapy

In prospective observational studies of mostly nondiabetic women, estrogen replacement therapy has been associated with a significant decrease in risk for CHD. About one-third of the beneficial effects of hormones in these studies has been estimated to be caused by changes in lipid levels, specifically reductions in LDL cholesterol and increases in HDL cholesterol. Oral estrogen given alone raises HDL levels by 10–20% by increasing apo A-I synthesis and decreasing hepatic lipase activity. Estrogen alone also lowers LDL cholesterol ~20% by increasing LDL receptor number on cells, particularly in the liver. Another benefit relates to the ability of estrogen to lower lipoprotein (a) levels ~20%. A potentially negative effect of estrogen administration on diabetic dyslipidemia is the increase in plasma triglycerides that occurs via increased hepatic secretion of VLDL. Severe hyperlipidemia and pancreatitis have been observed in women with preexisting hypertriglyceridemia who were receiving oral estrogen treatment. Addition of a progestational agent has been associated with much less HDL raising, but also less triglyceride raising, compared with estrogen therapy alone.

Early studies with high-dose estrogen-containing oral contraceptives indicated that glucose intolerance could occur, probably in women with the metabolic syndrome. There was a fear that estrogen treatment could "induce" diabetes in predisposed women. However, three intervention trials have assessed hormone therapy in women with type 2 diabetes for treatment periods of 6–12 weeks. All three showed that isolated estrogen treatment lowered blood glucose levels and glycosylated hemoglobin levels without raising plasma insulin concentrations or causing insulin resistance. Lipid profiles were also improved, with lower LDL and higher HDL cholesterol levels, and with no significant rise in plasma triglycerides in two of the three studies. Interestingly, estrogen replacement therapy appears to improve postprandial lipemia in normal subjects despite its effect to raise fasting triglyceride levels. It appears that, overall, hormone replacement therapy in women with type 2 diabetes can induce favorable lipid changes (particularly if micronized progesterone is used as the progestational agent) and has no detrimental effect on glycemic control.

With that said, the recent results from HERS (Heart and Estrogen/Progestin Replacement Study), the WAVE (Women's Angiographic Vitamins and Estrogen) study, and the Womens' Health Initiative showed no benefit in women with or without prior myocardial infarction who received combined therapy with equine conjugated estrogens (Premarin) plus low-dose medroxyprogesterone (Provera). Although we await the results from the Womens' Health Initiative study arm that was treated with estrogen only, and resolution of the question of whether all progestins have the same effects, it is not appropriate at this time to use hormone replacement therapy as a way to reduce cardiovascular risk. Indeed, women with diabetes who require hormone replacement therapy for hot flashes or other nontreatable symptoms of systemic estrogen deficiency (osteoporosis should be treated with drugs specific for that problem) should understand that there may be an increased risk for cardiovascular disease and breast cancer.

SUMMARY

When rationally approached, the patient with diabetes and hyperlipidemia can be well managed through both lifestyle interventions and pharmacotherapy. Close guidance and monitoring is needed, however, in choosing the proper approach. A variety of options are available to improve plasma lipids and thus reduce risk of CHD. The key, however, based on many clinical trials, is that significant benefit can be obtained by aggressively lowering LDL cholesterol and raising HDL cholesterol/lowering triglycerides.

When specific lipid-altering therapy is indicated, the physician has effective and safe agents from which to choose. Despite the fact that the characteristic diabetic dyslipidemia is one of higher triglycerides, lower HDL cholesterol, and average or slightly higher than average LDL cholesterol levels, the evidence from clinical trials indicates that lowering LDL cholesterol should be a central priority. Treatment with statins, regardless of initial LDL cholesterol levels, will, based on the Heart Protection Study, reduce event rates significantly. Whether statin therapy should always be first is a question that cannot be answered with full confidence, but it seems prudent to say that at least 90% of patients with diabetes should get a statin as part of their overall cardioprotective therapy.

For the diabetes patient with isolated hypertriglyceridemia and low HDL cholesterol (with an LDL cholesterol <100 mg/dl), fibric acid derivatives could be an alternative as the first choice for drug therapy. In some cases, fibric acid derivatives will be all that is necessary. If the LDL cholesterol increases during fibrate treatment and goes above 100 mg/dl, the physician has several choices. First, a bile acid–binding resin could be added to the fibrate: this would lower LDL cholesterol without, in the presence of the fibrate, significantly affecting triglyceride levels. The second alternative would be to switch to an HMG-CoA reductase inhibitor: this would be the logical choice if the triglyceride elevation (before or during fibrate treatment) was only moderate (<250 mg/dl). Finally, the physician could add the reductase inhibitor to the fibrate. The latter combination is effective in correcting severe combined hyperlipidemia but carries an increased risk of myositis. We believe that this combination can be used successfully, particularly if the patient knows clearly that he or she must stop the medications, drink large quantities of liquids, and call a physician if diffuse, symmetric muscle pain occurs. The patient should have liver function tests obtained regularly with the use of fibrates or reductase inhibitors alone or in combination. The final choice, nicotinic acid, could be used in patients with severe, combined hyperlipidemia or extremely low levels of HDL cholesterol. Both short-acting and intermediate-release niacin preparations are efficacious when used with a statin, and the risk of myositis is extremely low with this combination.

In those patients who present with combined elevations of both LDL cholesterol and plasma triglycerides, an HMG-CoA reductase inhibitor is probably the most effective single agent. Again, niacin could also be used as a sole drug, with caution taken as described above. A fibric acid derivative can be added if triglycerides are not sufficiently reduced by either of those drugs alone.

Therapy for the diabetic patient with an isolated reduction in HDL cholesterol is not clearly defined. Fibrates have not been demonstrated to be very effective in raising HDL cholesterol levels in nondiabetic individuals with isolated reductions in HDL, although no similar studies have been carried out in patients with diabetes. Niacin may be more effective in elevating HDL cholesterol concentrations when they are low in the absence of hypertriglyceridemia, but all of the caveats of niacin use in diabetes would apply here as well. An alternative to raising HDL in these subjects would be to more aggressively treat LDL cholesterol levels, with the goal of reducing them to much less than 100 mg/dl. It must be clear, however, that there are no endpoint trials supporting any approach to isolated reductions in HDL cholesterol, either in nondiabetic individuals or patients with diabetes.

Finally, in those patients with diabetes who have isolated high levels of LDL cholesterol, either a bile acid resin or an HMG-CoA reductase inhibitor may be used primarily. The combination of these two agents has been shown to be effective in those individuals with extremely high levels of LDL cholesterol resistant to monotherapy. Triglyceride levels need to be observed closely in those patients placed on resins.

BIBLIOGRAPHY

American Diabetes Association: Dyslipidemia management in adults with diabetes (Position Statement). *Diabetes Care* 27 (Suppl. 1):S68–S71, 2004

Chesney CM, Elam MB, Herd JA, Davis KB, Garg R, Hunninghake D, et al.: Effect of niacin, warfarin, and antioxidant therapy on coagulation parameters in patients with peripheral arterial disease in the Arterial Disease Multiple Intervention Trial (ADMIT). *Am Heart J* 140:631–636, 2000

Ellen RLB, McPherson R: Long-term efficacy and safety of fenofibrate and a statin in the treatment of combined hyperlipidemia. *Am J Cardiol* 81:60B–65B, 1998

Expert Panel on Detection, Evaluation, and Treatment of High Blood Cholesterol in Adults: Executive summary of the third report of the National Cholesterol Education Program (NCEP) Expert Panel on Detection, Evaluation, and Treatment of High Blood Cholesterol in Adults (Adult Treatment Panel III). *JAMA* 285:2486–2497, 2001

Ginsberg HN: Lipoprotein physiology (Review). *Endocrinol Metab Clin North Am* 27:503–519, 1998

Ginsberg HN, Illingworth DR: Postprandial dyslipidemia: an atherogenic disorder common in patients with diabetes mellitus. *Am J Cardiol* 88:9H–15H, 2001

Goldberg RB, Mellies MJ, Sacks FM, Moye LA, Howard BV, Howard WJ, et al.: Cardiovascular events and their reduction with pravastatin in diabetic and glucose-intolerant myocardial infarction survivors with average cholesterol levels: subgroup analysis in the Cholesterol and Recurrent Events (CARE) trial. *Circulation* 98:2513–2519, 1998

Grundy SM, Vega GL, McGovern ME, Tulloch BR, Kendall DM, Fitz-Patrick D, et al.: Diabetes Multicenter Research Group: efficacy, safety, and tolerability of once-daily niacin for the treatment of dyslipidemia associated with type 2 diabetes: results of the assessment of diabetes control and evaluation of the efficacy of niaspan trial. *Arch Intern Med* 22:1568–1576, 2002

Haffner SM: Management of dyslipidemia in adults with diabetes (Technical Review). *Diabetes Care* 21:160–178, 1998

Heart Protection Study Collaborative Group: MRC/BHF Heart Protection Study of cholesterol lowering with simvastatin in 20,536 high-risk individuals: a randomised placebo-controlled trial. *Lancet* 360:7–22, 2002

Hulley S, Grady D, Bush T, Furberg C, Herrington D, Riggs B, et al.: Randomized trial of estrogen plus progestin for secondary prevention of coronary heart disease in postmenopausal women: Heart and Estrogen/progestin Replacement Study Research Group. *JAMA* 280:605–613, 1998

Kannel WB, D'Agostino RB, Wilson PWF, Bleanger AJ, Gagnon DR: Diabetes, fibrinogen, and risk of cardiovascular disease: the Framingham experience. *Am Heart J* 120:672–676, 1990

Pyorala K, Pedersen TR, Kjekshus J, Faegerman O, Olsson AG, Thorgeirsson G: Cholesterol lowering with simvastatin improves prognosis of diabetic patients with coronary artery disease: a subgroup analysis of the Scandinavian Simvastatin Survival Study. *Diabetes Care* 20:614–620, 1997

Rubins HB, Robins SJ, Collins D, Fye CL, Anderson JW, Elam MB, et al.: Gemfibrozil for the secondary prevention of coronary heart disease in men with low levels of high-density lipoprotein cholesterol: Veterans Affairs High-Density Lipoprotein Cholesterol Intervention Trial Study Group. *N Engl J Med* 341:410–418, 1999

Tikkanen MJ, Laakso M, Ilmonen M, Helve E, Kaarsalo E, Kilkki E, et al.: Treatment of hypercholesterolemia and combined hyperlipidemia with simvastatin and gemfibrozil in patients with NIDDM: a multicenter comparison study. *Diabetes Care* 21:477–481, 1998

Writing Group for the Women's Health Initiative: Risks and benefits of estrogen plus progestin in healthy postmenopausal women: principal results from the Women's Health Initiative randomized controlled trial. *JAMA* 288:321–333, 2002

Dr. Ginsberg is the Irving Professor of Medicine and Director of the Irving Center for Clinical Research, Columbia University College of Physicians and Surgeons, New York, New York.

34. Antihypertensive Therapy

John Shin, MD, Valerie Goldburt, MD, MPH, James R. Sowers, MD, and Samy I. McFarlane, MD

Hypertension is a common comorbidity that affects 20–70% of patients with diabetes and accounts for up to 80% of cardiovascular disease (CVD) risk. In type 1 diabetes, hypertension is usually a manifestation of diabetic nephropathy, and hypertension and diabetic nephropathy appear to exacerbate each other. In type 2 diabetes, hypertension usually clusters with the other components of the metabolic syndrome, such as microalbuminuria, obesity, insulin resistance, dyslipidemia, and coagulation abnormalities (Table 34.1). Furthermore, the prevalence of hypertension and diabetes is almost twice as great in African Americans than in Caucasians, and both conditions are also more common among the ethnic minorities in the U.S. Hypertension substantially increases both macrovascular and microvascular complications of diabetes, including stroke, coronary artery disease, and peripheral arterial disease as well as retinopathy and nephropathy. Systolic blood pressure (BP) is an especially potent risk factor for microvascular and macrovascular disease in diabetic patients.

PATHOPHYSIOLOGY

Hypertension in patients with diabetes, compared with individuals without diabetes, has unique features, such as increased salt sensitivity, volume expansion, isolated systolic hypertension, loss of nocturnal dipping of BP and pulse, and increased propensity to proteinuria and orthostatic hypotension. Most of these features are considered risk factors for CVD (Table 34.1). An understanding of the pathogenesis of hypertension in the patient with diabetes and of the pharmacological effects of antihypertensive drugs in these individuals will help clinicians make rational therapeutic choices, such as the use of low-dose diuretics for treatment of volume expansion and angiotensin-converting enzyme (ACE) inhibitors or angiotensin II receptor blockers (ARBs) for reducing proteinuria. Furthermore, because of the propensity to orthostatic hypotension, standing BPs should be measured at each office visit. Because of the increased BP variability in these patients, ambulatory BP measurements or home BP monitoring may be particularly valuable.

Table 34.1 CVD Risk Factors Associated with Hypertension in Patients with Type 2 Diabetes

- Central obesity
- Family history
- Male sex or postmenopausal state
- Cigarette smoking
- Physical inactivity
- Insulin resistance/hyperinsulinemia
- Microalbuminuria
- Dyslipidemia: ↑ triglycerides, ↓ HDL, ↑ non-HDL cholesterol
- ↑ C-reactive protein
- Endothelial dysfunction
- ↑ Fibrinogen
- ↑ Plasminogen activator inhibitor 1
- ↑ Homocysteine
- ↓ Nocturnal dipping of BP and heart rate
- Salt sensitivity
- Left ventricular hypertrophy

PATIENT EVALUATION

1. Patients with diabetes are prone to BP lability; thus, BP measurement should be obtained every routine diabetes visit. Orthostatic measurements of BP should also be done; this will help assess the presence of autonomic neuropathy.

2. Next, 24-h ambulatory BP monitoring is helpful in identifying the loss of nocturnal dipping in BP and pulse in the presence of diabetic autonomic neuropathy and in elderly patients. Non-dipping of BP is associated with increased CVD risk (Table 34.1). This is an important consideration regarding the choice of the antihypertensive therapy and the use of medications that have a 24-h duration of action.

3. Once hypertension is documented, a thorough history and physical examination should be performed to assess end-organ damage and identify secondary causes of coexistent hypertension and diabetes (e.g., primary aldosteronism and renal artery stenosis).

4. Initial evaluation (Table 34.2): Assessment of the metabolic status of the patients before and after the use of antihypertensive therapy is important (e.g., monitoring serum potassium and creatinine before and after the use of an ACE inhibitor, ARB, or aldosterone antagonist). Evaluation of patients for the presence of albuminuria and left ventricular hypertrophy is also useful for determining baseline measurements for future follow-up and for aiding in the therapeutic choice of antihypertensive medications.

Table 34.2 Initial Evaluation

- Complete history and physical examination
- Complete blood count
- Serum creatinine and blood urea nitrogen
- Urinalysis
- Serum electrolytes
- Serum Mg^{2+}
- Serum uric acid
- Fasting lipid profile
- 24-h urine collection for total protein and creatinine clearance
- Electrocardiogram
- Chest X ray

THERAPEUTIC GOALS

Epidemiologic data suggest that a BP of >120/70 mmHg is associated with a higher CVD event rate and increased mortality in people with diabetes. Strong evidence also exists that therapy of hypertension in these patients effectively decreases CVD and microvascular disease. Furthermore, data from randomized controlled trials such as the United Kingdom Prospective Diabetes Study (UKPDS) and the Hypertension Optimal Treatment (HOT) trial showed improved outcomes with lower BP targets. The benefit of targeting diastolic BP of <80 mmHg was demonstrated in the HOT trial. Therefore, a BP goal of <130/80 mmHg is recommended by the Hypertension and Diabetes Executive Working Group of the National Kidney Foundation. This treatment goal is also adopted by both the American Diabetes Association and the Canadian Hypertension Society.

NONPHARMACOLOGICAL THERAPY

1. Weight reduction is the most important nonpharmacological modality in the management of most hypertensive patients with diabetes mellitus. Several controlled studies evaluated the relationship of weight loss and BP reduction. The loss of 1 kg body weight reduced mean arterial BP by ~1 mmHg. Furthermore, weight reduction can lead to improved blood glucose and lipid control as well as other health benefits.

2. Physical activity has been identified as an important nonpharmacological intervention in the management of patients with hypertension in general and in patients with diabetes in particular. Physical inactivity is one of the most important modifiable risk factors for CVD. In people with diabetes, regular exercise has been shown to improve glycemic control and promote a sense of well-being. Given the high risk of CVD in these patient populations, thorough evaluation with appropriate diagnostic studies should be performed before initiation of an exercise program to screen for the pres-

ence of macrovascular and microvascular complications that might be exacerbated by the physical activity program. Cardiac stress testing is recommended for diabetic patients older than the age of 35 years who are planning to begin a vigorous exercise program. An individualized physical activity plan could help minimize risk to the patient with cardiovascular complications.

3. Smoking cessation and restriction of alcohol consumption are recommended for all patients with diabetes. Smoking increases CVD risk, and excessive alcohol intake (more than three drinks daily) is associated with increased BP in the general hypertensive population. Furthermore, reduction of alcohol intake has been shown in randomized controlled trials to be associated with lowering of BP, with each reduction of one drink per day lowering systolic and diastolic BP by ~1 mmHg.

4. A diet high in potassium, fiber, and nonfat dairy products and relatively low in salt has been shown to reduce BP and other CVD risk factors.

PHARMACOLOGICAL THERAPY

General Considerations

To achieve the recommended BP target, many patients with diabetes will require three or more antihypertensive medications. The use of drug therapy must be in addition to, not a substitute for, nonpharmacological modalities. Furthermore, management of hypertension in people with diabetes should be integrated in the overall management of CVD. For example, achieving good glycemic control may preserve renal function, which in turn may contribute to better BP control. Emphasis on self-monitoring of blood glucose and BP will reinforce the concept of self-care and might increase the overall adherence to lifestyle changes such as exercise and weight loss, which in turn could lead to improved control of both blood glucose and BP.

Based on the results of randomized controlled trials, including the Antihypertensive and Lipid-Lowering Treatment to Prevent Heart Attacks Trial (ALLHAT), a treatment algorithm is suggested (Fig. 34.1) for management of hypertension in patients with diabetes.

Diuretic Therapy

Diuretic therapy is an important component of the management of hypertension in people with diabetes—a disease that is associated with volume expansion and higher systolic BP. Furthermore, ALLHAT, the largest hypertension clinical trial ever conducted (which included 42,418 patients with hypertension, of whom 36% had diabetes), showed no significant difference after 5 years of follow-up in the primary outcome of fatal coronary heart disease or nonfatal myocardial infarction among the groups treated with calcium-channel blockers (CCBs) and ACE inhibitors and those treated with a thiazide diuretic. Based on these results and considering the potential cost saving with the use of diuretics, a thiazide diuretic was recommended as an initial therapy by the ALLHAT investigators.

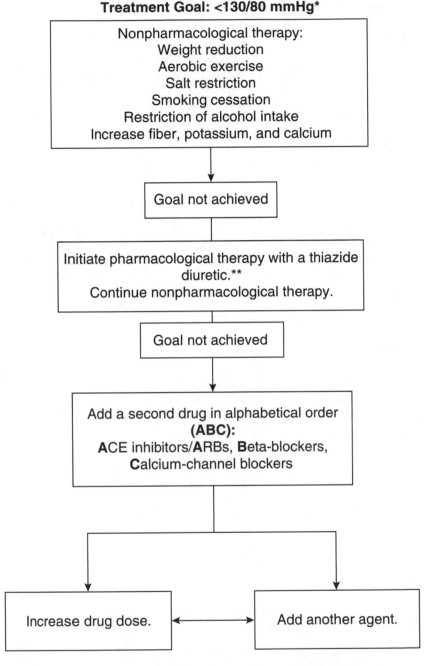

Treatment Goal: <130/80 mmHg*

Nonpharmacological therapy:
Weight reduction
Aerobic exercise
Salt restriction
Smoking cessation
Restriction of alcohol intake
Increase fiber, potassium, and calcium

Goal not achieved

Initiate pharmacological therapy with a thiazide diuretic.**
Continue nonpharmacological therapy.

Goal not achieved

Add a second drug in alphabetical order **(ABC)**:
ACE inhibitors/**A**RBs, **B**eta-blockers, **C**alcium-channel blockers

Increase drug dose. ⟷ Add another agent.

Figure 34.1 Antihypertensive therapy in people with diabetes. *In patients with >1 g proteinuria and renal insufficiency, the treatment goal is BP <125/75 mmHg. **Based on the results of ALLHAT (see text); in patients with serum creatinine >1.8 mg/dl, use a loop diuretic.

However, it is important to note again that three or more drugs are usually needed to control BP to the recommended target. In fact, 63% of patients in ALLHAT were on two or more medications by the end of the study. Also an important point to consider is the side effect profile of the diuretic therapy such as hypokalemia and the slightly higher serum cholesterol and glucose levels. Furthermore, in patients with renal impairment (serum creatinine >1.8 mg/dl), loop diuretics should be used (Fig. 34.1).

ACE Inhibitors

Data from randomized controlled trials such as the Captopril Prevention Project (CAPPP) and the MICRO-HOPE substudy of the Heart Outcome Prevention Evaluation (HOPE) trial have shown that ACE inhibitors provide cardiovascular benefits and may improve insulin resistance and prevent the development of diabetes. In patients with type 1 diabetes and proteinuria, the use of ACE inhibitors was associated with a 50% reduction in the risk of the combined endpoint of death, dialysis, and transplantation. Furthermore, ACE inhibitors provide considerable benefits in diabetes patients with heart failure. In the Studies Of Left Ventricular Dysfunction (SOLVD) trial, ACE inhibitors significantly reduced mortality and hospitalization from heart failure. With these clearly proven benefits, ACE inhibitors are favorable agents for patients with diabetes.

ARBs

ARBs are recommended for patients who cannot tolerate ACE inhibitors (usually because of cough) and in whom ACE inhibitor therapy is indicated. ARBs have been shown in randomized controlled trials to reduce the progression of renal disease in patients with diabetes and hypertension. These benefits were above and beyond those attributable to BP reduction.

Caution should be used when using ACE inhibitors and ARBs because worsening kidney function may occur if renal artery stenosis exists. Also, hyperkalemia may supervene or worsen in the presence of a hyporeninemic, hypoaldosteronemic state (type IV Renal Tubular Acidosis). Thus, monitoring electrolytes and creatinine is necessary during the first few weeks of treatment. The use of a thiazide diuretic may ameliorate hyperkalemia associated with the use of these agents.

β-Blockers

β-Blockers are useful antihypertensive agents in patients with diabetes. In the UKPDS, atenolol reduced microvascular complications of diabetes by 37%, strokes by 44%, and death related to diabetes by 32%.

Despite the potential adverse metabolic effects of β-blockers, these agents have been shown to have long-term favorable effects on CVD in patients with diabetes and hypertension. Therefore, β-blockers should be used particularly in diabetes patients with coronary artery disease and in patients post–myocardial infarction, where these agents have been shown to improve survival.

CCBs

Based on the results of ALLHAT mentioned above, with the null difference in the primary outcome between groups, the safety of CCBs was reaffirmed in this large study. The use of CCBs is particularly useful in achieving target BP, especially in patients with isolated systolic hypertension not responding to diuretic therapy.

α-Adrenergic Blockers

In ALLHAT, the α-adrenergic blocker doxazosin arm was stopped 2.5 years before the end of the study because of a 25% higher rate of combined cardiovascular events and a twofold increase in heart failure compared with the thiazide diuretic chlorthalidone. These results indicate that the initial therapy with doxazosin (and possibly other α_1-blockers) is definitely inferior to low-dose diuretic treatment for patients at high risk for CVD; therefore, these agents are no longer recommended in patients with diabetes.

BIBLIOGRAPHY

American Diabetes Association: Hypertension management in adults with diabetes (Position Statement). *Diabetes Care* 27 (Suppl. 1):S65–S67, 2004

Arauz-Pacheco C, Parrott MA, Raskin P: Treatment of hypertension in adults with diabetes. *Diabetes Care* 26 (Suppl. 1):S80–S82, 2003

Bakris GL, Williams M, Dworkin L, Elliott WJ, Epstein M, Toto R, Tuttle K, Douglas J, Hsueh W, Sowers J: Preserving renal function in adults with hypertension and diabetes: a consensus approach: National Kidney Foundation Hypertension and Diabetes Executive Committees Working Group. *Am J Kidney Dis* 36:646–661, 2000

Lewis EG, Hunsicker LG, Bain RP, Rohde RD, The Collaborative Study Group: The effect of angiotensin converting enzyme inhibition on diabetic nephropathy. *N Engl J Med* 329:1456–1462, 1993

McFarlane SI, Banerji M, Sowers JR: Insulin resistance and cardiovascular disease. *J Clin Endocrinol Metab* 86:713–718, 2001

McFarlane SI, Jacober SJ, Winer N, Kaur J, Castro JP, Wui MA, Gliwa A, Von Gizycki H, Sowers JR: Control of cardiovascular risk factors in patients with diabetes and hypertension at urban academic medical centers. *Diabetes Care* 25:718–723, 2002

McFarlane SI, Sowers JR: Hypertension in people with diabetes. In *Hypertension Primer*. 3rd ed. Dallas, TX, American Heart Association, 2003

Sowers JR, Epstein M, Frohlich ED: Diabetes, hypertension, and cardiovascular disease: an update. *Hypertension* 37:1053–1059, 2001

The ALLHAT Officers and Coordinators for the ALLHAT Collaborative Research Group: Major outcomes in high-risk hypertensive patients randomized to angiotensin-converting enzyme inhibitor or calcium channel blocker vs diuretic: the Antihypertensive and Lipid-Lowering Treatment to Prevent Heart Attack Trial (ALLHAT). *JAMA* 288:2981–2997, 2002

The Sixth Report of the Joint National Committee on Prevention, Detection, Evaluation, and Treatment of High Blood Pressure. *Arch Intern Med* 157:2413–46, 1997

UK Prospective Diabetes Study Group: Tight blood pressure control and risk of macrovascular and microvascular complications in type 2 diabetes: UKPDS 38. *BMJ* 317:703–713, 1998

Dr. Shin is Assistant Professor of Medicine; Dr. Goldburt is an intern; and Dr. McFarlane is an Associate Professor of Medicine and Fellowship Program Director at the State University of New York, Health Science Center at Brooklyn, Kings County Hospital Center and Brooklyn Veteran Administration Medical Center, Brooklyn, NY. Dr. Sowers is the Thomas W. and Joan F. Burns Missouri Chair in Diabetology; Director of the MU Diabetes and Cardiovascular Center; Associate Dean for Clinical Research; and Professor of Medicine, Physiology, and Pharmacology at the University of Missouri-Columbia, Columbia, MO.

35. Skin and Subcutaneous Tissues

JEAN L. BOLOGNIA, MD, AND IRWIN M. BRAVERMAN, MD

The cutaneous disorders discussed in this chapter are waxy skin and stiff joints, scleredema, diabetic dermopathy, necrobiosis lipoidica (diabeticorum), disseminated granuloma annulare, eruptive xanthomas, lipodystrophy, acanthosis nigricans, diabetic bullae, necrolytic migratory erythema (NME) (glucagonoma syndrome), and reactions to oral hypoglycemic drugs and insulin. Cutaneous infections (e.g., candidiasis and mucormycosis) and lower-extremity ulcerations are covered elsewhere (see Chapters 36 and 56).

PATHOPHYSIOLOGY

The underlying pathophysiology is theoretical in most of the cutaneous disorders associated with diabetes mellitus. In the skin lesions of necrobiosis lipoidica and diabetic dermopathy, there is histological evidence of microangiopathy, and this presumably plays a role in the formation of lesions. In waxy skin associated with stiff joints, the thickened dermis may be the result of an increase in glycosylated insoluble collagen. The epidermal hyperplasia seen in lesions of acanthosis nigricans is thought to result from the action of circulating insulin on insulin-like growth factor receptors on keratinocytes and fibroblasts, whereas the epidermal necrosis seen in NME may be a reflection of glucagon-induced hypoaminoacidemia. Hypertriglyceridemia and eruptive xanthomas are presumably due to the effects of hypoinsulinemia on lipid metabolism in that they quickly resolve after insulin administration.

WAXY SKIN AND STIFF JOINTS (CHEIROARTHROPATHY)

Up to 30% of young patients (ages 1–28 years) with type 1 diabetes have limited mobility of the small and large joints, and in individuals with diabetes for >5 years, the severity of joint disease is correlated with microvascular complications. Involvement of the small joints of the hands can be easily demonstrated by the failure of the palmar surfaces of the interphalangeal joints to approximate (Fig. 35.1). Approximately 30% of patients with limited joint mobility have tight, thick, waxy skin over the backs of the hands that is difficult to tent. This increased thickness can be confirmed by high-resolution ultrasonography. However, thickened skin

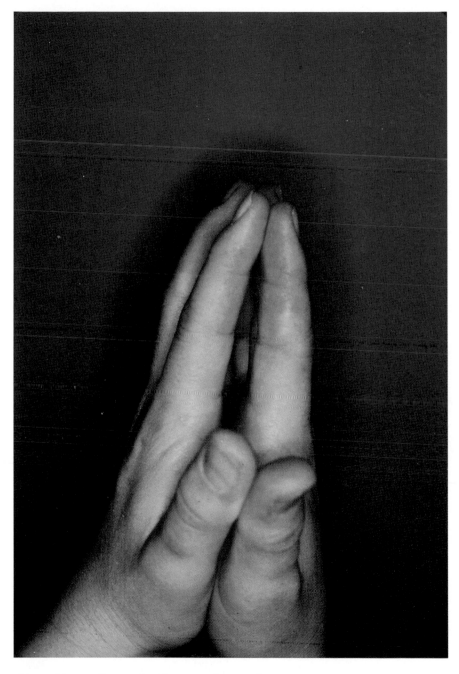

Figure 35.1 Failure of palmar surfaces of interphalangeal joints to approximate in a patient with stiff joints and waxy skin.

has been observed primarily in individuals with moderate to severe joint disease. Those skin findings may reverse with improved control of the diabetes; otherwise, there is no known treatment.

SCLEREDEMA

In scleredema, there is a thickening of the skin due to the deposition of glycosaminoglycans (in particular, hyaluronic acid) within the dermis. Areas of involvement may not be visually apparent, although they can develop a peau d'orange appearance as a result of prominent and depressed follicular openings (Fig. 35.2). The extent of involvement is best appreciated by palpation of the induration. Because scleredema is found most commonly on the upper back and posterior neck, the patient may be unaware of its presence. However, on physical examination, there is often decreased range of motion of the neck, especially dorsal extension. Less common sites of involvement include the face, upper arms, chest, lower back, and tongue. Rarely, there is cardiac, muscular, or esophageal involvement.

Scleredema has been associated with a monoclonal gammopathy or preceding streptococcal and viral infections as well as type 1 and type 2 diabetes (usually

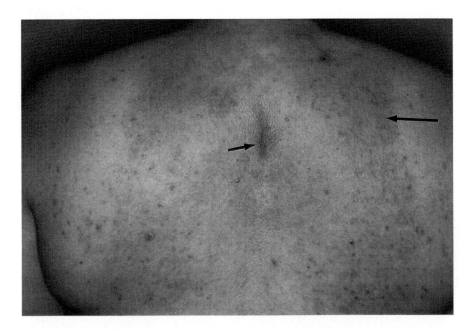

Figure 35.2 Scleredema of upper back with overlying erythema (*large arrow*) and development of peau d'orange appearance centrally (*small arrow*).

long standing). In the form seen in patients with diabetes, the induration may be accompanied by erythema (Fig. 35.2), which might be misdiagnosed as treatment-resistant cellulitis.

There is no consistently effective treatment for scleredema, although some cases, especially those in nondiabetic patients, may spontaneously resolve. In symptomatic patients, a 12-week course of PUVA [psoralens (8-methoxypsoralen, 0.4–0.6 mg/kg) plus ultraviolet A (UVA)] can be considered.

DIABETIC DERMOPATHY

Diabetic dermopathy is characterized by multiple hyperpigmented macules on the extensor surface of the distal lower extremities (Fig. 35.3). The individual lesions range in size from 0.5 to 2 cm, are oval or circular, and may have associated atrophy and scale. These skin changes have also been referred to as "shin spots" or "pigmented pretibial patches" and are thought to represent an abnormal response to trauma. In one series of 393 patients with type 2 diabetes, 12.5% had evidence of diabetic dermopathy, whereas in a second series of 173 patients (with both type 1 and type 2 diabetes), 40% had such lesions, in particular, individuals >50 years of age. These skin lesions may also be seen in individuals without evidence of glucose intolerance, albeit less often. In general, the dermopathy is asymptomatic except for its appearance, and no effective treatment has been described. However, a higher prevalence of neuropathy, retinopathy, nephropathy, and large-vessel disease has been reported in patients with diabetic dermopathy as compared with individuals without such skin lesions.

NECROBIOSIS LIPOIDICA (DIABETICORUM)

Necrobiosis lipoidica (NL) (diabeticorum) skin lesions are so named because of the presence of necrobiosis or degeneration of collagen in the dermis, the yellow color of most well-developed lesions due to carotene and lipid, and the association with diabetes mellitus. The disorder is characterized by red to red-brown to violet plaques that enlarge and frequently become yellow centrally. In addition, there is atrophy of the epidermis, which leads to shiny transparent skin and visualization of underlying dermal and subcutaneous vessels (Fig. 35.4). The most common location for NL is the shin (seen in 90% of patients), but lesions can also occur on the scalp, face, and arms. Plaques may ulcerate, especially those on the distal lower extremities.

NL is uncommon, occurring in 0.1–0.3% of the diabetes population, usually in the 3rd or 4th decade of life. However, there is some disagreement as to the proportion of patients with NL who actually have frank diabetes. The range that is usually cited is 40–65%, based primarily on clinical series from the 1950s and 1960s. In a more recent retrospective study of consecutive patients seen over a period of 25 years, only 7 (11%) of 65 patients with classic biopsy-proven NL had diabetes mellitus at presentation.

There is no well-established treatment for NL, but in small series, some success has been reported with topical corticosteroids (with or without occlusion),

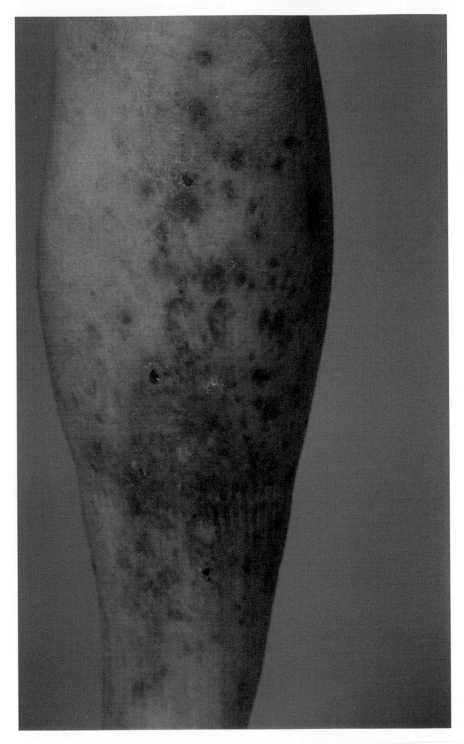

Figure 35.3 Hyperpigmented macules on shin of patient with diabetic dermopathy.

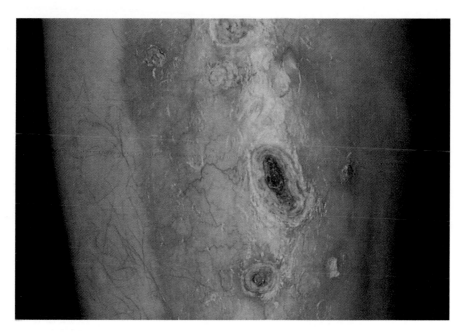

Figure 35.4 Necrobiosis lipoidica of anterior lower extremity with characteristic atrophy and visualization of underlying vessels.

pentoxifylline (400 mg three times per day), nicotinamide (500 mg three times per day), clofazimine (200 mg/day), and dipyridamole (50–75 mg three to four times per day) plus low-dose aspirin (325 mg/day). However, a double blind, placebo-controlled trial of the latter combination showed no significant benefit. Intralesional injections of corticosteroids (5 mg/ml triamcinolone acetonide) can be used to treat the active borders of the lesions. If ulceration occurs, the injections should be discontinued.

DISSEMINATED GRANULOMA ANNULARE

Granuloma annulare is characterized by annular or arciform plaques that form from the coalescence of skin-colored, pink, or red-brown papules (Fig. 35.5). The skin in the center of the lesion may be normal or erythematous in appearance. Most commonly, granuloma annulare has an acral distribution, but the lesions can be more numerous, papular, and located on the trunk as well as the extremities. The term generalized or disseminated granuloma annulare is used to describe the latter patients. The clinical diagnosis can be confirmed by performing a skin biopsy. A patient with generalized granuloma annulare should be screened for glucose intolerance, e.g., in one series of 100 patients with generalized granuloma

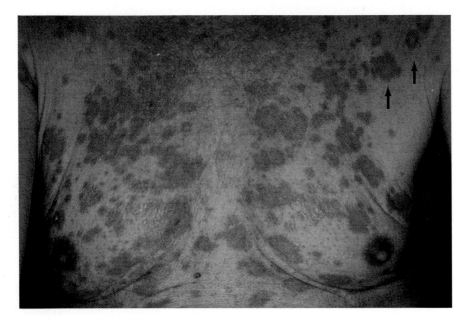

Figure 35.5 Generalized granuloma annulare. Annular shape of lesions is best seen on left shoulder.

annulare, 21% were shown to have diabetes. The etiology of granuloma annulare is unknown, and the treatment is empiric and includes topical and intralesional corticosteroids (5 mg/ml triamcinolone acetonide), niacinamide (500 mg three times per day), and in severe cases, PUVA two to three times per week or dapsone (50–100 mg/day).

XANTHOMAS

There are several types of cutaneous xanthomas, including eruptive, tendinous, tuberous, and planar, which are reflections of hypercholesterolemia and/or hypertriglyceridemia. Eruptive xanthomas can appear suddenly, and the lesions are usually 4–6 mm in diameter, firm, and yellow with a red base; the elbows, knees, buttocks, and sites of trauma are favored sites (Fig. 35.6). Biopsy findings are diagnostic and demonstrate collections of lipids within the dermis. The most common scenario for the appearance of eruptive xanthomas is hypertriglyceridemia in the setting of poorly controlled diabetes mellitus. Administration of insulin results in a decrease in the circulating levels of triglycerides, and the xanthomas quickly resolve. If the patient is not appropriately treated, the eruptive lesions can enlarge into tuberous xanthomas. Xanthelasma (plane xanthoma of the eyelids) is the least specific marker of hyperlipidemia in that 50% of the patients have normal lipid levels. In addition, there is no clear-cut association between diabetes and xanthelasma.

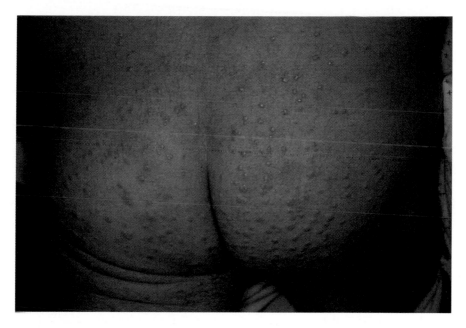

Figure 35.6 Eruptive xanthomas on buttocks of patient with poorly controlled diabetes mellitus.

LIPODYSTROPHY

Although the diseases outlined in this section are referred to as lipodystrophies, the patients have primarily lipoatrophy, and the lipoatrophy is divided into two major forms: total (generalized) and partial. In the generalized form, the entire body is involved. The onset is congenital (at birth or during infancy) in the inherited (autosomal recessive) form of the disease and during the 1st to 3rd decades of life in the sporadic form. In contrast, partial lipoatrophy usually involves the face, neck, arms, and upper trunk (above the waist); is usually sporadic; and has its onset from childhood to early adulthood. Occasionally, partial lipoatrophy affects only areas below the waist. In biopsy specimens of areas of subcutaneous fat loss, the fat cells are present, but the cytoplasmic fat is absent.

Both forms of lipoatrophy, total and partial, are associated with insulin-resistant diabetes mellitus. Patients with total lipoatrophy also have accelerated somatic growth and bone maturation, increased muscle mass, hypertriglyceridemia, and fatty infiltration of the liver. In addition, those with congenital total lipoatrophy have hyperpigmentation, acanthosis nigricans, and generalized hirsutism. In contrast, ~40–50% of those with acquired partial lipoatrophy have evidence of membranoproliferative glomerulonephritis, often in association with hypocomplementemia.

ACANTHOSIS NIGRICANS

In acanthosis nigricans, velvety tan to dark-brown plaques are seen on the sides of the neck, axillae, and groin (Fig. 35.7). Additional sites of involvement include the extensor surface of the small joints of the hand, the elbows, and the knees. Acanthosis nigricans can be a reflection of an underlying malignancy, usually adenocarcinoma of the gastrointestinal tract, but is more commonly associated with obesity.

The clinical spectrum in obese patients can range from euglycemia with mild hyperinsulinemia and tissue resistance to insulin-requiring diabetes mellitus. Acanthosis nigricans is also a cutaneous manifestation of the insulin-resistant syndromes, types A and B, as well as women with the HAIR-AN syndrome (hyperandrogenism, insulin resistance, acanthosis nigricans). In obese patients, weight loss and improvement of tissue resistance to insulin has improved their acanthosis nigricans. Otherwise, treatment is limited to topical agents such as tretinoin (0.05–0.1%), urea (10–25%), and α-hydroxy acids (lactic and glycolic), which can improve the cosmetic appearance.

BULLOSIS DIABETICORUM

The spontaneous formation of bullae in a primarily acral location (feet and distal lower extremities more than forearms and hands) is an uncommon manifestation of diabetes mellitus. The lesions arise from normal noninflamed skin and range

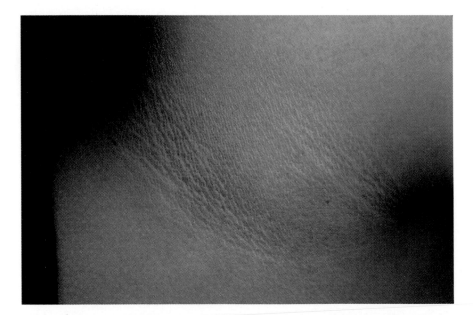

Figure 35.7 Velvety dark-brown plaques on lateral neck of patient with acanthosis nigricans.

in size from a few millimeters to several centimeters (Fig. 35.8). The blisters are usually tense and contain clear viscous fluid that is sterile. There is no history of antecedent trauma, and the lesions may recur. Two major forms exist and are distinguished by the site of blister formation: *1*) the blister is intra-epidermal and heals without scarring, or *2*) it is subepidermal and may heal with atrophy and mild scarring. Both types are found predominantly in middle-aged to elderly patients with long-standing diabetes who often have evidence of peripheral neuropathy. Other than local care (e.g., drainage and topical antibiotics to prevent secondary infection), there is no specific recommended treatment.

NECROLYTIC MIGRATORY ERYTHEMA

Patients with NME have bright erythematous patches that are most frequently seen in the girdle area (lower abdomen, groin, buttocks, and thighs), perioral region, and extremities (Fig. 35.9). The cutaneous finding that distinguishes NME from other migratory eruptions is the presence of superficial bullae at the active borders. Because the bullae rapidly break, only denuded areas and crusts may be observed clinically. These areas then heal with superficial desquamation as the erythema advances.

Histologically, swollen and necrotic keratinocytes are seen in the superficial layers of the epidermis, findings similar to those seen in acrodermatitis enteropathica. In addition to the cutaneous eruption, the patients frequently have glossitis, anemia, weight loss, and diarrhea, as well as diabetes mellitus.

Most patients with classic NME have an α-cell tumor of the pancreas and markedly elevated serum glucagon levels (a variant termed "necrolytic acral erythema" is a cutaneous marker of liver disease). Removal of the pancreatic tumor can result in prompt resolution of the cutaneous eruption. In inoperable cases, intermittent peripheral infusions of amino acids and fatty acids, subcutaneous injections of the long-acting somatostatin analog octreotide acetate, or transcatheter arterial embolization of hepatic metastases can lead to improvement.

DRUG REACTIONS TO ORAL HYPOGLYCEMIC AGENTS AND INSULIN

Administration of oral hypoglycemic agents can lead to commonly recognized drug reactions such as pruritus, urticaria, morbilliform eruptions, and erythema multiforme. Phototoxic (dose-related exaggerated sunburn) and photoallergic (idiosyncratic eczematous dermatitis in a photodistribution) eruptions are additional potential cutaneous side effects and are related to the sulfur moiety found in these compounds. A unique reaction is the chlorpropamide alcohol flush, which is similar to the disulfiram alcohol flush.

The cutaneous reactions to insulin can be divided into localized, generalized, and lipoatrophy/lipohypertrophy. The localized reactions include pruritus, erythema, induration, and, occasionally, ulceration at the insulin injection site. Allergic local reactions vary from the immediate formation of an urticarial lesion at the injection site to the appearance of a pruritic papule or nodule 24–48 h after the injection. The latter lesions represent a delayed hypersensitivity reaction and, as

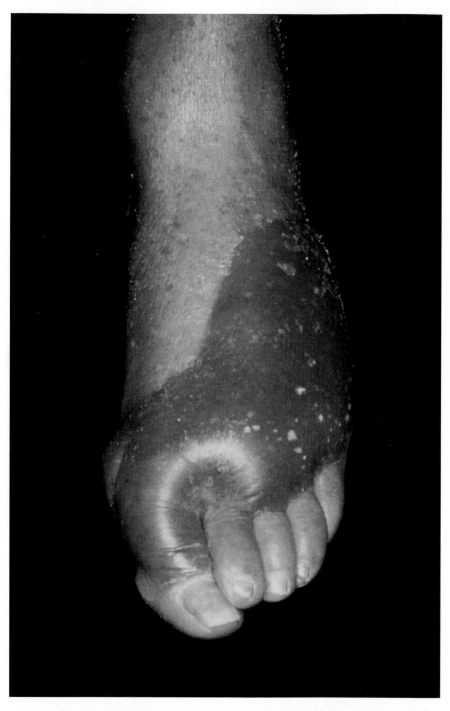

Figure 35.8 Tense large bulla on dorsum of foot characteristic of bullosis diabeticorum. From Braverman 1998.

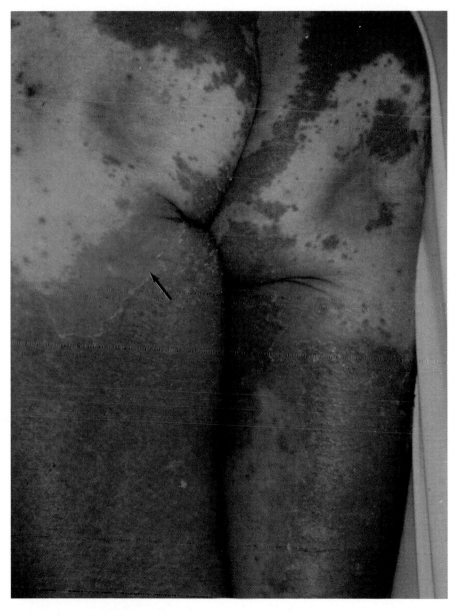

Figure 35.9 Angular erythematous patches on buttocks and thighs of patient with glucagonoma of the pancreas; arrow, peripheral desquamation. From Braverman.

such, heal slowly over a week or more and often leave residual hyperpigmentation. They frequently cease to form after several weeks or months. The primary treatment of persistent localized reactions is a switch to purer forms of insulin; if this is unsuccessful, the possibility of an allergy to the zinc, protamine, or preservative such as paraben in the preparation should be considered as well as small quantities of natural latex rubber antigens from the insulin injection materials.

Generalized systemic reactions are uncommon and are characterized by pruritus, urticaria/angioedema, and serum sickness–like illnesses. The risk of a systemic reaction to insulin is related to the source and purification of the insulin, with bovine insulin having the highest incidence and human insulin the lowest. Treatment options for individuals already receiving human insulin include desensitization and use of the insulin analog lispro. Lipoatrophy at injection sites is seen with subcutaneous administration and is much less common with monocomponent or recombinant human insulin. Improvement in the areas of subcutaneous fat loss has been reported after injection of human insulin into the edge of the lipoatrophy. In patients already receiving human insulin, the use of a jet injector may prove beneficial. Lipohypertrophy (i.e., an increase in the amount of subcutaneous fat) can also be seen at the site of insulin injection. Treatment consists of rotation of injection sites and perhaps liposuction and the use of lispro.

BIBLIOGRAPHY

Bolognia JL, Braverman IM: Cutaneous complications of type 1 diabetes. In *Type 1 Diabetes: Etiology and Treatment.* Sperling MA, Ed. Totowa, NJ, Humana Press, 2003, p. 485–499

Braverman IM: *Skin Signs of Systemic Disease.* 3rd ed. Philadelphia, Saunders, 1998

Jabbour SA: Cutaneous manifestations of endocrine disorders: a guide for dermatologists. *Am J Clin Dermatol* 4:315–331, 2003

Jelenick JE: *The Skin in Diabetes.* Philadelphia, Lea & Febiger, 1986

Perez MI, Kohn SR: Cutaneous manifestations of diabetes mellitus. *J Am Acad Dermatol* 30:519–531, 1994

Rosenbloom AL, Silverstein JH, Lezotte DC, Richardson K, McCallum M: Limited joint mobility in childhood diabetes mellitus indicates increased risk for microvascular disease. *N Engl J Med* 305:191–194, 1981

Shemer A, Bergman R, Linn S, Kantor Y, Friedman-Birnbaum R: Diabetic dermopathy and internal complications in diabetes mellitus. *Int J Dermatol* 37:113–115, 1998

Dr. Bolognia and Dr. Braverman are Professors of Dermatology at the Yale University School of Medicine, New Haven, CT.

36. Infections

MARTIN KRAMER, MD, AND MARY ANN BANERJI, MD, FACP

Host immune defenses are altered in patients with diabetes. Hyperglycemia and acidosis alter the functions of phagocytic cells and result in changing their movement toward the site of an infection and impairing their microbiocidal activity. Subtle alterations in cell-mediated immunity predispose the patient to tuberculosis, coccidioidomycosis, and cryptococcosis. The host's metabolic state in diabetes also favors the specific nutritional requirements of some microbes. High glucose concentrations in blood and body fluids promote the overgrowth of certain fungal pathogens—particularly *Candida* species and *Zygomycetes*. *Zygomycetes* also grow more rapidly in an acidotic environment. Finally, mechanical factors largely contribute to the increased susceptibility of patients with diabetes to infections (Table 36.1). Treatment of infection in a patient with diabetes involves both antibiotic therapy and aggressive maintenance of good glycemic control. Table 36.2 provides an empiric antimicrobial treatment scheme for the management of the more common infections affecting diabetes patients. More specific details are described in subsequent sections.

There are now ample clinical data suggesting that hyperglycemia increases the risk for potentially serious infections. A recent study involving patients in an intensive care unit demonstrated that intensive insulin treatment that maintained blood glucose levels between 80 and 110 mg/dl (4.4 and 6.1 mmol/l) resulted in a significant decrease in mortality when these patients were compared with a control group with hyperglycemia. The largest decrease involved (autopsy-proven) deaths due to multiple end-organ failure with a septic focus. Thus, it is likely that good glycemic control will decrease the incidence and possibly the severity of infections.

SUPERFICIAL TISSUE INFECTIONS

Minor trauma to tissues affected by vascular insufficiency often initiates superficial tissue infection. In addition, peripheral sensory neuropathy leads to the occurrence of an insensibility to minor injuries, which delays care. Infection may take the form of a cellulitis, soft tissue necrosis, draining sinus, or osteomyelitis. Although the feet are most commonly involved in these infections, a similar process can occur in the skin beneath pressure points. In both situations, tissue undermining can be extensive.

Table 36.1 Mechanical Factors Contributing to Infections in Patients with Diabetes

Physiological Change	Disease Process	Result
Ischemic changes	Chronic diabetic vascular disease	Mixed bacterial foot infections
Depressed cough reflex	Cerebrovascular insults	Pneumonia
Impaired bladder emptying	Autonomic neuropathy	UTIs
Fecal incontinence	Autonomic neuropathy	Cutaneous maceration
Impaired mobility	Various abnormalities	Pressure sores

Diabetic Foot Infections

Diabetic foot infections with ulcers can be broadly divided into two categories: non–limb-threatening and limb-threatening.

Non–limb-threatening infections

Non–limb-threatening infections are associated with shallow ulcers, minimal cellulitis, minimal or no tissue necrosis, and no systemic symptoms. Treatment involves wound care and oral antibiotics. Gram-positive bacteria such as group A streptococci, *Staphylococcus aureus*, and possibly coagulase-negative staphylococci are usually involved. Oral antibiotics that are reasonable to use include dicloxacillin, cephalexin, amoxicillin/clavulanate, or clindamycin. Maintaining good control of glucose levels is very important. Frequent observation is necessary to ensure that healing occurs.

Limb-threatening infections

Limb-threatening infections are associated with ulcers that are usually deep; the infection extends to the subcutaneous tissue or deeper with significant tissue necrosis and systemic symptoms. Patients must be hospitalized, and surgical evaluation (and often intervention) is essential. The bacteriology of these infections includes the gram-positive bacteria mentioned above, gram-negative bacteria (e.g., *Escherichia coli* and *Pseudomonas aeruginosa*), and anaerobic bacteria (e.g., *Bacteroides fragilis* and *Peptostreptococcus* species). Deep wound cultures and gram stains (preferably scrapings or curettage of tissue) should be done to determine therapy. In addition to determining the bacteriology, antimicrobial susceptibility must be determined in view of the increasing antimicrobial resistance of gram-negative and gram-positive bacteria (i.e., methicillin-resistant *S. aureus* [MRSA]). Empiric intravenous antibiotic therapy is directed at the presumed organisms mentioned above. Examples of such regimens include piperacillin/tazobactam,

Table 36.2 Empiric Antimicrobial Treatment

Organ System	Usual Organism	Primary	Alternate
Urinary Tract			
Bacteruria			
Asymptomatic male or female		No treatment	
Acute uncomplicated cystitis/urethritis	*E. coli, Staph Saphrophyticus*	Fluoroquinolone	Trimethoprim/sulfamethoxazole Ampicillin/clavulanate Vancomycin
	Enterococci	Ampicillin	
Acute pyelonephritis Hospitalized	*E. coli*	Fluoroquinolones Third-generation cephalosporin	Ticarcillin/clavulanate 3 or piperacillin/ tazobactam
	Enterococci	Ampicillin	Vancomycin
Perinephric abscess (drainage as required)			
With pyelonephritis	*E. coli*	Treat as for pyelonephritis	
With *S. aureus* bacteremia	*S. aureus*	Nafcillin *or* oxacillin	Cephazolin Vancomycin
Gall Bladder			
Cholecystitis	*Enterobacteriaceae* *Enterococci, Bacteroides*	Piperacillin/tazobactam Ampicillin/sulbactam Ticarcillin/clavulanate	Ceftazidime *plus* metronidazole Aztreonam *plus* clindamycin Ampicillin *plus* gentamicin with or without metronidazole
If life-threatening		Imipenem/cilastatin *or* meropenem	
Emphysematous	Polymicrobial including *Clostridium* species	Imipenem/cilastatin *or* meropenem	

(Continued)

Table 36.2 Empiric Antimicrobial Treatment (*Continued*)

Organ System	Usual Organism	Primary	Alternate
Ear, Nose, and Throat			
Rhinocerebral mucormycosis	*Mucor* and *Rhizopus* species	Amphotericin B	
Invasive otitis externa	*Pseudomonas aeruginosa*	Ciprofloxacin Ceftazidime	Imipenem/cilastatin Meropenem Piperacillin
Foot			

Non-limb-/life-threatening
Mild, previously untreated*
	S. aureus, streptococci	Clindamycin,
		  cephalosporin
		Amoxicillin/
		  clavulanate	

Chronic	Polymicrobial:
	  S. aureus, strep,
	  E. coli, *Proteus*, *Klebsiela/*
	  Anaerobes (e.g., *B. fragilis*)
		Ampicillin/sulbactam
		Piperacillin/tazobactam
		Ticarcillin/clavulanate
		Clindamycin *plus*
		  ceftriaxone or
		  cefotaxime	

Limb-/life-threatening	Polymicrobial: as above	Imipenem/cilastatin *or*
		  meropenem *plus*
		  vancomycin	

Soft Tissue			
Necrotizing fasciitis	Group A streptococcus, *Clostridia* species Polymicrobial	Penicillin G *plus* clindamycin Imipenem/cilastatin Meropenem	

*Shallow and no ischemia, abscess, or osteomyelitis. All antibiotic use and dosing should take into account renal and hepatic function, clinical circumstance, contraindications, and drug toxicity. These are examples of regimens likely to be effective. Other regimens may also be effective in specific circumstances. Examples of fluoroquinolones with enhanced activity are gatifloxacin, levofloxacin, ciprofloxacin, and moxifloxacin; examples of third-generation cephalosporins are ceftriaxone and cefotaxime.

ticarcillin/clavulanate, imipenem/cilastatin, or meropenem. There are many other potentially effective regimens. Any regimen used should take into account features such as local antimicrobial susceptibility data (i.e., the prevalence of MRSA), drug toxicity, and contraindications.

Patients with diabetes are more susceptible to developing severe necrotizing/ gangrenous infections. These may be monomicrobial (i.e., caused by *Streptococcus* species, primarily β hemolytic streptococcus such as group A) or polymicrobial. Immediate surgical intervention is warranted. Broad spectrum antibiotic therapy (see above) is indicated for polymicrobial infection. In group A streptococcal necrotizing fasciitis (which may result in streptococcal toxic shock syndrome [TSS]), both high-dose penicillin and clindamycin should be used. There are anecdotal data that intravenous immune globulin may be beneficial in treating streptococcal TSS.

MALIGNANT OTITIS EXTERNA

Malignant otitis externa is an infection usually caused by *P. aeruginosa* that occurs almost exclusively in patients with diabetes. It is a chronic erosive process that initially involves the soft tissue and cartilage around the external auditory canal. There is pain and drainage of purulent material and progressive destruction as the process progresses into the temporal and petrous bones and mastoids. The infection progresses regardless of tissue planes and ultimately reaches cranial nerves, the meninges, and/or the sigmoid sinus. Paralysis of nerves 7, 9, 10, 11, and possibly 12 may occur. Treatment consists of local debridement of necrotic tissue and prolonged therapy with anti-pseudomonal antibiotics. Because osteomyelitis is usually present, the course of therapy should be at least 4–6 weeks. Useful antimicrobial agents are listed in Table 36.2.

URINARY TRACT INFECTIONS

Women with diabetes have a two- to fourfold higher incidence of bacteriuria than nondiabetic women and diabetic men. *E. coli* and other gram-negative bacteria cause most urinary tract infections (UTIs). Hematogenous infection is most commonly caused by *S. aureus*. In contrast to nondiabetic women, women with diabetes have frequent involvement of the upper urinary tract (43–80% of cases). Acute pyelonephritis has a similar presentation in diabetic patients, and the response to therapy is likewise similar. A failure to respond to appropriate therapy raises the possibility of complications, including perinephric abscess, renal papillary necrosis, emphysematous cystitis, or emphysematous pyelonephritis. These complications need to be rapidly diagnosed and aggressively treated.

When upper urinary tract infection is suspected, patients should be hospitalized and treated with intravenous antibiotics and hydration. If there is poor response after 3–4 days of therapy, the above-mentioned complications should be sought using radiological investigations. The usual duration of therapy in uncomplicated infection with intravenous and subsequent oral antibiotics is 14 days.

Asymptomatic bacteruria is common in women with diabetes. There is no evidence that therapy of asymptomatic bacteruria is beneficial because relapse rates are high and therapy does not prevent the development of symptomatic UTIs. *Candida* UTIs are usually associated with indwelling bladder catheters or anatomic abnormalities. Less commonly, hematogenous spread occurs. *Candida* UTIs rarely occur otherwise. The presentation of *Candida* UTIs is similar to that of bacterial cystitis. Paranchymal involvement may result in pyelonephritis, abscess formation, or the development of fungus balls (which may also cause obstruction). Treatment consists of removal of the urinary catheters and/or the correction of anatomic abnormality. Symptomatic infection can be treated with fluconazole. There is no clear benefit to treating asymptomatic infection.

ABDOMINAL INFECTIONS

Emphysematous cholecystitis occurs with an increased frequency in patients with diabetes. Approximately 35% of the cases occur in patients with diabetes, and emphysematous cholecystitis is associated with increased mortality in 15% of patients with diabetes compared with <4% of individuals without diabetes. The presentation is similar to that of uncomplicated cholecystitis. The presence of crepitations, clinical deterioration, or failure to improve with conservative therapy should lead to radiological evaluation. Surgical intervention, in addition to broad spectrum antimicrobial therapy, may be lifesaving.

FUNGAL INFECTIONS

Mucormycosis (Zygomycosis)

Much less common but much more devastating is infection caused by the agents of mucormycosis (primarily the *Zygomycetes*). The syndrome most often seen in patients with diabetes is rhinocerebral mucormycosis. This is an invasive process caused by the mycelia of the genera *Mucor, Absidia, Rhizopus, Cunninghamella,* and others. The conidia of the organisms are unable to regenerate if ingested by normal macrophages, and the organisms are essentially nonpathogenic in the normal host. The growth of *Rhizopus* is inhibited by normal human serum. However, these fungi can grow rapidly in the presence of high concentrations of glucose and in an acid environment. Both conditions prevail in the patient with ketoacidosis. In such patients, these organisms are able to germinate at the site of infections (usually the nares and the sinuses) and to begin a rapid necrotizing process that characterizes rhinocerebral mucormycosis. Within a few days, the process may extend from a small eschar on the nasal septum to involve the paranasal sinuses and orbit. The infection proceeds without regard for tissue planes. It can track into the brain within a few days, and the result is often lethal if not diagnosed and treated at an early stage.

Diagnosis is by prompt aggressive surgical biopsy, including tissues deep to the area of necrosis. *Zygomycetes* are different from other fungi in that they stain better with hematoxylin and eosin than with methenamine silver. Identification of irregular pleomorphic nonseptate branching hyphae is pathognomonic. *Zygomycetes* must be differentiated from *Aspergillus*, which is the most similar in appearance. The hyphae of *Aspergillus* do not stain well with hematoxylin and eosin. Treatment of zygomycosis infection includes correction of ketoacidosis, vigorous and repeated surgical debridement, and antifungal therapy with amphotericin B; azole antifungal drugs are not effective against *Zygomycetes*.

PULMONARY INFECTIONS

It is not clear whether diabetes is associated with an increased incidence of pneumonia. However, the spectrum of pneumonia is different in patients with diabetes. There is an increased frequency of infections with gram-negative bacteria (e.g., *Klebsiella* and *E. coli*), *S. aureus*, *Mycobacterium tuberculosis*, and certain fungi such as *Aspergillus*, *Mucor*, *Cryptococcus*, and *Coccidiodes*. Other infections caused by *Streptococcus pneumoniae* (especially bacteremia), the influenza virus, and *Legionella* may be associated with increased morbidity and mortality. This spectrum of pulmonary infections needs to be considered with regard to diagnosis, (empiric) treatment, and clinical follow-up to ensure that the infection is resolving appropriately. Table 36.3 outlines an empiric approach to antimicrobial treatment for pulmonary infections.

Prevention of pneumonia should be addressed in all patients with diabetes. The Advisory Committee on Immunization Practices recommends that all patients with diabetes be vaccinated once with the pneumococcal vaccine and annually with the influenza vaccine. All patients with diabetes should undergo tuberculin skin testing to diagnose latent tuberculosis infection. The risk of a diabetes patient with a positive skin test developing active tuberculosis is two- to fourfold greater than that for a patient without diabetes with the same positive test. Patients with diabetes with a positive tuberculin skin test ≥10 mm should be strongly considered for preventive chemotherapy once active tuberculosis is excluded.

BIBLIOGRAPHY

Bartlett JG, Dowell SF, Mandell LA, File TM, Musher DM: Practice guidelines for the management of community acquired pneumonia in adults. *Clin Infect Dis* 31:347–382, 2000

Blumberg HM, Burman WJ, Chaisson RE, Daley CL, Etkind SC, Friedman LN, Fujiwara P, Grzemska M, Hopewell PC, Iseman MD, Jasmer RM, Koppaka V, Menzies RI, O'Brien RJ, Reves RR, Reichman LB, Simone PM, Starke JR, Vernon AA: American Thoracic Society/Centers for Disease Control and Prevention/Infectious Disease Society of America: Treatment of tuberculosis. *Am J Respir Crit Care Med* 167:603–663, 2003

Calvert HM, Yoshikawa T: Infections in diabetes. *Infect Dis Clin North Am* 15:407–421, 2001

Table 36.3 Empirical Selection of Antimicrobial Agents for Treating Patients with Community-Acquired Pneumonia

Outpatients

Generally preferred agents are (not in any particular order) as follows: doxycycline, a macrolide, or a fluoroquinolone.
Selection considerations:
- These agents have activity against the most likely pathogens in this setting, which include *Streptococcus pneumoniae, Mycoplasma pneumoniae,* and *Chlamydia pneumoniae.*
- Selection should be influenced by regional antibiotic susceptibility patterns for *S. pneumoniae* and the presence of other risk factors for drug-resistant *S. pneumoniae.*
- Penicillin-resistant *pneumococci* may be resistant to macrolides and/or doxycycline.
- For older patients or those with underlying disease, a fluoroquinolone may be a preferred choice; some authorities prefer to reserve fluoroquinolones for such patients.

Hospitalized patients

General medical ward
Generally preferred agents are as follows: an extended spectrum cephalosporin combined with a macrolide or a β-lactam/β-lactamase inhibitor combined with a macrolide or a fluoroquinolone (alone).

Intensive care unit
Generally preferred agents are as follows: an extended spectrum cephalosporin* or β-lactam/β-lactamase inhibitor† plus either fluoroquinolone‡ or macrolide§.
Alternatives or modifying factors are as follows:
- Structural lung disease: anti-pseudomonal agents (piperacillin, piperacillin/tazobactam, carbapenem, or cefepime) plus a fluoroquinolone (including high-dose ciprofloxacin)
- β-lactam allergy: fluoroquinolone with or without clindamycin
- Suspected aspiration: fluoroquinolone with or without clindamycin, metronidazole, or a β-lactam/β-lactamase inhibitor

Adapted from Bartlett et al. *Extended-spectrum cephalosporin: cefotaxime or ceftriaxone; †β-lactam/β-lactamase inhibitor: ampicillin/sulbactam or pipercillin/tazobactam; ‡fluoroquinolone: gatifloxacin, levofloxacin, moxifloxacin, or other fluoroquinolone with enhanced activity against *S. pneumoniae* (for aspiration pneumonia, some fluoroquinolones show in vitro activity against anaerobic pulmonary pathogens, although there are no clinical studies to verify activity in vivo); §macrolide: azithromycin, clarithromycin, or erythromycin.

Harding GKM, Zhanel GG, Nicolle LE, Cheang M, for the Manitoba Diabetes Urinary Tract Infection Study Group: Antimicrobial treatment in diabetic women with asymptomatic bacteriuria. *N Engl J Med* 347:1576–1583, 2002

Joshi N, Caputo GM, Weitekamp, Karchmer AW: Infections in patients with diabetes mellitus. *N Engl J Med* 341:1906–1912, 1999

Karchmer AW, Gibbons G: Foot infections in diabetes: evaluation and management. *Curr Clin Top Infect Dis* 14:1–22, 1994

Van den Berghe G, Wouters P, Weekers F, Verwaest C, Bruyninckx F, Schetz M, Vlasselaers D, Ferdinande P, Lauwers P, Bouillon R: Intensive insulin therapy in critically ill patients. *N Engl J Med* 345:1359–1367, 2001

Dr. Kramer is Associate Professor of Clinical Medicine from the Division of Infectious Diseases and Dr. Banerji is Associate Professor of Medicine from the Division of Endocrinology, SUNY Downstate Medical Center, Brooklyn, NY.

37. Visual Loss

LLOYD PAUL AIELLO, MD, PhD, LLOYD M. AIELLO, MD,
AND JERRY D. CAVALLERANO, OD, PhD

To achieve the goal of preserving vision, patients at risk of visual loss from diabetes must be identified and directed to experienced ophthalmologists for timely laser photocoagulation.

CLINICAL CONSIDERATIONS

All patients with diabetes should be advised that proven methods are in place to preserve vision. These methods include regular comprehensive eye and retinal examination; intensive control of blood glucose (as evaluated by glycated hemoglobin A1C levels); control of coexisting medical complications such as hypertension, kidney disease, and/or dyslipidemia; and appropriate and timely laser surgery when indicated for diabetic macular edema or diabetic retinopathy. As a routine part of the health history, all patients with diabetes should be asked if they have any visual symptoms (Table 37.1), such as

- any loss of visual acuity (either at a distance or near)
- fluctuation of vision
- floating spots in field of view
- flashing lights in field of view
- any metamorphopsia or apparent warping of straight lines
- diplopia (double vision)

There are numerous etiologies for reduced vision—some benign and some requiring immediate treatment. In general, patients who report floating spots in their view, flashing lights, or the sensation of a curtain or veil crossing their vision should be referred for immediate ophthalmological attention because they may be reporting the symptoms of a vitreous hemorrhage, retinal detachment, or retinal hole. Patients reporting metamorphopsia may have significant macular edema or traction in the macular area and should be referred for prompt ophthalmological evaluation, preferably within 1 week.

Fluctuating vision is frequently the result of poor blood glucose control. Elevated blood glucose levels may lead to a myopic shift, enabling presbyopic individuals to read without their glasses, while their distance vision becomes blurred.

Table 37.1 Visual Symptoms in Diabetic Patients Requiring Further Evaluation and Treatment

Symptom	Possible Etiology	Management Strategy	Ocular Evaluation
Blurred vision	Poorly controlled diabetes Cataract Macular edema	Control diabetes; no new glasses prescription for 4–6 wk Referral for comprehensive ocular examination	Prompt
Double vision	Diabetic mononeuropathy Other etiology	Neuroophthalmologic and neurological evaluation	Urgent
Floaters	Vitreous hemorrhage Retinal detachment Retinal hole	Complete ocular evaluation	Urgent
Ocular pain	Corneal abrasion Neovascular or angle-closure glaucoma Iritis	Complete ocular evaluation	Urgent

For some who never wore glasses, distance vision may become blurred, and for those with hyperopia, glasses may no longer be needed for clear distance vision. Blurred vision can also be a symptom of macular edema, cataract, or other ocular conditions. In general, if the vision clears with a pinhole, the condition is most likely refractive and referral is less urgent.

Patients complaining of pain in or above the eye should be evaluated for possible neovascular or angle-closure glaucoma, especially if there is a loss of corneal reflex, irregularity in shape and response of the pupil, or acute redness of the eye. Also, a painful or red eye may reflect a corneal abrasion or corneal erosion. In most cases, patients with anterior-segment complaints should be promptly examined with a slit-lamp biomicroscope to rule out any form of glaucoma, a foreign body, a corneal abrasion, or iritis. Tonometry to measure intraocular pressure is also advisable. Emergency referral to an ophthalmologist may be critical.

Patients with new-onset double vision require neuroophthalmic and often neurological evaluation. Any patient who shows neovascularization of the optic nerve head or elsewhere in the retina or hard exudates or microaneurysms in the macula area should be promptly referred for complete ophthalmological evaluation. If proliferative retinopathy is present, immediate referral is warranted (Table 37.2).

Because diabetic eye disease currently cannot be prevented, strategies address avenues to delay the onset and slow the progression of eye disease and ensure proper management of proliferative retinopathy and diabetic macular edema when these conditions are present. All patients should be informed of the potential

Table 37.2 Ocular Signs Requiring Referral for Management

Sign	Management
Retinal neovascularization	Immediate referral for comprehensive ocular examination and possible laser surgery
Vitreous hemorrhage	Immediate referral for comprehensive ocular examination and possible laser and/or vitrectomy surgery
Hard exudates or microaneurysms in macular area	Timely (1–2 wk) referral for comprehensive ocular examination and possible laser surgery for clinically significant macular edema
Cataract	Referral for comprehensive ocular examination depending on patient history, symptoms, and examination

ocular complications of diabetes and should be advised to have a comprehensive annual eye examination with pupil dilation and appropriate referral for management and treatment as indicated to preserve vision.

BIBLIOGRAPHY

Aiello LP, Cahill MT, Wong JS: Systemic considerations in the management of diabetic retinopathy. *Am J Ophthalmol* 132:760–766, 2001

Aiello LP, Gardner TW, King GL, Blankenship G, Cavallerano JD, Ferris FL III, Klein R: Diabetic retinopathy. *Diabetes Care* 21:143–156, 1998

Cavallerano JD: A review of non-retinal ocular complications of diabetes mellitus. *J Am Optom Assoc* 61:533–543, 1990

Early Treatment Diabetic Retinopathy Study Research Group: Early photocoagulation for diabetic retinopathy. ETDRS report number 9. *Ophthalmology* 98:766–785, 1991

Early Treatment Diabetic Retinopathy Study Research Group: Photocoagulation for diabetic macular edema. ETDRS report number 1. *Arch Ophthalmol* 103:1796–1806, 1985

The effect of intensive diabetes treatment on the progression of diabetic retinopathy in insulin-dependent diabetes mellitus. The Diabetes Control and Complications Trial. *Arch Ophthalmol* 113:36–51, 1995

Ferris FL III, Davis MD, Aiello LM: Treatment of diabetic retinopathy. *N Engl J Med* 341:667–678, 1999

Ferris FL III: Results of 20 years of research on the treatment of diabetic retinopathy. *Prev Med* 23:740–742, 1994

UK Prospective Diabetes Study (UKPDS) Group: Intensive blood-glucose control with sulphonylureas or insulin compared with conventional treatment and risk of complications in patients with type 2 diabetes (UKPDS 33). *Lancet* 352:837–853, 1998

Dr. Lloyd Paul Aiello is Assistant Director, Beetham Eye Institute, Joslin Diabetes Center; Head, Section of Eye Research, Joslin Diabetes Center; and Associate Professor of Ophthalmology, Harvard Medical School, Boston, MA. Dr. Lloyd M. Aiello is Director and Dr. Cavallerano is Staff Optometrist and Assistant to the Director, Beetham Eye Institute, Joslin Diabetes Center, Boston, MA.

38. Ocular Complications

Lloyd Paul Aiello, MD, PhD, Lloyd M. Aiello, MD,
and Jerry D. Cavallerano, OD, PhD

Diabetic retinopathy and diabetic macular edema (DME) affect individuals with both type 1 and type 2 diabetes. Type 1 diabetes patients, however, experience more frequent and severe ocular complications. In fact, after 5 years of diabetes, 23% of type 1 diabetes patients have retinopathy. After 10 years, this prevalence increases to almost 60%, and after 15 years, 80% have retinopathy. Proliferative diabetic retinopathy (PDR)—the most threatening form of the disease—is present in 25% of patients with type 1 diabetes after 15 years and often remains asymptomatic beyond the optimal stage for treatment. Patients with type 2 diabetes may have retinopathy at the time of diagnosis. Type 2 diabetes patients who take insulin for 5–10 years have about a 2% incidence of PDR. This rate increases to >50% in insulin-taking type 2 diabetes patients who have had diabetes for >20 years. Adherence to intensive blood glucose control regimens, as demonstrated by the Diabetes Control and Complications Trial and the United Kingdom Prospective Diabetes Study, may alter the rates of onset and progression of PDR.

An estimated 700,000 Americans have PDR, and 500,000 have DME. The annual projected incidence of new cases of PDR and DME is 65,000 and 75,000, respectively. About 8,000 new cases of blindness a year in the U.S. are caused by complications from diabetes.

Diabetic retinopathy is often asymptomatic in its most treatable stages. Unfortunately, only ~55% of the diabetes population receives adequate ophthalmic care. Early detection and treatment of diabetic retinopathy are critical. Laser surgery can ameliorate the devastating effects of diabetic retinal disease, particularly when laser surgery is initiated promptly once indicated. Laser surgery is generally required before significant vision loss has occurred. Timely laser photocoagulation can reduce the risk of severe visual loss (best vision of 5/200 or worse) from high-risk PDR by ~60%, thus lowering the overall risk of such loss to <4%. Timely laser surgery of DME can reduce the risk of moderate visual loss (a doubling of the visual angle, e.g., 20/20 reduced to 20/40) by 50%. Vitrectomy can restore useful vision to some people who have lost vision because of diabetes and prevent vision loss when retinal traction threatens detachment of the macula. Emphasis must therefore be placed on early detection of retinal disorders, with appropriate referral for management and treatment. In addition, careful control of blood glucose levels and concurrent systemic conditions such as hypertension, renal disease, and dyslipidemia is critical.

DIABETIC RETINOPATHY

Pathophysiology

Elevated blood glucose levels result in structural, physiological, and biochemical changes that alter cellular metabolism, retinal blood flow, and retinal capillary competency. Classic clinical pathological findings characterize diabetic retinopathy. Clinically, these processes are manifested as either PDR, nonproliferative diabetic retinopathy (NPDR), or DME (Table 38.1):

- decreased retinal blood flow
- impaired vascular autoregulation
- loss of retinal pericytes
- outpouchings of the capillary walls to form microaneurysms
- closure of retinal capillaries and arterioles
- increased vascular permeability of retinal capillaries
- proliferation of new vessels, with or without vitreous hemorrhage
- development of fibrous tissue

Table 38.1 Clinical Manifestations of Retinopathy

NPDR
- Mild—one or both of the following:
  - Few scattered retinal microaneurysms and hemorrhages
  - Hard exudate
- Moderate—one or more of the following:
  - More extensive retinal hemorrhages and/or microaneurysms
  - Mild IRMAs
  - Early venous beading
- Severe to very severe—one or more of the following:
  - Severe hemorrhages and/or microaneurysms in all four quadrants
  - Venous beading in at least two quadrants
  - More extensive IRMAs in at least one quadrant

PDR
- Early
  - Minimal NVD <1/4 disk area without preretinal or vitreous hemorrhage
    or
  - NVE without preretinal or vitreous hemorrhage
- High-risk
  - NVD ≥1/4 disk area with or without preretinal or vitreous hemorrhage
    or
  - NVD <1/4 disk area in extent accompanied by fresh hemorrhage
    or
  - NVE ≥1/2 disk area with preretinal or vitreous hemorrhage

IRMA, intraretinal microvascular abnormalities; NVD, new vessels on the optic disk; NVE, new vessels elsewhere on the retina. DME may occur at any level of diabetic retinopathy, although it is more common with more advanced retinopathy.

- contraction of vitreous and fibrous proliferation with subsequent retinal traction and detachment

These and other processes of diabetic retinopathy may affect the macula, significantly altering function and reading vision. Such processes include:

- DME: a collection of intraretinal fluid in the macular area with or without lipid exudates and with or without cystoid changes
- nonperfusion of parafoveal capillaries with or without intraretinal fluid
- traction in the macula exerted by contraction of fibrous tissue proliferation resulting in dragging of the retinal tissue, surface wrinkling, or detachment of the macula
- intraretinal or preretinal hemorrhage in the macula
- lamellar or full-thickness retinal hole formation
- combinations of the above

DME can be associated with any stage of diabetic retinopathy. Proper evaluation requires stereoscopic examination of the macula with slit-lamp biomicroscope and/or fundus photography. Loss of vision from diabetes usually results from nonresolving vitreous hemorrhage, PDR leading to fibrous tissue formation and subsequent traction retinal detachment, or DME.

Clinical Care

Proper management of diabetic retinopathy has been influenced by extensive research, including results of five major clinical trials. These studies helped establish the minimum standard of eye care for diabetes patients to preserve vision and reduce the threat of visual loss from diabetes.

The Diabetic Retinopathy Study (DRS) (1971–1975) definitively established the beneficial effects of scatter (panretinal) laser photocoagulation for PDR. The Early Treatment Diabetic Retinopathy Study (ETDRS) (1979–1990) demonstrated the benefit of focal laser treatment for DME and provided insight into the most appropriate timing for retinal laser surgery. The study also demonstrated that the use of 650 mg aspirin/day is unlikely to have any effect on the progression of diabetic retinopathy. The Diabetic Retinopathy Vitrectomy Study (1977–1987) established early guidelines on the timing of surgical intervention after visual loss from vitreous hemorrhage. The Diabetes Control and Complications Trial (1983–1993) demonstrated that intensive control of blood glucose levels in patients with type 1 diabetes mellitus, resulting in at least a 1% drop in glycosylated hemoglobin levels, reduces the risk of onset of any diabetic retinopathy, the progression of retinopathy, and the need for laser surgery. The United Kingdom Prospective Diabetes Study (UKPDS) (1977–1999) found similar results of intensive blood glucose control for patients with type 2 diabetes. Additionally, the UKPDS found that more intensive control of blood pressure, with either a β-blocking agent or an angiotensin-converting enzyme inhibitor, reduced the risk of progression of retinopathy.

In addition to demonstrating the value of scatter (panretinal) laser photocoagulation in preserving vision, the DRS identified specific retinal lesions that pose a significant threat for severe visual loss (visual acuity reduced to the 5/200 level).

These lesions comprise high-risk PDR, which indicates a need for immediate referral to a retinal specialist for prompt scatter photocoagulation (Table 38.1).

To determine ways to further reduce this risk, the ETDRS was designed to test the effects of a daily dose of 650 mg aspirin, laser surgery for DME, and the most appropriate timing and method of scatter laser treatment for PDR. The ETDRS determined the following:

- Focal laser surgery is effective to treat clinically significant DME.
- Scatter laser photocoagulation reduces the risk of severe visual loss, whether applied slightly before or at the development of high-risk PDR. For patients with type 2 diabetes, however, there is a clear advantage to earlier treatment (i.e., before high-risk PDR), particularly if severe NPDR or worse is present.
- Aspirin treatment does not alter the progression of diabetic retinopathy.

Diagnosis

Retinopathy rarely occurs before 5 years' duration of type 1 diabetes. After 10 years, however, at least some degree of retinopathy is present in 60% of the diabetes population, and the figure approaches 100% by 15–17 years. It is unusual for PDR to occur before 10 years of diabetes but PDR is present in 26% of type 1 diabetes patients after 15 years. After 20 years, PDR is present in ~56% of the type 1 diabetes population.

In type 2 diabetes, diabetic retinopathy is present in ~20% of cases at diagnosis, and this figure increases to 60–85% after 15 years. PDR is present in 3–4% of patients in <4 years, and after 15 years, it is present in 5–20% of the type 2 diabetes population. Thus, patients with type 2 diabetes are more likely to have diabetic retinopathy at diagnosis and are more likely to develop diabetic retinopathy sooner after diagnosis than patients with type 1 diabetes.

NPDR

Mild NPDR, characterized by microaneurysms with or without occasional blot hemorrhages, is virtually ubiquitous after 15–17 years of diabetes. Microaneurysms may resolve slowly with time or show little or no change. Older microaneurysms may acquire a yellowish white appearance, imitating the appearance of hard exudates. Dot hemorrhages and microaneurysms can be considered clinically as one type of lesion. They are frequently indistinguishable from one another by ophthalmoscopic examination without fluorescein angiography, but such invasive testing is not warranted at this stage of retinopathy unless macular edema threatening central vision is present. Rare flecks of hard exudates, representing small white or yellowish white deposits generally with sharp borders, may be present in the intermediate layers of the retina. Hard exudates are lipid deposits leaked from microaneurysms or compromised capillary beds and may be present at any stage of NPDR and PDR.

The microaneurysms represent outpouchings of blood vessel walls, possibly secondary to weakness of the capillary wall from loss of pericytes or from increased intraluminal pressure or due to endothelial proliferation. Patients with mild NPDR can safely be followed every 9–12 months unless macular edema is present (Table 38.1).

Moderate NPDR is characterized by more significant retinal lesions. These lesions represent not only changes in vascular and perivascular tissue, but also changes within the retina associated with the effects of relative retinal hypoxia and circulatory changes. More abundant retinal hemorrhages and microaneurysms are present (Fig. 38.1). Early venous caliber abnormalities may also be present, reflected clinically as tortuous vasculature with varying lumen size. Venous caliber abnormalities may be caused by either sluggish blood flow, blood vessel wall weakening, or hypoxia.

Another vascular change observed in moderate NPDR is intraretinal microvascular abnormalities (IRMAs) (Fig. 38.2). IRMAs are a type of intraretinal neovascularization. Cotton-wool spots may also be present at this stage and represent stasis of axoplasmic flow in the nerve fiber layer of the retina caused by hypoxia after microinfarcts of retinal capillaries. Cotton-wool spots tend to disappear as NPDR becomes more severe.

Patients with moderate NPDR have more significant retinal disease. These patients are at greater risk for progression to vision-threatening retinopathy and should be followed every 4–6 months.

Severe NPDR is characterized by an abundance of nonproliferative lesions that include venous beading (Fig. 38.3), IRMAs (Fig. 38.2), and extensive hemor-

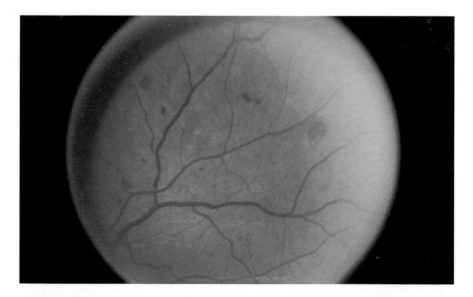

Figure 38.1 The severity and extent of hemorrhages or micro-aneurysms in all four quadrants constitutes severe NPDR. Standard photograph 2A.

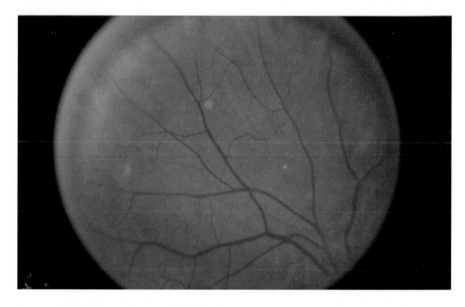

Figure 38.2 The extent of IRMAs in one or more quadrant constitutes severe NPDR. Standard photograph 8A.

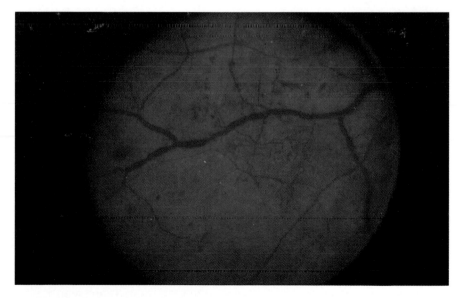

Figure 38.3 Venous beading in two or more quadrants constitutes severe NPDR. Standard photograph 6B.

rhages and microaneurysms (Fig. 38.1). The progression to severe NPDR represents more widespread retinal ischemia, but frank new-vessel growth on the retina is not present. Consultation with an ophthalmologist experienced in the management of diabetic eye disease for possible early laser surgery is urgent, particularly if extenuating circumstances exist (e.g., hypertension, renal disease, or pregnancy) or if the patient seems to be noncompliant or careless about follow-up examination. Rates of progression to high-risk PDR approach 45–50% in 2 years and 75% in 5 years if untreated. Patients with type 2 diabetes may be candidates for scatter laser photocoagulation at this time (i.e., before developing high-risk PDR).

PDR

PDR represents a severe form of retinopathy. It is characterized by the growth of new vessels on the optic disk or within 1 disk diameter of the optic disk (NVD), the growth of new vessels elsewhere on the retina (NVE), vitreous or preretinal hemorrhage, or preretinal fibrous tissue proliferation. These vessels grow over the retinal surface and on the posterior surface of the vitreous. They are fragile and rupture easily, causing preretinal and vitreous hemorrhage. The vessels can rupture spontaneously, even while a person is asleep, or with vigorous exercise, straining, coughing, and sneezing.

High-risk PDR puts a person at significant risk of visual loss (Table 38.1). The DRS revealed a 25–40% risk of severe visual loss over a 2-year period if high-risk PDR is present. Scatter laser treatment can reduce this risk by ~60%. High-risk PDR is characterized by any one of the following lesions:

- NVD greater than standard photo 10A of the modified Airlie House classification of diabetic retinopathy (i.e., NVD that covers more than one-fourth to one-third of the disk area) (Fig. 38.4)
- NVD less than standard photo 10A if preretinal or vitreous hemorrhage is present
- NVE greater than or equal to one-half of the disk area if preretinal or vitreous hemorrhage is present

Patients with high-risk PDR are candidates for immediate scatter laser photocoagulation. These patients should be referred immediately for laser treatment by a retinologist or ophthalmologist skilled in the treatment of diabetic retinopathy. These patients generally should not wait more than a few days for laser surgery.

The ETDRS demonstrated that scatter laser treatment applied when a person approaches or reaches high-risk PDR can reduce the 5-year risk of severe visual loss to <4%. In full scatter treatment, ~1,200–2,000 lesions are applied to the posterior pole. Two or more sessions are normally required to complete the treatment. The treating ophthalmologist applies the 500-µm laser burns ~500 µm apart. Major retinal vessels and scarred areas are avoided.

The response to full scatter photocoagulation varies depending on the retinal and medical status of the patient. There may be *1*) regression of active neovascularization, *2*) persistent neovascularization without further progression, *3*) continued growth of the neovascularization, and/or *4*) recurrent vitreous hemorrhage. Careful follow-up evaluation by the treating ophthalmologist with additional scat-

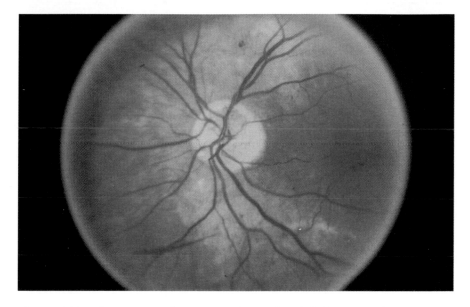

Figure 38.4 The extent of new vessels on the disk (greater than or equal to one-fourth of the disk area) with or without preretinal or vitreous hemorrhage constitutes high-risk diabetic retinopathy. Standard photograph 10A.

ter or local laser photocoagulation may be indicated, especially if continued new-vessel growth or recurrent vitreous hemorrhage occurs.

Fibrous tissue proliferation may lead to traction, which may cause a retinal detachment. If a view of the posterior pole is obscured by vitreous hemorrhage, ultrasound examination may be necessary. Nonresolving vitreous hemorrhage and traction retinal detachments, particularly those threatening detachment of the macula, may be indications for vitrectomy surgery.

PDR usually progresses through an active phase, followed by remission. In the remission phase, fibrous tissue will form, usually along abnormal vessels but also between the retina and posterior vitreous surface. A goal of scatter laser surgery is to shorten the active phase of retinopathy, leading to remission before major vitreous hemorrhage or fibrous tissue proliferation compromises vision. Patients who undergo scatter laser surgery for PDR may have activation of retinopathy in the future and may require further laser treatments.

Laser photocoagulation is not without potential complications. The DRS documented a minor decrease in visual acuity levels and peripheral visual fields, particularly in eyes treated with the xenon-arc photocoagulator, a system no longer in use. Today, scatter photocoagulation is performed with an argon laser. These risks need to be weighed against the potential benefits of laser surgery.

Many factors affect the progression of retinopathy in type 1 diabetes patients, including duration of diabetes, retinopathy status, pregnancy, the use of diuretics, and glycosylated hemoglobin levels. In type 2 diabetes patients, the age of the patient, severity of retinopathy, glycosylated hemoglobin levels, diuretic usage, lower intraocular pressure, smoking, and lower diastolic blood pressure may be risk factors. Extent of diabetes control, hypertension, kidney disease, cholesterol level, and anemia are documented risk factors for the progression of diabetic retinopathy.

DME

DME can be present at any stage of retinopathy and is a leading cause of moderate visual loss from diabetes. DME is a collection of fluid or thickening in the macula. Hard exudates within the macula area, nonperfusion of the retina inside the temporal vessel arcades, or any combination of these lesions may also be present. Patients with or suspected to have DME should be referred to an ophthalmologist for evaluation for clinically significant DME because laser photocoagulation is frequently indicated. Clinically significant DME is macular edema that involves or threatens the center of the macula and is characterized by any of the following retinal lesions:

- retinal thickening at or within 500 μm from the center of the macula
- hard exudates at or within 500 μm from the center of the macula if accompanied by thickening of the adjacent retina
- a zone or zones of thickening greater than or equal to one disk area in size, any portion of which is less than or equal to one disk diameter from the center of the macula

Patients with clinically significant DME should be referred to an experienced retinologist or ophthalmologist. The urgency for treatment of DME is not as acute as for high-risk PDR, but consultation and referral should occur within 1 month.

DME can only be adequately evaluated through dilated pupils and with stereoscopic examination of the macula. Stereo fundus photography is an important adjunct examination for patients who have or are suspected to have DME.

Patients with clinically significant DME are candidates for focal laser photocoagulation. The goal of treatment is to maintain acuity at approximately the same level as before treatment by preventing or limiting further leakage in the retina and allowing the leakage already present to reabsorb. With fluorescein angiography when possible, the ophthalmologist will determine whether treatable lesions are present and apply focal or grid laser surgery. Focal treatment is applied to focal leaks contributing to DME. Grid treatment is applied to areas of diffuse leakage or areas of nonperfusion in the macula area.

The ETDRS demonstrated that, in eyes with clinically significant macular edema, the risk of moderate visual loss was 50–60% less for eyes treated with focal laser compared with eyes assigned to deferral of treatment. Focal photocoagulation reduced the risk of moderate visual loss, increased the chance of visual improvement, decreased retinal thickening, and was not associated with any major adverse effects.

NONRETINAL OCULAR COMPLICATIONS

The ocular manifestations of diabetes that receive the most attention are those related to diabetic retinopathy and macular edema, because these changes are usually responsible for the most devastating visual threat from diabetes. Diabetic eye disease, however, represents an end-organ response to a systemic medical condition. Consequently, all structures of the eye are susceptible to the deleterious effects of diabetes. Following are some of the ocular problems in addition to retinopathy that are associated with diabetes:

- mononeuropathies of cranial nerves III, IV, or VI
- higher incidence of glaucoma
- earlier and more rapidly progressing cataracts
- susceptibility to corneal abrasions and recurrent corneal erosions
- early presbyopia
- blurred or fluctuating vision

Lenticular Opacities

Cataracts may occur at a younger age and progress more rapidly in the presence of diabetes. Cataracts are 60% more common in people with diabetes. This increased risk of cataract development occurs in both type 1 and type 2 diabetes populations.

Reversible lenticular opacities related to diabetes mellitus can occur in different layers of the lens and are most frequently related to poor glycemic control. The so-called true diabetic cataracts are usually bilateral and are characterized by dense bands of white subcapsular spots that look like snowflakes or fine needle-shaped opacities. Because diabetic cataracts are related to prolonged periods of severe hyperglycemia and untreated diabetes, they are now seldom seen in the U.S. and other industrialized countries.

Management of diabetic cataracts involves the same treatment strategies as management of age-related cataracts. For visual impairment not requiring surgery, optimum refraction for maximum visual acuity is recommended. Glare-control lenses and the use of sunglasses may relieve cataract-induced visual symptoms. Fortunately, cataract extraction with intraocular lens implantation is 90–95% successful in restoring useful vision, but the surgery has potential complications unique to diabetes. Intraocular lens implants provide the most natural postsurgical refractive correction. Careful patient education and consultation with the cataract surgeon is indicated.

A further consideration for the diabetes patient requiring cataract surgery involves the status of diabetic retinopathy. Diabetes is associated with an increased incidence of postoperative neovascularization on the iris (NVI) and neovascular glaucoma (NVG) after cataract extractions, regardless of the degree of retinopathy before surgery. If active PDR is present before cataract surgery, the risk of subsequently developing NVI, NVG, and vitreous hemorrhage is greater.

To provide appropriate preoperative care, physicians must determine diabetic retinopathy status before cataract extraction. Scatter laser photocoagulation is indicated for patients with high-risk PDR. With cataracts developing in the presence of severe NPDR or PDR without high-risk PDR, early laser treatment may be indicated. Laser treatment may be required a few days after surgery if active PDR is present.

Glaucoma

Open-angle glaucoma is 1.4–2.0% more common in the diabetes population. The prevalence of glaucoma increases with age and duration of diabetes, but medical therapy for open-angle glaucoma is generally effective. Argon-laser trabeculoplasty may normalize intraocular pressures in some patients if medical therapy proves ineffective. Treatment of open-angle glaucoma for the diabetes patient is essentially the same as for the nondiabetic patient.

NVG is a severe problem and sometimes occurs in eyes with severe diabetic retinopathy or retinal detachments or occasionally after cataract surgery. NVG results from a proliferation of new vessels on the surface of the iris. These vessels are usually first observed at the pupillary border. If the new vessels progress, a fine network of vessels and fibrous tissue may grow over the iris tissue and into the filtration angle of the eye. This growth results in peripheral anterior synechiae, and closure of the angle by this fibrovascular network results in NVG. In some cases, intraocular pressure may be elevated before angle involvement because of protein and cellular leakage from the proliferative vessels. Occasionally, iris neovascularization may be present in the filtration angle while not observed at the pupillary border.

NVG may be difficult to manage and generally requires aggressive treatment. Treatment modalities for NVI and NVG include the following:

- scatter laser photocoagulation
- goniophotocoagulation
- topical antiglaucoma drugs
- topical steroids
- topical atropine
- systemic antiglaucoma drugs
- cyclodestructive procedures
- filtration surgery
- a combination of these therapies

Early recognition and prompt retinal photocoagulation may help ameliorate this otherwise frequently devastating condition.

EXAMINATION CRITERIA AND FREQUENCY

Patients with diabetes mellitus should be examined *1*) at least within 3–5 years of diagnosis once a patient is ≥10 years of age for individuals diagnosed younger than age 30 years (generally type 1 diabetes) and at least yearly thereafter and *2*) at the time of diagnosis for individuals aged 30 years or older (generally type 2 diabetes) and at least yearly thereafter.

Pregnancy, nephropathy, hypertension, hypercholesterolemia, anemia, and other medical conditions may dictate more frequent examination. The presence of

DME and diabetic retinopathy greater than very mild NPDR indicates a need for more frequent examination. Tables 38.2 and 38.3 outline the examination schedule and guidelines for the care of diabetes patients.

VISUAL AND PSYCHOSOCIAL REHABILITATION

Patients with significant retinal disease or those who have lost vision from diabetic retinopathy should be encouraged to continue with regular eye care. Vitrectomy surgery can restore useful vision for some individuals who have lost sight from vitreous hemorrhages or fibrous tissue proliferation with traction retinal detachment. Proper refraction, visual rehabilitation (low-vision evaluation), optical aids, and other techniques and devices are available to enable a person to use even severely limited vision. Referral to visual rehabilitation specialists may be appropriate. Support groups for the visually impaired and organizations providing vocational rehabilitation exist in most areas. All practitioners should be familiar with appropriate referral sources for their patients with visual impairment.

Unlike many other eye conditions, diabetic retinopathy is not solely an eye problem but an end-organ response to a chronic systemic condition also affecting other organs (e.g., the heart and kidney). Multiple psychological and social issues may be present. Health care providers should be alert to these issues and assist in their appropriate management.

In its earliest stages, diabetic retinopathy causes no symptoms. Visual acuity may be excellent and, on evaluation and diagnosis, a patient may deny the presence of retinopathy. At this stage, the physician should initiate a careful program of education and follow-up. If the retinal disease progresses, visual acuity may be compromised by DME or episodes of vitreous hemorrhage. Difficulty in the work or home environment may result. Fear of blindness and other complications of diabetes, including death, may also develop.

If the visual acuity drops to 20/200 or worse, a patient may remain in a stage of uncertainty until the retinopathy is in quiescence secondary to either laser treatment or vitreoretinal surgery. Once the retinopathy is in remission and the vision

Table 38.2 Eye Examination Schedule

Age of Diabetes Onset (yr)	Recommended Time for First Examination	Routine Minimum Follow-Up*
0–29	3–5 yr after onset†	Annually
≥30	At diagnosis	Annually
During pregnancy	During first trimester	At discretion of the ophthalmologist but often each trimester and 6–8 wk postpartum

Adapted from Fong 2003.
*Abnormal findings dictate more frequent follow-up examinations (Table 38.3).
†Once ≥10 yr of age, <3–5 yr if in immediate postpubescent stage.

Table 38.3 Management Recommendations

Status of Retina	Follow-Up (mo)	Color Fundus Photography	Fluorescein Angiography	Laser
Normal or minimal NPDR	12	No	No	No
Mild to moderate NPDR without DME	6–12	Rarely	No	No
Mild to moderate NPDR with clinically insignificant DME	4–6	Occasionally	Rarely	No
Mild to moderate NPDR with CSME	3–4	Yes	Yes	Yes
Severe to very severe NPDR	3–4	Yes	Yes, if CSME	Consider
Non–high-risk PDR	2–3	Yes	Yes, if CSME	Consider
High-risk PDR	2–4	Yes	Yes, if CSME	Yes
High-risk PDR not amenable to photocoagulation	1–6	If possible	No	In connection with vitrectomy if indicated

CSME, clinically significant macular edema. Adapted from the American Academy of Ophthalmology: *Preferred Practice Patterns for Diabetic Retinopathy.* San Francisco, CA, American Academy of Ophthalmology, 1998.

stable, the patient is in a position to accept his or her situation and to make the appropriate psychological and social adjustments. At this time, visual and vocational rehabilitation is usually more successful.

Communication among all members of a patient's health care team is of paramount importance in dealing with the physical and psychological stresses of visual loss from diabetes.

BIBLIOGRAPHY

Aiello LP, Cahill MT, Wong JS: Systemic considerations in the management of diabetic retinopathy. *Am J Ophthalmol* 132:760–776, 2001

Aiello LM, Cavallerano J, Aiello LP: Diagnosis, management and treatment of nonproliferative diabetic retinopathy and macular edema. In *The Principles and Practices of Ophthalmology: The Harvard System.* Philadelphia, Saunders, 2000, p. 1900–1914

Aiello LP, Gardner TW, King GL, Blankenship G, Cavallerano JD, Ferris FL III, Klein R: Diabetic retinopathy (Technical Review). *Diabetes Care* 21:143–156, 1998

American Diabetes Association: Retinopathy in diabetes (Position Statement). *Diabetes Care* 27 (Suppl. 1):S84–S87, 2004

Early Treatment Diabetic Retinopathy Study Research Group: Early photocoagulation for diabetic retinopathy: ETDRS report no. 9. *Ophthalmology* 98:766–785, 1991

Early Treatment Diabetic Retinopathy Study Research Group: Effects of aspirin treatment on diabetic retinopathy: ETDRS report no. 8. *Ophthalmology* 98:757–765, 1991

Early Treatment Diabetic Retinopathy Study Research Group: Fundus photographic risk factors for progression of diabetic retinopathy: ETDRS report no. 12. *Ophthalmology* 98:823–833, 1991

Early Treatment Diabetic Retinopathy Study Research Group: Photocoagulation for diabetic macular edema: ETDRS report no. 1. *Arch Ophthalmol* 103:1796–1806, 1985

Ferris FL III: Early photocoagulation in patients with either type I or type II diabetes. *Trans Am Ophthalmol Soc* 94:505–537, 1996

Javitt JC, Aiello LP, Bassi LJ, Canner JK: Detecting and treating diabetic retinopathy: financial and visual savings associated with improved implementation of current guidelines. *Ophthalmology* 98:1565–1574, 1990

Klein R, Klein BEK, Moss SE, Davis MD, DeMets DL: The Wisconsin Epidemiologic Study of Diabetic Retinopathy. II. Prevalence and risk of diabetic retinopathy when age at diagnosis is less than 30 years. *Arch Ophthalmol* 102:520–526, 1984

Klein R, Klein BEK, Moss SE, Davis MD, DeMets DL: The Wisconsin Epidemiologic Study of Diabetic Retinopathy. III. Prevalence and risk of diabetic retinopathy when age at diagnosis is 30 or more years. *Arch Ophthalmol* 102:527–532, 1984

Dr. Lloyd Paul Aiello is Assistant Director, Beetham Eye Institute, Joslin Diabetes Center; Head, Section of Eye Research, Joslin Diabetes Center; and Associate Professor of Ophthalmology, Harvard Medical School, Boston, MA. Dr. Lloyd M. Aiello is Director and Dr. Cavallerano is Staff Optometrist and Assistant to the Director, Beetham Eye Institute, Joslin Diabetes Center, Boston, MA.

39. Drug-Induced Renal Dysfunction in Diabetes Patients

ALI J. OLYAEI, PHARMD, ANGELO M. DEMATTOS, MD,
AND WILLIAM M. BENNETT, MD

D rug-induced acute renal failure is a major cause of morbidity and mortality among patients with diabetes. The limited epidemiologic data available suggests that the most important factor in treating drug-induced acute renal failure in diabetes patients involves implementation of preventive strategies to reduce the incidence of drug-induced renal dysfunction among these patients. Drug-induced renal failure is manifest as acute tubular necrosis (ATN), prerenal renal failure, acute-onset chronic renal failure, and finally obstructive renal failure. In a prospective, multicenter, longitudinal study from 13 hospitals in Madrid, Spain, the most frequent causes of renal failure were ATN (45%), prerenal renal failure (21%), acute-onset chronic renal failure (12.7%), and obstructive renal failure (10%). The overall mortality rate was ~45% higher in patients with acute renal failure compared with other hospitalized patients.

Two major factors make the kidneys a major target for drug toxicity. First, the kidneys receive a high fraction (20–25%) of cardiac output relative to their weight (0.4%); therefore, a high concentration of drugs transit through the kidneys. Second, the renal countercurrent-concentrating mechanism for water also concentrates drugs and drug metabolites within the filtered tubular fluid. Thus, local concentrations of these substances in contact with renal epithelium may exceed those in peripheral blood.

It is important to be cautious when prescribing nephrotoxic agents and to be aggressive and prompt in diagnosing renal dysfunction. Identifying patients at risk for drug-induced nephrotoxicity and using caution when prescribing nephrotoxic agents attenuates nephrotoxicity. In diabetes patients, there is often subclinical preexisting renal dysfunction, even when blood urea nitrogen (BUN) and serum creatinine levels are within the normal range.

These laboratory tests are insensitive to pathological processes (e.g., diabetes-related macrovascular or microvascular disease) until substantial kidney damage is present. This is particularly true in the hypertensive diabetes patient. Therefore, early recognition is essential for prevention of permanent kidney damage.

SEVERAL FACTORS THAT AFFECT PRESCRIBING DRUGS FOR THE DIABETES PATIENT

Approximately 40% of all drugs are excreted through the kidneys. Subclinical and clinical diabetic nephropathy reduces renal blood flow and the glomerular filtration rate. The reduced renal function is an important risk factor for drug toxicity. About 40% of these cases occur in the elderly. Renal changes that occur with diabetes include nephrosclerosis (a thickening of the intrarenal vascular intima), sclerogenous changes of the glomeruli, and infiltration of chronic inflammatory cells and fibrosis in the stroma. Diabetes may also alter renal tubular functions, impairing handling of water, sodium, acid, and glucose. These pathophysiological changes caused by diabetes may increase the risk of prerenal acute renal failure, volume depletion, ATN, and postrenal azothemia. Impaired renal function ultimately alters the pharmacokinetics and pharmacodynamics of many drugs administered to diabetes patients. Furthermore, alteration in pharmacokinetics and pharmacodynamics may further increase the risk of drug-induced renal failure.

In diabetes patients, if proteinuria is present without other clinical diagnoses, diabetic nephropathy can be assumed. Diabetic retinopathy almost invariably indicates some degree of nephropathy. In a patient with a history of upper urinary tract infections, bladder dysfunction, or kidney stones, the clinician should be suspicious of renal papillary necrosis and underlying interstitial renal disease. For these diabetes patients, a measured or estimated creatinine clearance is essential to avoid overdosage or drug toxicity. The estimated clearance relates the serum creatinine to the patient's body habitus and age by the following:

$$\text{estimated creatinine clearance} = \frac{(140 - \text{patient age})\,(\text{body weight in kg})}{2\,(\text{serum creatinine in mg/dl})}$$

This formula is the most accurate estimated renal function in patients, with the exception of individuals with significant edema, ascites, or pregnancy. In female patients, the final value should be multiplied by 0.85. Note also that not all renal dysfunction in diabetes is due to the underlying diabetic renal disease (i.e., diabetes patients are as susceptible as nondiabetic individuals to glomerulonephritis or interstitial nephritis). A careful urinary sediment examination to exclude hematuria, cellular casts, and pyuria helps to exclude other processes in these patients.

NEPHROTOXINS

Radiographic Contrast Media

Radiocontrast-induced renal failure accounts for 20% of acute renal failure cases in the hospital setting. Diabetes patients are at a greater risk of renal dysfunction when exposed to radioconstrast media. In most diabetes patients, diagnostic procedures (e.g., intravenous pyelography, angiography, computed tomography) are performed with iodinated dyes. Contrast agents, including the newer nonionic dyes, are promptly excreted by the kidney and can produce acute increases in BUN and creatinine. In patients with normal renal function, iodinated contrast media have limited nephrotoxicity and rarely lead to significant renal failure or dialysis. However, patients with diabetic nephropathy or preexisting renal impairment are at a greater risk of radiocontrast-induced renal failure. In addition, diabetes patients with a medical history of congestive heart failure (class III or IV), with reduced effective arterial volume (e.g., nephrotic or cirrhotic), or who receive other nephrotoxic agents are at greater risk for radiocontrast nephrotoxicity. Contrast nephrotoxicity may be clinically important in patients with other factors simultaneously affecting the renal response to contrast or in whom acute renal failure would seriously affect their clinical prognosis. The major known risk factors for contrast nephropathy have in common preexisting renal disease and excessive loads.

In some patients, contrast-associated renal failure results in permanent impairment of renal function, with few requiring dialysis. Virtually all of these patients will have preexisting renal disease. Contrast-associated nephropathy is rarely the only etiologic factor in acute renal insufficiency, but the patients at greatest risk are clearly those with diabetic nephropathy and chronic renal failure.

Clinical presentation. The clinical presentation is nonspecific, with a rise in serum creatinine within the first 24 h after exposure. Urinalysis may indicate formed elements of epithelial cells, casts, and debris. Contrast-associated nephropathy is defined as a change in serum creatinine of ≥50% from baseline or an absolute increase of 1 mg/dl (88.4 µmol/l). Serum creatinine peaks within 3–5 days of the study, and oliguria is observed in only 30% of patients. Formed elements in urinary sediment, although frequent, are insensitive markers of injury and are of little diagnostic value. Although the fractional excretion of sodium is frequently low, it has little prognostic value because most patients recover from contrast nephropathy without clinical consequences. The most practical way to evaluate a patient in the absence of oliguria is to monitor serum creatinine daily in high-risk patients, especially if risk factors are present (Table 39.1).

The pathogenesis of contrast nephrotoxicity is most likely related to a combination of direct tubular injuries and renal ischemic vascular constriction. Existing data indicate a limited role for the newer low-osmolality media for the prevention of nephrotoxicity.

Prevention and management. When selecting an imaging study, use the least invasive procedure that will provide adequate diagnostic information. Prophylac-

Table 39.1 Clinical Risk Factors for Contrast Nephropathy

- Diabetes mellitus
- Abnormal baseline serum creatinine
- Preexisting renal disease
- Large amount of contrast material
- Several studies performed within a short time interval

tic use of acetylcysteine has been associated with a significant reduction in radiographic contrast agent–induced renal insufficiency in patients with abnormal renal function. Acetylcysteine, 600 mg orally, should be administrated before the radiocontrast agent in two daily oral doses on the day before and the day of contrast agent administration. In one study, the overall rate of acute contrast agent–induced renal failure was 2% in the acetylcysteine-treated group and 21% in the control group.

In addition, the following recommendations should be used for patients whose serum creatinine is ≥1.5 mg/dl (≥135 μmol/l) at baseline: 6 h before using the radiocontrast agent, start normal saline at a 75–100 ml/h infusion for a total of 500 ml. Normal saline should be continued during and for 6 h after the procedure. This regimen has been validated by controlled studies, and it appears to be as safe and as good as using vasodilating pharmacological agents.

In patients taking metformin, this drug should be discontinued before or at the time of radiology studies using iodinated contrast media and should not be reinstituted for 48 h. In all patients, renal function should be assessed and be in the normal range before reinstituting metformin. Administration of radiocontrast agents in metformin-treated patients has been associated with lactic acidosis, which can ultimately lead to acute renal failure.

Finally, many clinicians recommend the use of nonionic, low-osmolar contrast agents in diabetes patients with renal insufficiency to further reduce the risk of significant renal ischemia. Pharmacoeconomic evidence justifies the considerable cost of the newer agents for diabetes patients.

Nonsteroidal Anti-Inflammatory Drugs

Nonsteroidal anti-inflammatory drugs (NSAIDs) are widely used for the treatment of chronic arthritic diseases such as osteoarthritis and rheumatoid arthritis. Conventional NSAIDs nonspecifically inhibit both cyclooxygenase (COX)-1 and COX-2 isoforms. The anti-inflammatory and analgesic benefits of NSAIDs result from the inhibition of COX-2, whereas the increased rates of gastrointestinal (GI) complications are attributed to the inhibition of the COX-1 isoform. GI toxicity has been a significant problem for many patients using NSAIDs, especially for geriatric patients who consume these agents for extended periods of time. GI complications, including episodes of serious bleeding, are recognized with the use of oral NSAIDs. Much of this information comes from case-control or cohort studies, which have shown an incidence of such events to occur in ~2–6% of treated patients per year.

The adverse effects of NSAIDs on the kidneys are usually confined to the clinical setting of relative renal hypoperfusion (volume depletion, diuretic therapy, and renal impairment) such as that frequently coexisting with diabetes. In diverse conditions such as congestive heart failure, cirrhosis, nephrosis, or diuretic use, there are increases in angiotensin II, catecholamines, and vasopressin. Both angiotensin II and vasopressin stimulate production of vasodilatory prostaglandins and prostacyclin, which balance the vasoconstrictor actions of these agonists. Administration of NSAIDs causes selective inhibition of prostaglandin synthesis; an unmodulated vasoconstrictor response to angiotensin II, vasopressin, and catecholamines; and a reduction in renal blood flow and glomerular filtration rate. In addition to patients who have edema-forming states, others notably at risk include individuals with atherosclerotic cardiovascular disease and patients with volume depletion.

Clinical presentation. Clinical renal syndromes associated with NSAID use include a spectrum of drug-induced renal failure: hemodynamically mediated acute renal dysfunction, allergic interstitial nephritis with nephrotic syndrome, hyperkalemia due to hyporeninemic hypoaldosteronism, and sodium retention with diuretic resistance. The most common clinical presentation of NSAID-induced dysfunction is hemodynamically mediated acute renal dysfunction in patients with the aforementioned preexisting conditions of relative renal ischemia. NSAIDs frequently reduce the antihypertensive efficacy of diuretic agents, whereas the combination of NSAIDs with triamterene or other diuretics is additive and may produce a particularly severe form of acute renal failure.

Until further studies demonstrate the safety of rofecoxib in patients at risk of cardiovascular complications, caution should be exercised when using rofecoxib for the treatment of arthritis in diabetes patients. In rofecoxib safety studies, the overall incidence of vascular thrombotic events was 1.8% in the rofecoxib group and 0.6% in the naproxen group ($P < 0.002$). Myocardial infarction occurred in 0.5% of the patients randomized to rofecoxib and in 0.1% of those treated with naproxen ($P < 0.01$). These findings raise concerns about cardiovascular safety and the benefits of rofecoxib in patients with ischemic heart disease. Recently, the U.S. Food and Drug Administration required amendments to the rofecoxib package insert to reflect the enhanced cardiovascular risk associated with the use of this agent. It is also important to note that there is no clinical evidence that linked celecoxib and valdecoxib to higher incidence of thromboembolic events. Recently, investigators have shown a high incidence of cardiovascular complications in patients (50–84 years of age) taking rofecoxib (>25 mg daily). In this study, non-NSAID users ($n = 202,916$) were compared with individuals who used ibuprofen ($n = 59,007$), naproxen ($n = 70,384$), celecoxib ($n = 22,337$), <25 mg rofecoxib ($n = 20,245$), and >25 mg rofecoxib ($n = 3,887$). Although high-dose rofecoxib patients had lower cardiovascular risks than nonselective NSAID or celecoxib (low or high dose) users, the overall rate of cardiovascular complications was 1.7 times more likely than that of nonusers, other NSAID users, or celecoxib users. New users of high-dose rofecoxib were 2.2 times more likely than celecoxib users to have major complications.

In addition, diabetes patients with renal dysfunction are at particular risk of hyperkalemia when taking NSAIDs (Table 39.2). Elderly patients are at particularly high risk for problems with these agents, possibly because they use these drugs three times more frequently than patients <60 years of age.

Another common clinical presentation is that of acute interstitial nephritis with nephrotic-range proteinuria. There seems to be no clinical situation that predisposes the patient to this reaction. Onset may be weeks or months after starting NSAID therapy and is marked by proteinuria of ≥3 g/24 h. It is usually reversible on discontinuation of the NSAID. However, in the occasional patient who fails to respond promptly with a return to normal creatinine levels, a short course of high-dose steroids (e.g., 60 mg prednisone given over 3 days, with rapid tapering over the next week) can speed recovery of the filtration rate.

Table 39.2 Drug Interactions in Diabetes Patients That Predispose to Serious Hyperkalemia

Drug	Mechanism
β-Blockers	Inhibit renin-angiotensin system; block β-agonist movement of K+ into cells
Amiloride	Blocks renal K+ secretion
Triamterene	Blocks renal K+ secretion
Trimethoprim	Blocks renal K+ secretion
Spironolactone	Blocks renal K+ secretion by blocking aldosterone action
ACE inhibitors and receptor blockers	Inhibit conversion of angiotensin I to angiotensin II or angiotensin II action
NSAIDs	Inhibit prostaglandin-mediated renin responses
Cyclosporine	Blocks renal K+ secretion

ACE, angiotensin-converting enzyme; NSAIDs, nonsteroidal anti-inflammatory drugs.

Finally, renal abnormalities are associated with analgesic use and abuse in amounts >2 kg cumulatively. This can add to the papillary ischemia that occurs in some diabetes patients with bladder dysfunction and urinary tract infections. There is loss of renal concentrating capacity and the presence of electrolyte-wasting syndromes (e.g., renal sodium wasting, hyperkalemic renal tubular acidosis). Analgesic-associated nephropathy should be suspected in middle-aged women with diabetes who complain of recurrent headaches or back pain. Although many will deny intake, some confess to taking aspirin, acetaminophen, or combination analgesics in amounts of more than four to six tablets per day. NSAIDs alone can cause chronic renal failure. The treatment of choice is withdrawal of the agents. For chronic analgesic abuse, the entity will not be reversible, but many patients will plateau at their current level of function. Avoidance of these drugs in high-risk patients and the careful monitoring of serum creatinine are beneficial.

Antibiotics and Anti-Infective Agents

Most antimicrobials in clinical use have a low nephrotoxic potential except for the rare idiosyncratic acute interstitial nephritis produced by penicillin, sulfonamide, and cephalosporin derivatives. Others, e.g., amphotericin B, acyclovir, pentamidine, the aminoglycosides, are significantly nephrotoxic.

Aminoglycoside antibiotics. Aminoglycosides are valuable therapeutic agents for the treatment of serious gram-negative infections. However, 10–15% of all therapeutic courses are complicated by reversible renal dysfunction, even when peak and trough serum levels are kept within the desired therapeutic range. In addition, even in therapeutic concentrations, both cochlear and vestibular toxicity may occur in patients with impaired renal function. Both nephrotoxicity and ototoxicity are frequent, particularly in diabetes patients with preexisting renal dysfunction. Various risk factors that predispose the patient to the development of aminoglycoside nephrotoxicity have been identified (Table 39.3).

Aminoglycosides may affect the structure and function of proximal tubular cells. They predominantly impair tubular epithelium and cause obstruction of tubular lumens. The nephrotoxicity of aminoglycosides is linked to the number of cationic charges. Aminoglycosides with the highest charges are more nephrotoxic (neomycin), whereas those with fewer cationic charges are less nephrotoxic (streptomycin). Among the clinically available aminoglycosides, the spectrum of nephrotoxicity is as follows: gentamicin > tobramycin > amikacin > netilmicin. Monitoring of peak and trough serum concentrations will ensure efficacy, whereas elevation of the trough level, showing drug accumulation, will often precede a rise in the less sensitive serum creatinine measurements. Nonoliguric renal insufficiency is the most common manifestation of aminoglycoside nephrotoxicity. In general, most patients are able to maintain urine output >500 ml/day. Less common are various isolated tubular syndromes, e.g., nephrogenic diabetes insipidus, Fanconi syndrome, and renal potassium or magnesium wasting. Fortunately, severe oliguric renal failure requiring dialysis is rare from aminoglycosides alone. A drug-induced concentrating defect characterized by polyuria and secondary thirst stimulation precedes the detectable rise in BUN and serum creatinine that will occur in as many as 30% of hospitalized patients given >5–7 days of aminoglycoside treatment. Granular casts and mild proteinuria occur frequently but are not of diagnostic assistance. The renal histological picture associated with aminoglycoside nephrotoxicity is one of patchy proximal tubular necrosis. In addition, in patients who satisfy the clinical criteria for aminoglycoside nephrotoxicity, cellular autophagocytosis has been observed with electron microscopy.

Aminoglycosides are often necessary for managing the diabetes patient. Alternative antibiotics with gram-negative coverage should be prescribed whenever possible in patients with diabetic nephropathy to prevent aminoglycoside nephrotoxicity. Fluoroquinolones are excellent alternatives to aminoglycosides in diabetes patients with impaired renal function. When the use of aminoglycosides is required, a loading dose should be sufficient to achieve high peak levels to maximize bacterial killing. In patients with renal function, the elimination half-life of

Table 39.3 Risk Factors for Aminoglycoside Nephrotoxicity

- Long duration of treatment (>5 days)
- Recent courses of aminoglycoside therapy
- Age >60 yr
- Concomitant nephrotoxins
- Volume depletion
- K^+ depletion
- Mg^{2+} depletion
- Preexisting renal dysfunction
- Liver disease

aminoglycosides is normally 2 h. The elimination half-life is markedly prolonged as renal function falls. Maintenance-dose intervals should be carefully extended in patients with existing renal dysfunction when aminoglycosides are required. Extending the interval between doses is safer than reducing the size of individual doses in patients with renal insufficiency. Recent data indicate that once-daily aminoglycoside dosing may be less nephrotoxic for a given total daily dose. Finally, in patients at risk for aminoglycoside-induced renal failure, all correctable risk factors should be minimized.

Amphotericin B. Amphotericin B is a polyene antibiotic with activity against a broad spectrum of fungi. However, elevated serum creatinine has been reported in up to 80% of patients given amphotericin B. Amphotericin-induced nephrotoxicity is dose and duration dependent. Renal failure is inevitable in patients with cumulative doses >3 g per treatment in adults. In addition, the previous doses of amphotericin B should be considered in calculating cumulative dose of amphotericin B. Diabetes patients, the elderly, and particularly patients with depleted extracellular volume are at a greater risk of nephrotoxicity.

The rate of nephrotoxicity is relatively constant during amphotericin B treatment. For each 10-mg increase in the mean daily amphotericin B dose, the adjusted rate of renal toxicity increases by a factor of 1.13 (95% CI 1.02–1.25). The major risk factors for amphotericin B–induced renal impairment include a mean daily amphotericin B dose of ≥35 mg, male sex, weight ≥90 kg, chronic renal disease, and the use of amikacin or cyclosporine.

Clinical presentation. The usual clinical presentation of amphotericin B nephrotoxicity is characterized by defects in renal tubular function. Occasionally, this condition will progress to nonoliguric renal failure. Modest proteinuria associated with a relatively normal urinary sediment is the initial finding. Frank azotemia is preceded by hypokalemia, renal tubular acidosis, and impaired urinary concentrating capacity. In addition, the presence of a magnesium-wasting syndrome is a prominent feature of amphotericin B nephrotoxicity. Repetitive courses of amphotericin B may cause permanent impairment of renal function. Frequent monitoring of serum creatinine is recommended. If toxicity occurs, a lipid-based amphotericin B formulation should be considered. A doubling of the baseline serum creatinine is indicative of serious nephrotoxicity.

Sodium supplementation in the form of intravenous saline can be used as a safe and effective means of reducing the risk of amphotericin nephrotoxicity to ~10%. Sodium (150 meq/day) can be administered as follows: 500 ml normal saline 30 min before amphotericin B administration and a second 500 ml given during the 30 min after completion of the amphotericin B infusion. The goal is to achieve a urinary sodium excretion of 250–300 mmol/day. Lipid-based amphotericin B may allow larger doses with a higher therapeutic index. Several unique lipid-based amphotericin B delivery systems have been developed in an attempt to attenuate nephrotoxic complications of amphotericin B. The incorporation of amphotericin B within a lipid matrix, in theory, facilitates targeted delivery of an active drug to sites of inflammation or infection while limiting distribution into mammalian membranes. Currently, three different lipid-based amphotericin products are marketed in the U.S.: Amphotericin B Colloidal Dispersion (ABCD, Amphotec), Amphotericin B Lipid Complex (ABLC, Abelcet), and Liposomal Amphotericin B (L-Amph, AmBisome). All three lipid formulations have to some extent demonstrated an enhanced safety profile compared with conventional amphotericin B. However, Liposomal Amphotericin B (AmBisome) has shown a significantly lower incidence of nephrotoxicity than other lipid-based amphotericin B preparations. Voriconazole is an excellent alternative to amphotericin B in patients with impaired renal function.

Angiotensin-Converting Enzyme Inhibitors

With emerging evidence that treatment of systemic hypertension and concomitant lowering of intraglomerular pressure has a beneficial effect on the course of renal disease in diabetes, angiotensin-converting enzyme (ACE) inhibitors have been advocated as the antihypertensive therapeutic class of choice when microalbuminuria is first detected. Although these compounds are generally well tolerated, acute renal dysfunction can occur in the presence of atherosclerotic vascular disease involving the main renal arteries or in any other situation where renal hemodynamics are maintained by angiotensin-mediated constriction of postglomerular vessels.

Other examples of the clinical conditions that predispose patients to renal complications of ACE inhibitors include severe congestive heart failure, diuretic-induced extracellular volume depletion, or stenosis of an artery to a solitary kidney. A chemistry panel should be checked on all patients within 5–7 days of drug initiation, particularly individuals >50 years of age and those with any predisposing condition. If renal dysfunction occurs, dosage reduction or reduction of any concomitantly administered diuretic dosage usually improves renal hemodynamics. Although the overall incidence of transient elevation of serum creatinine is lower in the angiotensin II receptor blockers recipients, the same renal considerations apply with angiotensin II receptor blockers as with ACE inhibitors.

Immunosuppressive Drugs

Cyclosporine and tacrolimus are frequently used to prevent kidney transplant rejection as well as rejection in other solid organ transplants. Nephrotoxicity is the primary side effect of kidney transplant therapy, which is most often performed in diabetes patients. Cyclosporine produces drug- and dosage-related renal dysfunction characterized by rises in BUN, creatinine, and usually blood pressure. This phenomenon is due to the intrarenal hemodynamic effects of these agents to cause afferent arteriolar vasoconstriction. These effects are reversible when the drug dose is reduced. In kidney transplant patients, it is difficult to distinguish renal dysfunction secondary to the immunosuppressive drug from transplant rejection. This issue may only be resolved by a transplant biopsy. In addition to acute renal dysfunction, cyclosporine may produce hyperkalemic metabolic acidosis, hyperuricemia and gout, and hypomagnesemia. Furthermore, chronic use of cyclosporine may result in chronic nephropathy characterized by slowly progressive chronic renal dysfunction. Therefore, early attempts to use cyclosporine in patients with early-onset diabetes is not a viable clinical strategy. Cyclosporine and tacrolimus therapy must be carefully monitored through blood levels. Once the patient is stable, the blood levels may be obtained every 3–4 months, but after transplantation, achieving a stable dose and total exposure to the drug so that toxicity is minimized and effectiveness is maximized is usually done by transplant specialists. Many drug interactions that occur with cyclosporine can precipitate nephrotoxicity. Drugs that inhibit cyclosporine's liver metabolism include the following:

- diltiazem
- verapamil
- erythromycin
- ketoconazole
- fluconazole

Although the drug interactions for tacrolimus are less well documented, the dose should be adjusted downward if any of these agents are used concomitantly. On the other hand, when inducers of drug metabolism (e.g., anticonvulsants, rifampicin, or isoniazid) are introduced into therapy, cyclosporine and tacrolimus blood levels may be reduced, thus exposing the patient to increased risk of rejection.

BIBLIOGRAPHY

Bates DW, Su L, Yu DT, Chertow GM, Seger DL, Gomes DR, et al.: Mortality and costs of acute renal failure associated with amphotericin B therapy. *Clin Infect Dis* 32:686–693, 2001

Bennett A: Anti-inflammatory drugs, cyclooxygenases and other factors. *Exp Opin Pharmacother* 2:1–2, 2001

Bennett WM, Henrich WL, Stoff JS: The renal effects of non-steroidal anti-inflammatory drugs: summary and recommendations. *Am J Kidney Dis* 28:556–562, 1996

Bennett WM, Swan SK: Nephrotoxic acute renal failure. In *Acute Renal Failure*. Lazarus M, Brenner B, Eds. New York, Churchill Livingstone, 1993, p. 357–359

Crofford LJ: Specific cyclooxygenase-2 inhibitors: what have we learned since they came into widespread clinical use? *Curr Opin Rheumatol* 14:225–230, 2002

Costa S, Nucci M: Can we decrease amphotericin nephrotoxicity? (Review) *Curr Opin Crit Care* 7:379–383, 2001

deMattos AM, Olyaei AJ, Bennett WM: Mechanisms and risks of immuno-suppressive therapy. In *Immunologic Renal Diseases*. Neilson EG, Couser WG, Eds. Philadelphia, Lippincott-Raven, 1997, p. 861–885

Gerlach AT, Pickworth KK: Contrast medium-induced nephrotoxicity: patho-physiology and prevention. *Pharmacotherapy* 20:540–548, 2000

Girmenia C, Gentile G, Micozzi A, Martino P: Nephrotoxicity of amphotericin B desoxycholate. *Clin Infect Dis* 33:915–916, 2001

Lanas A: Clinical experience with cyclooxygenase-2 inhibitors (Review). *Rheumatology* 41 (Suppl. 1):16–22, 2002

Luber AD, Maa L, Lam M, Guglielmo BJ: Risk factors for amphotericin B-induced nephrotoxicity. *J Antimicrob Chemother* 43:267–271, 1999

Murphy SW, Barrett BJ, Parfrey PS: Contrast nephropathy. *J Am Soc Nephrol* 11:177–182, 2000

Pflueger A, Larson TS, Nath KA, King BF, Gross JM, Knox FG: Role of adenosine in contrast media-induced acute renal failure in diabetes mellitus. *Mayo Clinic Proc* 75:1275–1283, 2000

Quader MA, Sawmiller C, Sumpio BA: Contrast-induced nephropathy: review of incidence and pathophysiology. *Ann Vasc Surg* 12:612–620, 1998

Rudnick MR, Berns JS, Cohen RM, Goldfarb S: Contrast media-associated nephrotoxicity. *Semin Nephrol* 17:15–26, 1997

Strand V, Hochberg MC: The risk of cardiovascular thrombotic events with selective cyclooxygenase-2 inhibitors. *Arthritis Rheum* 47:349–355, 2002

Swan SK: Aminoglycoside nephrotoxicity. *Semin Nephrol* 17:27–33, 1997

Swan SK, Bennett WM: Drug dosing guidelines. In *Renal Failure in Current Practice of Medicine*. Glassock RJ, Ed. Philadelphia, Current Medicine, 1996, p. 29.1–29.11

Textor SC: Renal failure related to angiotensin-converting enzyme inhibitors. *Semin Nephrol* 17:67–76, 1997

Drs. Olyaei and deMattos are Associate Professors of Medicine, Division of Nephrology and Hypertension, Oregon Health and Science University, Portland, OR. Dr. Bennett is Director of Solid and Cellular Transplantation, Legacy Good Samaritan Hospital, Portland, OR.

40. Diabetic Nephropathy

Ralph A. DeFronzo, MD

D iabetic nephropathy represents the most common cause of end-stage renal failure in the United States and accounts for ~40% of all new patients entering end-stage renal disease (ESRD) programs. Over the last decade (1990–2000), both the prevalence and incidence of ESRD in the U.S. have approximately doubled, and nephropathy due to type 2 diabetes accounts for the great majority of the increase. Increased longevity due to more aggressive treatment of cardiovascular risk factors and decreased cardiovascular death allows diabetic nephropathy to run its full course in patients with type 2 diabetes. The treatment cost of diabetic patients with ESRD is approximately $16 billion and consumes about 6% of the Medicare budget. Although dialysis and transplantation prevent death from uremia, the 5-year survival rate in diabetic patients with ESRD is much worse than that in nondiabetic patients and approaches 20%. Therefore, it is important to recognize the earliest stages of diabetic nephropathy and to institute appropriate therapy. Once overt proteinuria (urinary albumin excretion >300 mg/day) has become established, relentless progression to ESRD is inevitable.

Diabetic nephropathy develops in ~50% of patients with type 1 diabetes mellitus who have had diabetes for 20 years. Clinically significant renal disease is less common in type 2 diabetes mellitus, occurring in 15–20% of individuals. However, in certain populations with an increased prevalence of type 2 diabetes mellitus, e.g., Native Americans, Hispanics, and African Americans, the prevalence of renal disease is much greater and approaches that in populations with type 1 diabetes mellitus. Caucasians have the lowest prevalence of diabetic nephropathy among the major ethnic groups.

PATHOGENESIS

A rational approach to the therapy of diabetic renal disease depends on a thorough understanding of its pathogenesis. Factors that have been implicated in the development of diabetic nephropathy are briefly reviewed (Table 40.1). Essentially all diabetic patients, both type 1 and type 2, who develop renal insufficiency demonstrate evidence of poor glycemic control, as documented by persistently elevated fasting plasma glucose (>160–180 mg/dl [>8.8–10.0 mmol/l]) and glycated hemoglobin A1C (A1C) (>8.0%) levels. The product of the mean A1C and the duration

Table 40.1 Etiologic Factors in the Development of Diabetic Renal Disease

- Poor glycemic control (fasting plasma glucose >140–160 mg/dl [>7.7–8.8 mmol/l]); A1C >7–8%
- Genetic factors
- Hemodynamic abnormalities (increased RBF and GFR, elevated intraglomerular pressure)
- Systemic hypertension
- Insulin resistance syndrome (metabolic syndrome)
- Inflammation (highly sensitive C-reactive protein, fibrinogen, NFκB)
- Altered vascular permeability
- Excessive protein intake
- Metabolic disturbances (abnormal polyol metabolism, formation of advanced glycation end products, increased cytokine production)
- Release of growth factors
- Abnormalities in carbohydrate/lipid/protein metabolism
- Structural abnormalities (glomerular hypertrophy, mesangial expansion, glomerular basement membrane thickening)
- Disturbances in ion pumps (increased Na^+-H^+ pump and decreased Ca^{2+}-ATPase pump)
- Hyperlipidemia (hypercholesterolemia and hypertriglyceridemia)
- Activation of protein kinase C

of diabetes is the best predictor of diabetic nephropathy. The results of the Diabetes Control and Complications Trial (DCCT) (intensive insulin therapy in type 1 diabetes), the Japanese Intervention Study (intensive insulin therapy in type 2 diabetes), and the United Kingdom Prospective Diabetes Study (UKPDS) (intensive therapy with oral agents and/or insulin in type 2 diabetes) have conclusively demonstrated that tight glycemic control serves as primary prevention for all microvascular complications, including nephropathy, retinopathy, and neuropathy. These observations are consistent with a meta-analysis of numerous smaller studies.

Genetic factors are also important, and diabetic nephropathy, as well as hypertension, clearly aggregates in families of both people with type 1 diabetes and people with type 2 diabetes. Although these genetic factors cannot be reversed, a strong family history of renal involvement should alert the physician to pay closer attention to the monitory signs of renal involvement. Although several genes and chromosomal regions have been linked to diabetic nephropathy, no causal association between any gene and diabetic renal disease has yet been documented.

Hemodynamic abnormalities play a major role in the pathogenesis of diabetic nephropathy. Poor glycemic control is associated with a rise in renal blood flow (RBF) and glomerular filtration rate (GFR), the latter resulting from both renal hypertrophy and increased sensitivity of the efferent arteriole to angiotensin II. Efferent arteriolar vasoconstriction causes an increase in intraglomerular pressure, which, if it persists over a long period of time, contributes to the demise in renal function by directly injuring the glomerulus and causing glomerular nephrosclerosis.

These hemodynamic abnormalities are exacerbated by excessive protein intake. Systemic hypertension per se directly causes renal damage and will exacerbate local renal hemodynamic abnormalities.

Metabolic disturbances, including abnormal polyol metabolism, formation of advanced glycosylation end products, and disturbances in collagen metabolism, which develop secondary to poor glycemic control, also have been implicated in the pathogenesis of diabetic nephropathy. Release of growth factors and various cytokines, including transforming growth factor-β, insulin-like growth factors (IGFs), vascular endothelial growth factor (VEGF), and abnormalities in carbohydrate/lipid/protein metabolism contribute to the development of structural abnormalities (glomerular hypertrophy, mesangial expansion, and glomerular basement membrane thickening) that characterize diabetic nephropathy. An increase in Na^+-H^+ pump activity has been demonstrated in some diabetic patients with renal disease, and this has been implicated in the development of systemic hypertension, cardiomegaly, and accelerated atherosclerosis. Recent studies have demonstrated a strong correlation between the development of proteinuria and the insulin resistance syndrome (also called the metabolic syndrome, dysmetabolic syndrome, and syndrome X) in both type 1 and type 2 diabetic patients. A link between circulating markers of inflammation (highly sensitive C-reactive protein and fibrinogen) and intracellular inflammatory proteins/transcription factors (nuclear factor κβ [NFκβ]) also has been demonstrated in both animals and humans with diabetic nephropathy. Much evidence has implicated protein kinase C (PKC)-β as an important mediator of diabetic nephropathy and diabetes-induced vascular dysfunction.

NATURAL HISTORY OF DIABETIC NEPHROPATHY

The natural history of renal disease has been well characterized in both patients with type 1 and type 2 diabetes mellitus who are destined to develop renal insufficiency.

- At initial diagnosis, there are no renal histological abnormalities, but RBF and GFR are elevated (Fig. 40.1).
- Within 3 years, histological changes (increased mesangial matrix material, glomerular and tubular basement membrane thickening, and arteriolar hyalinosis) of diabetic nephropathy are evident, but GFR and RBF remain elevated.
- Over the subsequent 10–15 years, there is progressive histological damage, but renal hyperfiltration persists and there are no laboratory clues to suggest the presence of renal involvement.
- Approximately 15 years after the diagnosis of diabetes, albuminuria (>300 mg/day) is detected, and the elevated rates of RBF and GFR have returned to normal (Fig. 40.1). This ominous sign heralds the onset of progressive renal insufficiency, which is highly variable from individual to individual (decrement in GFR = 2–20 ml/min/year, with a mean decrement of 12 ml/min/year). Once overt albuminuria develops (>300 mg/day), no intervention has been shown to prevent the eventual

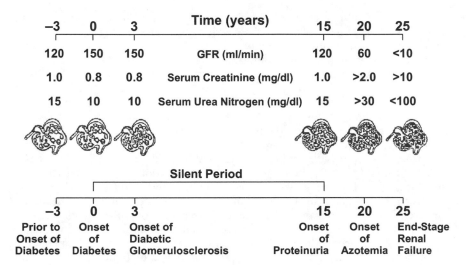

Time (years)						
−3	0	3		15	20	25
120	150	150	GFR (ml/min)	120	60	<10
1.0	0.8	0.8	Serum Creatinine (mg/dl)	1.0	>2.0	>10
15	10	10	Serum Urea Nitrogen (mg/dl)	15	>30	<100

Silent Period

−3	0	3	15	20	25
Prior to Onset of Diabetes	Onset of Diabetes	Onset of Diabetic Glomerulosclerosis	Onset of Proteinuria	Onset of Azotemia	End-Stage Renal Failure

Figure 40.1 Natural history of diabetic nephropathy (see text). Adapted from DeFronzo.

progression to ESRD, although pharmacological therapy can slow the rate of GFR decline.
- Within 5 years after the onset of albuminuria, ~50% of patients experience a 50% reduction in GFR and a doubling of serum creatinine.
- Within a mean of another 5 years, 50% of these patients progress to ESRD. By 20 years, >75% of diabetic patients with overt albuminuria will have progressed to ESRD.

Albuminuria

At or just before onset of overt or clinical albuminuria (>300 mg/day), most patients develop hypertension, and the increase in blood pressure markedly accelerates the progression of renal disease. Effective treatment of the hypertension has been documented to slow but not prevent the progression to ESRD. Once clinically detectable albuminuria has developed, tight glycemic control cannot prevent the development of renal insufficiency. Moreover, it remains unproven that tight glycemic control can even slow the progression of renal disease once clinical albuminuria has been reached. However, it is important to maintain an A1C <6.5–7.0% to retard the progression of diabetic retinopathy and neuropathy.

Microalbuminuria

Before the onset of overt or clinical albuminuria, there is a preclinical stage of diabetic nephropathy (also called incipient diabetic nephropathy) characterized by microalbuminuria (Table 40.2). Nondiabetic individuals do not excrete

Table 40.2 Definition of Microalbuminuria

	Urinary Albumin Excretion Rate		Urine Albumin-Creatinine Ratio (µg/mg)
	mg/day	µg/min	
Normoalbuminuria	<30	<20	<30
Microalbuminuria	30–300	20–200	30–300
Clinical or macroalbuminuria	>300	>200	>300

The mean value for urinary albumin excretion rate in normal individuals is 10 ± 3 mg/day or 7 ± 2 µg/min.

>10–20 mg/day of albumin in their urine. However, routine laboratory tests do not detect these small amounts of albuminuria unless the albumin excretion is ≥300 mg/day. Thus, there is a range of albumin excretion (30–300 mg/day or 20–200 µg/min) that is distinctly abnormal yet is not detectable by routine tests. This range is referred to as microalbuminuria and is the first laboratory evidence of diabetic renal disease. Fortunately, microalbuminuria can be detected with more sophisticated techniques (e.g., radioimmunoassay or an enzyme-linked immunosorbent assay). If assays for microalbuminuria are not readily available, screening with reagent tablets for microalbuminuria may be carried out because they show good sensitivity (95%) and specificity (93%). All positive tests by reagent strips or tablets should be confirmed by more specific methods.

It is advisable to determine microalbuminuria in a timed urine collection (i.e., 24 h) because this allows simultaneous measurement of creatinine clearance. However, the urine albumin-to-creatinine ratio (microalbuminuric range 30–300 µg/mg creatinine) is nearly as good as a timed urine collection.

Most importantly, tight glycemic control with insulin and treatment with angiotensin-converting enzyme (ACE) inhibitors during the microalbuminuric stage have been shown to prevent the progression of microalbuminuria to overt clinical albuminuria in both type 1 and type 2 diabetes subjects. No study has demonstrated that tight glycemic control can slow the progression to ESRD once the urine albumin excretion exceeds ~300 mg/day. Therefore, it is essential that all type 1 diabetic patients be screened yearly for microalbuminuria, starting 5 years after the time that diabetes is diagnosed. Type 2 diabetic patients should be screened yearly for microalbuminuria starting at diagnosis because these individuals may have had their disease for many years before their initial encounter with the physician.

Recent studies have demonstrated that it may be possible to detect individuals who are at risk of developing overt nephropathy even before the onset of microalbuminuria, as detected by currently available assays. In healthy nondiabetic individuals, all filtered albumin is reabsorbed by the proximal tubule either by 1) a rapid transtubular pathway or 2) cellular uptake, followed by lysosomal degradation into peptide fragments that are returned to the bloodstream. In diabetic patients who are destined to develop renal disease, these peptide fragments are excreted into the urine, where they can be quantitated by HPLC (Microalbumin

Plus; AusAm Biotechnologies, Santa Monica, CA). This methodology also detects microalbuminuria (intact albumin molecule) that is not measured by currently available assays, because the tertiary structure of the albumin molecule has been altered. In a study of type 1 diabetic patients, Microalbumin Plus, on average, detected albumin in the urine 4 years before the onset of microalbuminuria (as determined by currently available methods), making it possible to initiate therapy at an earlier stage in the natural history of diabetic nephropathy.

Type 2 Diabetes Mellitus

The natural history of diabetic nephropathy in individuals with type 2 diabetes who are destined to develop ESRD closely mimics that in type 1 diabetic patients, but there are several important differences:

- Clinically detectable albuminuria is common at the time of diagnosis, but a smaller percentage (5–10%) of Caucasian patients with type 2 diabetes mellitus progress to ESRD by 20 years.
- The incidence of progression of microalbuminuria to renal insufficiency is much higher (15–20%) in African Americans, Mexican Americans, and Asian subjects and exceeds 50% in certain Native American tribes.
- In all individuals with type 2 diabetes, regardless of ethnic background, microalbuminuria is a strong predictor of death from stroke or myocardial infarction.
- Approximately 80% of individuals with type 2 diabetes die from atherosclerotic cardiovascular complications within 10 years after the onset of microalbuminuria.
- Microalbuminuria is strongly associated with the insulin resistance syndrome.

EVALUATION OF LOSS OF RENAL FUNCTION

Every diabetic patient who develops proteinuria or a rise in serum creatinine concentration should have a thorough evaluation to define the cause of renal failure. It is unwise to assume that all diabetic subjects who experience deterioration in renal function have diabetic nephropathy. It is unusual for individuals with diabetic nephropathy to have more than three to five red blood cells per high-powered field, and the presence of more than five red blood cells per high-powered field should suggest another cause of renal disease. Similarly, it is uncommon to see a reduction in GFR due to diabetic nephropathy in the absence of heavy proteinuria. It also has been stated that it is unusual to observe diabetic nephropathy without retinopathy. However, in a series of 347 type 2 diabetic patients with albuminuria (>300 mg/day), of whom 93 (27%) had no evidence of diabetic retinopathy, kidney biopsy revealed diabetic glomerulosclerosis in 69% of these 93 individuals. The remaining 31% had a variety of renal diseases that dictated very different therapeutic approaches than normally would be used to treat diabetic nephropathy.

A comprehensive evaluation should exclude other causes of renal disease. In general, they can be divided into prerenal, postrenal, and intrarenal (glomerulonephritis, tubulointerstitial disease, and vasculitis).

History and Physical Examination

The history and physical examination should focus on

- drugs taken (nonsteroidal anti-inflammatory drugs and analgesics)
- toxin exposure
- administration of radiographic contrast media
- hereditary diseases
- history of renal disease
- allergic manifestations
- skin rash
- arthritis
- fever
- involvement of other organ systems

Intravascular volume and cardiac status should be assessed to ensure that renal perfusion is adequate. Symptoms of urinary tract obstruction, especially in men, or neurogenic bladder should be elicited. A history of oliguria suggests another cause of renal failure.

In type 1 diabetic patients, clinical evidence of renal disease is extremely rare within the first 5 years after the diagnosis of diabetes and is uncommon (<5–10%) within the first 10 years. This is not true in type 2 diabetes, because the true onset of diabetes is difficult to document, and many patients may have had their disease for ≥5 years before their diabetes was diagnosed.

Albuminuria is the hallmark of diabetic nephropathy and, in its absence, the diagnosis should not be made. Diabetic retinopathy usually accompanies diabetic nephropathy. However, ~70% of diabetic patients with albuminuria and without evidence of retinopathy still turn out to have diabetic glomerulosclerosis on renal biopsy.

Laboratory Assessment

Urinalysis. Urinalysis in diabetic nephropathy is usually benign. Occasional erythrocytes may be seen. Numerous erythrocytes or erythrocyte casts indicate glomerulonephritis. The presence of leukocytes and bacteria implies urinary tract infection, and a urine culture should be obtained. If renal tubular epithelial cells accompany leukocytes, one of the tubulointerstitial causes of renal disease should be suspected. Heavy proteinuria is consistent with diabetic renal disease or glomerulonephritis. The absence of proteinuria virtually excludes diabetic nephropathy. Numerous uric acid or calcium crystals should suggest renal calculus disease.

Serum chemistries and blood tests. Serum urea nitrogen and creatinine concentrations help exclude prerenal and postrenal causes of renal failure. In intrinsic renal disease, they rise in parallel in a ratio of 10–15:1. A disproportionate rise in serum urea nitrogen should suggest intravascular volume depletion, congestive heart failure, and/or urinary tract obstruction. Hyperkalemia and hyperchloremic metabolic acidosis, in the absence of a significant increase in the serum creatinine concentration (<3–4 mg/dl [<265–354 µmol/l]), suggests the presence of interstitial nephritis or hypoaldosteronism. The latter is common in diabetic nephropathy. Specific renal tubular defects in potassium and hydrogen ion secretion (in the absence of hypoaldosteronism) also occur in diabetic patients with nephropathy. Serum calcium and uric acid concentrations should be measured to rule out hypercalcemic and uric acid nephropathy, respectively.

Peripheral eosinophilia suggests an allergic interstitial nephritis. In patients with suspected glomerulonephritis, total serum complement and C3, antinuclear antibody, antistreptolysin O titer, antiglomerular basement membrane antibody titer, and cryoglobulins should be obtained. A very high erythrocyte sedimentation rate suggests vasculitis. Microangiopathic hemolytic anemia and thrombocytopenia are observed in hemolytic uremic syndrome and thrombotic thrombocytopenic purpura.

Other diagnostic maneuvers. Renal ultrasound is a simple noninvasive method to exclude urinary tract obstruction without the necessity of injecting radio contrast dye. It also allows quantification of kidney size. Small kidneys imply chronic advanced renal disease. Patients with early diabetic nephropathy have normal or, more commonly, increased kidney size. Radionuclide imaging with radiolabeled technetium allows assessment of RBF. If, after a thorough evaluation, the cause of the renal failure remains undefined, a renal biopsy should be considered. Because diabetic nephropathy is generalized and involves all parts of all glomeruli, the diagnosis cannot be missed. Diabetic nephropathy is characterized by

- an increase in mesangial matrix material
- glomerular basement membrane thickening
- hyalinosis of the afferent and efferent arterioles
- thickened tubular basement membranes
- tubular atrophy
- interstitial fibrosis

The renal histology also allows differentiation between vasculitis versus glomerulonephritis versus interstitial nephritis and provides information concerning the specific etiology of glomerulonephritis or tubulointerstitial nephritis.

TREATMENT OF MICROALBUMINURIA

Microalbuminuria represents the earliest stage of diabetic nephropathy that can be detected clinically, although a new urine test (Microalbumin Plus) may allow the physician to detect degraded albumin fragments and a structurally altered intact albumin molecule at an even earlier stage. Type 1 diabetic patients with microalbuminuria have a 15- to 20-fold increase in the incidence of developing albuminuria after 10 years; the incidence of clinically overt albuminuria after 10 years in type 2 diabetic individuals is increased 5- to 10-fold. In individuals with type 2 diabetes, microalbuminuria is less predictive of eventual diabetic nephropathy than in individuals with type 1 diabetes, but it is a powerful predictor of cardiovascular mortality, and 80% of microalbuminuric type 2 diabetic patients die within 10 years. At initial onset of microalbuminuria, less than one-third of type 1 diabetic patients are hypertensive, but the incidence of hypertension increases as the severity of the microalbuminuria progresses. In type 1 diabetic patients, microalbuminuria is related closely to the presence of renal disease. More type 2 diabetic patients are hypertensive at the time that they present with micro-albuminuria. The elevation in blood pressure also may be related to underlying diabetic nephropathy, be due to coexisting essential hypertension, or be secondary to a myriad of other secondary causes, such as renal vascular disease. As micro-albuminuria worsens, there is a progressive increase in the incidence of hypertension in both type 1 and type 2 diabetic patients.

Because of the significant day-to-day variation (~40–50%) in urinary micro-albumin excretion, at least two baseline determinations (positive for microalbu-minuria) should be obtained to establish the diagnosis. This also provides a more accurate baseline against which to judge the efficacy of subsequent therapeutic interventions. Several factors can increase the urinary albumin excretion rate:

- stress
- systemic or urinary tract infection
- acute metabolic decompensation
- fever
- exercise
- hypertension
- cardiac failure

These confounding medical disorders must be resolved before measuring the albumin excretion rate.

Glycemic Control

Strict glycemic control (and treatment of hypertension, if present) is the most critical factor in treating diabetic patients during the microalbuminuric stage. Type 1 diabetic patients in the highest quartile for hyperglycemia have a 4- to 5-fold increased risk of developing overt albuminuria and eventually renal insufficiency compared with individuals in the lowest quartile. Hyperglycemia also predicts the development of clinical albuminuria in individuals with type 2 diabetes. In every animal model of diabetes, tight glycemic control has been shown to prevent the development of renal disease. No study has demonstrated that normalization of the plasma glucose profile can alter the relentless progression to ESRD in type 1 diabetic patients with clinical albuminuria or renal insufficiency. However, several prospective studies (e.g., the DCCT) have shown that tight glycemic control with insulin, which maintains the A1C below 7.0–7.5%, prevents the development of clinical albuminuria in type 1 diabetic patients with microalbuminuria (Fig. 40.2). Moreover, tight glycemic control prevents the progression of normoalbuminuria to microalbuminuria (i.e., primary prevention) in type 1 diabetic patients without microalbuminuria. Although some concern has been raised about extrapolation of the DCCT results to type 2 diabetic patients, both the Japanese (Kumamoto) intervention study and the Wisconsin Epidemiologic Study of Diabetic Retinopa-thy have demonstrated the importance of normoglycemia or near-normoglycemia in the prevention of microvascular complications (renal and retinal) in type 2 diabetic subjects.

These studies indicate that strict glycemic control, if implemented early enough, can halt the progression of microalbuminuria to clinical albuminuria and thus prevent the development of ESRD. Based on these observations, type 1

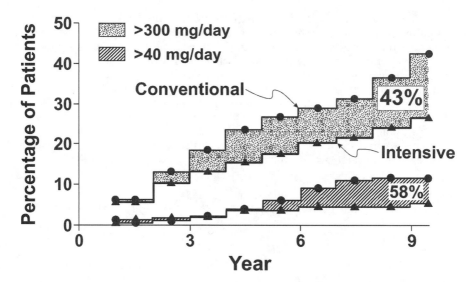

Figure 40.2 Effect of conventional versus intensive glycemic control on urinary albumin excretion rate in type 1 diabetic patients with normoalbuminuria and microalbuminuria. Tight glycemic control significantly reduced development of microalbuminuria in normoalbuminuric patients (primary prevention) and slowed the progression from microalbuminuria to overt albuminuria (secondary prevention). Adapted from The DCCT Research Group.

diabetic patients with a normal urinary albumin excretion rate and especially individuals with microalbuminuria should be aggressively treated with insulin to maintain as near normal a glycemic profile as possible and to achieve an A1C value <6.5–7.0% and ideally <6.0% (Table 40.3). Such intensive therapy requires a highly motivated patient, multiple insulin injections, and home glucose monitoring, because the risk of hypoglycemia is significant.

In type 2 diabetic patients, similar glycemic control should be achieved with diet, exercise, oral agents (i.e., sulfonylureas, metformin, pioglitazone, rosiglitazone, acarbose, repaglinide, and nateglinide), and, if necessary, insulin. The benefits of tight glycemic control to reduce urinary albumin excretion may require 1–2 months to become evident. However, the UKPDS has demonstrated that intensive glycemic control reduces the risk of developing microalbuminuria and overt nephropathy in type 2 diabetic patients.

Dietary Protein

In both diabetic and nondiabetic models of renal disease, a high-protein diet exacerbates and a low-protein diet ameliorates the progression of chronic renal disease. Many studies in humans have demonstrated that a low-protein diet slows

Table 40.3 Treatment of Diabetic Patients with and Without Microalbuminuria and with Overt Diabetic Nephropathy

	No Micro-albuminuria	Micro-albuminuria	Clinical Albuminuria/Renal Insufficiency
Glycemic control (A1C)	<6–7%	<6–7%	<7–8%
Blood pressure*			
Systolic/diastolic (mmHg)	120–130/80	120–130/80	120–130/80
Mean arterial pressure (mmHg)	90–95	90–95	90–95
Dietary protein intake (g/kg/day)	≥1.0–1.2	0.8–1.0	0.6–0.8†

*If the diabetic patient's normal blood pressure before the onset of hypertension is known and is <120–130/80–85 mmHg, this should be established as the therapeutic end point.
†If the patient is on an angiotensin-converting enzyme inhibitor, dietary intake can be higher (0.8–1.0 g/kg/day).

the decline of GFR in patients with all types of chronic renal disease, including diabetic nephropathy. When dietary protein is restricted to 0.6–0.8 g/kg body weight/day in patients with diabetic nephropathy, the rate of decline in GFR is blunted and urinary albumin excretion is diminished. In microalbuminuric diabetic patients with normal renal function, a low-protein diet reduces urinary albumin excretion without any change in GFR. Based on these observations, moderate protein restriction of 0.8–1.0 g/kg/day is advocated in diabetic patients with overt microalbuminuria (Table 40.3). Replacement of animal protein with vegetable protein is recommended because this has the same effect as a low-protein diet in slowing the rate of GFR decline in diabetic patients. Patients with normal renal function and no microalbuminuria should avoid a high-protein diet and substitute vegetable protein for animal protein. In diabetic patients receiving ACE inhibitors and calcium-channel blockers, clinical trials (Modified Diet in Renal Disease Study) have not documented a beneficial effect of a low-protein diet. This observation suggests that treatment with an ACE inhibitor provides near-maximum protection against diabetic renal disease and that addition of a low-protein diet provides little if any further protection.

Antihypertensive Therapy

Hypertension is a characteristic feature of diabetic nephropathy and is the most important factor known to accelerate the progression of renal failure. In type 1 diabetes, the onset of hypertension characteristically occurs at onset of microalbuminuria or shortly thereafter. In type 2 diabetes, hypertension may occur at any time and more closely parallels the patient's age and obesity index. However, once microalbuminuria develops in type 2 diabetic patients, the incidence of hypertension increases significantly. Multiple factors (e.g., diabetic nephropathy, increased total-body sodium content, sympathetic nervous system overactivity-enhanced responsiveness to angiotensin II and norepinephrine, impaired insulin-mediated vasodilation, endothelial dysfunction and impaired nitric oxide generation, and increased circulating levels of vasoconstrictors) contribute to the development of hypertension. Treatment of hypertension at or before the microalbuminuric stage can prevent the development of microalbuminuria or arrest its progression, respectively. In contrast, treatment of hypertension at the stage of clinical albuminuria can only slow the rate of deterioration of renal function.

Early and aggressive antihypertensive therapy has been shown to dramatically extend the median life expectancy in type 1 diabetic patients, with a reduction in mortality from 94% to 45% and a decrease in the need for dialysis/transplantation from 73% to 31% 16 years after the development of nephropathy. In the Steno study, comprehensive management of hyperglycemia, hypertension, dyslipidemia, and other cardiovascular risk factors reduced the risk of nephropathy, retinopathy, and autonomic neuropathy by 39%, 42%, and 37%, respectively, and reduced the risk of cardiovascular disease (myocardial infarction, stroke, revascularization, amputation, and cardiovascular death) by 47%.

Antihypertensive therapy should begin at the earliest indication of a rise in blood pressure and should be aggressive. The most prudent goal is to lower the patient's blood pressure to the level present before the onset of proteinuria and/or renal insufficiency. For many patients, especially if they are young, this level may be less than the standard value of 120–130/80 mmHg. If the patient's normal blood pressure is unknown, the recommended goal should be 120–130/80 mmHg (Table 40.3). This level corresponds to a mean arterial blood pressure of 90–95 mmHg. Caution is advised in elderly hypertensive patients who may have underlying cerebrovascular and cardiovascular disease.

It should be emphasized, however, that early in the microalbuminuric stage, many diabetic patients will not be hypertensive, but they still require treatment with "antihypertensive" medications (e.g., ACE inhibitors and angiotensin receptor blockers [ARBs]). The therapeutic approach to such individuals is discussed in a subsequent section.

Nonpharmacological Treatment

Nonpharmacological intervention consists of weight loss, especially in obese type 2 diabetic patients, regular physical activity (walking 2–3 miles/day at 15–20 min/mile, four to five times per week), and salt restriction (4–5 g/day or 68–85 meq/day). These lifestyle changes can be very effective in reducing blood pressure. In addition, weight loss and exercise increase insulin sensitivity, enhance glycemic control, and improve dyslipidemia. If these nonpharmacological measures do not normalize blood pressure, pharmacological intervention is indicated.

The ideal antihypertensive agent should not only lower blood pressure but reverse the specific pathophysiological derangements responsible for hypertension, slow or halt the progression of renal disease, and be metabolically neutral (i.e., not aggravate insulin resistance, hyperinsulinemia, or dyslipidemia, all of which have been implicated in the accelerated atherosclerosis that characterizes type 1 diabetes and especially type 2 diabetes). Patients should monitor their blood pressure daily at home, and the physician should adjust the blood pressure medication at weekly intervals until normotension is achieved.

Pharmacological Therapy

ACE inhibitors. This class of drugs most closely approximates the ideal antihypertensive agent. ACE inhibitors

- decrease peripheral vascular resistance by inhibiting the production of angiotensin II
- lower intraglomerular pressure
- prevent glomerular hypertrophy
- reduce proteinuria and microalbuminuria
- slow the rate of GFR decline
- provide protection against cardiovascular disease (Heart Outcomes Prevention Evaluation study)
- improve insulin sensitivity

Numerous studies have shown that ACE inhibitors halt the progression of microalbuminuria or cause a reduction in the rate of progression of microalbuminuria in both type 1 and type 2 diabetic patients. The most abundant data have been obtained with captopril and enalapril. Similar but less extensive data have been accumulated with the other ACE inhibitors. There are three primary mechanisms by which the ACE inhibitors decrease microalbuminuria and preserve renal function.

1. They decrease the vasoconstrictor effect of angiotensin II on the efferent arteriole, leading to a reduction in intraglomerular pressure.
2. They inhibit glomerular hypertrophy and reduce mesangial matrix proliferation.
3. They decrease systemic blood pressure. Although the reduction in systemic blood pressure accounts for the majority of the protective effect of the ACE inhibitors, this class of antihypertensive agent clearly has effects that extend beyond its blood pressure–lowering action.

ACE inhibitors also improve insulin sensitivity, ameliorate hyperinsulinemia, and promote a more favorable serum lipid profile by reducing LDL cholesterol and triglyceride levels and increasing HDL cholesterol. The beneficial effects of ACE inhibitors on insulin sensitivity and serum lipids have been best demonstrated with captopril.

ACE inhibitors may cause hyperkalemia, especially in patients with type IV renal tubular acidosis, i.e., the hypoaldosteronism syndrome. In some patients (i.e., those with renal artery stenosis, especially if bilateral, severe congestive heart failure, or advanced renal insufficiency), the GFR may be highly dependent on angiotensin II–mediated efferent arteriolar tone, and ACE inhibition may cause a precipitous decline in GFR. In patients who are prone to develop hyperkalemia and/or deterioration in renal function, the decline in GFR is observed shortly after starting the drug. Therefore, patients who are treated with an ACE inhibitor should have their serum potassium and creatinine concentrations checked ~1 week after initiation of therapy.

Currently available ACE inhibitors and specific dosages are listed in Table 40.4.

Angiotensin receptor blockers. There are two types of angiotensin receptors in humans: AT_1 and AT_2. Most of the clinical effects of angiotensin II are mediated

Table 40.4 Recommended Antihypertensive Agents for Hypertensive Diabetic Patients

Drug	Usual Dose (range in mg)	Significant Side Effects	Other Considerations
ACE inhibitors			
Captopril	25–50 mg 2–3×/day	Rash	Can improve insulin sensitivity, glucose tolerance, and plasma lipid levels. If total daily dose of enalapril and benazepril is ≥20 mg, split into two daily doses.
Enalapril	5–40 mg/day	Neutropenia	
Benazepril	10–40 mg/day	Proteinuria	
Fosinopril	10–40 mg/day	Hyperkalemia	
Lisinopril	5–40 mg/day	Decline in GFR	
Ramipril	2.5–20 mg/day		
Quinapril	5–40 mg/day		
ARBs			
Losartan	25–100 mg/day	Decline in GFR	Does not increase plasma bradykinin levels
Irebesartan	150–300 mg/day	Hyperkalemia	Not associated with cough
Candesartan	8–32 mg/day		
Valsartan	80–320 mg/day		
Telmisartan	40–80 mg/day		
Eprosartan	400–800 mg/day		
Ca^{2+}-channel antagonists			
Verapamil	40–120 mg 3×/day	Increases serum digoxin level	Long-lasting formulations of these drugs are available. Calcium-channel blockers have no significant adverse effects on glucose or lipid metabolism.
		Negative inotropic effect	
		May cause AV block	
Diltiazem	30–90 mg 3×/day	Constipation	
		May cause AV block	
Nicardipine	20–40 mg 3×/day	Peripheral edema	
Nifedipine	10–30 mg 3×/day	Peripheral edema	
Isradipine	2.5–10mg 2×/day	Peripheral edema	

Diuretics

Hydrochlorthiazide	12.5–50 mg/day	Hyponatremia	Thiazides are not effective when GFR decreases to <40–50 ml/min.
Chlorthiazide	50–200 mg/day	Hypokalemia	
Chlorthalidone	12.5–50 mg/day	Glucose intolerance	
Metolazone	2.5–10 mg/day	Increased LDL cholesterol and triglycerides	
Furosemide	20–80 mg/day up to 40–160 mg 2×/day		Higher doses of furosemide may be required when nephrotic syndrome and/or renal insufficiency are present.
Ethacrynic acid	25–100 mg/day up to 50–200 mg 2×/day	Decreased HDL cholesterol	
Bumetanide	0.5–2 mg/day up to 1–4 mg 2×/day	Insulin resistance	

β₁-Selective antagonists

Metoprolol	50–100 mg 2×/day	May cause AV block	At higher doses, β₁-selectivity is lost, bronchospasm may be precipitated, hypoglycemia may occur, and symptoms of hypoglycemia are masked.
Atenolol	50–100 mg/day	May exacerbate congestive heart failure	

Central adrenergic antagonists

Clonidine	0.1–0.6 mg 2×/day	Drowsiness	Rebound hypertension may occur if these drugs are stopped abruptly.
Guanabenz	4–16 mg 2×/day	Dry mouth	

Peripheral α₁-antagonists

Prazosin	1–2 mg 2–3×/day	Orthostatic hypotension	These drugs can improve insulin sensitivity and plasma lipid profile.
Terazosin	1–5 mg/day at bedtime	First-dose phenomenon of syncope	
Doxazosin	2–8 mg/day at bedtime		

Vasodilators

Apresoline	10–50 mg 3–4×/day	Headache	Minoxidil is very effective in patients with refractory hypertension and renal insufficiency.
Minoxidil	5–30 mg 2×/day	Reflex tachycardia	
		Excess hair growth	

ACE, angiotensin-converting enzyme; ARBs, angiotensin II receptor blockers; AV, arteriovenous.

via activation of the AT_1 receptor. Not all diabetic patients treated with ACE inhibitors reach blood pressure goals, and some have persistent albuminuria/microalbuminuria despite treatment with multiple antihypertensive agents, including maximum doses of ACE inhibitors. This has led to the suggestion that pathways other than ACE may be responsible for angiotensin generation, especially in tissues and blood vessels. It also has been suggested that chronic ACE inhibition may lead to the accumulation of angiotensin I and stimulation of the angiotensin II subtype 1 (AT_1) receptor, despite maximum doses of ACE inhibitors. On the other hand, the ACE inhibitors, but not ARBs, lead to an increase in plasma levels of bradykinin, a potent vasodilator. These concerns have led to the development of a new class of antihypertensive agents, the angiotensin II receptor (subtype 1) blockers (ARBs).

There have been four major trials with ARBs in diabetes: two in patients with microalbuminuria and two in individuals with overt nephropathy. In the Irbesartan Microalbuminuria Type 2 Diabetes in Hypertensive Patients (IRM2) trial, irbesartan demonstrated a dose-dependent (150 and 300 mg/day) reduction in the progression of microalbuminuria to overt albuminuria over a period of 2 years in type 2 diabetic patients (Fig. 40.3). Similarly, in the Microalbuminuria Reduction with Valsartan (MARVAL) trial, valsartan produced a clear reduction in microalbuminuria at 6 months in type 2 diabetic patients, whereas the calcium-channel blocker amlodipine had no effect on microalbuminuria. Both antihypertensive agents had similar effects to reduce blood pressure.

Two large trials have examined the efficacy of ARBs in type 2 diabetic patients with overt nephropathy. In the RENAAL (Reduction of Endpoints in NIDDM with

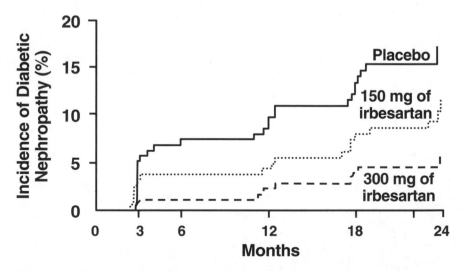

Figure 40.3 Effect of angiotensin receptor blockade on the development of overt albuminuria (≥300 mg/day) in type 2 diabetic patients with microalbuminuria.

the Angiotensin II Antagonist Losartan) trial, losartan at a dose of 50–100 mg/day (in addition to standard antihypertensive therapy) versus placebo significantly reduced the time required to double the serum creatinine and the risk of progression to ESRD requiring dialysis or kidney transplantation. However, there was no difference in all-cause or cardiovascular mortality between the losartan and placebo groups. In the Irbesartan Type 2 Diabetic Nephropathy Trial (IDNT), irbesartan (titrated to 300 mg/day) was compared with amlodipine (10 mg/day) and placebo (all in addition to conventional antihypertensive therapy). Irbesartan significantly reduced the composite index (time required to double the serum creatinine, onset of ESRD, and all-cause mortality) compared with both amlodipine and placebo. Amlodipine compared with placebo had no significant effect on the composite index.

No study has directly compared the beneficial effects on renal function of the ACE inhibitors versus ARBs in diabetic patients with microalbuminuria or overt albuminuria. However, comparison of the published trials does not indicate any benefit of one class, ACE inhibitors versus ARBs, over the other. Several small studies have examined the effect of adding an ARB to an ACE inhibitor in diabetic patients with persistent albuminuria, and the results have been inconsistent. Some studies have failed to demonstrate any additional effect on albuminuria, whereas others have shown a small, further reduction in albuminuria.

Calcium-channel antagonists. In hypertensive diabetic patients, the intracellular calcium concentration is increased, which is thought to be related to decreased activity of Ca^{2+}-ATPase. An increase in intracellular calcium enhances the pressor responsiveness to vasoactive hormones such as angiotensin II and norepinephrine. This pathophysiological derangement provides the rationale for the use of Ca^{2+}-channel antagonists. These agents are quite effective in reducing blood pressure in hypertensive diabetic patients. The calcium-channel blockers have been shown to decrease proteinuria and improve renal function in diabetic patients with microalbuminuria or overt albuminuria. However, it is unclear whether this renal protective effect is above and beyond their blood pressure–lowering effect. Short-acting dihydropyridines, particularly nefedipine, have been shown to aggravate proteinuria in some studies and probably should be avoided. calcium-channel blockers do not adversely affect the plasma lipid profile or impair glucose tolerance, although several studies carried out in small numbers of diabetic patients suggest that nifedipine may aggravate the insulin resistance. Peripheral edema may occur during therapy.

After ACE inhibitors and ARBs, calcium-channel blockers are the drug of choice in the treatment of hypertensive diabetic patients with microalbuminuria (or overt albuminuria or renal insufficiency). Diltiazem, a benzothiapine, and verapamil, a phenylalkylamine, are preferred. Dihydropyridine calcium-channel blockers, such as nifedipine, should be avoided. Specific dosages of currently available calcium-channel blockers are listed in Table 40.4.

Diuretics. Diabetic patients with hypertension have an increase in total-body sodium content, which is aggravated when proteinuria and renal insufficiency develop. Increased intracellular sodium content enhances the vascular responsiveness to angiotensin II and norepinephrine. Based on the central role of sodium retention in diabetic hypertension, diuretic therapy is a rational therapeutic option. However, thiazides, when used in high doses (≥ 25–50 mg/dl), can cause deterioration in glucose tolerance, worsening of preexisting insulin resistance, an increase in LDL cholesterol and triglyceride levels, and a decrease in HDL cholesterol.

The effect of thiazide diuretics on the progression of early or advanced diabetic nephropathy has not been studied. Furosemide in combination with β-adrenergic blockers has been shown to slow the rate of decline of GFR in type 1 diabetic patients. Thiazide diuretics have been shown to be effective in reducing the risk of stroke and coronary heart failure in subjects both with and without diabetes. In elderly individuals with isolated systolic hypertension, thiazides also have been shown to reduce cardiovascular morbidity.

In diabetic patients with evidence of sodium overload, diuretic therapy almost always becomes a necessary component of the therapeutic regimen. Blood glucose and lipid levels should be monitored closely after the start of diuretic therapy, because impaired glucose tolerance and dyslipidemia are common when doses of hydrochlorothiazide exceed 12.5–25 mg/day. Concomitant use of captopril has been shown to offset the deleterious effect of diuretics on glucose tolerance and serum lipids. Diuretics also have the undesirable side effect of hypokalemia, which can increase peripheral vascular resistance and cause arrhythmias. Periodic determination of serum electrolyte concentrations and appropriate KCl supplementation can effectively correct this side effect.

The choice of diuretic agents and their recommended dosage are shown in Table 40.4. When the serum creatinine concentration is >1.8–2.0 mg/dl (>159–177 μmol/l), thiazides become ineffective and the more powerful loop diuretics furosemide and ethacrynic acid are required to promote diuresis. Potassium-sparing diuretics (i.e., spironolactone, triamterene, and amiloride) should be used with caution in diabetic patients, who may have underlying hypoaldosteronism.

β-*Adrenergic blockers.* β-Blockers have been shown to effectively reduce blood pressure and slow the progression of diabetic nephropathy. In the UKPDS, antihypertensive treatment with an ACE inhibitor was compared with the β-blocker metoprolol. Both drugs were equally effective in reducing blood pressure, and there were no differences in the incidence of microalbuminuria or proteinuria between the two treatment groups. However, the prevalence of nephropathy in this population was low, and it is unlikely that there were sufficient events to show the superiority of either drug over its comparator. In two other randomized trials in diabetic patients with proteinuria, β-blockers and ACE inhibitors produced similar reductions in proteinuria.

β-Blockers predispose to hypoglycemia, impair recovery from hypoglycemia, exacerbate hypoglycemic unawareness (especially in patients with autonomic neuropathy), inhibit insulin secretion in type 2 diabetic patients, cause hyperkalemia by impairing extrarenal potassium uptake, exacerbate insulin resistance and hyperinsulinemia, worsen glucose tolerance, and induce adverse changes in the plasma lipid profile. Consequently, β-adrenergic antagonists are not advocated as first-line drugs for the treatment of diabetic hypertension. β-Blockers may be warranted in combination with other agents in patients with progressive renal insufficiency and severe hypertension that is unresponsive to multiple-drug therapy.

Hypertensive diabetic patients with angina also may be treated with β-blocking agents, but the plasma glucose and lipid profile should be monitored closely after institution of such therapy. β-Blockers should be used in the post–myocardial infarction period because they are the only class of drugs that has been shown to decrease mortality from sudden death.

When β-adrenergic antagonists must be used, β_1-blockers (rather than non-selective β_1, β_2-antagonists such as propranolol, nadolol, timolol, and pindolol) are recommended, because they have quantitatively less prominent metabolic side effects. The recommended doses of atenolol and metoprolol are shown in Table 40.4. Both of these agents lose their β-selectivity at higher doses.

Vasodilators. If an adequate response to combined therapy with ACE inhibitors, ARBs, calcium-channel blockers, and diuretics is not achieved, a peripheral vasodilator can be added (Table 40.4). In diabetic patients with renal failure and severe refractory hypertension, minoxidil is particularly effective. The major side effect of minoxidil is hair growth.

Adrenergic antagonists. Several central adrenergic antagonists (aldomet, clonidine, and guanabenz) and peripheral β_1-antagonists (prazosin, doxazosin, and terazosin) are available for the treatment of hypertension in diabetic patients (Table 40.4). α-Antagonists enhance insulin sensitivity, leading to improvement in glucose tolerance and lower plasma lipid levels. They also have been shown to reduce microalbuminuria and to have beneficial effects on glucose tolerance, dyslipidemia, and microalbuminuria. There are no long-term studies examining the effect of the α-adrenergic antagonists on the prevention of diabetic nephropathy. It is surprising that the long-term benefit of this class of drugs has not been more closely examined in diabetic patients with albuminuria and/or diminished GFR. Of concern is the recent publication that the doxazosin arm of the ALLHAT (Antihypertensive and Lipid-Lowering Treatment to Prevent Heart Attack Trial) was stopped early because of an increased incidence of cardiovascular events (specifically congestive heart failure) in the α-adrenergic group.

TREATMENT OF MICROALBUMINURIA WITHOUT HYPERTENSION

Tight glycemic control and modest protein restriction should be instituted as described above (Table 40.3). Which antihypertensive agent to use and how the dose should be adjusted needs amplification, because, at the time that microalbuminuria is initially diagnosed, the majority of diabetic patients are not hypertensive.

In diabetic patients with microalbuminuria and normal blood pressure, the natural history of progression to overt albuminuria and eventual development of impaired renal function is no different than that in hypertensive microalbuminuric patients, with the obvious exception that hypertension hastens the onset of clinical albuminuria. Therefore, aggressive treatment with a drug that has a specific renal protective effect is indicated.

Only two classes of antihypertensive drugs, ACE inhibitors and ARBs, have been shown to specifically reverse hemodynamic alterations (i.e., efferent arteriolar vasoconstriction and increased intraglomerular pressure) that characterize diabetic nephropathy. Because most of the data have been accumulated with ACE inhibitors; because this class of drugs improves insulin sensitivity, glucose tolerance, and dyslipidemia; and because generic ACE inhibitors are more cost-effective,

ACE inhibitors are the drugs of choice for the treatment of microalbuminuria. If cough presents a problem, an ARB can be used. If hyperkalemia or deterioration in renal function develops, a non-dihydropyridine Ca^+-blocker can be substituted. From the standpoint of efficacy, ARBs have been shown to be as effective as ACE inhibitors in treating microalbuminuria, although there are many fewer studies with the ARBs. ARBs are considerably more expensive than ACE inhibitors, especially generic ACE inhibitors.

Captopril and enalapril have been most extensively studied in the treatment of microalbuminuria. Their use is described to illustrate the general approach. Once microalbuminuria has been documented, the patient should be started on a low dose of captopril (12.5 mg three times per day) or enalapril (5 mg/day). The patient should return in 4–8 weeks for a repeat determination of microalbuminuria. If no microalbuminuria is present at the follow-up visit, the dose of ACE inhibitor should be held constant. The patient should return in 6 months and yearly thereafter if no microalbuminuria is detected on follow-up visits. In microalbuminuric diabetic patients in whom the ACE inhibitor normalizes or significantly reduces the microalbumin excretion rate, the drug cannot be discontinued, since this will result in a return of the microalbuminuria to pretreatment levels.

If microalbuminuria is present in an unchanged or decreased amount 4–8 weeks after starting the ACE inhibitor, the dose of captopril (25 mg three times per day) or enalapril (10 mg/day) should be doubled, and a repeat determination of microalbuminuria should be performed in 4–8 weeks. This procedure should be repeated every 4–8 weeks. The dose of captopril or enalapril should be increased by 12.5 mg three times per day or 5 mg/day every 4–8 weeks until the microalbuminuria disappears completely, decreases but remains stable in three consecutive urine determinations, or side effects of the medication are encountered. If microalbuminuria decreases but does not disappear despite maximum-dose ACE inhibitor therapy, the following options should be considered: *1*) add a calcium-channel blocker (non-dihydropyridine) to the ACE inhibitor, or *2*) add an ARB to the ACE inhibitor. Neither of these combined therapies has been proven efficacious in preventing diabetic nephropathy in long-term clinical trials.

TREATMENT OF DIABETES WITH OVERT ALBUMINURIA AND/OR RENAL INSUFFICIENCY

Glycemic Control

In diabetic patients with clinical albuminuria and especially in patients with established renal insufficiency (serum creatinine >1.8 mg/dl [>159 μmol/l]), tight glycemic control has not been shown to slow the progression of renal disease. Moreover, patients with renal insufficiency are difficult to control, and hypoglycemia occurs more frequently because of decreased insulin clearance, impaired glucose counterregulation, and hypoglycemic unawareness related to autonomic neuropathy. Diabetic patients with macroalbuminuria and especially patients with an elevated serum creatinine concentration often have underlying cardiovascular disease. Therefore, the physician should strive for moderate glycemic control with A1C levels in the 7.0–8.0% range. Although less stringent glycemic control is recommended for diabetic patients with established renal disease, such patients remain at high risk for developing diabetic retinopathy.

Caution should be interjected about diabetic patients with modestly increased levels of clinical albuminuria (300–500 mg/day), because it is not known precisely at what level of albuminuria tight glycemic control ceases to be effective in preventing and/or slowing the progression of diabetic nephropathy. Because some of these patients with low levels of clinical albuminuria (300–500 mg/day) may benefit from normalization/near-normalization of blood glucose levels, tight glycemic control (A1C <7.0%) should be pursued in this group as well. A reasonable goal in diabetic patients with a urinary albumin excretion rate >500 mg/day, with or without renal insufficiency, is to maintain the A1C in the 7.0–8.0% range and the fasting plasma glucose concentration at ≤140 mg/dl (≤7.7 mmol/l).

Antihypertensive Therapy

The general approach, therapeutic goals, and choice of antihypertensive agents are essentially the same as described earlier for diabetic patients without renal insufficiency and clinical albuminuria (Table 40.4). In many patients, blood pressure will be normalized, yet significant albuminuria will persist. In such individuals, ACE inhibitors or ARBs can be increased progressively until the albuminuria has disappeared (an unlikely occurrence) or has declined significantly but remains stable despite escalation of the dose of antihypertensive medication or until hypotension or other side effects limit further dose increases. However, it is essential that the blood pressure be reduced to optimal levels (120–130/80 mmHg). In most diabetic patients with overt diabetic nephropathy, this will require combination therapy with multiple antihypertensive agents.

Protein Restriction

The therapeutic approach and benefits of dietary protein restriction in slowing the decline in renal function in patients with overt albuminuria and renal insufficiency are similar to those described earlier. However, the large multicenter Modified Diet in Renal Disease Study demonstrated that a low-protein diet (0.58 g/kg) failed to slow the rate of decline in renal function over a 36-month follow-up period in patients with renal failure secondary to diabetes (3% of the total group) or to nondiabetic causes (97% of the total group). The failure of this study to demonstrate any benefit of a low-protein diet on preservation of renal function is in contrast to previously published studies with much fewer patients.

Any beneficial effect of the low-protein diet in the Modified Diet in Renal Disease Study probably was obscured by the concomitant use of antihypertensive medications, which were taken by ~80% of the participants. In particular, 44% of the study patients were on an ACE inhibitor, and this class of drugs has a specific renal protective effect in patients both with and without diabetes. Based on these results, it seems prudent to recommend only modest protein restriction (0.9–1.0 g/kg/day) in diabetic subjects who are taking an ACE inhibitor, while reserving more severe protein restriction (0.6 g/kg/day) for patients who are not receiving antihypertensive medications. It is our experience that severe protein restriction is poorly tolerated by most diabetic patients and that adherence to such a diet for more than 3–6 months is unusual.

Finally, all diabetic patients with hypertension and overt albuminuria and/or renal insufficiency (serum creatinine >1.6–1.8 mg/dl [>133–159 µmol/l]) should be referred to a nephrologist or a diabetes specialist who has expertise in treating diabetic nephropathy. If the patient's blood pressure fails to normalize with the above approach or if evidence of hypertensive organ-system damage (i.e., retinopathy, congestive heart failure, or nephropathy) is present, referral to a nephrologist/diabetes specialist is indicated. Accelerated or malignant hypertension is cause for immediate referral and hospitalization for parenteral antihypertensive treatment.

MONITORING RENAL FUNCTION

In type 1 diabetic patients without microalbuminuria and normal renal function at the time of initial diagnosis, a repeat determination for microalbuminuria and creatinine clearance should be performed yearly, starting after 5 years' duration of disease, because microalbuminuria and renal dysfunction are distinctly uncommon within the first 5 years of diabetes (Fig. 40.4 and Table 40.5).

In type 2 diabetic patients without microalbuminuria, repeat determinations of microalbuminuria and serum creatinine or creatinine clearance should be performed yearly from the time that the patient is first diagnosed, because most of these individuals will have had their disease for many years.

In diabetic patients with microalbuminuria, overt albuminuria, or renal insufficiency, serum creatinine, urea nitrogen, and electrolyte concentrations and 24-h urine creatinine and protein/albumin excretion rates should be obtained every 6 months, or more frequently based on the response to treatment.

URINARY TRACT INFECTION

Urinary tract infections occur more frequently in individuals with diabetes than in the general population. Glucosuria provides an excellent culture medium for bacterial growth, whereas hyperglycemia impairs the migration of white blood cells from the vasculature to tissue sites of infection and interferes with their phagocytic activity. Impaired bladder function or benign prostatic hypertrophy in males can lead to urinary stasis, and the residual urine volume fosters bacterial replication. All diabetic patients should have a urinalysis on each visit to the physician. If white blood cells or bacteria are noted, a urine culture should be performed, and appropriate antibiotic therapy should be instituted based on sensitivity testing. It is not uncommon to find unusual, drug-resistant organisms in diabetic patients, especially if there is a history of recurrent urinary tract infection and previous antibiotic therapy. Failure to treat bladder infection in a timely fashion can lead to ascending infection and pyelonephritis. Kidney infection in a diabetic patient is a serious medical problem that requires hospitalization with broad-spectrum intravenous antibiotic therapy.

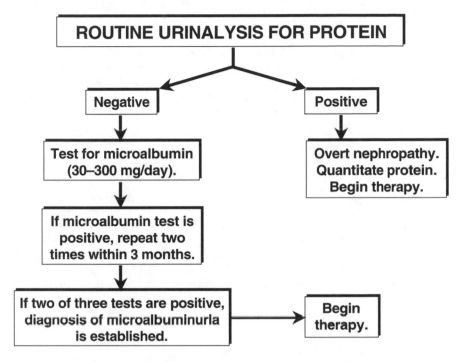

Figure 40.4 Screening for microalbuminuria. Adapted from the American Diabetes Association.

Table 40.5 Monitoring Renal Function in Postpubertal Diabetic Patients

Test	Initial Evaluation	Follow-Up*
Urine microalbumin determination	After initial glycemic control (within 3 mo of diagnosis)	Type 1 diabetes: yearly after 5 yr Type 2 diabetes: yearly from time of diagnosis
Creatinine clearance	At initial diagnosis	Every 1–2 yr until GFR <100 ml/min/1.73 m², then yearly or more frequently*
Serum creatinine	At initial diagnosis	Yearly or more frequently depending on rate of decline in renal function

*More frequent evaluation is indicated in diabetic patients with creatinine clearance <70–80 ml/min or serum creatinine >1.6–1.7 mg/dl (>133–146 μmol/l).

NEUROGENIC BLADDER

Neurogenic involvement of the bladder can cause urinary tract obstruction and a rapid, irreversible decline in renal function if it is not recognized and treated. The suspicion of neurogenic bladder should be heightened in patients with peripheral neuropathy and especially in patients with other manifestations of autonomic dysfunction. Clinical symptoms include

- a weak urinary stream
- frequent voiding of small amounts of urine
- loss of sensation of bladder fullness
- recurrent urinary tract infections

The diagnosis can be made by demonstration of a large postvoid residual (>150 ml) after bladder catheterization and confirmed by a cystometrogram, which reveals a large, atonic bladder with decreased force of contraction after distension with sterile water. Patients with neurogenic bladder should be instructed in the manual Crede voiding maneuver and should empty their bladder every 8 h. If this conservative measure proves ineffective, urecholine (10–15 mg orally three times per day) or phenoxzbenyamine (10–40 mg orally three times per day) can be tried.

PAPILLARY NECROSIS

Impaired blood flow to the medullary tissues can lead to anoxic damage and eventually necrosis of the papilla. If the papilla sloughs, it can obstruct the renal pelvis, and the patient will present with flank pain and a clinical picture that mimics a renal calculus. Hematuria will be present. The diagnosis can be established with a renal ultrasound or an intravenous pyelogram, if necessary. If the patient is afebrile and does not appear toxic, symptomatic treatment with analgesics and hydration is usually sufficient for the papilla to be passed. If, however, the obstruction persists, especially if there is accompanying infection, antibiotic therapy and surgical intervention may be necessary.

HYPERKALEMIA

Hyperkalemia is common in diabetic patients with long-standing nephropathy and can result from disturbances in both extrarenal and renal potassium metabolism. Insulin, aldosterone, and epinephrine all enhance potassium uptake by extrarenal tissues. These hormones are often deficient in diabetic patients. In addition, the hypertonicity that occurs secondary to hyperglycemia causes a shift in potassium from an intracellular to an extracellular environment. Hyperglycemia usually is accompanied by insulin deficiency (absolute or relative), thus exacerbating the osomotically driven shift of potassium out of cells. Concomitant metabolic acidosis, secondary to either aldosterone deficiency or chronic renal failure, will exacerbate the hyperkalemia as H^+ moves into cells to be buffered in exchange for potassium. Diabetic patients with nephropathy often have the syndrome of hypoaldosteronism, which impairs renal potassium excretion. The deficiency in aldosterone is magnified when concomitant renal failure is present and tubular mass is reduced sufficiently to impair potassium secretion. Metabolic acidosis also exerts a direct effect to impair renal tubular potassium secretion.

Treatment of hyperkalemia involves redistribution of potassium into cells and augmentation of urinary potassium excretion. The insulin regimen should be optimized to restore normoglycemia. This redistributes potassium back into cells and may improve the defect in aldosterone secretion in some patients. Metabolic acidosis should be corrected with sodium bicarbonate (1.8–4.8 g/day [or 24–64 meq/day]). The maintenance dose should be adjusted empirically, based on the change in plasma bicarbonate concentration. Correction of acidosis will redistribute potassium into cells and relieve the inhibition of renal potassium secretion. In patients with hypoaldosteronism, renal tubular potassium secretion becomes dependent on sodium and fluid delivery to the distal nephron segments. Therefore, an adequate intake of salt and water is essential to maintain renal perfusion and GFR. Dietary potassium intake should be reduced to <60 meq/day. In most patients, these conservative measures will be sufficient to restore normokalemia. If significant hyperkalemia (≥6.0 meq/l) persists, especially if there are electrocardiographic or neuromuscular signs of hyperkalemia, institution of 0.1–0.2 mg/day Florinef should be considered. In many patients with hyperkalemia secondary to hypoaldosteronism, the renal tubular cell is refractory to Florinef, and higher doses may be required. However, sodium retention and congestive heart failure may occur with these higher doses, and the risks may outweigh the benefit of therapy. In such cases, Florinef should be discontinued and more severe dietary potassium restriction instituted. In some patients, it may be necessary to continue the Florinef and start diuretic therapy to prevent sodium retention. Drugs that predispose to the development of hypoaldosteronism (nonsteroidal anti-inflammatory agents, ACE inhibitors, ARBs, β-adrenergic blockers, or heparin) or that inhibit renal tubular potassium secretion (spironolactone, triamterene, or amiloride) should be avoided in the hyperkalemic diabetes patient.

BIBLIOGRAPHY

Agarwal R: Add-on angiotensin receptor blockage with maximized ACE inhibition. *Kidney Int* 59:2282–2289, 2001

American Diabetes Association: Nephropathy in diabetes (Position Statement). *Diabetes Care* 27 (Suppl. 1):S79–S83, 2004

Arauz-Pacheco C, Parrott MA, Raskin P: The treatment of hypertension in adult patients with diabetes. *Diabetes Care* 25:134–147, 2002

Bakris GL, Williams M, Dworkin L, Elliott WJ, Epstein M, Toto R, Tuttle K, Douglas J, Hsueh W, Sowers J, for the National Kidney Foundation Hypertension and Diabetes Executive Committee Working Group: Preserving renal function in adults with hypertension and diabetes: a consensus approach. *Am J Kidney Dis* 36:646–661, 2000

Bennett PH, Haffner S, Kasiske BL, Keane WF, Mogensen CE, Parving HH, Steffes MW, Striker GE: Screening and management of microalbuminuria in patients with diabetes mellitus: recommendations to the Scientific Advisory Board of the National Kidney Foundation from an ad hoc committee of the Council on Diabetes Mellitus of the National Kidney Foundation. *Am J Kidney Dis* 25:107–112, 1995

Brenner BM, Cooper ME, De Zeeuw D, Keane WF, Mitch WE, Parving H-H, Remuzzi G, Snapinn SM, Zhang Z, Shahinfar S, for the RENAAL Study Investigators: Effects of losartan on renal and cardiovascular outcomes in patients with type 2 diabetes and nephropathy. *N Engl J Med* 345:861–869, 2001

Bressler R, DeFronzo RA: Drugs and diabetes. *Diabetes Reviews* 2:53–84, 1994

Chaturvedi N, Bandinelli S, Mangili R, Penno G, Rottiers RE, Fuller JH: Microalbuminura in type 1 diabetes: rates, risk factors and glycemic threshold. *Kidney Int* 60:219–227, 2001

Christensen PK, Larsen S, Horn T, Olsen S, Parving H-H: Causes of albuminuria in patients with type 2 diabetes without diabetic nepropathy. *Kid Int* 58:1719–1731, 2000

Cooper ME: Interaction of metabolic and haemodynamic factors in mediating experimental diabetic nephropathy. *Diabetologia* 44:1957–1972, 2001

DeFronzo RA: Diabetes and the kidney. In *Diabetes Mellitus: Management and Complications.* Olefsky JM, Sherwin RS, Eds. New York, Churchill Livingstone, 1985, p. 169

Diabetes Control and Complications Trial Research Group: The effect of intensive treatment of diabetes on the development and progression of long-term complications in insulin-dependent diabetes mellitus *N Engl J Med* 329:977–986, 1993

Feldt-Rasmussen B, Borch-Johnsen K, Decker T, Jensen G, Jensen JS: Microalbuminuria: an important diagnostic tool. *J Diabetes Complications* 8:137–145, 1994

Festa A, D'Agostino R Jr, Howard G, Mykkanen L, Tracy RP, Haffner SM: Inflammation and microalbuminuria in nondiabetic and type 2 diabetic subjects: The Insulin Resistance Atherosclerosis Study. *Kidney Int* 58:1703–1710, 2000

Fried LF, Orchard TJ, Kasiske BL, for the Lipids and Renal Disease Progression Meta-Analysis Study Group: Effect of lipid reduction on the progression of renal disease: a meta-analysis. *Kidney Int* 59:260–269, 2001

Flyvberg A: Putative pathophysiological role of growth factors and cytokines in experimental diabetic kidney disease. *Diabetologia* 43:1205–1223, 2000

Gaede P, Vedel P, Larsen N, Jensen GVH, Parving H-H, Pedersen O: Multifactorial intervention and cardiovascular disease in patients with type 2 diabetes. *N Engl J Med* 348:1925–1927, 2003

Heart Outcomes Prevention Evaluation (HOPE) Study Investigators: Effects of ramipril on microvascular outcomes in people with diabetes mellitus: results of the HOPE study and MICRO-HOPE substudy. *Lancet* 355:253–259, 2000

Hovind P, Rossing P, Tarnow L, Smidt UM, Parving H-H: Progression of diabetic nephropathy. *Kidney Int* 59:702–709, 2001

Hovind P, Rossing P, Tarnow L, Smidt UM, Parving H-H: Remission and regression in the nephropathy of type 2 diabetes when blood pressure is controlled aggressively. *Kidney Int* 60:277–283, 2001

Klahr S, Levey AS, Beck GJ, Caggiula AW, Hunsicker L, Kusek JW, Striker G: The effects of dietary protein restriction and blood pressure control on the progression of chronic renal disease. *N Engl J Med* 330:877–884, 1994

Klein R: Hyperglycemia and microvascular and macrovascular disease in diabetes. *Diabetes Care* 18:258–268, 1995

Kshirsager AV, Joy MS, Hogan SL, Falk FJ, Colindres RE: Effect of ACE inhibitors in diabetic and nondiabetic chronic renal disease: a systemic overview of randomized placebo-controlled trials. *Am J Kidney Dis* 35:695–707, 2000

Lacourchere Y, Belanger A, Godin C, Halle J-P, Ross S, Wright N, Marion J: Long-term comparison of losartan and enalapril on kidney function in hypertensive type 2 diabetics with early nephropathy. *Kidney Int* 58:762–769, 2000

Laffel LMB, McGill JB, Gans DJ, the North American Microalbuminuria Study Group: The beneficial effect of angiotensin-converting enzyme inhibition with captopril on diabetic nephropathy in normotensive IDDM patients with microalbuminuria. *Am J Med* 99:497–504, 1995

Lewis EJ, Hunsicker LG, Bain RP, Rohde R, Raz I: The effect of the angiotensin converting enzyme inhibition on diabetic nephropathy. *N Engl J Med* 329:1456–1462, 1993

Lewis EJ, Hunsicker LG, Clarke WR, Berl T, Pohl MA, Lewis JB, Ritz E, Atkins RC, Rohde R, Raz I, for the Collaborative Study Group: Renoprotective effect of the angiotensin receptor antagonist irebesartan in patients with nephropathy due to type 2 diabetes. *N Engl J Med* 345:851–860, 2001

Microalbuminuria Captopril Study Group: Captopril reduces the risk of nephropathy in IDDM patients with microalbuminuria. *Diabetologia* 39:587–593, 1996

Mogensen CE: How to protect the kidney in diabetic patients with special reference to IDDM. *Diabetes* 46 (Suppl. 2):S104–S111, 1997

Mogensen CE, Poulsen PL: Epidemiology of microalbuminuria in diabetes and in the background population. *Curr Opin Nephrol Hypertens* 3:248–256, 1994

Nelson RG, Bennett PH, Beck GJ, Tan M, Knowler WC, Mitch WE, Hirschman GH, Myers BD, the Diabetic Renal Disease Study Group: Development and progression of renal disease in Pima Indians with noninsulin-dependent diabetes mellitus. *N Engl J Med* 335:1636–1642, 1996

Ohkubo Y, Kishikawa H, Araki E, Miyata T, Isami S, Motoyoshi S, Kojima Y, Furuyoshi N, Shichir M: Intensive insulin therapy prevents the progression of diabetic microvascular complications in Japanese patients with noninsulin dependent diabetes mellitus: a randomized prospective 6 year study. *Diabetes Res Clin Pract* 28:103–117, 1995

Orchard TJ, Chang Y-F, Ferrell RE, Petro N, Ellis DE: Nephropathy in type 1 diabetes: a manifestation of insulin resistance and multiple genetic susceptibilities? Further evidence from the Pittsburgh Epidemiology of Diabetes Complication Study. *Kidney Int* 62:963–970, 2002

Parving H-H, Lehnert H, Brochner-Mortensen J, Gomis R, Andersen S, Arner P, for the Irebesartan in Patients with Type 2 Diabetes and Micro-albuminuria Study Group: The effect of irbesartan on the development of diabetic nephropathy in patients with type 2 diabetes. *N Engl J Med* 345:870–878, 2001

Ravid M, Brosh D, Levi Z, Bar-Dayan Y, Ravid D, Rachmani R: Use of enalapril to attenuate decline in renal function in normotensive, normoalbuminuric patients with type 2 diabetes mellitus. *Ann Intern Med* 128:982–988, 1998

Ravid N, Savin H, Jutrin I, Bental T, Katz B, Lishner M: Long-term stabilizing effect of angiotensin-converting enzyme inhibition on plasma creatinine and on proteinuria in normotensive type II diabetic patients. *Ann Intern Med* 118:577–581, 1993

Ritz E, Rychlik I, Locatelli F, Halimi S: End-stage renal failure in type 2 diabetes: a medical catastrophe of worldwide dimensions. *Am J Kidney Dis* 34:795–808, 1999

Rossing K, Jensen BR, Christensen PK, Parving H-H: Dual blockage of the renin-angiotensin system in diabetic nephropathy. *Diabetes Care* 25:95–100, 2002

Russo LM, Bakris GL, Comper WD: Renal handling of albumin: a critical review of basic concepts and perspective. *Am J Kidney Dis* 39:899–919, 2002

Taal MW, Brenner BM: Renoprotective benefits of RAS inhibition: from ACEI to angiotensin II antagonists. *Kidney Int* 57:1803–1817, 2000

Torffvit O, Agardh C-D: The impact of metabolic and blood pressure control on incidence and progression of nephropathy: a 10-year study of 385 type 2 diabetic patients. *J Diabetes Complications* 15:307–313, 2001

U.S. Renal Data System: *USRDS 2001 Annual Data Report: Atlas of End-Stage Renal Disease in the United States.* Bethesda, MD, National Institute of Diabetes and Digestive and Kidney Diseases, 2001

Wang PH, Lau J, Chalmers TC: Meta-analysis of effects of intensive blood-glucose control on late complications of type I diabetes. *Lancet* 341:1306–1309, 1993

Dr. DeFronzo is a Professor of Medicine and Chief of the Diabetes Division at the University of Texas Health Science Center, San Antonio, TX.

41. Chronic Kidney Disease

ELI A. FRIEDMAN, MD

End-stage renal disease (ESRD) resulting from diabetic nephropathy is manifested by ~30% of individuals with type 1 diabetes and afflicts an undefined but probably equivalent subset of people with type 2 diabetes. Currently, in the U.S., Japan, and industrialized Europe, diabetes mellitus is the leading cause of ESRD, surpassing glomerulonephritis and hypertension. As listed by the U.S. Renal Data System in 2003, of 406,081 U.S. patients receiving either dialytic therapy or a kidney transplant on December 31, 2001, 142,963 had diabetes (a prevalence rate of 35.2%). Furthermore, during 2001, of 96,295 new (incident) cases of ESRD, 42,813 (44.5%) were listed as having diabetes. An additional 10% of incident ESRD patients had diabetes, although that was not the disease listed as having caused their renal failure, and a further 6% had the diagnosis of diabetes established during their first year of treatment for ESRD, raising the total proportion of diabetes patients with ESRD to ~60% after 1 year. The actual reported lower prevalence for diabetes patients with ESRD is explained by their sharply higher death rate during ESRD therapy.

After years of hyperglycemia (usually accompanied by hypertension) and hyperlipidemia, diabetic nephropathy may reduce renal function to the extent that life is no longer possible without replacement therapy (i.e., hemodialysis, peritoneal dialysis, or kidney transplantation). Kidney malfunction in diabetes typically follows a well-demarcated sequence of microalbuminuria preceding proteinuria that in turn is followed by azotemia over several years to a decade or longer. Chronic renal failure (CRF), however, may develop suddenly because of a vascular catastrophe (atheroembolic disease), sustained hypotension complicating coronary artery surgery or another major surgery, or treatment with a nephrotoxic drug or antibiotic.

Microalbuminuria, a 24-h urinary albumin excretion rate of 20–200 μg/min (30–300 mg/24 h), is a laboratory finding predictive of subsequent nephropathy. The upper limit corresponds approximately to a total urinary protein concentration of 0.5 g/l, the hallmark of clinical nephropathy. Increased mortality is observed in both type 1 and type 2 diabetes patients who have microalbuminuria. The usual course of diabetic nephropathy, however, entails months to years of a nephrotic syndrome (proteinuria >3.5 g/day, hypoalbuminuria, hyperlipidemia, and anasarca) followed by azotemia, which signals the onset of CRF. ESRD is the typical termination of CRF. Severe CRF induces myriad extrarenal diverse symptoms, physical signs, and abnormal laboratory values that, in the aggregate, constitute the uremic syndrome. Appropriate therapy for the microalbuminuric and/or proteinuric individual with diabetes will retard progression of nephropathy, sometimes delaying ESRD for years.

Untreated uremia results in orange-yellow skin discoloration, easy bruisability, wasting of muscle and fat, and a blunted, dull affect stressed by a reversed diurnal sleep pattern. Anemia, acidosis, and azotemia are the cardinal laboratory findings in CRF. Agonal ESRD may present with fibrinous pericarditis and pericardial tamponade, bowel ulceration (colitis, gastritis), and neurological syndromes (grand mal seizures, transient cortical blindness, motor nerve paralysis). When treated by hemodialysis, peritoneal dialysis, or kidney transplantation, life extension for several years to as long as more than 2 decades is attainable for many individuals with diabetes who develop ESRD.

THERAPY

Every person with diabetes and a kidney syndrome should understand the overall strategy for care, termed "a life plan." Management approaches to diabetic nephropathy have three main objectives:

1. Detect and eliminate potentially reversible factors that can decrease renal functional reserve.
2. Preserve the glomerular filtration rate (GFR) by modulating blood pressure, metabolic control, and dietary protein intake. The choice of antihypertensive medications should include (unless precluded by drug toxicity such as hyperkalemia and/or an incapacitating dry cough) either an angiotensin-converting enzyme (ACE) inhibitor or a receptor blocker because of their renoprotective effects.
3. Prepare the patient and his or her family for kidney replacement therapy while preserving work, school, or home activities when uremia supervenes. These decisions include:
   - scheduling treatment of comorbid extrarenal conditions, especially diabetic retinopathy, heart disease, and peripheral arterial disease
   - feasibility of an intrafamilial kidney transplant
   - selection of dialysis technique (peritoneal or hemodialysis) when a renal transplant is unlikely
   - election of locale (home or facility) if hemodialysis is chosen
   - identifying markers indicating that ESRD therapy must be initiated

When constructing an individual's life plan, every opportunity should be taken to fortify the patient for coming arduous components of kidney replacement therapy. An intensive patient educational program under the auspices of a nurse educator should include consideration of normal and abnormal renal function and descriptions of dialysis and kidney transplantation. Provision of literature from the American Association of Kidney Patients and introductions to patients currently undergoing ESRD therapy is often helpful in minimizing stress. Key components of therapy are given in Table 41.1.

Table 41.1 Therapy for Azotemic Diabetes Patients

1. Discontinue nephrotoxic drugs, limit exposure to radiocontrast agents.
2. Detect and treat urinary infection.
3. Correct electrolyte imbalance.
4. Establish a daily log to record weight, blood pressure, and blood glucose excursions.
5. Decrease excess extracellular volume (anasarca) by combining metolazone (10–40 mg) with 40–240 mg furosemide in a twice-daily regimen until a stable "dry weight" is obtained. Record and monitor daily weight as well as self-measured daily blood glucose values. Report unusual weight increases (fluid retention) or decreases (excess diuretic effect) to physician.
6. Expand plasma volume if contracted.
7. Control hypertension, striving for continuous blood pressure levels <125/75 mmHg. Include ACE inhibitor or receptor blocker, as tolerated.
8. With the assistance of a nutritionist, construct acceptable diet, restricting dietary protein to ≤40–60 g/day.
9. Correct hyperlipidemia by diet or pharmacological means using a standard hypolipidemic regimen plus a statin drug.
10. Control hyperphosphatemia by diet and calcium-based phosphate binders (calcium carbonate).
11. Reduce hyperuricemia if >12 mg/dl or at lower values if symptomatic gout occurs.
12. Add 1.2–4.8 g/day oral bicarbonate for severe acidosis, especially for renal tubular acidosis.
13. Administer synthetic vitamin D, with careful attention to avoid overshooting to hypercalcemia.
14. For symptomatic anemia, when hematocrit is <30%, after excluding blood loss and other extrarenal causes, administer recombinant erythropoietin 50–150 units/kg s.c. three times per week, maintaining iron stores as needed. Consider darbepoetin alfa given once weekly subcutaneously in equivalent or reduced dosage.
15. Avoid volume depletion, radiocontrast media, nephrotoxic drugs, and bladder catheterization.

Preserving Renal Functional Reserve

Caution when using nephrotoxic drugs will avoid superimposed iatrogenic injury. Drugs that should not be administered to patients with azotemia include nitrofurantoin, spironolactone, amiloride, triamterene, metformin, and phenformin. Abruptly deteriorating renal function may be the consequence of interstitial nephritis (not directly induced by diabetes) caused by captopril, cimetidine, methicillin sodium, allopurinol, phenylhydantoin, nonsteroidal anti-inflammatory drugs, or furosemide. The ACE inhibitors benazepril, captopril, cilazapril, enalapril, enalaprilat, fosinopril, lisinopril, moexipril, perindopril, quinapril, ramipril, and trandolapril may reversibly worsen azotemia and precipitate hyperkalemia and incapacitating nonproductive cough in up to 20% of individuals with diabetes. Rapidly expanding application of angiotensin receptor blockers including losartan, valsartan, irbesartan, and candesartan to regulate hypertensive blood pressure, reduce proteinuria, and slow the course of nephropathy may also trigger renal functional deterioration and, less often, nonproductive cough. Dosage reductions according to residual GFR of cyclophosphamide, cimetidine, clofibrate, digoxin, and many antibiotics (particularly aminoglycosides) are required for azotemic patients.

Because of the risk of urinary infection, bladder catheterization in an azotemic diabetes patient should be restricted to the few instances when the information to be gained is unobtainable by other means. Easing the measurement of daily urinary output is insufficient justification for an indwelling bladder catheter.

There is serious risk of worsening renal insufficiency when radiographic contrast medium is administered to diabetes patients with serum creatinine levels >2.5 mg/dl (>227.3 μmol/l). Under circumstances where radiographic contrast medium must be given, e.g., before a limb arterial bypass, prior hydration with half-normal saline and mannitol infusion (25 g in 2 liters 0.45% saline solution) may protect against renal injury. Early trials in small numbers of diabetes patients suggest that pretreatment with N-acetylcysteine (600 mg orally twice daily) coupled with hydration with saline solution will preempt contrast medium injury (see Chapter 39).

Minimizing the Rate of GFR Loss

The rate of renal functional decline in diabetic nephropathy is slowed by normalization of hypertension and dietary protein restriction (see Chapter 40). In microalbuminuric individuals who are not hypertensive, treatment with an ACE inhibitor has been shown to reduce the rate of increase in albumin excretion. Thus, regardless of blood pressure level, every individual with type 1 or type 2 diabetes should be treated with an ACE inhibitor when microalbuminuria is discovered. For individuals who cannot tolerate ACE inhibitors because of drug allergy, nonproductive cough, or a rise in serum potassium or creatinine concentration, a trial with an angiotensin receptor blocker will achieve the same objective of retarding the course of nephropathy.

Preservation of bone integrity is the objective of treatment with intestinal phosphate binders. Hypertension due to diabetic nephropathy is often associated with intravascular volume expansion and anasarca resulting from hypoalbuminemia consequent to nephrotic-range proteinuria. Reduction of the intravascular and extracellular excess fluid is a vital component of blood pressure control. Diuresis can usually be effected by graded doses of furosemide (40–120 mg twice per day). Metolazone (5–40 mg once or twice per day) induces diuresis even when the creatinine clearance has fallen to <10 ml/min. Close observation of the patient, with recording of daily weight, is mandatory when prescribing a potent diuretic regimen. Once edema is reduced, doses of metolazone and furosemide should be decreased while monitoring daily weight to avoid dehydration and vascular collapse. As GFR declines to <15 ml/min, patient compensation straddles a narrow range between dehydration and extracellular volume overload—the difference in weight between the two extremes may be as little as 3–6 kg, underscoring the necessity for recording daily weight. GFR stabilization by intensified antihypertensive treatment is possible in patients with overt diabetic nephropathy, even if renal function is markedly impaired. For hypertension resistant to diuretics, ACE inhibitors, and calcium-channel blockers, a trial-and-error regimen of vasodilators and β-blockers may be attempted.

When successive trials of ACE inhibitors, angiotensin receptor blockers, calcium-channel blockers, vasodilators, α-blockers, as well as β-blockers fail to attain satisfactory blood pressure regulation, minoxidil in doses of 2.5–70 mg/day almost always reduces blood pressure to <140/90 mmHg. Careful observation of minoxidil-treated patients for tachycardia and fluid retention is required and managed by the addition of diuretics and β-blockers. Single daily doses of long-acting antihypertensive drugs such as nifedipine (a calcium-channel blocker) and lisinopril (an ACE inhibitor) facilitate patient compliance over that attained with multidose regimens.

Dietary protein restriction may retard renal injury that ends as glomerulosclerosis. Trials in small groups of patients with progressive renal disorders, including diabetic nephropathy, show that a diet containing 40–60 g/day protein (with or without addition of essential amino acids or their precursor α-keto derivatives) slows renal functional loss. Appreciating that the benefit of protein restriction on the progress of diabetic nephropathy is unproven, the prudent physician may nevertheless opt to prescribe a diet containing <80 g/day dietary protein while suggesting modest protein restriction (40–60 g/day).

Maintenance of the Metabolic Environment

Perturbed lipid metabolism is characteristic of diabetes patients with nephropathy, especially when accompanied by a nephrotic syndrome. Hypertriglyceridemia and low levels of HDL are typical of azotemic patients with diabetic nephropathy; the risk of coronary artery disease expressed as the ratio of total cholesterol to HDL cholesterol is elevated. Partial correction of these lipid abnormalities may be affected by weight reduction in obese individuals with a low-fat diet, nicotinic acid, atorvastin, benzafibrate, fluvastin, gemfibrozil, lovastatin, pravastatin, probucol, or simvastatin.

As the GFR falls below 20 ml/min, hyperphosphatemia may cause reciprocal hypocalcemia and hyperparathyroidism. Hyperphosphatemia can be controlled by limiting phosphate intake to 500–800 mg/day; dairy products are high in phosphate content. Premeal ingestion of intestinal phosphate-binding drugs, e.g., aluminum hydroxide and aluminum carbonate or magnesium hydroxide (1–2 g three times per day), and calcium supplementation (calcium carbonate 1–3 g three times per day) will lower the serum phosphate concentration to 5 mmol/l. Unfortunately, when reducing the serum phosphate concentration to normal, treatment with phosphate binders may be complicated by hypermagnesemia, hypercalcemia, aluminum-induced vitamin D–resistant bone disease, and neurological disorders. Aluminum toxicity is also associated with a syndrome of dementia and anemia. For these reasons, a calcium-based phosphate binder is the first choice, and aluminum gels are no longer used.

Hypocalcemia in the absence of marked hyperphosphatemia is effectively treated by daily administration of 1,25-dihydroxyvitamin D_3. Treatment with this vitamin early in the course of progressive renal insufficiency prevents renal bone disease and reverses secondary hyperparathyroidism.

In advanced diabetic nephropathy, attention to the amount of dietary sodium and potassium is important as the GFR falls below 15 ml/min. A small subset of diabetes patients—those with concurrent interstitial renal disease—may lose large quantities of urinary sodium, similar to salt-wasting individuals with Addison's disease. In contrast, most azotemic individuals with diabetes predominantly have glomerular disease, which causes retention of salt and water. Defining a correct dietary salt prescription for the individual patient requires a process of trial and error termed "salt balancing." Daily weights are the keystone to the regimen, which begins with a diet made up of 40 g protein and 2 g salt. The salt waster's weight will decrease, necessitating supplementation with sodium bicarbonate tablets (600 mg) given up to four times per day. With continued weight loss, the amount of sodium bicarbonate is increased by increments of 1.2 g day until a stable weight results. At the other extreme, the nephrotic salt retainer may evince pulmonary congestion and peripheral edema with the initial 2 g salt prescription, in which case, furosemide (40–80 mg three times per day) is added.

Dietary potassium restriction is rarely required before the daily urine output falls below 1 liter or the patient is under treatment with drugs that impair K^+ excretion (e.g., an ACE inhibitor). Hyperkalemia <6 meq/l can usually be managed by reducing dietary intake of K^+, especially in citrus juices. More severe K^+ retention requires administration of a cation-exchange resin (e.g., sodium polystyrene sulfonate). A trial discontinuance of ACE inhibitors and other K^+-retaining drugs is a key step in managing hyperkalemia.

Anemia in diabetes patients with reduced renal function is mainly the consequence of diminished renal secretion of erythropoietin. In patients with ESRD who are sustained by hemodialysis or peritoneal dialysis, correction of typical anemia (20–25% to 32–38%) is effected by thrice-weekly subcutaneous injections of recombinant erythropoietin (2,000–8,000 units). Indications for erythropoietin administration in predialysis patients include advanced anemia (hematocrit <31%), coronary artery disease, and inordinate fatigue. Raising erythrocyte mass in the azotemic individual with diabetes is an important component of sustaining daily activities before developing ESRD. Broad use of erythropoietin indicates that correction of anemia in predialysis patients achieves substantive benefit in terms of life quality, ability to continue employment, and subjective assessment of severity of illness. Introduction of darbepoetin alfa, a genetically engineered form of human erythropoietin that can be injected subcutaneously as infrequently as once every 2 weeks, has simplified the regimen, although high cost continues to be an impediment to universal acceptance of the need for raising hematocrit levels to normal. Comprehensive management of declining renal function involves:

- normalization of hypertensive blood pressure
- correction of hyperlipidemia
- reduction of hyperphosphatemia with phosphate binders
- administration of synthetic 1,25-dihydroxyvitamin D_3
- raising hematocrit with recombinant erythropoietin

During progressive loss of GFR, periodic (monthly to weekly as GFR falls) measurements of weight, glycated hemoglobin, hematocrit, blood urea nitrogen, serum creatinine, serum lipids, serum potassium, and serum calcium should be performed at each visit. Insulin and other small peptide hormones are partially degraded by the kidney. On reduction of GFR to ~25 ml/min, insulin catabolism within the kidney lessens to the extent that progressively intensive hypoglycemic episodes may interfere with metabolic control in a previously stable individual. When the serum creatinine level increases to >5 mg/dl (>442 µmol/l), the need for kidney replacement therapy is urgent.

HEMODIALYSIS

Maintenance hemodialysis is the kidney replacement regimen used for >80% of people with diabetes who develop ESRD in the U.S. Performance of maintenance hemodialysis requires vascular access to the circulation. Creation of the standard access—an internal arteriovenous fistula in the wrist—is usually more difficult in a patient with diabetes than in a nondiabetic person because of systemic atherosclerosis. For many diabetes patients with peripheral vascular calcification and/or atherosclerosis, establishment of an access for hemodialysis necessitates use of synthetic (Dacron) prosthetic vascular grafts. In both sexes and in all age-groups, survival of individuals with diabetes treated with maintenance hemodialysis is distinctly inferior to that of nondiabetic patients. Presently, the added value of daily hemodialysis is under evaluation as a means of enhancing quality of life, reducing the need for erythropoietin and antihypertensive drugs, and improving nutritional status, as judged by a rising serum albumin concentration. The main concerns in delivering maintenance hemodialysis for diabetes patients are listed in Table 41.2.

PERITONEAL DIALYSIS

Peritoneal dialysis has been used effectively to sustain life in 8–15% of individuals with diabetes who develop ESRD. Continuous ambulatory peritoneal dialysis

Table 41.2 Concerns in Conducting Maintenance Hemodialysis

- Choice and surgical creation of vascular access
  1. Internal arteriovenous fistula
  2. Bovine carotid arteriovenous heterograft
  3. Teflon arteriovenous graft
- Metabolic regulation
  1. Frequent fingerstick glucose measurements (insulin-treated diabetes)
  2. Fractional insulin doses or insulin pump (type 1 diabetes)
  3. Reeducate about diet and exercise
- Normalize weight
- Propensity to hypotension
  1. Minimize intradialytic weight gain
  2. Bicarbonate dialysate
  3. Gradual ultrafiltration for fluid extraction during hemodialysis
- Preservation of vision
  1. Collaboration with ophthalmologist
  2. Lowest effective heparin dosage during hemodialysis
  3. Two or more pillows for head elevation during active retinopathy
- Preservation of lower extremities
  1. Wearing heel booties
  2. Collaboration with podiatrist
- Obstipation complicating use of phosphate binders
  1. Prescribe detergent with antacid gel for phosphate sorption
  2. Metoclopramide stimulates bowel motility and is taken before meals, non-glucose containing stool softeners such as psyllium seed husks (Metamucil) a soluble plant fiber that is often labeled a laxative, but is not. Fibers become gelatinous and sticky in water, are not absorbed in the small bowel and are broken down in the large bowel becoming a food source for bacteria in the colon.
- Depression
  1. Membership in patient self-help organizations
  2. Enlisting patient, patient's family, and social support givers in overall planning

(CAPD), a self-treatment, has grown rapidly in application because of its advantages (compared with home hemodialysis) of rapid training, reduced cardiovascular stress, and avoidance of heparin (Table 41.3); home hemodialysis requires 3–16 weeks of training. As a facilitating procedure for peritoneal dialysis, an intraperitoneal catheter is sewn in place several days before CAPD is begun. Motivated diabetes patients, including those who are blind, are able to learn to perform CAPD at home within 10–15 days. In practice, patients exchange 2–3 liters of commercially prepared sterile dialysate four to five times per day. Insulin, antibiotics, and other drugs are added by the patient to each dialysate exchange.

Simplification of peritoneal dialysate exchanges has been brought about by use of a mechanical cycler in the therapeutic variation called continuous cyclic peritoneal dialysis (CCPD). Both CAPD and CCPD subject the diabetes patient to the constant risk of peritonitis and a gradual decrease in peritoneal surface area. Peritonitis has an incidence rate of about once every 10 months of peritoneal dialysis.

KIDNEY TRANSPLANTATION

Kidney transplantation is the preferred therapeutic option for selected patients with ESRD due to diabetic nephropathy. Both patient survival and degree of rehabilitation in diabetic transplant recipients are sharply superior to results attained by dialytic therapy. With cyclosporine or tacrolimus as the main immunosuppressive drugs coupled with induction therapy including monoclonal antilymphocyte antibodies, kidney transplantation has improved progressively to the extent that patient survival at 1 and 2 years is equivalent in recipients with and without diabetes, whereas kidney graft survival is ~10% lower in individuals with

Table 41.3 Continuous Ambulatory Dialysis for Diabetes Patients

- Advantages
  1. Rapid establishment as home therapy
  2. Partner not essential, although required for home hemodialysis
  3. Few profound hypotensive episodes compared with hemodialysis
  4. Insulin regimen simplified by direct addition to dialysate
  5. Enthusiastic patient acceptance of freedom from machine
  6. Minimal stress to cardiovascular system; no extracorporeal circulation
- Disadvantages
  1. Intra-abdominal catheter related
  2. Pain, bleeding, dialysate leak
  3. Obstruction of intraperitoneal catheter
  4. Perforation of abdominal viscus during catheter insertion
- Mechanical
  1. Abdominal hernia
  2. Hydrothorax, ascites
- Peritoneal
  1. Peritonitis
  2. Peritoneal thickening (sclerosis) and loss of dialyzing surface
- Neuropsychiatric
  1. Depression over daily necessity for multiple exchanges
  2. Boredom with regimen and altered self-image
  3. Time required for multiple daily fluid exchanges

diabetes than in nondiabetic recipients at 2 years. Newer immunosuppressive drugs in clinical trials, including rapamycin, sirolimus, lefunomide, and mycophenolate mofetil, offer promise of still further reduced allograft rejection with less nephrotoxicity.

Kidney replacement therapy is more difficult to initiate and sustain, and the course is stressful in diabetes patients because of excessive morbidity and mortality imparted by extrarenal disease. Variables in selecting therapy are presented in Table 41.4. Preparation for a kidney transplant in a diabetes patient, for example, requires careful cardiac evaluation to detect and treat coronary artery disease, the major cause of death in the azotemic diabetes patient. A dobutamine or exercise stress test with thallium imaging will suffice, if normal, as a prelude to a kidney or kidney-pancreas transplantation. Cardiac catheterization and corrective coronary artery bypass grafting or intracoronary stent placement will preempt unanticipated death from heart disease during the posttransplant period.

Consultations with an ophthalmologist and a podiatrist familiar with abnormalities of the diabetic eye and foot, respectively, are also desirable during transplant evaluation. Assistance from other specialists, including a gastroenterologist and neurologist, is usually required before kidney replacement therapy. Unappreciated gastroparesis may interfere with regimens contingent on relating the timing of food ingestion to insulin injections. Once discovered, metoclopramide given in doses of 5–10 mg before meals usually corrects gastric hypomotility.

REFERRAL TO A RENAL SPECIALIST

First referral to a nephrologist is advisable when urinary protein excretion is constant at >500 mg/day. Initial renal evaluation will be directed toward quantifying renal reserve by measuring GFR and excluding causes of nephropathy other than diabetes. Resorting to percutaneous renal biopsy is indicated when the renal syndrome is atypical for diabetes: absence of retinopathy, associated gross hematuria, or pyuria. Subsequent nephrology consultations at yearly intervals will chart progress of renal functional loss, increase in proteinuria, and regulation of blood pressure. The use of synthetic vitamin D and erythropoietin to manage hyperphosphatemia (hypocalcemia) and anemia should be guided by a kidney specialist. Once azotemia is noted (serum creatinine concentration >1.5 mg/dl in men and >1.2 mg/dl in women), the frequency of contact with a nephrologist should increase to bimonthly, and later, monthly. When it is anticipated that dialytic therapy or a kidney transplantation will be needed within 6 months (serum creatinine ≥5 mg/d [442 μmol/l]), the main responsibility for management should shift to the collaborating nephrologist. Provision of comprehensive care in which collaborating specialists are orchestrated by a team-leading nephrologist is a central theme of successful management of advanced diabetic nephropathy.

BIBLIOGRAPHY

Abbott KC, Bakris GL: What have we learned from the current trials? *Med Clin North Am* 88:189–207, 2004

Table 41.4 Comparison of Options in Kidney Replacement Therapy in Diabetes

Variable	Peritoneal Dialysis	Hemodialysis	Kidney Transplant
Extensive extrarenal disease	No limitation	No limitation except where hypotension interdicts sufficient extracorporeal blood flow	Excluded in cardiovascular insufficiency, liver failure, active hepatitis, bone marrow depression, active malignancy
Geriatric patients (>65 yr)	No age restriction	No age restriction	Arbitrary exclusion of older patients; age cutoff (65–75 yr) determined by some programs
Complete rehabilitation	Rare, if ever, unless high residual GFR	Very few individuals unless high residual GFR	Common as long as allograft functions at GFR >40 ml/min, contingent on proactive approach to eye, heart, and vascular disease
Death rate	Much higher than for nondiabetic peritoneal dialysis patients	Much higher than for nondiabetic hemodialysis patients	About the same as nondiabetic transplant recipients for the first 2 yr, then increases
First-year patient survival	~75%	~75%	95–98%
Survival to second decade	Rare; only 4% alive after 10 yr	Unusual <5% living after 10 yr	About one in five recipients of a living related donor kidney survive 10 yr; a lower subset of cadaver donor kidney live 10 yr.
Progression of complications	Usual and unremitting; hyperglycemia and hyperlipidemia accentuated	Usual and unremitting	Interdicted by functioning pancreas + kidney. Macro- and microvasculopathy progress in recipients of renal allografts. Regression of neuropathy reported.
Special advantage	Can be self-performed; rapid training; avoids swings in solute and intravascular volume level	Can be self-performed; extraction of solute and water in hours	Cures uremia; freedom to travel; offers best survival and superior rehabilitation

(continued)

**Table 41.4 Comparison of Options in Kidney Replacement
Therapy in Diabetes (*Continued*)**

Variable	Peritoneal Dialysis	Hemodialysis	Kidney Transplant
Disadvantage	Peritonitis, hyper-insulinemia, hyperglycemia, hyperlipidemia; long hours of treatment; more days hospitalized than either hemodialysis or transplant patients	Blood access a hazard for clotting, hemorrhage, and infection; cyclical hypotension, weakness; aluminum toxicity, amyloidosis	Cosmetic disfigurement from corticosteroids and cyclosporine; hypertension; personal expense for cytotoxic drugs; induced malignancy; HIV transmission. Corticosteroids and tacrolimus aggravate glycemic control.
Patient acceptance	Variable, after initial enthusiasm, usual compliance with passive tolerance for regimen	Variable, often noncompliant with dietary, metabolic, or antihypertensive component of regimen	Buoyant during periods of good renal allograft function; joyful when pancreas transplant establishes euglycemia
Bias in comparison	Delivered as first choice by enthusiasts, but in U.S., substantially higher mortality than for hemodialysis; in Canada, peritoneal dialysis has lower mortality than hemodialysis	Treatment by default; often complicated by inattention to progressive cardiac and peripheral arterial disease	Kidney transplant programs preselect patients with fewest complications; exclusion of those >45 yr for pancreas + kidney simultaneous grafting obviously favorably biasing outcome
Relative cost	Approximately $58,100 annually for 1997–2001 according to U.S. Renal Data System	Approximately $60,000 annually for 1997–2001 according to U.S. Renal Data System	Pancreas + kidney engraftment most expensive uremia therapy for diabetes (more than $140,000); kidney transplant alone approximately $24,000 annually for 1997–2001 according to U.S. Renal Data System

Berman DH, Friedman EA, Lundin AP: Aggressive ophthalmological management in diabetic ESRD: a study of 31 consecutively referred patients. *Am J Nephrol* 12:344–350, 1992

Biesenback G, Janko O, Zazgornik J: Similar rate of progression in the predialysis phase in type I and type II diabetes mellitus. *Nephrol Dial Transplant* 9:1097–1102, 1994

Coyle D, Rodby RA: Economic evaluation of the use of irbesartan and amlodipine in the treatment of diabetic nephropathy in patients with hypertension in Canada. *Can J Cardiol* 20:71–79, 2004

Diaz-Sandoval LJ, Kosowsky BD, Losordo DW: Acetylcysteine to prevent angiography-related renal tissue injury (the APART trial). *Am J Cardiol* 89:356–358, 2002

Johnson DW: Evidence-based guide to slowing the progression of early renal insufficiency. *Intern Med J* 34:50–57, 2004

Kaplan NM: Management of hypertension in patients with type 2 diabetes mellitus: guidelines based on current evidence. *Ann Intern Med* 135:1079–1083, 2001

Klahr S, Morrissey J, Hruska K, Wang S, Chen Q: New approaches to delay the progression of chronic renal failure. *Kidney Int* 61 (Suppl. 80):23–26, 2002

Knudsen ST, Poulsen PL, Hansen KW, Ebbehoj E, Bek T, Mogensen CE: Pulse pressure and diurnal blood pressure variation: association with micro- and macrovascular complications in type 2 diabetes. *Am J Hypertens* 15:244–250, 2002

Lane JT: Microalbuminuria as a marker of cardiovascular and renal risk in type 2 diabetes mellitus: a temporal perspective. *Am J Physiol Renal Physiol* 286:F442–450, 2004

Nangaku M: Mechanisms of tubulointerstitial injury in the kidney: final common pathways to end-stage renal failure. *Intern Med* 43:9–17, 2004

Parving HH, Chaturvedi N, Viberti G, Mogensen CE: Does microalbuminuria predict diabetic nephropathy? *Diabetes Care* 25:406–407, 2002

Patient Registration Committee, Japanese Society for Dialysis Therapy: An Overview of Regular Dialysis Treatment in Japan (as of 31 December 2001). *Ther Apher* 8:3–32, 2004

Remuzzi G, Schieppati A, Ruggenenti P: Clinical practice: nephropathy in patients with type 2 diabetes. *N Engl J Med* 346:1145–1151, 2002

Rippin JD, Barnett AH, Bain SC: Cost-effective strategies in the prevention of diabetic nephropathy. *Pharmacoeconomics* 22:9–28, 2004

Ruilope LM, Segura J: Losartan and other angiotensin II antagonists for nephropathy in type 2 diabetes mellitus: a review of the clinical trial evidence. *Clin Ther* 25:3044–3064, 2004

Sferra L, Kelsberg G, Dodson S: Do ACE inhibitors prevent nephropathy in type 2 diabetes without proteinuria? *J Fam Pract* 53:68–69, 2004

Song JC, White CM: Clinical pharmacokinetics and selective pharmacodynamics of new angiotensin converting enzyme inhibitors: an update. *Clin Pharmacokinet* 41:207–224, 2002

U.S. Renal Data System: *USRDS 2003 Annual Data Report Atlas of End-Stage Disease in the United States.* Bethesda, MD, National Institutes of Health, National Institute of Diabetes and Digestive and Kidney Diseases, 2003

Dr. Friedman is Distinguished Teaching Professor of Medicine and Chief of the Division of Renal Diseases at the Downstate Medical Center, Brooklyn, NY.

42. Painful or Insensitive Lower Extremity

ANDREW J. M. BOULTON, MD, FRCP

Peripheral neuropathy is the most common cause of leg pain in patients with diabetes. Another common etiology is intermittent claudication as a consequence of peripheral arterial disease. Whereas sensory neuropathy is usually the precipitant of painful symptoms, other neuropathic syndromes may also result in pain (Table 42.1). Reduced sensation to sensory stimuli including pain, temperature, touch, and vibration in the feet and lower parts of the legs in diabetes patients is invariably a result of sensory neuropathy and may go unnoticed by patients for years unless specifically tested for and demonstrated. Paradoxically, some patients may experience spontaneous painful or paresthetic symptoms while concurrently having marked loss of sensation on neurological examination—a condition described as the "painful/painless leg." The explanation for this not uncommon finding is that the sensory nerves to the feet are severely diseased and fail to conduct stimuli. Proximally, however, spontaneous electrical activity in diseased peripheral axons is interpreted by the patient as pain and is perceived in the area (i.e., the foot) that the nerve used to innervate.

PATHOPHYSIOLOGY

The true causes of diabetic neuropathy remain enigmatic. However, evidence from large trials such as the Diabetes Control and Complications Trial and the United Kingdom Prospective Diabetes Study clearly implicate chronic hyperglycemia as the prime abnormality that results in many of the mechanisms summarized in Table 42.2.

EPIDEMIOLOGY

Peripheral sensory neuropathy is common, affecting up to 50% of older type 2 diabetes patients. The average endocrine practice with a mixed age range of patients would expect a neuropathy prevalence of ~33%. Neuropathy is more prevalent with increasing age and duration of diabetes (Table 42.3). Of 100 patients with sensory neuropathy, up to 50 may be asymptomatic and only 10 would be expected to have significant symptoms that require treatment.

Table 42.1 Conditions that Result in Pain in Lower Limbs of Diabetes Patients

---

- Sensory neuropathy
  - □ Acute sensory
  - □ Chronic sensorimotor
- Entrapment neuropathy
  - □ Meralgia paresthetica
- Proximal motor neuropathy (amyotrophy)
- Peripheral arterial disease
  - □ Intermittent claudication
  - □ Rest pain

DIAGNOSIS

Because up to half of all patients with diabetic distal sensory neuropathy may experience no symptoms, the diagnosis cannot be made by history alone. Careful clinical examination of the feet is indicated in all patients at least on an annual basis.

History

Take a careful history, inquiring about pain, discomfort, or numbness in the legs. Patients with no spontaneously volunteered symptoms might, if asked, describe numbness or say that their "feet feel dead." Remember, diabetic neuropathy is a diagnosis of *exclusion* of other causes. Atypical features that might suggest a nondiabetic cause of neuropathy include rapid progression, foot drop, back or neck pain, marked asymmetry, weight loss, and family history.

EXAMINATION

A careful inspection of the feet is indicated. In long-standing sensorimotor neuropathy, small muscle wasting may be seen. Dry skin suggests coexisting sympa-

---

Table 42.2 Proposed Pathogenetic Mechanisms for Neuropathy

- Hyperglycemia
- Nonenzymatic glycation
- Oxidative stress
- Ischemic/hypoxic factors
- Nerve Growth Factor (NGF) abnormalities
- Polyol pathway activation
- Immunological abnormalities

Table 42.3 Risk Factors for Neuropathy

- Age
- Duration of diabetes
- Glycemic control
- Cholesterol/triglyceride level
- Hypertension
- Other microvascular complications
- Smoking

thetic dysfunction. Look for ulcers, deformities, or Charcot changes. Simple neurological assessment ideally would include:

- pinprick sensation
- light touch
- vibration (use a 128-Hz tuning fork at the apex of the hallux)
- ankle reflexes
- pressure sensation (use a 10-g monofilament)

All these tests should be performed bilaterally, and the patient should be observed walking after the shoes have been inspected. Patients with severe sensory loss but no symptoms are often unsteady during normal gait because of the loss of proprioception.

The diagnosis of diabetic neuropathy is normally a clinical one. Quantitative assessment of sensory modalities and electrophysiological studies may help to define the severity of the neuropathy but will not distinguish between neuropathy due to diabetes or other causes (Table 42.4). It is particularly important to exclude malignant disease. For example, an older male diabetes patient who smokes and has typical neuropathic symptoms and signs coupled with weight loss might well have a paraneoplastic syndrome associated with a bronchogenic carcinoma, giving rise to the neurological symptoms and signs.

Table 42.4 Other Causes of Peripheral Neuropathy

- Malignant disease
- Toxins (e.g., alcohol)
- Uremia
- Infections (e.g., HIV)
- Metabolic disorders (e.g., uremia, hypothyroidism)
- Iatrogenic agents (e.g., cytotoxic drugs, isoniazid)
- Inflammatory disease (e.g., chronic inflammatory demyelinating polyneuropathy)

PAINFUL NEUROPATHY

As stated above, the differential diagnosis of pain in the diabetic leg includes a number of conditions (Table 42.1), the most common of which is sensory neuropathy.

Sensory Neuropathy

Distal sensory neuropathy includes the common chronic sensorimotor variety and the relatively rare acute sensory neuropathy. The symptoms are of similar character and commonly comprise burning discomfort, pain of an electrical nature, stabbing, prickling, pricking, and shooting or stabbing pains symmetrically in the feet and lower legs. Pins and needles (novocaine like) and other dysesthetic symptoms are also common. All these symptoms are prone to nocturnal exacerbation with characteristic bedcloth hyperesthesia.

Patients with troublesome nocturnal symptoms may benefit from getting up and walking around, in contrast to enduring ischemic rest pain. They may occasionally immerse their legs in cold water to relieve the burning discomfort.

Acute sensory neuropathy tends to follow periods of metabolic instability (such as ketoacidosis) or a sudden change of metabolic control, such as after rapid improvement of control after starting insulin (insulin neuritis). Symptoms are severe, signs are few, and the prognosis for disappearance of symptoms is good (in a matter of weeks or months).

Chronic sensorimotor neuropathy is the most common variety of diabetic neuropathy and is of insidious onset with symptoms that wax and wane. Although symptoms are sensory, as described above, signs are both sensory and motor, with small muscle wasting and absent reflexes, hence "sensorimotor neuropathy."

The symptoms of this type of neuropathy were well described by Dr. Pavy of London in 1884 as being "of a burning and unremitting character." These symptoms may last intermittently for years but gradually tend to improve; this improvement is often accompanied by progressive sensory loss, leaving the patient at risk of insensitive foot injuries.

Entrapment Neuropathy

Entrapment of the lateral cutaneous nerve of the thigh can give rise to localized neuropathic symptoms in its area of innovation, the lateral area of the midthigh. This pain is localized and usually unilateral, in contrast to symmetrical distal sensory neuropathy. It is known as "meralgia paresthetica."

Amyotrophy (Proximal Motor Neuropathy)

As described in Chapter 43, amyotrophy typically affects older male type 2 diabetes patients with neuropathic pain in the thigh region together with proximal motor weakness.

Peripheral Arterial Disease

Claudication, a classic symptom of peripheral arterial disease, should not be confused with neuropathic pain. It is usually described as a cramping in the calf muscles, induced by exercise and relieved by rest without changing positions.

TREATMENT OF PAINFUL SENSORY NEUROPATHY

Many patients with severely painful conditions believe that they have malignant disease; thus, reassurance that this is not the case and that treatment is available for these symptoms, which may well resolve in due course, is an important part of management. The first step in symptom management is to stabilize glycemic control. There is increasing evidence that blood glucose flux may exacerbate neuropathic pain, so avoiding swings of glycemia from hypoglycemia to hyperglycemia may help. Insulin is not always needed in type 2 diabetes patients if control is satisfactory on oral agents. Most patients will also require some form of pharmacotherapy for the painful symptoms, as summarized in Table 42.5.

Tricyclic drugs remain the first-line therapy because they have proven efficacy in several randomized trials. Their pain-relieving effects are usually apparent in a matter of days, in contrast to their antidepressant actions. The predictable side effects of drowsiness and anticholinergic symptoms (particularly dry mouth) limit their use, and a significant minority of patients cannot tolerate them at all. To avoid these effects, start with a low dose given at bedtime (25 mg) and build up gradually until symptoms are relieved.

Gabapentin is the most useful of the anticonvulsant agents, again with efficacy confirmed in randomized trials. Lamotrogine also shows promise as a useful treatment for symptomatic neuropathy.

Among the other listed drugs, tramadol, an opioid-like centrally acting synthetic nonnarcotic analgesic, has also been shown to be efficacious in the man-

Table 42.5 Drug Treatment of Neuropathic Symptoms

Agent/Group	Drug	Daily Dosage	Side Effects
Tricyclics	Amitriptyline	25–150 mg hs	Drowsiness
	Imipramine	25–150 mg hs	Anticholinergic
Anticonvulsants	Gabapentin	900–3,000 mg divided	Central side effects: dizziness,
	Lamotrogine		somnolence
	Carbamazepine	Up to 800 mg divided	
Anti-Arrhythmics	Mexilitene	Up to 450 mg divided	Gastrointestinal and neurologic complaints
Opioid-Like	Tramadol	50–400 mg divided	Nausea, constipation, drowsiness

hs, bedtime.

agement of neuropathic pains, although only short-term (up to 6 months) use is recommended. Topical agents such as capsaicin may be helpful in cases of localized pain, and acupuncture has been shown to be of use in a long-term open study.

THE INSENSITIVE FOOT

Any patient found on clinical examination to have reduced sensation to modalities such as vibration, touch, or pain must be considered to be at risk of insensitive injury. Methods to avoid further complications such as ulceration or Charcot neuroarthropathy should be actively pursued in such individuals. These typically include education in personal foot care, regular visits to a podiatrist, more frequent visits to the physician, and advice on footwear. Further management of individual problems is considered in Chapter 56.

SUGGESTED READINGS/BIBLIOGRAPHY

Abbott CA, Carrington AL, Ashe H, Bath S, Every LC, Griffiths J, Hann AW, Hussein A, Jackson N, Johnson KE, Ryder CH, Torkington R, Van Ross ER, Whalley AM, Widdows P, Williamson S, Boulton AJ: The North-West Diabetes Foot Care Study: incidence of, and risk factors for, new diabetic foot ulceration in a community-based patient cohort. *Diabet Med* 19:377–384, 2002

Boulton AJM: Current and emerging treatments for diabetic neuropathy. *Diabetes Reviews* 7:379–386, 1999

Boulton AJM, Connor H, Cavanagh PR (Eds.): *The Foot in Diabetes.* 3rd ed. New York, Wiley, 2000

Boulton AJM, Gries FA, Jervell JA: Guidelines for the diagnosis and outpatient management of diabetic peripheral neuropathy. *Diabet Med* 15:508–514, 1998

Bowker JH, Pfeifer MA (Eds.): *Levin & O'Neal's The Diabetic Foot.* 6th ed. St. Louis, MO, Mosby, 2001

Veves A (Ed.): *Clinical Management of Diabetic Neuropathy.* Totowa, NJ, Humana Press, 1998

Dr. Boulton is Visiting Professor of Medicine, University of Miami School of Medicine, Miami, FL; Professor of Medicine, University of Manchester; and Consultant Physician, Manchester Royal Infirmary, Manchester, U.K.

43. Diabetic Monoradiculopathy/ Amyoradiculopathy

AARON VINIK, MD, PhD, AND ANAHIT MEHRABYAN, MD

Peripheral neuropathies in diabetes comprise a variety of peripheral nerve afflictions. Of the various subgroups, length-dependent distal symmetric polyneuropathy (DSPN) is the most common type of peripheral nerve damage. However, all anatomical parts of the peripheral nervous system may be affected by diabetes, and this creates difficulties in proper diagnosis and selection of optimal therapy. The focal and multifocal neuropathies are confined to the distribution of single or multiple peripheral nerves, and their involvement is referred to as mononeuropathy or mononeuritis multiplex. A focal neurological deficit in the nerve distribution at the brachial or lumbosacral plexus is known as diabetic plexopathy or, when at the nerve roots, as radiculopathy. Each neurological abnormality has a different pathogenesis, mode of onset, course of disease, signs and symptoms, and associated laboratory and clinical information from that of DSPN, and if this is understood and recognized, then response to treatment can be quite salutary. Table 43.1 distinguishes the features of classic DSPN from those of the asymmetric mono-/polyneuropathies.

FOCAL NEUROPATHIES (MONONEURITIS) AND ENTRAPMENT SYNDROMES

Focal neuropathies are distinguished by their presentation and distribution of clinical symptoms (Table 43.2). They have the following characteristics:

- focal (asymmetric unilateral or bilateral muscle weakness)
- painful (pain is one of the most disabling features)
- acute or subacute (all signs and symptoms develop in a few days to 2 months)
- self-limited (spontaneous complete recovery or significant improvement of clinical signs is the rule)

Mononeuropathies are due to a vasculitis with subsequent ischemia or infarction of nerves. They heal spontaneously, usually within 6–8 weeks. Common mononeuropathies involve cranial nerves 3, 4, 6, and 7 and thoracic and peripheral nerves including the peroneal, sural, sciatic, lateral cutaneous nerve of the thigh, femoral, ulnar, and median. Their onset is acute and associated with pain, and their course is self-limiting, resolving over a period of 6 weeks. Mononeuropathies

Table 43.1 Differentiation of Distal Symmetric Polyneuropathy from Mono-/Amyoradiculopathies

	DSPN	Mono-/Amyoradiculopathies
Onset	Insidious	Acute/subacute
Distribution	Distal, length dependent	Proximal, asymmetric
Leading signs and symptoms	Mild to moderate sensory symptoms (negative or positive) and mild motor symptoms	Severe sensory (positive pain) and motor (weakness and atrophy) symptoms
Course of disease	Slow progression	Monophasic
Glycemic control	Dependent	Independent
Duration of diabetes	Dependent	Independent
Association with retinopathy and nephropathy	Associated	Not associated

must, however, be distinguished from entrapment syndromes, which start slowly, progress, and persist without intervention (Table 43.3).

Common entrapment syndromes involve the following:

- median nerve with impaired sensation in the first three fingers and positive Tinel sign over the wrist
- ulnar nerve with decreased sensory perception in the little and ring fingers and Tinel sign over the ulnar canal at the elbow (ulnar entrapment)
- lateral cutaneous nerve of the thigh with pain in the upper anterior aspect of the thigh and hyper- or hypoesthesia in the nerve distribution (the condition is known as meralgia paresthetica, and the nerve is trapped under the inguinal ligament)
- peroneal nerve with pain in the outer anterior aspect of the tibial region and weakness during dorsiflexion of the foot
- median and lateral plantar nerves with decreased sensation in the inside and outside of the feet, respectively (medial and lateral plantar entrapments)

Table 43.2 Common Mononeuropathies

Cranial	3rd, 4th, 6th, 7th
Thoracic	Mononeuritis multiplex
Peripheral	Peroneal
	Sural
	Sciatic
	Femoral
	Ulnar
	Median

Table 43.3 Comparison of Features of Mononeuritis and Entrapment

	Mononeuritis	Entrapment
Onset	Sudden	Gradual
Pain	Acute	Chronic
Multiplex	Occurs	Rare
Course	Resolves	Persists without intervention
Treatment	Physical therapy	Rest, splints, steroid and local anesthetic injections, surgery

The entrapment neuropathies are highly prevalent in diabetes patients. One in every three patients has one, and they should be actively sought in every patient with signs and symptoms of neuropathy because the treatment may be surgical.

In mononeuropathies, such as peroneal palsy, where weakness is a prominent feature, physical therapy may be necessary to maintain good muscle tone and prevent contractures.

MONONEUROPATHIES

Painful Ophthalmoplegia

Severe retro- and periorbital pain with radiation into the frontal and temporal areas is the first symptom of painful ophthalmoplegia. Diplopia due to ocular mononeuropathy or partial lesion of all oculomotor nerves follows the acute pain syndrome resembling either retro-orbital infection or acute brain pathology. Sparing of the pupillary reaction is a very important sign in differentiating diabetic ophthalmoplegia (DO) from structural ophthalmoplegia. DO is self-limited, and spontaneous recovery occurs over a period of 6–8 weeks. The lesion is a vascular occlusion to an interfascicular neuron, and other fascicles take over the function. It is imperative to distinguish DO from the other causes of painful ophthalmoplegia because it is a common presentation of orbital, and paraorbital, diseases as well as brainstem catastrophes. Posterior communicating aneurysm rupture can be distinguished because it presents with loss of the pupillary reaction to light and accommodation, and this is spared in diabetic oculomotor palsy. Other causes of painful ophthalmoplegia, such as cavernous sinus thrombosis, orbital infection, cranial arteritis, primary or metastatic tumors, Tolosa-Hunt syndrome, and Gradenigo's syndrome, should be excluded because they require active intervention as opposed to DO.

Diabetic Thoracoabdominal Neuropathy

Diabetic thoracoabdominal neuropathy is characterized by manifestations of symptoms and signs along single or multiple intercostals nerves. Pain is the leading complaint and often results in unnecessary surgical treatment, especially in low thoracic root involvement, when acute abdominal pathology can be suggested. Pain in thoracoabdominal neuropathy is mostly burning and tingling in character and associated with hyperesthesia and allodynia. It resembles herpetic pain or sunburn-type pain and is rarely followed by numbness and hypoesthesia in the corresponding dermatomes. Profound anterior or anterior-lateral abdominal and thoracic involvement is characteristic, whereas back pain is atypical. Muscle weakness is also common. It is prominent with lower thoracic root affliction and creates a "false" hernia with bulging of the abdominal muscles because of loss of tone. Superficial pain and hyperesthesia in combination with painless deep palpation can be useful diagnostic criteria to exclude underlying visceral involvement. The course of the disease and prognosis are the same as in the proximal neuropathies.

ENTRAPMENT SYNDROMES

Carpal Tunnel Syndrome

Carpal tunnel syndrome (CTS) occurs twice as frequently in a diabetic population than in a healthy population. Its increased prevalence in diabetes may be related to repeated undetected trauma, metabolic changes, or accumulation of fluid or edema within the confined space of the carpal tunnel. It is more common in females and in obese individuals (BMI >30 kg/m^2) and affects the dominant hand. It occurs in 2% of the general population, 14% of diabetic subjects without diabetic proximal neuropathy (DPN), and 30% of diabetes subjects with DPN. It peaks at around 40–60 years of age, and an increased wrist index is a risk factor. CTS used to be associated with work-related injury but now seems to be common in people in sedentary positions and is probably related to the use of keyboards and typewriters. Dentists are particularly prone to CTS. Smoking appears to be an important risk factor for entrapments, and systemic disorders such as hypertension, hypothyroidism, rheumatoid arthritis, and acromegaly all contribute to its occurrence. If recognized, the diagnosis can be confirmed by an electrophysiological study. The unaware physician seldom realizes that symptoms may spread to the whole hand or arm in CTS, and the signs may extend beyond those subserved by the nerve entrapped. Tinel sign for median nerve (percussion at the wrist) is positive in 61% and Phalen's test (wrist flexion) in only 46%. Thus, the very nature of the trouble goes unrecognized, and an opportunity for successful therapeutic intervention is often missed. Electromyogram–nerve conduction velocity (EMG-NCV) can be particularly useful in distinguishing CTS from DSPN and the double crush syndrome of C7-8 radiculopathy. The high sensitivity and specificity of a nerve conduction study makes it the most valuable diagnostic method for diagnosing CTS (80% positive). Moreover, it is the only technique to establish subclinical cases and differentiate CTS from DSPN. Impaired nerve conduction at the wrist over the median nerve with normal ulnar nerve conduction is characteristic of CTS. Combined entrapment of the median and ulnar nerves can mimic DSPN and can only be distinguished by an EMG-NCV with nerve stimulation in the palm.

Treatment of CTS involves rest, splinting the wrist in a neutral position, use of a diuretic to reduce edema, liberal use of nonsteroidal anti-inflammatory agents, and injections of steroids and local anesthetics under the ligament. Surgical release may be required in cases unresponsive to these medical measures.

Ulnar Nerve Entrapment

The second common entrapment syndrome is that of the ulnar nerve (ulnar nerve entrapment). Sensory symptoms and weakness of the fourth and fifth fingers, accompanied by hypothenar atrophy, are the typical signs of ulnar nerve entrapment. Etiology of ulnar nerve entrapment includes trauma, arthritis, and systemic diseases (less often than in CTS). As in CTS, conduction through the elbow is decreased. A C8-T1 radiculopathy must be excluded. Response to local injections is less rewarding than in CTS, and surgical release is only of value if done early, before there is wasting of the interosseous muscles.

Peroneal Nerve Entrapment

Peroneal nerve entrapment at the level of the fibula head is the most common entrapment syndrome in the lower limbs and is due to the ease of external compression of the peroneal nerve under general anesthesia, when crossing the legs (especially in older people while sleeping), and with weight loss. It needs to be distinguished from an L5 radiculopathy with foot drop. Tripping and fractures are a consequence of impaired peroneal nerve function, especially in older people.

Tarsal Tunnel Syndrome

Tarsal tunnel syndrome (TTS) is a painful lower limb entrapment. Passing through the tarsal tunnel, the tibial nerve innervates only muscles of the sole, and clinical signs are mostly sensory. Foot pain may be severe, burning, or worse on standing and walking; Tinel sign on the underside of the medial malleolus, with atrophy of the sole muscles, is typical. Weakness is rare because most of the small foot muscles (flexor hallucis longus) are not damaged in TTS. NCV can be informative in the case of a normal plantar response from one leg and an abnormal response from the symptomatic side in unilateral TTS. TTS is not difficult to diagnose clinically when DSPN is not severe and NCV is moderately abnormal. Mild symmetric peroneal and tibial NCV abnormality with intact ankle jerks and sensation of the dorsal aspect of the foot with the above-mentioned clinical signs are the most important diagnostic features of TTS. When neuropathy is severe, diagnosis may be impossible.

The mainstays of nonsurgical treatment are avoiding use of the joint, placing a splint in a neutral position for day and night use, and using anti-inflammatory medications and targeted injections of local anesthetics and steroids. Surgical treatment consists of sectioning the offending ligament. The decision to proceed with surgery should be based on several considerations, including severity of symptoms, appearance of motor weakness, and failure of nonsurgical treatment.

Diabetic Proximal Neuropathy

DPN is one of the most unpleasant and disabling conditions of diabetes. It was first reported by Bruns and Garland as subacute proximal leg weakness with moderate pain, and the term "diabetic amyotrophy" was coined by Garland in 1961 to emphasize prominent thigh muscle affliction. Based on clinical and neurophysiological findings, the same condition was described variably as "diabetic femoral neuropathy," "diabetic polyradiculopathy," "proximal motor neuropathy," and "diabetic lumbosacral plexopathy." Despite this diversity of terminology and some disagreement on the complement and severity of symptoms and signs, DPN is now a well-known and established entity. DPN presents clinically with the following features:

- It primarily affects the elderly (>64 years of age) and almost exclusively affects males.
- It can be gradual or abrupt in onset.
- It begins with jabbing, knifelike pain with hyperesthesia and allodynia, usually in the anterior thigh region spreading to the rear end and down the leg. It usually starts on one side and then spreads to the other.
- Sensory loss is atypical.
- Pain is followed by significant pelvifemoral muscle weakness (quadriceps, iliopsoas, hip adductors, hamstrings, and glutei), with predominantly thigh muscles involved; the inability to rise from a chair or rise from the kneeling position occurs.
- DPN begins unilaterally and spreads bilaterally.
- Knee reflexes are absent.
- It coexists with distal symmetric polyneuropathy.
- Patients include individuals with chronic inflammatory demyelinating polyneuropathy (CIDP), monoclonal gammopathy of unknown significance (MGUS), GM1 antibody syndrome, and inflammatory vasculitis as well as those with diabetes.
- It was formerly thought that DPN was often a self-limited condition and resolved spontaneously in 1.5–3.0 years.
- Current thinking is that DPN is an inflammatory condition with vasculitis or immune-mediated nerve damage and can resolve within days on appropriate therapy.
- This condition is unrelated to blood glucose control and is not associated with triopathies.
- A more severe diffuse distal-proximal DSPN with strongly pronounced weight loss is known as "diabetic neuropathic cachexia," and weight loss may amount to as much as 10–20 kg.

Proximal motor neuropathy can be clinically identified based on proximal muscle weakness and muscle wasting with fasciculation and/or twitching of muscles. It may be symmetric or asymmetric in distribution. The condition is readily recognizable clinically, with prevailing weakness of the iliopsoas, obturator, and adductor muscles, together with relative preservation of the gluteus maximus and minimus, and hamstrings. Individuals affected have great difficulty rising out of chair unaided and often climb up their bodies (Gowers' Maneuver). Heel or toe standing is surprisingly good. In the classic form of diabetic amyotrophy, axonal loss is the predominant process, and the condition coexists with DSPN. However, this accounts for <9% of cases. Electrophysiological evaluation reveals lumbosacral plexopathy. In contrast, 91% of cases are due to a demyelinating condition, and there is an 11-fold greater risk of chronic inflammatory demyelinating polyneuropathy in people with diabetes, and 12% of diabetes patients develop some form of MGUS or monosialoganglioside neuropathy (GM1). If demyelination predominates and the motor deficit affects proximal and distal muscle groups, the diagnosis of CIDP, MGUS, vasculitis, and GM1 syndrome should be considered. The clinical differences between these syndromes is given in Table 43.4. It is important to divide proximal syndromes into these two subcategories because the autoimmune and inflammatory variants respond dramatically to intervention, whereas amyotrophy runs its own course over months to years. Until more evidence is available, we consider them as separate syndromes.

DIAGNOSIS

It has been difficult to establish the exact site of the lesion, but recent studies labeled DPN as "diabetic lumbosacral polyradiculoplexus neuropathy," pointing to the multifocal proximal nerve involvement. Indeed, the most important conditions to exclude are the proximal myopathies (e.g., carcinoid, thyrotoxicosis, Cushing's or steroid treatment, and carcinoma). Lumbosacral outlet syndrome must also be excluded on an anatomical basis and usually requires magnetic resonance imaging with contrast. Bilateral painless proximal motor weakness is common in the genetically determined myopathies, motor neuron disorders, and neuromuscular junction lesions. The clinical picture usually serves to distinguish them from DPN. EMG findings are typical. A detailed EMG examination and blood work including immunoelectrophoresis, antibodies to nerve structures, and paraneoplastic antibodies are necessary to establish that the primary demyelination in diabetes is due to MGUS, CIDP, vasculitis, or a paraneoplastic syndrome. If doubt remains as to the diagnosis, then a cerebrospinal fluid tap combined with immunohistochemical evaluation of an obturator nerve biopsy will usually establish the diagnosis. An EMG is helpful in distinguishing these syndromes, since diabetes per se lowers amplitudes. CIDP and MGUS cause severe demyelination and prolong conduction velocities, and specific nerve root entrapments in the lumbosacral outlet can be identified. These investigations make it possible to direct therapy to the appropriate condition.

THERAPIES FOR PROXIMAL NEUROPATHIES

Treatment of proximal neuropathies can now be rational and based on the nature of the underlying pathogenesis. The following is an outline of what is available, and specific details can be found in the publications cited in the Bibliography.

Table 43.4 Distribution (%) of Symptoms and Signs of Proximal Neuropathies in Diabetes

Clinical Presentation	Vasculitis	CIDP	MGUS	Diabetes
DSPN (motor/sensory)	3	91	100	67
Distal (asymmetric)	27	9	0	0
Multifocal	70	0	0	33

Vasculitis: Withdraw drugs and treat with steroids or immunosuppressive agents.
CIDP: Give intravenous immunoglobulin (1.0 g/kg) on 2 consecutive days and repeat at 2-week intervals for three treatments. Further treatment depends on the response. Plasmapheresis and immunosuppressive therapy (steroids and azathioprine) are alternative treatments.
MGUS: Undergo plasmapheresis.
Diabetes: Achieve glycemic control.
Sacral outlet syndrome: Undergo physical therapy/surgery.

BIBLIOGRAPHY

Barohn RJ, Sahenk Z, Warmolts JR, Mendell JR: The Bruns-Garland syndrome (diabetic amyotrophy). *Arch Neurol* 48:1130–1135, 1991

Chia L, Fernandez A, Lacroix C, Adams D, Plante VSG: Contribution of nerve biopsy findings to the diagnosis of disabling neuropathy in the elderly: a retrospective review of 100 consecutive patients. *Brain* 119:1091–1098, 1996

Dawson DM: Entrapment neuropathies of the upper extremities. *N Engl J Med* 329:2013–2018, 1993

Krendel DA, Costigan DA, Hopkins LC: Successful treatment of neuropathies in patients with diabetes mellitus. *Arch Neurol* 52:1053–1061, 1995

Leedman PJ, Davis S, Harrison LS: Diabetic amyotrophy: reassessment of the clinical spectrum. *Aust N Z J Med* 18:768–773, 1988

Vinik AI, Holland MT, LeBeau JM, Liuzzi FJ, Stansberry KB, Colen LB: Diabetic neuropathies. *Diabetes Care* 15:1926–1975, 1992

Vinik AI, Milicevic Z: Recent advances in the diagnosis and treatment of diabetic neuropathy. *Endocrinologist* 6:443–461, 1996

Dr. Vinik is Professor of Medicine at the Eastern Virginia Medical School and Director of the Diabetes Research Institute in Norfolk, VA. Dr. Mehrabyan is a neurologist from Armenia who is participating in an American Diabetes Association mentorship.

44. Gastrointestinal Disturbances

AARON I. VINIK, MD, ANAHIT MEHRABYAN, MD, AND DAVID A. JOHNSON, MD

Gastrointestinal (GI) disturbances caused by autonomic neuropathy are common and often a disabling complication of diabetes. Between 20% and 40% of patients with diabetes mellitus develop dysfunction of the autonomic nervous system. This may be a functional disturbance, as occurs with severe hyperglycemia or ketoacidosis, or a consequence of autonomic neuropathy. Diabetes mellitus can affect every part of the GI tract (i.e., the esophagus, stomach, small intestine, and colon). Thus, the GI manifestations are quite variable and include the following:

- dysphagia
- abdominal pain
- nausea
- vomiting
- malabsorption
- fecal incontinence
- diarrhea
- constipation

The clinical spectrum of these complaints can range from relatively silent to life-threatening. This chapter focuses on the clinical features, pathophysiology, diagnosis, and treatment of GI disturbances in diabetes patients.

PATHOGENESIS

GI complications of diabetes appear to be more common in patients with long-standing disease and poorly controlled blood glucose levels. The most prevalent GI complication is a motility disturbance of the viscera, which is generally the result of widespread autonomic neuropathy. Clinical symptoms of enteric diabetic neuropathy are more common in patients with long-standing diabetes, poor glucose control, increased age, and symptoms of peripheral or cardiovascular autonomic neuropathy.

The clinical features of certain diabetic enteropathies resemble those caused by surgical resection of the nerve plexus supplying that organ. Unfortunately, convincing morphological demonstration of gross neuropathology in human diabetic enteropathy is lacking, and correlation of GI symptoms with other signs of end-organ neuropathic damage is sometimes poor. Further complicating the understanding of this condition is a relatively high incidence of affective anxiety disorders in diabetic patients with GI symptoms that often resemble those of autonomic dysfunction. Microangiopathic changes, as seen in the retina or kidney, do not seem to cause disease in the GI tract.

Disturbed release of gut hormones may play some role in the symptom complex and the pathogenesis of GI complications of diabetes. These are conflicting, however. Cholinergic neuromuscular transmission in the myenteric plexus of the intestinal tract may be diminished. Additionally, failure of gut muscle to react appropriately on neurostimulation may be the result of relative deficiencies of stimulatory neurotransmitters such as motilin, neuropeptide Y, and methionine-enkephalin. Defective postprandial release of pancreatic polypeptide has also been demonstrated in diabetes patients with autonomic neuropathy but may only reflect loss of vagal integrity.

Metabolic abnormalities such as hyperglycemia and electrolyte imbalances undoubtedly play at least a contributory role in the disruption of GI motility in patients with diabetes. Clinically, this is most apparent when diabetic ketoacidosis occurs and the typical features of anorexia, nausea, vomiting, or abdominal pain develop. As the metabolic derangements are controlled, the GI symptoms resolve. It is well demonstrated that acute hyperglycemia inhibits GI motility. Some of the motor disturbances described with diabetes may therefore be directly related to glycemic control and are functional, and the integrity of the autonomic nervous system is intact.

ESOPHAGEAL DYSFUNCTION

Esophageal motor disorders have been described in 75% of patients with diabetes. Esophageal dysfunction is so common in patients with diabetic autonomic neuropathy that its absence in patients with GI symptoms casts doubt on the diagnosis of diabetic enteropathy. Motor abnormalities include impairment of peristaltic activity with double peak and tertiary contractions or impaired peristalsis and diminished lower esophageal sphincteric pressures. These factors may further predispose the patient to gastroesophageal reflux disease, particularly in the setting of impaired gastric emptying.

Esophageal disturbances may be asymptomatic, although dysphagia has been described in up to one-third of patients. The presence of esophageal dysfunction in individuals with diabetes in the absence of symptoms suggests an underlying sensory autonomic diabetic neuropathy, similar to that observed with painless myocardial infarction. Interestingly, neuropsychiatric profiles of diabetes patients with abnormalities of esophageal motility have shown that abnormal contractions are more frequent during episodes of anxiety and depression. Esophageal dysfunction is of particular concern with ingestion of drugs such as oral bisphosphonates, which may cause ulceration, perforation, bleeding, and mediastinitis.

Patients with diabetes are prone to *Candida* esophagitis. This should be suspected where pharyngeal thrush is evident or clinical symptoms of odynophagia or dysphagia exist.

GASTRIC DYSFUNCTION

With the advent of electrogastrography, it has now been established that functional disturbances such as arrhythmias, tachygastria, bradygastria, pylorospasm, and hypomotility may occur in patients with diabetes. Organic lesions include gastroparesis, antral dilatation and obstruction, ulceration, inflammation, and bezoar formation.

Gastroparesis diabeticorum can be detected in 25% of patients with diabetes. This is usually clinically silent, although severe diabetic gastroparesis is one of the most debilitating of all the GI complications of diabetes. The prevalence of gastric motility abnormalities ranges from 20% to 30%. Physiology of gastric emptying largely depends on vagus nerve function, which may be grossly disturbed in diabetes. Liquid emptying is controlled by the proximal stomach (fundus) and depends on the volume of gastric contents. With impaired vagal function, the proximal stomach is less relaxed, and liquid emptying may actually be increased in diabetes patients. Solid-phase emptying is effected by powerful contractions of the distal stomach (antrum). These contractions, known as phase 3 contractions, grind and mix solid food into particles of <1 mm in size, which then pass through the pylorus into the duodenum. Phase 3 contractions of the interdigestive migratory motor complex are frequently absent in diabetes patients. This results in poor antral grinding and emptying, which may result in gastric retention. Furthermore, there may be disordered integration of gastric and duodenal motor function resulting from disturbances in receptor relaxation of the stomach. Pylorospasm may occur because of disturbed contractility, which causes a functional resistance to gastric outflow. Impaired gastric emptying puts the patient at particular risk for gastric bezoar formation.

The exact pathophysiology of gastric motor disturbances is not certain. It is clear that vagal parasympathetic function disturbances may occur. The release of the peptide motilin, which regulates GI motility, is under vagal control. Motilin stimulates the initiation of phase 3 motor activity of the migrating motor complex of the stomach in patients with gastroparesis. High levels of this peptide have been reported in patients with gastroparesis. High motilin levels may therefore be partly compensatory. Further support is the observation that motilin levels fall in patients who have gastroparesis and receive treatment with prokinetic agents. Hyperglycemia itself may cause delayed gastric emptying in both healthy individuals and individuals with diabetes.

Symptoms

Typical symptoms of gastroparesis (Table 44.1) include the following:

- nausea
- vomiting
- early satiety
- abdominal bloating
- epigastric pain
- anorexia

Table 44.1 GI Disturbances in Diabetes

Condition	Symptom	Treatment
Esophageal dysfunction	Dysphagia	Metoclopramide
Gastroparesis	Nausea, vomiting, early satiety, anorexia, epigastric pain	Blood glucose control Care with hypoglycemia Bethanecol Metoclopramide Domperidone Tegaserod
Hemorrhagic gastritis	Repeated vomiting and hematemesis (ketoacidosis and gastroparesis)	Erythromycin Clonidine, levosulpiride Treat cause
Cholelithiasis	Gallstone biliary colic, cholecystitis	Dissolution therapy, lithotripsy, or surgery
Pancreatic insufficiency	None (steatorrhea)	Enzyme replacement
Diabetic diarrhea	Paroxysmal, nocturnal, painless, explosive diarrhea	Gluten-free diet, pancreatic enzymes, antibiotics, cholestyramine, diphenoxylate, loperamide, Sandostatin (Octreotide, Sandoz)
Fecal incontinence	Soiling without awareness	Treat diarrhea Biofeedback training
Constipation	Infrequent bowel actions, abdominal pain	Improve toilet habits Increase fluid intake Psyllium, Metoclopramide, mistoprostil
Liver dysfunction	Abdominal pain	Test for hepatitis C Control blood glucose Lower lipids Stop hepatotoxic drugs

Classically, patients with gastroparesis have emesis of undigested food consumed many hours or even days previously. Postprandial vomiting is a rule, but more subtle presentation such as morning nausea or even nonproductive retching may also occur. Even with mild symptoms, gastroparesis interferes with nutrient delivery to the small bowel and therefore disrupts the relationship between glucose absorption and exogenous insulin administration. This may result in wide swings of glucose levels and unexpected episodes of postprandial hypoglycemia. Gastroparesis should therefore always be suspected in patients with erratic glucose control. It may, in its most troublesome form, cause chronic nausea and anorexia, punctuated by bouts of prolonged emesis requiring hospitalization for dehydration and uncontrolled hyperglycemia. Inexplicably, symptoms are variable and may fluctuate markedly over a period of weeks to months.

Chronic gastritis and gastric atrophy have been noted with a high prevalence in patients with diabetes. The role of *Helicobacter pylori* is not clear. This organism seems to play a minor role, if any, in disturbances in the upper alimentary tract of patients with diabetes. Interestingly, there is a significantly lower incidence of *H. pylori* infections in diabetes patients with delayed gastric emptying compared with individuals with normal emptying. Furthermore, gastric atrophy and hypochloridia are not uncommon, especially with type 1 diabetes, and there is the potential predisposition for bacterial overgrowth. Chronic gastritis and gastric atrophy are often associated with significant titers of antiparietal antibodies and antithyroid antibodies. This partly explains the high incidence of pernicious anemia and hypothyroidism in patients with diabetes. Awareness of these associations is necessary to appropriately direct replacement therapies. Acute hemorrhagic gastritis is common in patients with repeated emesis of gastroparesis or ketoacidosis. Additionally, bleeding may develop from Mallory-Weiss tears, particularly in patients with repetitive emesis.

Diagnosis

Upper-GI symptoms should not be attributed to gastroparesis until conditions such as gastric ulcer, duodenal ulcer, severe gastritis, and gastric cancer have been excluded. An upper-GI endoscopy or high-quality barium series should be performed. The finding of retained food in the stomach after an 8- to 12-h fast, in the absence of obstruction, is diagnostic of gastroparesis. The lack of this finding, however, does not rule out the diagnosis.

Nuclear medicine scintigraphy is the gold standard for evaluation of gastric emptying. This involves ingestion of a standard radiolabeled meal and provides a useful means to not only diagnose but objectively follow patients' response to therapy. Newer noninvasive imaging tests have also been developed recently. Magnetic resonance imaging and percutaneous electrogastrography hold promise for future clinical application. Gastroduodenal manometrics may be helpful in select patients (e.g., symptomatic patients with apparently normal emptying to look for pylorospasm or incoordinate gastric and duodenal motility). This test is generally cumbersome, available only in a few research centers interested in motility disorders, and at this point does not dictate therapeutic strategies.

Treatment

Initial treatment of diabetic gastroparesis should focus on blood glucose control. Hyperglycemia, even acute, may interfere with gastric contractility. Physiological control of blood glucose levels may improve gastric motor dysfunction. Overregulation of blood glucose control should be avoided when gastric emptying is impaired because of the danger of severe hypoglycemia resulting from a variable pattern of gastric emptying. Patients who complain of early satiety and bloating may benefit from a low-fat, low-fiber diet and several small meals throughout the day. Fiber, vegetables, and poorly digestible solids should be avoided because of their predisposition to gastric bezoar formation.

Pharmacological therapy is usually necessary in patients with clinically significant gastroparesis. Evaluation of ancillary medications is critical before treating with prokinetic medications. Any drugs with anticholinergic potential that may further decrease gastric emptying should be withdrawn. Avoidance of medications such as carafate or psyllium may help to decrease gastric bezoar potential.

Metoclopramide

Metoclopramide is a dopamine antagonist that stimulates acetylcholine release in the myenteric plexus. This drug acts centrally on the chemoreceptor triggers in the floor of the fourth ventricle, which provides an important anti-emetic activity. Controlled trials documenting the efficacy of metoclopramide have been unable to consistently show an improvement in gastric emptying rate. This drug is given at a dose of 10–30 mg 1 h before meals and at bedtime. For patients with severe impairment of gastric emptying, use of the elixir form seems to be more effective. In addition, metoclopramide can be given subcutaneously, allowing for a more sustained effect in complicated patients. Intravenous administration of this medication may be helpful in hospitalized patients. Administration of a 25-mg rectal suppository dose of metoclopramide has been effective in some patients.

The effectiveness of this drug typically wanes because of a tachyphylaxis effect, so its efficacy is short-lived (<6 months) in most patients. However, patients may respond after reintroduction of the medication after a period of withdrawal.

Side effects of metoclopramide include drowsiness, lethargy, and depression, especially at higher doses. If Parkinson-like tremor occurs, medication should be discontinued immediately. Galactorrhea and breast tenderness may occur because of increased prolactin secretion caused by metoclopramide. Metoclopramide may lower the seizure threshold in patients with epilepsy and should be used with extreme caution in these patients.

Domperidone

Domperidone is similar to metoclopramide in that it is a dopamine antagonist, but it has little action on acetylcholine release in the myenteric plexus. It does not cross the blood-brain barrier and thus has limited side effects. It does reach the hypothalamus, which is outside the barrier. The dose is 20–40 mg taken 1 h before meals and at bedtime. Domperidone stimulates prolactin secretion and may cause breast tenderness and galactorrhea. Intravenous administration of domperidone causes cardiac dysrhythmias. Domperidone appears to be most useful for patients who have responded well to metoclopramide but are unable to take it because of side effects. Domperidone is free of tachyphylaxis with long-term treatment, and improvements in gastric emptying persist for 6 months to 1 year.

Erythromycin

The macrolide erythromycin and its derivatives duplicate the action of motilin, which is responsible for the migrating motor complex activity, by binding to and activating motilin receptors. Intravenous administration of this antibiotic enhances the emptying rate of both liquids and solids. The effects are not as dramatic with oral therapy, although clinical efficacy has been demonstrated with erythromycin in a dose of 250 mg 0.5 h before meals. Substitution of the enteric-coated form may be better tolerated in some patients. Erythromycin has the downside of creating antibiotic-related resistance problems. However, it appears to be an effective therapeutic alternative to more established forms of treatment in patients with diabetic gastroparesis, especially when other drugs have failed. Newer erythromycin derivatives that have potentially less antibiotic and more prokinetic effectiveness are being investigated.

Levosulpiride

Levosulpiride is a new prokinetic drug that is a selective antagonist for D_2-dopamine receptors. Recent studies have suggested that this medication, given at a dosage of 25 mg three times a day orally for 6 months, shows maintained improvement in gastric emptying and improved glycemic control in diabetes subjects with gastroparesis. Further studies are forthcoming. The drug is not yet freely available.

Clonidine

Clonidine is a specific α_2-adrenergic receptor antagonist used to control diabetic diarrhea. A recent study has demonstrated significant improvement in diabetes patients with chronic refractory symptoms of bloating, nausea, and vomiting. Patients were treated with 0.1 mg clonidine two or three times a day. This preliminary work suggests that improvement of adrenergic influences on GI motility may play a role in diabetic gastroparesis. Therefore, clonidine may be helpful in select cases, but dosing must be cautious because of the danger of orthostatic hypotension.

Tegaserod

Tegaserod, a new selective 5-HT4 agonist, has been shown to improve gastric emptying in diabetes patients with gastroparesis. Clinical studies have demonstrated stimulation of GI tract motility and improvement of visceral sensitivity in irritable bowel syndrome, which is associated with abdominal pain, bloating, and constipation.

Tegaserod (6 mg orally twice daily) increases colonic motility and proximal colonic filling, accelerates orocecal transit, and improves esophageal acid clearance. Preclinical studies have demonstrated the antinociceptive effects of Zelnorm (tegaserod), which are supposedly the result of pain threshold alteration. Binding selectively to one subclass of serotonin receptors, tegaserod does not create adverse effects on the cardiovascular system. Tegaserod can be administered safely in liver and renal impairment.

Severe disabling symptoms refractory to pharmacological therapy may require surgical intervention. Percutaneous gastrostomy for gastric decompression and a jejunostomy feeding tube have been helpful in some patients. More radical surgeries including gastrostomy, pyloroplasty, and jejunostomy may be necessary in certain patients to ensure adequate nutrition and gastric decompression. Such procedures have generally been disappointing and are rarely recommended.

BILIARY DISEASE

Earlier data suggesting that patients with diabetes have a higher incidence of cholelithiasis (reported incidence 1.5 times that of the normal population) are controversial. The high incidence of type 2 diabetes in populations at risk for cholelithiasis (i.e., women, obese people, and patients with hyperlipoproteinemia) makes it difficult to identify diabetes as an independent risk factor. Most recent studies have suggested gallstone disease is multifactorial, and it is an independent risk factor only in females with type 2 diabetes.

Theoretically, diabetic autonomic neuropathy predisposes patients to gallstone formation because diminished gallbladder contractility leads to stasis. This stasis causes the bile to become supersaturated with cholesterol, which predisposes to stone formation. The role of prophylactic cholecystectomy in diabetes patients with asymptomatic gallstones is controversial. More recent studies have assessed the outcome of acute cholecystitis in patients with diabetes mellitus and suggest there is no incremental risk of morbidity or mortality. Accordingly, there seems to be no role for routine prophylactic cholecystectomy in diabetes patients with cholelithiasis.

Medical treatment for cholesterol gallstones with dissolution therapy may be an alternative to surgery in patients with symptomatic gallstones. Laparoscopic cholecystectomy, however, will probably have fewer and fewer applications in symptomatic cholelithiasis. Medical therapy is being investigated to attempt to augment abnormal gallbladder motility with the intent to decrease bile stasis. Levosulpiride D_2, a dopamine antagonist, has shown preliminary effectiveness in augmenting gallbladder emptying in patients with diabetic cholecystoparesis.

PANCREAS

Exocrine pancreatic function is reduced in >50% of patients with type 1 diabetes. The degree of impairment progresses with greater duration of the disease. This may be the consequence of chronic insulin deficiency and resultant autonomic neuropathy. Clinically significant pancreatic insufficiency is rare, however, because 90% of exocrine function must be lost before steatorrhea occurs.

Diabetes and pancreatic cancer are known to be associated, but the cause of the association and whether diabetes is a risk factor for pancreatic cancer remain controversial. Pancreatic cancer may occur with increased frequency among patients with long-standing diabetes (>5 years). It is important to recognize that new-onset diabetes in older patients without a family history of diabetes may develop as the "form fruste" of pancreatic cancer or a neuroendocrine tumor (e.g., somatostatinoma) and is presumably caused by the tumor itself.

LIVER DISEASE

Certain types of liver disease are usually associated with glucose intolerance or diabetes. The liver is the principal organ responsible for insulin metabolism. Approximately 50% of the insulin secreted by the pancreas is removed by the first passage through the liver. In the presence of cirrhosis, there is decreased extraction by the liver, and the peripheral circulating insulin is increased. Despite this increase, hyperglycemia is common, suggesting that peripheral insulin resistance coexists. Consistent with this hypothesis is the finding that peripheral monocytes have been obtained from patients with cirrhosis and shown to have fewer insulin receptors. The specific mechanism responsible for the decreased cellular receptor number and resultant insulin resistance is not known.

Glucose intolerance or diabetes may be a reflection of underlying liver disease associated with diabetes. For example, hemochromatosis is a disorder of iron metabolism that is frequently associated with glucose intolerance. Excess iron is deposited in the liver, pancreatic islets, and other organs. As a result, diabetes mellitus and hepatic fibrosis and cirrhosis may be manifestations of progressive disease.

Autoimmune forms of chronic active liver disease are also associated with diabetes characterized by inheritance of specific HLA alleles. The relative risk for diabetes is increased threefold in individuals who carry the HLA-B8 allele and approximately fourfold in those carrying the HLA-Dw3 allele. Both of these alleles are found twice as often in patients with autoimmune chronic active hepatitis.

Liver disease may be evident in the absence of other recognizable hereditary factors. In particular, hepatic steatosis has been reported in 30–80% of individuals with diabetes. Accumulation of triglycerides may occur by any or a combination of the following factors:

- increased uptake from peripheral fatty acids
- increased fatty triglyceride synthesis (either carbohydrates or nonesterified fatty acids)
- reduced hepatic oxidation of fat
- increased formation of VLDL
- reduced hepatic release of newly formed VLDL

Hepatic steatonecrosis is characterized by large fat-droplet deposition associated with hepatic fibrosis and may lead to cirrhosis in some patients. Progressively more patients with nonalcoholic steatohepatitis are being recognized. Modifiable factors include control of diabetes, lipids, and obesity.

Recent evidence has associated the hepatitis C virus infection with diabetes. Glucose intolerance is particularly common in patients with chronic hepatitis C. Testing for hepatitis C infection in diabetes patients with abnormal liver-related enzymes is therefore mandatory. Studies to date have not found particular epidemiological factors for hepatitis C infection in diabetes or a direct role for hepatitis C in the development of diabetes.

Individuals with diabetes are at increased risk for hepatitis not only as a consequence of diabetes but as a consequence of medical management of their disease. Iatrogenic liver disease can occur with oral hypoglycemic agents such as chlorpropamide. This drug may result in a cholestatic or granulomatous liver injury. Similar reactions have been seen with tolbutamide and with troglitazone. Primary hepatocellular injury has also been found with hypolipidemic drugs such as lovastatin.

SMALL INTESTINE

Diarrhea may be evident in 20% of diabetes patients, particularly those with known autonomic neuropathy. Motor disturbances of the small intestine do not entirely explain the pathogenesis of diarrhea. Predisposition of bacterial overgrowth may induce diarrhea. Additionally, because adrenergic nerves stimulate intestinal reabsorption of fluids and electrolytes, decreased adrenergic tone may contribute to pathogenesis. Small-bowel malabsorption of bile salts may induce diarrhea via a colonic stimulatory effect.

There is frequency of the HLA-DR3 genotype in insulin-dependent diabetes, which explains why many patients also have celiac disease. Appropriate recognition of this condition is critical to effect the necessary dietary restriction of gluten. Serological screening with anti-endomysial and antigluten antibodies is 95% sensitive and specific for celiac disease. Small-bowel biopsy should be considered for any patient for whom this diagnosis is a possibility.

Exocrine pancreatic insufficiency may occur. Patients with diabetes have impaired responses to stimulation with duodenal infusion of amino acids or intravenous secretin or cholecystokinin. Pancreatic exocrine insufficiency rarely becomes severe enough to contribute to malabsorption. However, in patients with diarrhea, it is prudent to replace pancreatic enzymes.

Autonomic neuropathy may cause diarrhea by its effects on gut motility and/or enterocyte absorption. Although gut dysmotility makes sense and has been the most widely accepted explanation for diabetic diarrhea, motility testing and small-bowel transit studies have produced variable and inconsistent results. Adrenergic nerve dysfunction interferes with normal electrolyte and fluid absorption by the enterocyte.

Evaluation of diarrhea in a patient with diabetes should begin with a good history. Care should be taken to exclude medication-related diarrhea. Sorbitol may be implicated as an additive to medications and diabetic foods. Biguanides may also be responsible for diarrhea in some patients. The patient should be asked about particular dietary exacerbants (e.g., milk products suggesting lactose intolerance). Diarrhea that resolves with fasting suggests an osmotic diarrhea caused by ingested substances. In contrast, diarrhea that continues in the absence of ingestion, as with nocturnal awakening, is more suggestive of a secretory-type process, and neuroendocrine causes should be pursued. Stools should be obtained for occult blood examination for ova and parasites, fecal leukocytes, and qualitative fecal fat.

Patients with large-volume diarrhea and those with positive assessment of qualitative fecal fat should be further studied with a 72-h fecal fat collection. This must be done while ingesting a 100-g fat diet. Screens for malabsorption should be done in patients who have diminished albumin stores or low serum carotene levels. A D-xylose test is a good screen for small-bowel malabsorptive disorders. Serum B_{12} level should be considered in patients with suspected diarrhea involving the distal small bowel because the primary absorption area is in the ileum. Erythrocyte folate levels are particularly elevated in patients with bacterial overgrowth and should be checked in the appropriate setting. Directed investigation of the small intestine by small-bowel biopsy and/or radiographic studies should be done in patients with protracted symptoms. Pancreatic function testing should be considered in patients with steatorrhea. Proctosigmoidoscopy and possibly full colonoscopy with biopsies of the right and left colon and rectum to exclude microscopic or collagenous colitis or amyloid should also be considered. Empiric therapeutic trials of antibiotics, gluten-free diet, and pancreatic enzymes may less accurately define the diagnosis but can be considered when facilities for detailed study are not available.

Evaluation of stool electrolytes is helpful in separating osmotic from secretory-type diarrheas. A calculated osmolality based on 2(stool Na + stool K) subtracted from the calculated serum osmolality of 290 gives the calculated osmotic gap. Patients with osmotic diarrhea typically have an osmotic gap >50 and more frequently >100. Patients with an osmotic gap of <50 should be considered for secretory diarrheal workup. This includes evaluations for carcinoid, glucagonoma, gastrinoma, VIPoma, and prostaglandin-producing tumors.

Treatment of diabetic diarrhea should address the specific etiology. Celiac sprue and pancreatic insufficiency should be treated with gluten-free diet and pancreatic enzyme supplements, respectively. A trial of antibiotics is appropriate if bacterial overgrowth is found or cannot be ruled out (Table 44.2). Hydrophilic dietary supplements such as psyllium may be useful if diarrhea alternates with constipation. Care should be taken, however, in patients with a tendency toward gastric bezoar, which may be aggravated by high-residue diets. Chelation of bile salts with cholestyramine may reduce the bile acid component of diarrhea. Standard synthetic opiates such as diphenoxylate and loperamide are potent, nonaddicting antidiarrheal agents and should be tried early in the course. Care must be exercised not to produce obstipation and impaction.

Because GI adrenergic function is impaired in diabetic autonomic neuropathy, adrenergic agonists should stimulate intestinal reabsorption of fluids and electrolytes. Clonidine may reverse adrenergic nerve dysfunction and improve diarrhea. This agent also has potent antimotility effects, which may partly explain symptomatic improvement in some patients. Initial treatment should begin with 0.1 mg two or three times a day, increased to 0.4–0.6 mg titrating up over several days. Because the antihypertensive effects of clonidine are mediated through the

Table 44.2 Drug Therapy for Diabetic Diarrhea

Drug	Starting Dose
Psyllium (sugar-free)	1 tsp to 1 Tbsp 1–3 times/day
Kaolin + pectin (mixture)	2 Tbsp 2 times/day
Cholestyramine	1 packet (4 g) 1–6 times/day
Tetracycline	250 mg 4 times/day
Ampicillin	250 mg 4 times/day
Pancreatic enzymes	2–4 tablets or capsules with meals and snacks
Diphenoxylate	2.5 mg 2 times/day
Loperamide	2 mg 2 times/day
Clonidine	0.2 mg 2 times/day
Sandostatin	50–100 µg 3 times/day

central nervous system, diabetes patients with severe autonomic neuropathy may not experience worsening of preexisting postural hypotension, which may actually improve. If the medication is withdrawn, it should be done slowly to avoid rebound hypertension.

The long-acting somatostatin analog octreotide is effective in some refractory patients. Octreotide probably inhibits the release of gastroenteropancreatic endocrine peptides, which may be a pathogenic factor responsible for diarrhea and electrolyte imbalance in diabetes patients. Recent studies with this agent in patients with intestinal pseudo-obstruction and bacterial overgrowth suggest that it may increase gut transit and decrease abdominal distention-related complaints. The initial dose is 50–100 µg three to six times a day as needed. Adverse effects of this agent include pain at the site of injection, which can be reduced by warming the syringe by hand and then injecting slowly over 2–3 min. Additional symptoms include abdominal cramps, bloating, and flatulence. Diabetic diarrhea may be worsened by this agent, usually because of steatorrhea, which may respond to pancreatic enzyme supplements. The drug is expensive and should be reserved for patients with severe refractory symptoms.

CONSTIPATION

Constipation is the most common GI complication, affecting nearly 25% of diabetes patients and >50% of individuals with diabetic autonomic neuropathy. Myoelectric studies of the colon have demonstrated diminished motility in response to ingestion of a standard meal (gastrocolonic reflux). Cholinergic agents stimulate colonic motility, suggesting a defect in neural control of the smooth muscle. Colonic smooth muscle is capable of responding to cholinergic stimulation; therefore, neuroprokinetic agents may be effective.

Severe constipation may be complicated by ulceration, perforation, and fecal impaction. Barium studies pose a risk to patients with underlying visceral myopathy, so barium-related impaction must be avoided. Aggressive catharsis should be used in patients undergoing barium studies such as GI series or enema. Fecal impaction may also cause overflow diarrhea and incontinence and must be considered in the differential underlying constipation of diabetic diarrhea. Long-standing constipation with straining predisposes to stretch injury of the nerves to the anal sphincter, which may lead to fecal incontinence through reduced sphincteric pressure. Precipitous change in bowel habits should prompt colonic evaluation to exclude the possibility of an obstructive lesion such as stricture or neoplasm.

Anorectal manometry may be useful in evaluating the rectal anal inhibitory reflex. This test is helpful in distinguishing colonic hypomotility from rectosigmoid dysfunction causing outlet obstructive symptoms. Biofeedback and/or patient training with regard to defecation may be directed with this technique.

Colonic segmental transit time may be derived by mean segmental transit radiopaque markers that are ingested orally. Sequential X rays on alternate days demonstrate passage of these radiopaque markers through the right and left colon and rectosigmoid area. This provides objective measurement of bowel transit and helps define patient complaints, both at baseline and in response to therapy.

Treatment for constipation should begin with emphasis on good bowel habits, which include regular exercise and maintenance of adequate hydration and fiber consumption. Many constipated patients respond to a high–soluble fiber diet supplemented with daily hydrophilic colloid (1–2 Tbsp psyllium) one to three times a day. This is best given with a meal. The patient should avoid psyllium just before bedtime because its efficacy is compromised. Osmotic agents such as sorbitol or lactulose (1–2 Tbsp three or four times a day) may be helpful. These doses can be titrated to effect. The intermittent use of saline or osmotic laxatives (e.g., 30 ml milk of magnesia or antacids) may be required for patients with more severe symptoms. Stimulatory laxatives should be avoided because of their tendency to damage the colonic myenteric plexus with long-term use. Magnesium-containing agents must be used with caution if renal insufficiency exists. Metoclopramide, 10–20 mg, 0.5 h before meals and qhs may help patients with intractable constipation because of its effects on colonic smooth muscle. Additionally, 200 μg mistoprostil three or four times a day is effective in patients with protracted constipation through its influence on the migrating motor complex.

FECAL INCONTINENCE

Fecal incontinence may be associated with severe diabetic diarrhea or constitute an independent disorder of anorectal dysfunction. Incontinent diabetes patients have decreased basal sphincteric pressure, suggesting abnormal internal and external anal sphincter function. The threshold of recognition of rectal distension in incontinent diabetes patients appears to be higher and not related to differential rectal compliance, suggesting impaired afferent function. External sphincteric function is impaired in some cases.

Patients who have had any rectal trauma are at increased risk for fecal incontinence. This mostly occurs in women who may have sustained a rectal tear during childbirth. Rectal foreign body insertion may further decrease the sphincteric tone.

Assessing the volume of incontinence in diabetes patients is essential. Large-volume diarrhea and incontinence suggest more of a pancolonic or small-bowel cause than an isolated anorectal dysfunction.

Anorectal function can be evaluated by anorectal manometry and a test of continence for solids and liquids. Anorectal manometry profiles the maximum basal sphincter pressure in the maximum "squeeze" sphincter pressure. In addition, the rectal anal inhibitory reflex is measured by inflation of a balloon in the rectum. This causes a reflex relaxation in the internal anal sphincter. Identification of rectal dysfunction allows for therapy including biofeedback treatment, which attempts to improve rectal distention sensing as well as sphincteric function in patients with an intact rectal sensation.

ABDOMINAL PAIN

Autonomic neuropathy may present with abdominal pain. Consideration should be given to diagnoses of acute cholecystitis, pancreatitis, gastroparesis, and diabetic ketoacidosis. Patients will occasionally present with severe epigastric pain not attributable to any of these conditions. When signs of neuropathy are present, the most likely diagnosis is diabetic abdominal radiculopathy. Symptoms of severe anorexia and weight loss are easily confused with gastroparesis or pancreatic disease such as neoplasia. For unclear reasons, symptoms typically resolve after many months. The diagnosis may be established by an abnormal electromyograph of the anterior abdominal wall muscles compared with an electromyograph of the thoracic paraspinal muscles. Analgesics, antiepileptic drugs (e.g., gabapentin, tegretol), or amitriptyline may help in select patients. Transcutaneous stimulation devices or nerve root injection may also be helpful in intractable cases.

BIBLIOGRAPHY

Annese V, Lombardi G, Frusciante V, Germani U, Andrulli A, Bassotti G: Cisapride and erythromycin prokinetic effects in gastroparesis due to type I (insulin-dependent) diabetes mellitus. *Aliment Pharmacol Ther* 11:599–603, 1997

Camilleri M: Gastrointestinal manifestations of diabetes mellitus: overview. *Eur J Gastroenterol Hepatol* 7/8:709–710, 1995

Chapman BA, Wilson IR, Frampton CM, Chisholm RJ, Stewart NR, Eagar GM, Allan RB: Prevalence of gallbladder disease in diabetes mellitus. *Dig Dis Sci* 41:2222–2228, 1996

Enck P, Frieling T: Pathophysiology of diabetic gastroparesis. *Diabetes* 46 (Suppl. 2):S77–S81, 1997

Farrell FJ, Keeffe EB: Diabetic gastroparesis. *Dig Dis* 13:291–300, 1990

Gillett HR, Ferguson A: Coeliac disease and insulin-dependent diabetes mellitus. *Lancet* 349:1698, 1997

Gray H, Wreghitt T, Stratton IM, Alexander GJ, Turner RC, O'Rahill S: High prevalence of hepatitis C infection in Afro-Caribbean patients with type II diabetes and abnormal liver function tests. *Diabet Med* 12:244–249, 1995

Grimbert S, Valensi P, Levy Marchal C, Perret G, Richardkt JP, Raffoux C, Trunchet S, Beangran M: High prevalence of diabetes mellitus in patients with chronic hepatitis C: a case control study. *Gastroenterol Clin Biol* 20:544–548, 1996

Haines ST: Treating constipation in the patient with diabetes. *Diabetes Educ* 21:223–232, 1995

Jacober SJ, Vinik Al, Narayan A, Strodel WE: Jejunostomy feeding in the management of gastroparesis. *Diabetes Care* 9:217–219, 1985

Jones KL, Horowitz M, Wishart MJ, Maddox AF, Harding PE, Chatterton BE: Relationships between gastric emptying, intragastric meal distribution, and blood glucose concentrations in diabetes mellitus. *J Nucl Med* 36:2220–2228, 1995

Lacy BE, Yu S: Tegaserod: a new 5-HT4 agonist. *J Clin Gastroenterol* 34:27–33, 2002

Locke GR: Epidemiology of gastrointestinal complications of mellitus. *Eur J Gastroenterol Hepatol* 7:711–716, 1995

Melga P, Mansi C, Ciuchi E, Giusti R, Sciaba L, Prando R: Chronic administration of levosulpiride and glycemic control in insulin dependent diabetes mellitus patients with gastroparesis. *Diabetes Care* 20:55–58, 1997

Nakabayashi H, Fujii S, Mawa U, Seta T, Takeda R: Marked improvement of diabetic diarrhea with the somatostatin analog octreotide. *Arch Intern Med* 154:1863–1867, 1994

Ogbonnaya KL, Arem R: Diabetic diarrhea: pathophysiology, diagnosis and management. *Arch Intern Med* 150:262–267, 1990

Perdichizzi G, Bottari M, Pallio S, Fera MT, Cerbane M, Barresi G: Gastric infection by *Helicobacter pylori* and antral gastritis in hyperglycemic obese and in diabetic subjects. *New Microbiol* 19:149–154, 1996

Reardon TM, Schnell GA, Smith OJ, Hubert TT: Critical therapy of diabetic gastroparesis. *J Clin Gastroenterol* 11:204–207, 1989

Rosa-e-Silva L, Troncon LE, Oliveira RB, Iazigi N, Gallo L Jr, Foss MC: Treatment of diabetic gastroparesis with oral clonidine. *Aliment Pharmacol Ther* 9:179–183, 1995

Rothstein RD: Gastrointestinal motility disorders in diabetes mellitus. *Am J Gastroenterol* 85:782–785, 1990

Saukkonen T, Savilahti E, Rijonen H, Ilonen J, Tuemillehto-Wolf E, Alcerblom HK: Coeliac disease: occurrence after clinical onset of insulin dependent diabetes mellitus. *Diabet Med* 13:464–470, 1996

Schpitz B, Sigal A, Kauffman Z, Dinbar A: Acute cholecystitis in diabetic patients. *Am Surg* 61:964–967, 1995

Sninsky CA: Gastrointestinal complications with diabetes mellitus. *Curr Ther Endocrinol Metab* 5:420–425, 1994

Sun WM, Katsinlos P, Horowitz M, Read NW: Disturbances in anorectal function in patients with diabetes mellitus and faecal incontinence. *Eur J Gastroenterol Hepatol* 8:1007–1012, 1996

Valdovinos MA, Camilleri M, Zimmermann BR: Chronic diarrhea and diabetes mellitus: mechanisms and an approach to diagnosis and treatment. *Mayo Clin Proc* 68:691–702, 1993

Vinik AI, Erbas T: Recognizing and treating diabetic autonomic neuropathy. *Cleve Clin J Med* 68:928–944, 2001

Vinik AI, Glowniak JV: Hormonal secretions in diabetic autonomic neuropathy. *N Y State J Med* 82:871–878, 1982

Vinik AI, Maser R, Mitchell B, Freeman R: Diabetic autonomic neuropathy. *Diabetes Care* 26:1553–1579, 2003

Vinik AI, Suwanwalaikorn S: Autonomic neuropathy. In *Current Therapy of Diabetes Mellitus.* DeFronzo R, Ed. St. Louis, MO, Mosby-Yearbook, 1997, p. 165–176

Virally-Monod ML, Guillausseau PJ, Assayag M, Teilmans D, Aizenberg C, Vassen-Mallus S, Imbertz C, Warnet A: Variable efficacy of octreotide in diabetic diarrhea. *Diabetes Metab* 22:356–358, 1996

Dr. Vinik is Professor of Medicine at the Eastern Virginia Medical School and Director of the Diabetes Research Institute in Norfolk, VA. Dr. Mehrabyan is a neurologist from Armenia who is participating in an American Diabetes Association mentorship. Dr. Johnson is Professor of Medicine at the Eastern Virginia Medical School in Norfolk, VA.

45. Bladder Dysfunction

CAI FRIMODT-MØLLER, MD, DMSC, FEBU

B ladder disturbances related to diabetes mellitus were recognized more than 40 years ago, but although much emphasis has been put on this subject, it is still ignored by many doctors as well as patients. A major reason for this is the lack of symptoms for a long period and then suddenly the patient experiences a quick progression of serious voiding problems.

ETIOLOGY AND PATHOPHYSIOLOGY

Urodynamic and urophysiological investigations have revealed loss of viscero-sensory innervation of the bladder, thus identifying a connection with peripheral neuropathy, which for many years has been known as a major symptom complex in diabetes mellitus. The patient loses his or her ability to record the "desire to void," which usually occurs at the filling rate of 300–400 ml in healthy subjects. The distension of the detrusor muscle (i.e., the bladder wall) gradually weakens the contractility of the detrusor, resulting in the inability to expel the urine contents of the bladder, which results in the development of urinary retention. From a pathophysiological point of view, the gradual loss of sensation blocks the viscoelastic and the viscous properties of the detrusor muscle, which results in a weakening of the bladder wall stiffness, thereby delaying reflexes to the afferent nerve paths. The viscero-motor pathways are patent, so the diabetes patient will be able to use his or her detrusor muscle capacity to expel urine. But when the ongoing stretching of the bladder wall continuously weakens the muscular filaments of the detrusor, the possibility of building up tension is lost. The end result will be a steady increase in residual urine and hypoactivity of the detrusor, and the patient will need to strain to support detrusor function.

CLINICAL FEATURES

Incidence and Prevalence

Incidence and prevalence of neurogenic bladder dysfunction in patients with diabetes are higher in type 1 diabetes patients (40–50%) than in type 2 diabetes patients (25%). Among patients with type 1 diabetes, there is a time period of

~10 years from the outbreak of the disease for the neurogenic disorders to develop. This time development is identical with the development of peripheral diabetic neuropathy. Roughly, the prevalence rate of diabetic bladder dysfunction is 1–3 per 1,000 people.

Sex and Age Distribution

No difference is seen in male and female populations regarding neurogenic bladder dysfunction. With regard to age, little information is available for children and adolescents. In the elderly population (>65 years old), the prevalence of neurogenic bladder disorders is equal in both sexes, but bladder dysfunction of non-neurogenic origin (for instance, benign prostatic hyperplasia) occurs significantly more frequently in the male population.

Symptoms

Symptoms have an insidious onset with gradual loss of bladder sensation. The patient seldom pays any attention to the growing interval between voidings, and the elderly male is quite happy not to be disturbed by nocturia. Although a number of patients with diabetes experience polyuria, they also report a reduced number of voidings per day (two to three during the day and zero to one during the night). Gradually, the symptoms become more serious as residual urine develops, and the patient will, on careful questioning, report having to strain during voiding, will record an impaired stream force, and will have an interrupted stream and a prolonged voiding act. Finally, he or she will have a feeling of retention or a feeling of lower abdominal distension. It is noteworthy that only ~25% of patients complain of their symptoms.

Clinical Findings

Findings of primary interest are *1*) measurement of residual urine, *2*) voiding-volume chart, and *3*) uroflowmetry. Residual urine is easily measured by ultrasound, which gives a rough estimate of the bladder content, where volumes <100 ml are acceptable but where repeated residual volumes >200 ml are pathological, either of neurogenic or obstructive origin.

An easy test to perform is to let the patient fill in a chart for voidings and voided volumes over 3 days. Important information can thus be obtained regarding the average voided volume, which is normally ~250–350 ml, but in diabetes patients, usually averages 500–600 ml.

Flow curves with a bell configuration and a peak flow >20 ml/s are regarded as normal, whereas a prolonged and flat flow curve with a peak flow <15 ml/s should raise suspicion.

Frequently, a mixture of findings occur among the noninvasive tests, and the only method of distinguishing between diabetic cystopathy and other types of bladder dysfunction is to perform a urodynamic investigation measuring the intravesical, abdominal, and detrusor pressures simultaneously with flow recording. An additional cystoscopy is often also required to study the bladder wall, the bladder-neck, and the prostatic part of the urethra. Whereas an obstruction of the bladder outlet will result in an increasing detrusor tension, which can be seen as trabeculation, the changes of the bladder wall in the patient with diabetes typically result in a flaccid folded bladder wall. Looking at the bladder outlet, the diabetes patient with neurogenic disturbances often presents a stiff narrow bladderneck and no prostatic enlargement. A patient with infravesical obstruction demonstrates either a stiff, closed bladderneck or occluding prostatic adenomas in the prostatic urethra.

DEFINITION

If the noninvasive tests demonstrate residual urine volumes >500 ml, voiding-volume charts show voiding intervals of 6–8 h and voided volumes >600 ml, and flow studies demonstrate bell-shaped flow curves with normal peak flows, a diabetic bladder with sensory loss is predictable. This neurogenic disorder is termed *diabetic cystopathy*.

DIABETIC CYSTOPATHY AND OTHER DISORDERS IN THE DIABETES PATIENT

There is a close relationship between diabetic cystopathy and peripheral neuropathy, where ~85% of patients with neurogenic bladder disorders also suffer from peripheral neuropathy and vice versa (Fig. 45.1). It should therefore be kept in mind

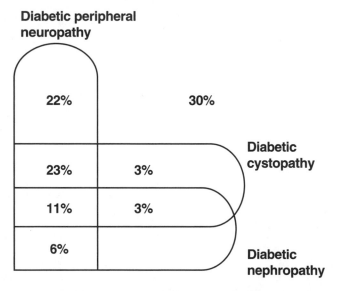

Figure 45.1 Venn diagram illustrating the interrelationship between diabetic peripheral neuropathy, diabetic cystopathy, and diabetic nephropathy in 116 diabetes patients.

that a patient presenting with symptoms of peripheral neuropathy (and where, for instance, examination of his or her vibratory threshold shows marked reduction) is at high risk of suffering from concomitant neurogenic dysfunction of the bladder.

Diabetic Nephropathy and Retinopathy

Diabetic nephropathy (in this study defined as persistent proteinuria) has a similar high relation to peripheral neuropathy (85%) and a lower but still significant 70% relation to diabetic cystopathy (Fig. 15.1).

Diabetic retinopathy, regardless of severity of illness, did not show any relation to diabetic cystopathy.

TREATMENT

The primary objective in dealing with diabetic cystopathy is to eliminate the high residual volume and to find means of replacing the irreversible sensory loss. Because the loss of sensation is permanent, the treatment must be followed to achieve lifelong control of the bladder.

The principles of nonsurgical management are as follows:

1. Schedule voiding every 3–4 h.
2. Perform triple voiding (i.e., repeated voidings 3–5 min after the primary voiding until no urine can be passed; straining is usually applied).
3. If residual urine exceeds 2–300 ml following the above-mentioned regimens and the uroflowmetry curve is in the lower peak flow level, treatment with α-adrenergic blockers should be administered.
4. If residual urine exceeds 500 ml, clean, intermittent catheterization is recommended one to three times daily, with the frequency of catheterizations depending on the amount of residual urine and whether the patient has symptomatic bacteriuria. In the case of asymptomatic bacteriuria, there is no need for prophylactic chemotherapy. However, if the patient has symptomatic bacteriuria, prophylaxis with a bacteriostatic antibiotic drug is recommended.

If these methods are ineffective, the urologist might have to resort to surgical intervention—bladderneck incision/resection to relieve the patient of any risk of outlet obstruction.

In patients with urodynamically disclosed obstruction, surgery is inevitable. A temporary medical treatment with α-blocking agents should be tried, but long-term medical treatment is not recommendable. Whether transurethral resection or transurethral microwave treatment is used is up to the urologist. Prostatic stents in a diabetes patient with increased risk of bacteriuria should be avoided, because a foreign body (i.e., a stent) has a high risk of developing symptomatic bacteriuria.

Earlier recommendations of using bethanecol chloride as a parasympathomimetic drug in the neuropathic bladder are not in effect today, partly because the side effects of the high doses of the drug create a lot of discomfort. Urodynamic investigations have demonstrated an increase in bladderneck tonus, thereby worsening the bladder outlet.

Another earlier recommendation to perform a reduction cystoplasty to reduce the bladder capacity has also been given up. Within a short time, the bladder will regain its former capacity.

TREATMENT RESULTS

The better diabetes is regulated, the greater the chance of avoiding neurological disturbances. The earlier the diabetic cystopathy is recognized, the better the results. A thorough urological investigation as early as possible is recommended, and if no outlet obstruction has been detected, the general practitioner or the diabetologist can proceed with the controls.

For a long period, prophylactic measures such as voiding around the clock with intervals of 3–4 h, double-triple voiding activities at every micturition, residual urine control by ultrasonography every third month, regular urine culturing to detect bacteriuria every 3 months, and an annual check of renal function by means of S-creatinine will reduce the risk of developing irreversible bladder dysfunction and probably also prevent end-stage renal disease.

If residual urine exceeds 500 ml at a minimum of two ultrasonic investigations, it is recommended that the patient perform intermittent self-catheterization at least once daily, probably before sleep and again in the morning. If the residual volume increases in spite of these measures, the patient will have to rely on catheterization every 4–5 h daily. Whenever any progression of bladder dysfunction is noted, the patient should be referred to the urologist for reinvestigation.

Last but not least, a close cooperation between the patient, his or her general practitioner, the diabetologist, and the urologist is crucial for success in avoiding or reducing the symptoms of diabetic cystopathy.

BIBLIOGRAPHY

Ellenberg M, Weber H: The incipient asymptomatic diabetic bladder. *Diabetes* 16:331–335, 1967

Faerman I, Maler M, Jadzinsky M, Alvarez E, Fox D, Zilbervarg J, Cibeira JB, Colinas R: Asymptomatic neurogenic bladder in juvenile diabetics. *Diabetologia* 7:168–172, 1971

Frimodt-Møller C: Diabetic cystopathy: a review of the urodynamic and clinical features of neurogenic bladder dysfunction in diabetes mellitus. *Dan Med Bull* 25:49–60, 1978

Kaplan SA, Te AE, Blaivas JG: Urodynamic findings in patients with diabetic cystopathy. *J Urol* 153:342–344, 1995

Sasaki K, Chancellor MB, Phelan MW, Yokoyama T, Fraser MO, Seki S, Kubo K, Kuman H, Groat WC, Yoshimura N: Diabetic cystopathy correlates with a long-term decrease in nerve growth factor levels in the bladder and lumbosacral dorsal root ganglia. *J Urol* 168:1259–1264, 2002

Ueda T, Yoshimura N, Yoshida O: Diabetic cystopathy: relationship to autonomic neuropathy detected by sympathetic skin response. *J Urol* 157:580–584, 1997

Dr. Frimodt-Møller is Chief Urologist at the Erichsen's Private Hospital, Copenhagen, Denmark.

46. Erectile Dysfunction

KENNETH J. SNOW, MD

It is well known that diabetes can affect sexual function in men. Although sexual dysfunction can include difficulties with excitement, erections, ejaculation, and pain, men are most likely to seek treatment for problems with erectile difficulties. Previously, the term "impotence" was used for all aspects of sexual dysfunction, which led to confusion. In 1992, the National Institutes of Health Consensus Conference recommended that the term "erectile dysfunction" (ED) be used to describe problems relating to penile erections and defined ED as the inability to achieve or maintain an erection long enough to permit satisfactory sexual intercourse.

PREVALENCE AND PATHOPHYSIOLOGY OF ED

Despite being a common problem in men, especially men with diabetes, the medical community has only recently begun to address the extent of sexual problems. The recent Massachusetts Male Aging Study, which evaluated nearly 1,300 men age 40–70 years, found some degree of erectile difficulty in 52% of these subjects. Studies report the incidence of ED in men with diabetes varying from 27.5% to 75%. As the age of the study population increased, the incidence increased, with up to 95% of men with diabetes over age 70 years having some degree of ED. In men with diabetes under the age of 30 years, 20% had ED.

For men with diabetes, the incidence of ED seems to be related to age, duration of diabetes, the level of glucose control as reflected by an elevated glycated hemoglobin A1C (A1C) level, and the presence or absence of diabetes complications. Macrovascular risk factors that often accompany diabetes, such as hypercholesterolemia, hypertension, and smoking, also contribute to the risk of ED. For most patients, the etiology of ED is due to multiple factors. Hypogonadism is not uncommon in men with diabetes and can contribute to ED.

There are a variety of medications that can affect erectile function. Table 46.1 lists some of the more commonly used medications. Thiazide diuretics and β-blockers have been shown to be associated with ED. Earlier β-blockers caused more difficulties than more recent β-blockers. Even local ophthalmological β-blockers may affect erections. Many drugs that affect the central nervous system may inhibit sexual function by direct action on the central neurological impulses or by the production of prolactin. Many over-the-counter drugs such as pseudoephedrine and certain antihistamines such as diphenhydramine and chlorpheniramine can affect ED as well.

Table 46.1 Commonly Used Drugs that Affect Erectile Function

Cardiovascular
    β-Blockers (especially propranolol, metoprolol, penbutolol, pindolol, timolol)
    Certain α-blockers (clonidine, guanfacine)
    α- and β-blockers (labetalol)
    α-Methyldopa
    Thiazide diuretics
    Older antihypertensives (reserpine, guanethidine, hydralazine)
    Spironolactone
    Digoxin
    Calcium-channel blockers (fairly low risk)

Central nervous system–acting drugs
    Antidepressants (including tricyclics and selective serotonin reuptake inhibitors
      [SSRIs])
    Antipsychotics
    Tranquilizers
    Anorexiants

Allergy related
    Corticosteroids
    Theophylline
    Bronchodilators

Antifungals
    Fluconazole, ketoconazole, itraconazole

Miscellaneous
    Metoclopramide, flutamide, clofibrate, gemfibrozil

Recreational
    Marijuana
    Alcohol

Nonprescription
    Antihistamines (chlorpheniramine, diphenhydramine, chlotrimeton)
    Decongestants
    Cimetidine

NORMAL AGING CHANGES

Some men seeking help for ED may only be having changes that are part of the aging process. As men age, they lose the ability to achieve spontaneous erections from visual sexual images or sexual fantasy. More direct genital stimulation (foreplay) may still lead to erections. In addition, with aging, distraction and fatigue are more likely to lead to erectile difficulties, and sexual activity needs to be attempted in a place with minimum distractions when the individual is not fatigued.

DIAGNOSTIC EVALUATION

History

    As part of the evaluation of ED, a careful history should be performed with an emphasis placed on history of sexual and reproductive functions as well as pertinent, related medical history (Table 46.2). The first issue that needs to be clarified is what exactly is the problem. Many patients may complain of impotence while the primary problem is decreased libido or ejaculatory problems. When dealing with ED, the duration of the problem and its presentation—whether sudden or gradual, with or without progression—provides information to suggest a greater or lesser likelihood of organic disease. The presence of nocturnal or morning erections suggests a psychogenic component to ED, although their absence does not dispute it, because morning erections decrease in frequency as men age.

Because poor blood glucose control increases the likelihood of ED, ascertain the patient's glycemic control as well as the presence of diabetes complications. Concomitant medical illnesses should be identified, with particular attention paid to medications used and the presence of vascular disease.

Psychological Considerations

If possible, the initial interview should be carried out with the sexual partner present. Whereas this arrangement may not always be possible, it is useful for the health care provider to observe the dynamics between the two individuals. ED can cause, or be caused by, problems in a relationship, and this knowledge can be useful in determining the course of evaluation and/or treatment. Significant numbers of men with ED and diabetes will have psychological problems. Referral to a mental health professional with expertise in sexual counseling is often helpful.

Physical Examination

When performing the physical examination, seek evidence of specific disease states relating to sexual function and carry out a more general screening to assess overall health (Table 46.2). Of particular importance is evidence of the following:

- normal virilization
- anatomical changes such as Peyronie's disease, hypospadias, or past injury
- testicular abnormalities

Table 46.2 Evaluation of Men with Diabetes and ED

History	Physical examination
Exact problem	Blood pressure
Onset	Cardiovascular examination
Duration	Neurological examination
Duration and control of diabetes	Breast examination
Diabetes complications	Genital examination
Other medical conditions	
Medications (prescription and nonprescription)	Diagnostic tests
	A1C, lipids, creatinine, liver function tests, hemoglobin, testosterone
Performance anxiety	
Social setting	
Relationship problems	
Health of partner	
Other stresses in patient's life	

- diffuse vascular disease
- diabetic neuropathies

An adequate evaluation of a man with ED cannot be performed without examination of the penis and testes.

Laboratory Measurements

The list of laboratory tests that are needed for a complete evaluation of ED starts with an assessment of overall health and, in particular for men with diabetes, an assessment of glucose control (A1C) and the presence of diabetes-related conditions (Table 46.2).

In nondiabetic patients, testosterone is not routinely measured unless the individual elicits either symptoms or signs of testosterone deficiency. In men with diabetes, however, low testosterone is more common, and frequently it is useful to screen for this as part of the initial evaluation. There is some debate of whether total or free testosterone should be measured. Total testosterone depends on the amount of testosterone that is bound to sex hormone–binding globulin (SHBG) as well as to albumin. SHBG increases with age, especially in men over age 55 years, making the total testosterone level less useful in this age-group. Also, testosterone will be affected by any significant change in serum proteins, such as that seen in the nephrotic syndrome. In the past, some have argued to check free testosterone to avoid this issue. Often though, the free testosterone assay is not accurate. A reasonable approach, especially if there is any concern regarding the reliability of the free testosterone assay, is to measure a total testosterone level, preferably in the morning when testosterone levels peak. Any low value should be confirmed with a repeat measurement. If there is a question of a protein-binding issue (i.e., if the patient is over 55 years or has nephrotic syndrome), obtain a direct measurement of SHBG and determine if there is any significant change in the level that is affecting total testosterone values.

If the testosterone is low, the next step is to measure the leutinizing hormone. An elevated level indicates primary testicular failure, whereas a normal or low level is seen in central hypogonadism. If the testosterone level is normal in a patient with a normal physical examination, no further laboratory evaluation is needed.

Nocturnal Penile Tumescence and Rigidity Monitoring

If the differentiation between organic and psychogenic ED is difficult to determine, measuring nocturnal penile activity may be beneficial. A portable home monitor, the RigiScan, can measure tumescence and rigidity while the patient sleeps in the privacy of his own home. Patients with ED of an organic origin should have an abnormal nocturnal tumescence study. Patients with psychogenic disease may still have nocturnal erections. Thus, the presence of normal nocturnal erections confirms a psychogenic etiology for ED.

Further Testing

Duplex ultrasound after the intracavernosal injection of papaverine or prostaglandin E1 can be used to monitor cavernosal artery pressure. Caution should be taken when interpreting these results, however, because decreased blood flow is seen in men with diabetes who have normal erectile function versus control subjects. There is still no substitute for a good history and examination of lower-extremity pulses and femoral bruits for diagnosing vascular disease. The patient's history and physical examination will generally disclose the presence of diabetic neuropathy.

TREATMENT

The first consideration in a man who has diabetes and ED is to achieve optimal control of his blood glucose while avoiding hypoglycemia. In addition, if the patient is on a drug that is known to affect erectile function, consider changing the medication to an agent less likely to be a problem. Even if the agent is not the entire cause for the ED, and full function does not resume, the medication may be contributing along with other factors. Patients with primary gonadal failure need permanent testosterone replacement. Treatment of testosterone deficiency will help ameliorate the symptoms of gonadal insufficiency—lethargy, depression, muscle weakness, anemia, and osteoporosis. Although men with primary gonadal failure and ED and no other medical problems will frequently respond to testosterone therapy, men with other medical problems such as diabetes and especially men with slightly low testosterone levels will usually not see a reversal of ED by supplementing with testosterone. The use of testosterone, however, may prove beneficial in conjunction with other therapies. Because testosterone may aggravate a preexisting prostate cancer, a digital rectal examination and a prostate-specific antigen test (PSA) should be performed before testosterone treatment. The rectal examination and PSA should be rechecked after 3–6 months of treatment. An abnormal examination or an increase in the PSA >1.5 ng/ml implies prostatic stimulation that warrants evaluation by a urologist. Hematocrit levels should also be checked regularly because of the risk of polycythemia, especially in smokers. A baseline hematocrit >52% or a rise to >54% is a contraindication to testosterone therapy.

If controlling blood glucose, changing medications, or replacing testosterone does not sufficiently reestablish normal sexual function, other methods should be considered. Because of the variety of therapies available, treatment for ED should be tailored to the patient's complaints, using the therapy most readily accepted by the patient. Patients who have no trouble attaining an adequate erection with foreplay but who lose the erection prematurely before ejaculation are said to have early detumescence or venous leakage. They do not need medications or devices to produce an erection but rather something to prevent detumescence. Rubber constriction devices such as rings of various sizes or adjusting constriction bands are available and are simple, safe, and inexpensive. The vast majority of patients with diabetes who have a significant neurovascular component as the cause of their ED should be started with oral therapy.

Oral Medications

Released in early 1998, sildenafil (Viagra) has revolutionized the treatment of ED. Sildenafil inhibits phosphodiesterase type 5 (PDE-5). During sexual stimulation, nitric oxide is released in the corpus cavernosum, which activates guanylate cyclase and results in increased levels of cyclic guanosine monophosphate (cGMP). This causes smooth muscle relaxation in the corpus cavernosum, allowing increased blood flow with tissue expansion. PDE-5 degrades cGMP, which allows the penis to return to its usual flaccid state. Inhibition of PDE-5 by sildenafil causes an increase in cGMP with subsequent increased vasodilation.

The drug is rapidly absorbed with peak serum levels ~30–120 min after taking it. Therefore, patients should be instructed to take the medication about 1 h before attempting intercourse and that sexual stimulation (foreplay) is necessary to attain an erection. Absorption of the drug is delayed with a fatty meal. The recommended starting dose of sildenafil is 50 mg 1 h before sexual activity. The dosage can be increased to 100 mg if needed or decreased to 25 mg if the side effects outlined below occur. A patient should not take more than one dose each day.

Sildenafil has been shown to improve erections in up to 70% of men with diabetes and ED. Patients with complete or near-complete loss of erectile function have a lower response rate. The most common side effects include headache, flushing, dyspepsia, and nasal congestion. The drug is contraindicated for patients taking nitrates because of the high likelihood of developing significant hypotension.

Concern has been raised regarding the cardiac safety of sildenafil. Studies have not shown sildenafil to increase the risk of a cardiac event. Physicians need to remember that patients with ED are more likely to have cardiac disease and that several of the risk factors for ED are also risk factors for coronary artery disease. In the diabetes population, this concern needs to be even higher because of the possibility of silent ischemia. If the physician has any concern regarding possible undiagnosed cardiac ischemia, cardiac stress testing should be performed before initiating therapy. A prescription for sildenafil should be considered on par with a prescription for initiation of a new exercise regimen, and appropriate cardiac precautions should be taken.

Vardenafil (Levitra) was approved for use in the U.S. in August 2003. This agent also works by inhibition of PDE-5. The drug reaches maximal concentration in 1 h. The starting dose is 10 mg with the option to increase to 20 mg. Dosages of 2.5 mg and 5 mg are available for patients on antiretroviral therapy or ketoconazole.

Vardenafil has been shown to improve erections in about 70% of men with diabetes and ED. Common side effects include headache, flushing, rhinitis, and dyspepsia. The drug is contraindicated for patients taking nitrates or α-blockers because of the risk of hypotension.

Tadalafil (Cialis) was approved for use in the U.S. in November 2003. This agent is the third PDE-5 inhibitor available. Its pharmacokinetics are quite different, with maximal concentration achieved 2 h (0.5–6.0 h) after taking the drug as it has a half-life of 24 h. Thus, the drug is less an option to take on demand but rather in anticipation of sexual activity later. The starting dose is 10 mg with options to increase to 20 mg or to decrease to 5 mg as needed.

Tadalafil has been shown to improve erections in up to 70% of men with diabetes and ED. Common side effects include headache, flushing, rhinitis, dyspepsia, and lower back pain. The latter is felt to be due to cross-reactivity with PDE-11 present in skeletal muscle. The drug is contraindicated with nitrates and with α-blockers, with the exception of tamulosin.

Differences exist in the potencies of these agents but whether this difference translates into more effective therapy remains to be seen. To date, no head-to-head, controlled trials have been performed.

For patients who do not respond to a PDE-5 inhibitor or who have a contraindication to its use, second-line therapy can involve intracavernosal injection therapy, intraurethral prostaglandin E1 therapy, or the use of a vacuum assistance device.

Intracavernosal Injection Therapy

The effectiveness of intrapenile injection with vasoactive substances was first demonstrated in 1983. Papavarine and phentolamine are used in combination. The addition of prostaglandin E1 was found to improve the results, with up to 90% of patients responding. Recently, the use of prostaglandin E1 alone has increased. It is the only intrapenile drug approved for use by the U.S. Food and Drug Administration. It does not appear to be as effective in diabetic ED (~50% success rate) as the mixtures. Acceptance of this therapy has been limited by the patient's willingness to perform intrapenile injections. Studies have revealed that half of all patients do not continue therapy by the end of 1 year. Penile scarring and priapism are potential complications.

Intraurethral Therapy

Prostaglandin E1 has been formulated into an intraurethral suppository that is absorbed into the corpora spongiosum of the glans penis and migrates rapidly into the corpora cavernosa. In men with diabetes, 40–60% will attain adequate erections with this therapy. Penile or scrotum pain and orthostatic hypotension are rare complications.

Vacuum Assistance Devices

Vacuum pumps are plastic cylinders that are placed over the penis. Air is evacuated from the cylinder, creating a negative pressure drawing venous blood into the penis. A ring is placed around the base of the penis to retain the erection. Satisfactory erections are obtained in ~75% of patients, and ~50% of patients have long-term satisfaction with the resulting sexual function. This method is safe but quite mechanical. Younger men and those patients who do not have a long-term relationship may find the technique cumbersome and embarrassing. Yet some couples use the procedure of pumping the device and placement of the ring as a form of foreplay and turn this negative factor into a positive one. Greater involvement of the partner in the decision process will often increase the likelihood for use of a vacuum assistance device.

Penile Implants

Penile implants were the first modern therapy for ED. There are two basic types. The simpler model is the semirigid rod. The second type, an inflatable rod, has more hardware that is placed in the penis and scrotum. Earlier models had a high rate of mechanical failure, but this rate has decreased significantly with engineering improvements. Satisfaction rates among men with diabetes and their partners are frequently quite high. With the development of newer therapies, the number of implants performed yearly has substantially decreased.

New Therapies

Apomorphine is now available in Europe for the treatment of ED. The drug is a D1/D2 dopamine agonist that acts centrally to improve erectile function without effects on libido. Administered sublingually, apomorphine has a rapid onset of action (~15 min). Efficacy is less than that seen with PDE-5 inhibitors. Nausea, yawning, and somnolence are the most common side effects. Its role in the treatment of ED in the U.S. remains to be seen.

When to Refer a Diabetes Patient with ED

After performing the initial evaluation, therapy may be started if the cause of ED is clear and the physician is comfortable with the use of oral therapy. If the cause is not clear or if therapy with an oral medication is not successful, the patient should be referred to a specialist for further treatment.

SUGGESTED READINGS

Drugs that cause sexual dysfunction: an update (Review). *Med Lett Drugs Ther* 34:73–78, 1992

Feldman HA, Goldstein I, Hatzichristou DG, Krane RJ, McKinley JB: Impotence and its medical and psychosocial correlates: results of the Massachusetts Male Aging Study. *J Urol* 151:54–61, 1994

Hakim LS, Goldstein I: Diabetic sexual dysfunction. *Endocrinol Metab Clin North Am* 25:379–400, 1996

Kaiser KE, Viosca SP, Morley JE, Mooradian AD, Davis SS, Korenman SG: Impotence and aging: clinical and hormonal factors. *J Am Geriatr Soc* 36:511–519, 1988

Lue TF: Erectile dysfunction. *NEJM* 342:1802–1813, 2000

Meuleman E, et al.: Clinical evaluation and the doctor-patient dialogue. In: *Erectile Dysfunction*. Plymouth, UK, Plymbridge Distributors, 2000; p. 115–138

Sharpless J, Snow K: Gender-specific issues. In *Joslin's Diabetes Deskbook*. Boston, MA, Joslin Diabetes Center, 2001, p. 473–50

Snow KJ: Erectile dysfunction: a review and update. *Formulary* In press.

Dr. Snow is Associate Chief of Adult Diabetes and Director of the Sexual Function Clinic, Joslin Clinic, Joslin Diabetes Center, Boston, MA.

47. Sexual Dysfunction in the Female Diabetes Patient

FELECIA RITTENHOUSE FICK, CRTT, RPA-C, AND DEBORAH J. LIGHTNER, MD

Diabetes affects the vascular, renal, and neurological systems, secondarily disturbing sexual function in the affected female at higher rates than in nondiabetic patients. Whereas many publications address various aspects of erectile dysfunction in men with diabetes, female sexual dysfunction, which is more prevalent than male sexual dysfunction, remains much less discussed and less studied. Patient modesty, health care provider time, and third-party insurance coverage may limit the evaluation of this important quality-of-life issue. We review herein the available information on this subject so that the female diabetic population might be better served.

GETTING STARTED: THE MEDICAL REVIEW

The key to helping the female diabetes patient is to address her sexual health during the history portion of the clinical visit. Health care providers are increasingly pressured to see more patients and spend less time with each one. This time constraint makes it difficult for providers to ask about a patient's sexual function. Health care providers may not be well versed on the right questions to ask and thereby are unable to establish by history the sexual dysfunction that is bothersome to the patient or the current treatment appropriate for this problem. Concern may exist that the provider is unable to offer help with these sensitive issues, but there are increasingly effective therapies available.

A sexual history should take only a few minutes and can be incorporated into the screening questions for abuse. As routine as it is to ask about the patient's safety, the health care provider can inquire about a patient's sexual function; it is an important component of quality of life. The questions should be specifically aimed at the four types of female sexual dysfunction that occur:

1. hypoactive sexual desire disorder, or decreased libido
2. female sexual arousal disorder
3. female orgasmic disorder
4. female sexual pain disorder

Each disorder occurs separately from the others. For example, a woman may have hypoactive sexual desire disorder but can be stimulated, aroused, and capable of a pleasurable and orgasmic experience. Alternatively, a patient with an arousal disorder, such as failure to lubricate, may be orgasmic if able to supply the lubrication with commercially available water-based lubricants. Specific questions might include, "Have you noticed a decrease in your sexual desire?" and "Do you think about sexual activity less often than you used to?" For arousal disorders, common in diabetes patients, specific questions might include, "Do you have difficulty staying aroused once you become sexually involved?" "Are your vaginal tissues dry during sexual experiences?" "Are you able to have an orgasm?" "Do you have pain with sexual activity?" and "Where does this occur?" Most important, in any sexual history, is the question of how significant this symptom is to the patient. Furthermore, sexuality changes with the life cycle, and decreased sexual desire or responsiveness may be normal during lactation, with certain medications and chemotherapy agents, or with the recent loss of a spouse. It is the patient's own degree of discomfort that should direct further investigation and therapy.

Health care providers may request that a patient return at another time for a longer appointment to fully address sexual concerns. Likewise, referral to another health care provider more conversant in sexual dysfunction may also be appropriate, and the patient should be so advised.

REFERRAL TO A SPECIALIST

The greatest continuity of care comes from the patient's primary care provider. If the primary care recommendations fail to adequately address the patient's sexual health, then a referral to a specialist should be considered. Specialists in female sexual dysfunction may include urologists, gynecologists, psychologists, or psychiatrists. Physician assistants who specialize in this area of medicine can also provide quality health care as well as long-term follow-up, which is important for this patient population. A team approach is especially helpful because sexual dysfunction is a multifaceted reflector of the patient's overall mental, physical, and emotional health.

PATHOPHYSIOLOGY AND RISK FACTORS

In one study, premenopausal women with type 1 diabetes did not report higher rates of desire, disorder, orgasmic dysfunction, or pain problems than healthy women with similar backgrounds. However, a recent animal study in diabetic female rat vaginas demonstrated thinning of vaginal epithelial cell layers (about half as many layers as in normal healthy rats), decreased vaginal submucosal vasculatures, and vaginal tissue fibrosis. This combination of adverse changes, if occurring in the female with diabetes, might lead to decreased vaginal lubrication, decreased arousal, and possible dyspareunia. Vaginal lubrication is a transudate of plasma and therefore requires a responsive genital vascular supply. Inability to increase blood flow to the genital organs that produce this normal transudate can result in dyspareunia. A decline in vaginal blood flow, therefore, may be related to sexual arousal disorders. Consistent with this, a study of females with type 1 diabetes demonstrated decreased levels of vaginal pulse amplitude (a measure of the responsiveness of genital blood flow) compared with healthy control subjects.

However, other measurements such as labial temperatures during sexual arousal did not show any difference between females with and without type 1 diabetes.

A recent comparison study of older women with type 2 diabetes and healthy age-matched control subjects revealed an increased prevalence of sexual dysfunction in the women with type 2 diabetes across all four diagnostic categories. It is possible that as the vagina loses elasticity and the blunted vasoactive responsiveness reduces lubrication, the effects of diabetes may become more apparent in the aging individual with diabetes. In the study mentioned, ~50% of the women with diabetes were postmenopausal. Additionally, could the associated obesity common in many women with type 2 diabetes result in hypoactive sexual desire disorder from a distortion of body image? A single study suggests that this may not be interrelated. In this group of females with type 1 diabetes, there was no correlation of female sexual dysfunction with either age or BMI.

THERAPEUTIC INTERVENTION

If a woman's sexual dysfunction is mild and of brief duration, practical and brief intervention by the health care team may be effective. Supportive therapy for life events can be curative of their distress. Other treatment options might include treatment for disturbed sleep and the multiple somatic manifestations of depression, if found. The cessation or replacement of any of the multiple drugs associated with secondary female sexual dysfunction can also be efficacious. These drugs include antihistamines, antihypertensives, anticholinergics, and any drug that causes related side effects or modifications in the central nervous system, including sedatives, hypnotics, pain medications, antiepileptic medications, and antidepressants. Patients with premature ovarian dysfunction may respond to hormonal supplementation. Arousal disorders secondary to atrophic vaginal tissues and poor vaginal lubrication may respond to low-level estrogen replacement in the form of a pill, a patch, or vaginal cream, with estrogen reversing vaginal atrophy generally within a 6-week treatment period. Vaginal lubricants are helpful in premenopausal women with diabetes or postmenopausal women who have risk factors preventing estrogen replacement. Although recent events suggest that androgen therapy may help improve female sexual dysfunction in women failing adequate estrogen replacement after a surgically induced menopause, there is *no* documented placebo-controlled trial demonstrating a therapeutic benefit of androgen for premenopausal women with hypoactive sexual desire or other sexual disorders. Beyond this, safe androgen replacement doses have not been established for women, and available formulations are largely dosed for the normally higher levels in men. A further caveat is that androgen supplementation is associated with adverse changes in lipid and liver function profiles and, if used in the postmenopausal female, should be cautiously used, monitored, and stopped if a therapeutic trial is not successful. Currently accepted androgen-estrogen combinations are indicated only for intractable menopausal symptoms.

Other therapies may involve behavioral modifications. To minimize introital localized coitally associated pain occurring with pelvic floor tension myalgia, a patient may find benefit in relaxation exercises for the pubococcygeal muscles of the pelvic floor. Pelvic floor tension myalgia can often be simply diagnosed in the patient with a compatible history by transvaginal palpation of the spastic and poorly relaxing levator muscles, reproducing coital discomfort. Women who have pain on penetration or with thrusting may modify coital positions, giving them more control (i.e., using the female superior position or having both partners lie on their sides). Vaginismus can also be significantly improved with behavioral techniques.

A decrease in orgasmic capacity may result from hypoactive desire, decreased or poorly sustained arousal, or physical discomfort during sex. Therefore, treatment of any of these problems may significantly improve orgasmic capacity. Before assuming that orgasmic disorder is related to diabetic neuropathy, the patient should be carefully asked whether or not she is still orgasmic with other genital stimulation (i.e., manually, with a vibrator, or by a partner). Many women, particularly with age, have a difficult time reaching orgasm from penile-vaginal thrusting alone. Women with orgasmic difficulty may simply require more adequate clitoral stimulation.

Lastly, concerns about infertility may adversely affect a couple's sex life. On the contrary, fear of pregnancy and sexually transmitted diseases can also interfere with sexual desire and activity and can be addressed specifically.

CONCLUSION

Questions regarding female sexual health should be a routine part of the history-taking, because female sexual dysfunction is common yet, without direct questioning, remains underreported by patients. Limited studies have shown that women with diabetes may have an increased risk of female sexual dysfunction over their normal age-matched healthy control subjects. Further research is clearly necessary, because the true prevalence of diabetes resulting in female sexual dysfunction is unknown. If female sexual dysfunction is uncovered, the type of dysfunction is used to direct therapy, with appropriate referrals made as necessary. The female diabetes patient will appreciate the improvement in her quality of life.

BIBLIOGRAPHY

Grady D: Postmenopausal hormones: therapy for symptoms only. *N Engl J Med* 348:1835–1837, 2003

Hays J, Ockene J, Brunner RL, Kotchen JM, Manson JE, Patterson RE, Aragaki AK, Shumaker SA, Brzyski RG, LaCroix AZ, Granke IA, Valanis BG: Effects of estrogen plus progestin on health-related quality of life. *N Engl J Med* 348:1839–1854, 2003

Jensen SB: Sexual dysfunction in insulin-treated diabetics: a six-year follow-up study of 101 patients. *Arch Sex Behav* 15:271–283, 1986

Leedom L, Feldman M, Procci W, Zeidler A: Symptoms of sexual dysfunction and depression in diabetic women. *J Diabetes Complications* 5:38–41, 1991

Schover LR, Jensen SB: *Sexuality and Chronic Illness: A Comprehensive Approach.* New York, Guilford, 1988

Schreiner-Engel P, Schiavi RC, Vietorisz D, Smith H: The differential impact of diabetes type on female sexuality. *J Psychosom Res* 31:23–33, 1987

Slob AK, Koster J, Radder JK, van der Werff ten Bosch JJ: Sexuality and psychophysiological functioning in women with diabetes mellitus. *J Sex Marital Ther* 16:59–69, 1990

Spector IP, Leiblum SR, Carey MP, Rosen RC: Diabetes and female sexual function: a critical review. *Ann Behav Med* 15:257–264, 1993

Tyrer G, Steel JM, Ewing DJ, Bancroft J, Warner P, Clarke BF: Sexual responsiveness in diabetic women. *Diabetologia* 24:166–171, 1983

Wincze JP, Albert A, Bansal S: Sexual arousal in diabetic females: physiological and self-report measures. *Arch Sex Behav* 22:587–601, 1993

Ms. Fick is a certified physician assistant and Dr. Lightner is Associate Professor of Urology in the Department of Urology, Mayo Clinic, Rochester, MN.

48. Postural Hypotension

ITALO BIAGGIONI, MD

Maintenance of upright posture is made possible by instantaneous cardio-vascular adaptation that depends primarily on an intact autonomic nervous system. When this system fails, as may occur with long-standing diabetes mellitus, orthostatic hypotension ensues. The incapacitating nature of orthostatic hypotension underscores the importance of cardiovascular autonomic reflexes for normal life. The cardiovascular autonomic neuropathy seen in patients with diabetes mellitus shares common features with primary autonomic failure. Because the latter has been extensively studied, some of the recommendations in this chapter were derived from our knowledge of this condition. Nonetheless, features pertinent to diabetic autonomic neuropathy are emphasized.

PHYSIOLOGY

When a healthy nondiabetic individual stands, up to 700 ml of blood pools in the legs and lower abdominal veins. Venous return decreases, resulting in a transient decline in cardiac output. The reduction in central blood volume and arterial pressure is sensed by cardiopulmonary volume receptors and arterial baroreceptors. Afferent signals from these receptors reach vasomotor centers in the brain stem. Efferent fibers from these centers reduce parasympathetic output and increase sympathetic outflow. Norepinephrine is released from postganglionic sympathetic nerve terminals at target organs, resulting in an increase in heart rate and cardiac contractility, partial restoration of venous return and diastolic ventricular filling by venoconstriction, and an increase in peripheral resistance by arteriolar vasoconstriction. As a net effect of these adaptive mechanisms, upright cardiac output remains reduced by 10–20% compared with supine, systolic blood pressure is reduced by 5–10 mmHg, diastolic blood pressure increases by 2–5 mmHg, mean blood pressure remains almost unchanged, and heart rate increases by 5–20 beats/min.

PATHOPHYSIOLOGY

Orthostatic hypotension is arbitrarily defined as a decrease in systolic blood pressure >30 mmHg or any fall in diastolic blood pressure on standing. It is best characterized clinically as any decrease in arterial blood pressure that produces symptoms such as light-headedness, blurry vision, and pain in the back of the neck, finally leading to transient loss of consciousness. Symptoms never occur while supine but usually occur shortly after standing and are always relieved immediately on sitting or lying down. Failure to meet these criteria should make us rule out other causes of syncope that may occur in diabetes patients (e.g., hypoglycemia, arrhythmias, transient ischemic attacks).

DIAGNOSIS

Subclinical cardiovascular autonomic neuropathy is relatively common, but overt orthostatic hypotension usually appears as a late complication. Spectral analysis of heart rate variability appears to be very sensitive in detecting cardiac autonomic impairment, but the diagnosis of cardiovascular autonomic neuropathy also can be done easily with simple measurements of heart rate and blood pressure (Table 48.1).

Whereas no single test completely differentiates patients with autonomic failure from age-matched control subjects, taken together, they provide a reliable indicator of the presence and severity of cardiovascular autonomic impairment.

Table 48.1 Assessment of Autonomic Function: Bedside Physiological Tests

Posture
- Measure blood pressure (BP) and heart rate (HR) after patient has been supine 15 min and standing 5 min.
- Express as supine–standing values.
- Normal response: systolic BP = –15 to 0 mmHg, diastolic BP = –5 to 5 mmHg, HR = 0 to 20 bpm

Sinus arrhythmia (SA) ratio
- Have patient breathe deeply six times per minute while monitoring HR in continuous strip.
- Measure longest R-R interval during expiration (R-R$_{exp}$) and shortest R-R interval during inspiration (R-R$_{insp}$). Take average of six breaths.
- SA ratio = R-R$_{exp}$/R-R$_{insp}$.
- Normal response: ≥1.2

Valsalva ratio
- Use a 6- to 12-ml syringe barrel as the mouthpiece connected to the sphygmomanometer.
- Ask patient to blow mercury column to 40 mmHg for 15 s while monitoring HR in continuous strip. Repeat four times. Make sure effort is barred by thorax and not mouth (e.g., by introducing a pin-sized leak in the mouthpiece).
- Measure shortest R-R during strain (R-R$_{strain}$) and longest R-R after release (R-R$_{release}$).
- Valsalva ratio = R-R$_{release}$/R-R$_{strain}$.
- Normal response: ≥1.4

Cold pressor test
- Measure baseline BP and HR. Have patient place hand in ice water for 1 min. Measure BP and HR at end of minute.
- Normal response: rise in systolic BP >15 mmHg

Patients with severe autonomic neuropathy lack the compensatory increase in upright heart rate and plasma norepinephrine that should accompany orthostatic hypotension. Autonomic neuropathy, however, is not always the cause of orthostatic hypotension in diabetes patients. The presence of orthostatic tachycardia usually indicates that the orthostatic hypotension may be triggered by potentially reversible factors in patients with borderline autonomic function (e.g., hypovolemia, pharmacological agents) (Table 48.2). Therefore, these autonomic function tests, or even the simple measurement of supine and upright heart rate, can provide important clinical information.

Two additional factors may precipitate hypotension in patients with autonomic failure. *1*) Meals lower blood pressure dramatically in patients with primary autonomic failure and therefore may provoke symptomatic postprandial orthostatic hypotension. *2*) Insulin lowers blood pressure in diabetes patients with autonomic neuropathy and has no effect in individuals without autonomic neuropathy. The frequency and magnitude of these problems may be small in most patients but may be of importance in a given patient.

PROGNOSIS

A mortality rate as high as 25% in 5 years has been reported in patients with diabetes and autonomic neuropathy. Cardiovascular autonomic neuropathy appears to be an independent risk factor for increased mortality. Patients with autonomic neuropathy frequently have other complications of diabetes, and this may also contribute to their poor prognosis. For example, these patients have silent myocardial ischemia and a prolonged QT interval, which may predispose them to sudden death.

TREATMENT

There is no specific therapy for cardiovascular autonomic neuropathy. Trials involving few patients have shown a slight delay in progression of autonomic neuropathy in patients receiving aldose reductase inhibitors. Data from the Diabetes Control and Complications Trial suggest that intensive insulin therapy may delay the progression of diabetic peripheral neuropathy. Intensive insulin therapy also produced a slight improvement in results of tests of autonomic function. On the other hand, patients with autonomic neuropathy appear to be at a

Table 48.2 Drugs that May Precipitate or Worsen Orthostatic Hypotension in Patients with Autonomic Failure

- Diuretics
- Tricyclic antidepressants
- Phenothiazides
- Venodilators (nitrates)
- Antihypertensives (α-blockers)
- Insulin

greater risk of developing severe hypoglycemia during insulin treatment, and this risk should be considered before intensive therapy is recommended for them. Conversely, hypoglycemia causes transient autonomic impairment that compromises counterregulatory mechanisms, with worsening subsequent hypoglycemic episodes. It is possible that hypoglycemia-induced autonomic failure may also impair orthostatic tolerance.

In general, a stepwise approach to treatment according to the severity of the symptoms is preferable (Table 48.3). These should be considered general guidelines, and treatment should be individualized. Some recommendations may actually be contraindicated in a given patient.

Nonpharmacological Therapy

In patients with persistent symptoms, conservative nonpharmacological therapy is indicated. Medical therapy includes the following (Table 48.3):

- Increase salt intake: Patients with autonomic failure may be unable to conserve sodium, and liberalization of sodium intake is generally recommended.
- Avoid supine diuresis: These patients have exaggerated nocturnal diuresis with relative hypovolemia and worsening of orthostatic hypotension early in the morning. Nocturnal diuresis can be reduced by elevating the head of the bed with 6- to 9-inch blocks.
- Decrease venous pooling: During the day, patients should wear waist-high custom-fitted elastic support stockings that will exert pressure on the legs and reduce venous pooling (some patients find them cumbersome to wear, and sensory neuropathy or vasculopathy may limit their use). Alternatively, abdominal binders can be tried.
- Avoid wearing support stockings while supine because they may contribute to diuresis and supine hypertension.

Table 48.3 Stepwise Approach to Management of Orthostatic Hypotension

1. Remove aggravating factors
   - Volume depletion
   - Anemia
   - Drugs*
   - Prolonged bed rest/deconditioning
   - Alcohol
2. Medical treatment
   - Liberalize salt intake, salt supplements
   - Head-up tilt during the night
   - Waist-high support stockings
   - Exercise as tolerated
3. Pharmacological treatment†
   - Fludrocortisone
   - Short-acting pressor agents

*See Table 48.2. †See Table 48.4.

Pharmacological Therapy

Some patients may require pharmacological therapy in addition to nonpharmacological therapy. At this stage, the goal of treatment is to minimize symptoms rather than to normalize an upright blood pressure:

- Fludrocortisone: Therapy is usually initiated with fludrocortisone acetate at a low dose (0.1 mg/day) and increased slowly to 0.4 mg/day if needed. A weight gain of 1–2 kg and mild ankle edema may be desirable in these patients. However, hypokalemia, supine hypertension, and pulmonary edema may occur, and patients must be monitored carefully. Fludrocortisone will not be effective unless it is given in conjunction with increased salt intake (e.g., sodium chloride tablets, 1 g with meals).
- Pressor agents: The goal in using these drugs is to provide patients with periods when they can remain upright rather than to try to keep severely afflicted patients symptom free throughout the day.

Most of the agents listed in Table 48.4, if effective in a given patient, will increase blood pressure for 2–3 h. In general, these agents are best given before periods of exertion as needed rather than at fixed (e.g., three times per day) intervals. This approach may reduce the likelihood of side effects and the development of tolerance that reduces their long-term efficacy. Patients should also avoid lying down for 4–5 h after taking these drugs to prevent supine hypertension. These drugs have negligible effects in healthy subjects; the increase in blood pressure seen in patients with autonomic failure is a reflection of their extreme hypersensitivity to most pressor and depressor agents. Therefore, treatment should be started at very small doses and should be individualized. This is best

Table 48.4 Pharmacological Agents in Treating Orthostatic Hypotension

Drug	Initial Dose	Side Effects	Contraindications
NaCl	2 g/day	Nausea, diarrhea	
Fludrocortisone (Florinef)	0.1–0.4 mg/day	Hypokalemia Supine hypertension	Congestive heart failure
Midodrine (Proamitine)	5–10 mg*	Scalp itching Goose bumps	
Pseudoephedrine	30–60 mg*	Nervousness, tachycardia	
Yohimbine (Yocon)	5.4 mg*	Nervousness, tremor	
Indomethacin (Indocin)	25 mg	Gastrointestinal discomfort	Peptic ulcer

Refer to more detailed sources for a complete list of side effects and contraindications. *A dose of these short-acting pressor agents, given before exertion, will improve orthostatic symptoms for 2–3 h. In general, administration of more than three doses per day is discouraged to avoid side effects and development of tolerance.

done by measuring blood pressure at 15- to 30-min intervals for 2–3 h after administration of the first dose of each drug. Some of these agents may be contraindicated in patients with other diabetes complications.

Treatment of Related Conditions

Autonomic failure can be associated with low-production anemia and inappropriately low serum erythropoietin levels. If other causes of anemia are ruled out, patients can be treated with recombinant erythropoietin (25–50 units/kg s.c. three times per week). Erythropoietin has been shown to improve upright blood pressure, and its use may be warranted for this reason alone rather than as a treatment for anemia.

Many patients may also have supine hypertension resulting from preexisting essential hypertension or as part of their autonomic failure. In occasional patients, significant hypertension may be present even in the seated position. During the day, supine hypertension is best managed by simply avoiding the supine position. At night, it is often necessary to give vasodilators at bedtime, after which the patient should be advised against getting up during the night without assistance. The following agents have been used with some success:

- very low doses of nitrates as transdermal preparations (e.g., 0.1–0.2 mg/h Nitro-Dur applied at bedtime and removed on arising)
- hydralazine hydrochloride (25–100 mg)
- calcium-channel blockers (e.g., 30 mg nifedipine)

Patients with angina may also be difficult to manage. Nitrates and other venodilators may produce dramatic hypotension in patients with autonomic failure. Conversely, angina may be precipitated by postural hypotension and relieved by resuming the supine position. β-Blockers may be an alternative treatment in these patients if no contraindication to their use exists. Propranolol (20–60 mg/day) and pindolol (15 mg/day) will probably not worsen orthostatic hypotension and may actually improve symptoms in some patients.

BIBLIOGRAPHY

Biaggioni I: Erythropoietin in autonomic failure. In *Primer on Autonomic Function.* Robertson D, Low PA, Polinsky RJ, Eds. San Diego, CA, Academic Press, 1996, p. 332–334

Davis SN, Mann S, Galassetti P, Neill RA, Tate D, Ertl AC, Costa F: Effects of differing durations of antecedent hypoglycemia on counterregulatory responses to subsequent hypoglycemia in normal humans. *Diabetes* 49:1897–1903, 2000

Jankovic J, Gilden JL, Hiner BC, Kaufmann H, Brown DC, Coghlan CH, Rubin M, Fouad-Tarazi FM: Neurogenic orthostatic hypotension: a double-blind, placebo-controlled study with midodrine. *Am J Med* 95:38–48, 1993

Low PA: Diabetic autonomic neuropathy. *Sem Neurol* 16:143–151, 1996

May O, Arildsen H: Assessing cardiovascular autonomic neuropathy in diabetes mellitus: how many tests to use? *J Diabetes Complications* 14:7–12, 2000

Orchard TJ, Lloyd CE, Maser RE, Kuller LH: Why does diabetic autonomic neuropathy predict IDDM mortality? An analysis from the Pittsburgh Epidemiology of Diabetes Complications Study. *Diabetes Res Clin Pract* 34 (Suppl.):S165–S171, 1996

Pagani M: Heart rate variability and autonomic diabetic neuropathy. *Diabetes Nutr Metab* 13:341–346, 2000

Stephenson JM, Kempler P, Cavallo Perin P, Fuller JH: Is autonomic neuropathy a risk factor for severe hypoglycaemia? The EURO-DIAB IDDM Complications Study. *Diabetologia* 39:1372–1376, 1996

Toyry JP, Nisjanen LK, Mantysaari MJ, Lansimies EA, Uusitupa MIJ: Occurrence, predictors, and clinical significance of autonomic neuropathy in NIDDM. *Diabetes* 45:308–315, 1996

Dr. Biaggioni is Professor of Medicine and Pharmacology at Vanderbilt University, Nashville, TN.

49. Heart Disease and Diabetes

Burton E. Sobel, MD

PATHOGENETIC MECHANISMS

Several different types of heart disease and pathogenetic mechanisms are encountered in patients with diabetes. Cardiomyopathy, with a predisposition to congestive heart failure after myocardial infarction, altered integrated ultrasonic backscatter, impaired myocardial energy metabolism, altered calcium cycling, and increased myocardial stiffness, may be a significant problem in the patient with diabetes.

Hypertension and its cardiac sequelae occur with syndromes of insulin resistance. Determinants may include altered endothelial cell (EC) function, potentially exacerbated by hyperglycemia and elevated concentrations of free fatty acids (FFAs) in blood, centrally altered sympathetic vasomotor tone, vessel wall stiffness secondary to advanced glycation end products (AGEs), and abluminal atheromatous changes. EC dysfunction is accompanied by altered expression of adhesion molecules, a prothrombotic state, increased vascular permeability, attenuation of insulin-induced vasodilation mediated by nitric oxide, and accumulation of AGEs that may play a pathogenetic role.

Type 2 diabetes (and to a lesser extent type 1 diabetes) is strongly associated with accelerated coronary atherosclerosis, a procoagulant state, impaired fibrinolysis, and altered smooth muscle cell (SMC) migration and proliferation. Hyperglycemia and elevated concentrations in blood of FFAs, LDL, and glycated and oxidized lipoproteins may impair EC barrier functions and contribute to extracellular matrix–associated accumulation of lipoproteins and glycated and oxidized metabolites. Increased EC and SMC production of procoagulants, adhesion molecules, chemotactic factors, cytokines, and growth factors facilitate adherence and penetration of circulatory monocytes into the neointima, where they become activated macrophages. SMC migration and proliferation and secretion of fibrous caps follow. Hyperglycemia, increased FFAs, and oxidation and glycation products can induce cell death within the tunica media of vessel walls with consequent evolution of plaques with large lipid cores, necrotic and apoptotic components, and thin fibrous caps, all of which predispose to plaque rupture.

A prothrombotic state predisposing to acute coronary syndromes (ACSs) results from an imbalance between coagulation and fibrinolysis. Insulin resistance typical of type 2 diabetes leads to inhibition of fibrinolysis mediated by increased synthesis of plasminogen activator inhibitor type 1 (PAI-1). Elevated concentrations of insulin, proinsulin, tumor necrosis factor-α, FFAs, and triglycerides may contribute. Hyperglycemia augments platelet activation.

Diabetes increases release of cytokines from macrophages as a result of oxidation (via oxygen-centered free radicals) and glycoxidation of proteins and nucleic acids, and accumulation of lipids and AGEs. Accumulation of AGEs in vessel walls traps immunoglobulins with consequent mechanical, biochemical, and receptor- and nonreceptor-mediated altered cellular function, proliferation, and accumulation of matrix. Formation of immune complexes with modified lipoproteins and elevated C-reactive protein is associated with diabetes and may accelerate atherosclerosis. Atherectomy specimens exhibit increased macrophage content and necrotic areas in lesions from patients with diabetes. Restenosis after percutaneous coronary intervention (PCI) is increased and associated with increased collagen. Patients with type 2 diabetes are at risk for sudden death and harbor plaques with increased necrotic cores. By contrast, plaques in type 1 diabetes are typified by increased fibrous tissue and fewer foam cells, which may reflect paradoxically protective phenomena.

A prothrombotic state accompanies both type 1 and type 2 diabetes. Insulin resistance (in type 2 diabetes) as well as hyperglycemia, elevated FFAs, and hypertriglyceridemia lead to increased concentrations of fibrinogen, coagulation factor VII, and PAI-1 in blood and atheroma. Conversely, decreased urokinase (the predominant plasminogen activator in tissue) in plaques and increases in platelet aggregation are typical. PAI-1 is increased in part because of the direct effects of insulin and proinsulin, VLDL, FFAs, and triglycerides on PAI-1 synthesis. Thiazolidinediones, insulin sensitizers, decrease both PAI-1 and carotid intimal-medial thickness.

PAI-1 is increased both in blood and in plaque in type 2 diabetes. It may decrease the capacity of vascular SMCs to migrate into the neointima and hence the secretion of thick fibrous caps that protect plaques against rupture. Potentiation of vulnerability to rupture may result from the dominance in plaques of lipids, macrophages, T-cells, and other structurally nonsupportive elements. In such plaques capped by thin fibrous caps, proteolysis in the shoulder regions initiated by mechanical stimuli, inflammation, and neuro-hormonal stress may precipitate plaque rupture and ACSs, including unstable angina and acute myocardial infarction.

Several markers of inflammation are present within plaques prone to precipitate ACSs, including cytokines, growth factors, C-reactive protein, and bacterial constituents. Macrophages laden with constituents from bacteria can carry antigens from organisms such as chlymadia and mycoplasma into the neointima whether or not they play a pathogenic role in atherogenesis.

CLINICAL CONSIDERATIONS

Diabetes and its predecessors (impaired glucose tolerance, insulin resistance, and obesity, among others) accelerate coronary artery disease (CAD). Mortality from CAD is twofold greater in people with type 2 diabetes. The incidence of ACS is increased in proportion to the duration and severity of type 2 diabetes. In elderly subjects, inadequate glycemic control (glycated hemoglobin A1C >7%) is associated with a 4.3-fold higher risk of mortality from CAD and a 2.2-fold increased risk of any cardiovascular event associated with CAD. More than 35% of patients >55 years of age who sustain acute myocardial infarction have diabetes and insulin resistance.

CORONARY LESIONS IN PATIENTS WITH TYPE 2 DIABETES

Unfortunately, culprit lesions responsible for ACS do not live alone. In fact, the entire coronary vasculature is abnormal in individuals with insulin resistance. The lesions are abluminal and do not necessarily obstruct blood flow. Thus, stress testing and other diagnostic modalities may yield negative diagnostic results. The abluminal, lipid-laden atheroma seen in diabetes are relatively devoid of vascular SMCs, ultrasonically distinguishable, and vulnerable to plaque rupture. Addressing the culprit lesion when an ACS does indeed occur will not thoroughly protect the patient. Reduction of generation of vulnerable plaques will be required.

Congestive heart failure should be treated conventionally with afterload and preload reduction with vasodilators, angiotensin-converting enzyme (ACE) inhibitors and/or angiotensin receptor blockers, diuretics, and judiciously titrated β-adrenergic receptor blockers. Decompensation may require a brain-type natriuretic peptide or cardiotonic agents. Symptomatic coronary disease should be treated conventionally as well, with β-blockers, vasodilators, calcium-channel blockers, and amelioration of exacerbating factors such as arrhythmia, anemia, obesity, thyrotoxicosis, and other comorbidities.

THERAPEUTIC CONSIDERATIONS

Many drugs used for noncardiovascular-targeted reasons may be cardioprotective as well. Thus, ACE inhibitors and angiotensin receptor blockers used for nephroprotection and treatment of hypertension can attenuate elevated NAD(P)H oxygenase activity (proinflammatory), elevated PAI-1, and myocardial fibrosis. Statins and fibrates are anti-inflammatory. Insulin sensitizers and metformin, an inhibitor of hepatic gluconeogenesis, lower PAI-1 and facilitate fibrinolysis. Metabolic control normalizes concentrations of FFAs and triglycerides, thereby decreasing synthesis of PAI-1. Aspirin exerts anti-inflammatory as well as antiplatelet effects.

MANAGEMENT OF DIABETES

Stringent glycemic control is imperative; so is amelioration of insulin resistance. Thus, in addition to sulfonylureas, insulin itself and its congeners, nateglinide, and metformin, peroxisome proliferator-activated receptor ligand agonists that can increase insulin sensitivity (glitazones) should be considered as potentially helpful vasculoprotective agents. Rapid-acting insulin agonists such as lispro, agonists of first-phase insulin secretion such as nateglinide, and inhibitors of glucose absorption (α-glucosidase inhibitors) can enhance metabolic control in addition to that achieved by rigorous lifestyle modification, control of diet, caloric restriction to achieve ideal weight, exercise, and smoking cessation. Hyperlipidemia and hypertension must be ameliorated. Elevated blood pressure is a particularly powerful determinant of cardiac complications.

In patients who do sustain an ACS, treatment of hyperglycemia and dyslipidemia is essential to enhance myocardial energy metabolism and glucose utilization in the presence of insulin resistance.

MANAGEMENT OF CORONARY ARTERIAL LESIONS

When it comes to managing coronary arterial lesions, several dilemmas confront clinicians. These include what to do about lesions in patients without cardiac symptoms, how to manage culprit lesions responsible for ACS, and how to prevent adverse reactions after PCI, known to be more common when type 2 diabetes is present.

Asymptomatic Coronary Lesions

Until recently, treatment of coronary lesions has focused on relieving obstruction to blood flow in epicardial coronary arteries. Percutaneous transluminal coronary angioplasty (PTCA), rotoblation, extraction atherectomy, laser dissolution, drug-eluting stents, and brachytherapy (all of which constitute PCI) are effective. They enhance myocardial perfusion and reduce morbidity associated with unstable CAD. However, patients with diabetes have not benefited commensurately.

Both Falk and Davies demonstrated that morbidity and mortality associated with CAD are often attributable to lesions that are not necessarily obstructive before the acute event but rather are attributable to vulnerable plaques that can now be recognized with intravascular ultrasound, magnetic resonance imaging, thermal analysis, and positron emission tomography. Lesions characterized by rich lipid cores (relative acellularity), thin fibrous caps, and abluminal rather than luminal incursion (i.e., vulnerable plaques) are the prominent cause of ACS in patients with diabetes. Because they occur throughout the coronary tree, attack of a culprit lesion alone with PCI or pharmacological thrombolysis is not sufficient to confer complete protection. The Bypass Angioplasty Revascularization Investigation 2 Diabetes (BARI 2D) trial is designed to determine whether the evolution of CAD can be modified favorably before such vulnerable plaques evolve.

Management of Culprit Lesions

Plaque that precipitates an ACS can be managed in patients with type 2 diabetes with PCI, pharmacological coronary thrombolysis, or a combination of the two. However, diabetes compromises the benefit conferred and increases the risk of complications and recurrent events. The relative adverse impact of diabetes on thrombolysis and PCI is not yet clear. What is likely is that the pivotal determinant of efficacy will not necessarily be the mode of intervention. Instead, the rapidity, completeness, and persistence of restoration of patency of an occluded coronary artery are likely to be paramount. Coronary artery bypass grafting (CABG) may be the preferred method for revascularization, especially in patients with diabetes who have distal and multiple obstructive lesions (see below).

It is not yet clear whether immediate revascularization in patients with type 2 diabetes who have only mild symptoms diminishes morbidity and mortality. Among patients who underwent initial PTCA in the initial BARI trial (BARI 1), subjects with diabetes experienced a greater increase in the percentage of jeopardized myocardium assessed angiographically compared with that in nondiabetic subjects, consistent with a higher long-term mortality after PTCA. One factor responsible was the increased incidence of restenosis.

Although stents diminish restenosis, their use is less salutary in patients with diabetes than in individuals without diabetes. Adverse outcomes associated with diabetes after PCI may reflect deleterious consequences of insulin or proinsulin on vessel walls. Thus, insulin sensitizers may be beneficial. No one would question the necessity of relieving obstructive coronary lesions that precipitate ACSs or refractory symptoms in patients with type 2 diabetes by implementing thrombolysis, PCI, or CABG. However, these interventions do not obviate the underlying and relentless progression of abluminal coronary atherosclerosis.

THE PROBLEM OF RESTENOSIS

Van Belle et al. (2001) found that diabetes leads to adverse outcomes long after implementation of PCI, including an increased incidence of both nonocclusive and occlusive restenosis. Their observations raise the question of whether surgery or PCI is the preferred initial treatment strategy for lesions requiring revascularization. The BARI 1 results (obtained before stents were available) indicate that patients with diabetes do less well after PTCA than after CABG, although the outcome is less favorable with either when diabetes is present, compared with that in individuals without diabetes. What is crucial is the management of the diabetes itself, such that attenuation of progression of vasculopathy is maximized. The BARI 2D trial is testing the hypothesis that insulin-sparing regimens may lead to less rapid progression of coronary vasculopathy with or without the intercession of coronary intervention.

We do not yet know whether immediate (as opposed to symptom-driven) revascularization in patients with type 2 diabetes with mild or absent symptoms of obstructive CAD is beneficial with respect to long-term cardiac morbidity and mortality. In one study of consecutively treated patients undergoing PTCA, restenosis was prominent in individuals with diabetes and was a major determinant of increased long-term mortality. In BARI 1 as well, long-term mortality was higher in patients with diabetes undergoing PTCA. Despite the advent of stents, results remain less salutary in patients with diabetes as opposed to those without diabetes. Adverse responses may reflect paradoxical reduction of intimal hyperplasia in restenotic regions of lesions compatible with increased intramural synthesis of PAI-1, possibly mediated in part by compensatory hyperinsulinemia. Insulin resistance and the associated elevated concentrations of PAI-1 in blood are associated with accelerated CAD whether or not frank diabetes exists. Such changes may be responsible for compositional changes in evolving lesions that predispose to plaque rupture, restenosis, or both. Insulin sensitizers reduce progression of carotid intimal-medial thickness in patients with diabetes and improve the maintenance of patency after coronary stenting.

CONCLUSION

Type 2 diabetes is the archetype of syndromes of insulin resistance and, in turn, the tip of an iceberg apparently responsible for accelerating coronary atherosclerosis. Vulnerable plaques prone to rupture and consequent precipitation of ACS accompany diabetes and insulin resistance. Such lesions are often abluminal and nonobstructive before the occurrence of a catastrophic event. Accordingly, prophylaxis and therapy should target the vessel wall itself, the culprit lesion, and maintenance of cardiac function before, during, and after an acute coronary event. Prevention is paramount. Insulin sensitizers are promising. Treatment of culprit lesions must be vigorous, but in the absence of concomitant therapy attenuating progression of intramural coronary atherosclerotic disease, it cannot be entirely sufficient. The response to PCI is less salutary in people with diabetes than in people without diabetes. The risk of restenosis is high, even with stents. Accordingly, attenuation of progression of coronary atherosclerotic disease by modification of insulin resistance, normalization of glycemia, and implementation of other potentially vasculoprotective measures is essential.

BIBLIOGRAPHY

Davies MJ, Bland M, Hangartner WR, Angellini A, Thomas AC: Factors influencing the presence or absence of acute coronary thrombi in sudden ischemic death. *Eur Heart J* 10:203–208, 1989

Eckel RH, Wassef M, Chait A, Sobel BE, Barrett E, King G, Lopes-Virella M, Reusch J, Ruderman N, Steiner G, Vlassaa H: Prevention Conference VI: Diabetes and Cardiovascular Disease: Writing Group II: Pathogenesis of atherosclerosis in diabetes. *Circulation* 105:138e–143e, 2002

Falk E: Morphologic features of unstable atherothrombotic plaques underlying acute coronary syndromes. *Am J Cardiol* 63:114E–120E, 1989

Falk E: Unstable angina with fatal outcome: dynamic coronary thrombosis leading to infarction and/or sudden death: autopsy evidence of recurrent mural thrombosis with peripheral embolization culminating in total vascular occlusion. *Circulation* 71:699–708, 1985

Jaffe AS, Spadaro JJ, Schechtman K, Roberts R, Geltman EM, Sobel BE: Increased congestive heart failure after myocardial infarction of modest extent in patients with diabetes mellitus. *Am Heart J* 108:31–37, 1984

Juhan-Vague I, Alessi MC, Vague P: Increased plasma plasminogen activator inhibitor 1 levels: a possible link between insulin resistance and atherothrombosis. *Diabetologia* 34:457–462, 1991

Libby P: Molecular bases of the acute coronary syndromes. *Circulation* 91:2213–2221, 1998

Moreno PR, Murcia AM, Palacios IF, Leon MN, Bernardi VH, Fuster V, Fallon JT: Coronary composition and macrophage infiltration in atherectomy specimens from patients with diabetes mellitus. *Circulation* 102:2180–2184, 2000

Perez JE, McGill JB, Santiago JV, Schechtman KB, Waggoner AD, Miller JG, Sobel BE: Abnormal myocardial acoustic properties in diabetic patients and their correlation with the severity of disease. *J Am Coll Cardiol* 19:1154–1162, 1992

Sobel BE: Acceleration of restenosis by diabetes: pathogenetic implications. *Circulation* 103:1185–1187, 2001

Sobel BE, Frye R, Detre KM: Burgeoning dilemmas in the management of diabetes and cardiovascular disease: rationale for the Bypass Angioplasty Revascularization Investigation 2 Diabetes (BARI 2D) trial. *Circulation* 107:636–642, 2003

Sobel BE, Taatjes DJ, Schneider DJ: Intramural plasminogen activator inhibitor type-1 (PAI-1) and coronary atherosclerosis. *Arterioscler Thromb Vasc Biol.* 23:1979–1989, 2003

Sobel BE, Woodcock-Mitchell J, Schneider DJ, Holt RE, Marutsuka K, Gold H: Increased plasminogen activator inhibitor type-1 in coronary artery atherectomy specimens from type 2 diabetic compared with nondiabetic patients: a potential factor predisposing to thrombosis and its persistence. *Circulation* 97:2213–2221, 1998

Van Belle E, Ketelers R, Bauters C, Perie M, Abolmaali K, Richard F, Lablanche JM, McFadden EP, Bertrand ME: Patency of percutaneous transluminal coronary angioplasty sites at 6-month angiographic follow-up: a key determinant of survival in diabetics after coronary balloon angioplasty. *Circulation* 103:1218–1224, 2001

Dr. Sobel is Amidon Professor and Chair, Department of Medicine, University of Vermont College of Medicine, Colchester, VT.

50. Noninvasive Cardiac Testing

JEFF P. STEINHOFF, MD, VENU MENON, MD, AND SIDNEY C. SMITH JR., MD

Diabetes mellitus quadruples the risk of developing atherosclerotic coronary heart disease, which is the leading cause of death in the diabetes population. Of the estimated 18 million Americans with diabetes, ~20% (or 3.6 million) are asymptomatic. In addition to presenting with premature coronary heart disease, patients with diabetes have markedly worse short- and long-term prognosis than their nondiabetic counterparts. The 7-year mortality rate for diabetes patients without prior myocardial infarction (MI) (20%) is similar to that of nondiabetic patients with a prior MI (19%). People with diabetes also have worse in-hospital mortality with MI, worse outcomes after treatment with thrombolysis, and worse prognosis after the development of cardiogenic shock. The likelihood of restenosis after percutaneous coronary intervention is increased in patients with diabetes, even when coronary stents are used. The presence of diabetes is particularly detrimental in women and negates the protective effect of female sex in the premenopausal period. Women with diabetes also display higher 28-day and 1-year mortality after MI than their nondiabetic counterparts.

Given the inherent risk of manifesting occult or established coronary heart disease, the American Diabetes Association recommends noninvasive cardiac testing to evaluate patients with symptoms suggestive of coronary heart disease or with an abnormal resting electrocardiogram. It is also suggested that screening testing may be performed in the following populations: 1) patients with a history of peripheral vascular disease or carotid disease; 2) patients who are sedentary, who over the age of 35 years, and who are planning to begin rigorous exercise; and 3) patients with more than two risk factors (hypertension, tobacco abuse, strong family history, elevated cholesterol, and micro- or macroalbuminuria). The following discussion will review the results of tests specifically designed to evaluate the heart. Tests such as the ankle-brachial index and the carotid Doppler ultrasound, which can identify the presence of peripheral arterial disease, a known marker for coronary heart disease, will not be covered in this section.

RESTING ELECTROCARDIOGRAM

The resting 12-lead electrocardiogram (ECG) is a safe, inexpensive, and easily available test. It may reveal diagnostic Q waves that indicate silent MI in this population. The rates of silent MI as diagnosed by a surface ECG in the Framingham study 30-year follow-up were 28% for men and 35% for women; however, diabetes has not conclusively emerged as an independent predictor of silent MI. Although insensitive, presence of ECG criteria for left ventricular hypertrophy is a relatively specific indicator for increased left ventricular mass in the adult population. Left ventricular hypertrophy is an adverse risk marker for future cardiovascular complications.

In patients being evaluated for an acute coronary syndrome, the presence of diagnostic ST elevation on the ECG is a marker for an occluded infarct related artery. These subjects require emergent consideration for primary reperfusion therapy with thrombolysis or primary percutaneous intervention. Patients with dynamic ST segment changes or resting ST depression on their ECG are also at high risk for subsequent death or MI or may require urgent revascularization.

RESTING ECHOCARDIOGRAM

The echocardiogram is a safe noninvasive ultrasound evaluation of the heart that provides useful information in the diabetes patient with suspected coronary heart disease. It can diagnose the presence of left ventricular contractile dysfunction, a powerful predictor of future cardiovascular risk. Patients with occult or manifest coronary heart disease may have wall motion abnormalities on this study, which are diagnostic for prior MI or consistent with ischemia in the territory of a coronary artery. Other forms of cardiomyopathy secondary to hypertension or microvascular disease may also become apparent. In addition, the echocardiogram provides invaluable information about valvular function and right ventricular function and provides an accurate estimate of pulmonary artery pressures.

EXERCISE TREADMILL TESTING

The standard exercise treadmill test (ETT) uses periodically increasing workloads such as treadmill speed and elevation to increase a patient's heart rate. The target heart is ≥85% of the age-predicted maximum heart rate. The age-predicted maximal heart rate in beats per minute is calculated as 220 minus the age of the patient in years. An ischemic response is often defined as ≥1 mm horizontal or downsloping ST depression at 60–80 ms after the J-point occurring during exercise or recovery. High-risk end points that warrant termination of the test include the following: ≥2 mm of ST segment depression, ST elevation in leads without prior Q waves, a drop in systolic blood pressure or inability to increase systolic blood pressure from baseline, severe limiting angina, multifocal premature ventricular beats, or ischemic changes within the first 3 min of the test.

Lee et al. (2001) evaluated the accuracy of ETT in 190 patients with diabetes. A total of 73 patients (38%) had ischemic findings. Subsequent coronary angiography revealed a sensitivity of 47%, a specificity of 81%, a positive predictive value of 85%, and a negative predictive value of 41%. Subjects with left ventricular hypertrophy and females were at high risk to develop false-positive ECGs. The stress ECG is also not interpretable in patients with left bundle branch block and pre-excitation. These patients should have concomitant imaging studies as part of their diagnostic evaluation. A significant proportion of patients with diabetes have morbid obesity, peripheral vascular disease, or peripheral neuropathy, which impede performance of exercise. A pharmacological stress study using adenosine, dipyridamole, or dobutamine should be considered in this subset.

STRESS ECHOCARDIOGRAPHY

Stress echocardiography combines ECG monitoring with echocardiographic evaluation of wall motion. It is often added to a standard ETT to increase the sensitivity and specificity and add incremental prognostic information. Inducible wall-motion abnormalities precede symptoms in the classic ischemic cascade. This is especially true in diabetes patients who may not have typical angina symptoms with exercise. Dobutamine stress echocardiography (DSE) can be used as an alternative to exercise, and the safety of this modality has been established. The response of the normal myocardial segment to exercise is to increase contractility, which is manifested by increased wall thickening of the segment. A biphasic response or a failure to augment contractility in a vascular territory is strongly suggestive of an underlying ischemic substrate. The extent of wall-motion abnormality and the inability of the ventricular cavity size to diminish are markers for high-risk anatomy. In addition, DSE is also able to distinguish between hibernating, stunned, and infarcted myocardial segments.

Kamalesh et al looked at mortality in 233 patients (98% male) with normal stress echocardiograms, of which 89 (37%) had diabetes. A high MI and cardiovascular death rate in diabetes patients with normal stress echocardiograms compared with nondiabetic subjects (6.0% vs. 2.7% per year) was reported. Marwick et al. prospectively evaluated a larger cohort of 937 diabetes patients after stress echocardiography. This cohort was 57% male, with a mean age of 59 ± 13 years. Although a normal stress echocardiogram was associated with a better prognosis, patients who had a normal exercise echocardiogram had markedly better outcomes (4%, 2-year mortality) compared with those patients with normal dobutamine echocardiograms (17%, 2-year mortality). In fact, the inability to exercise was the strongest prognostic factor for cardiovascular death and MI. In a cohort of 396 diabetes patients, Sozzi et al. (2003) found the event rate for death or MI was lower but not inconsequential in a normal DSE with 5%, 8%, and 10% at 1, 3, and 5 years, respectively. This evidence underscores the importance of aggressive risk factor treatment in all diabetes patients, regardless of a "negative" stress echocardiogram. People with diabetes who have an abnormal DSE result represent a subgroup at very high risk. The likelihood of cardiac death or MI with an abnormal DSE (fixed or ischemic response) resulted in a 7%, 18%, and 23% event rate at 1, 3, and 5 years, respectively. Similarly, Marwick's data in diabetic patients with established coronary heart disease showed 10%, 22%, and 38% mortality at 1, 3, and 5 years with a DSE demonstrating ischemia.

MYOCARDIAL PERFUSION IMAGING

Myocardial perfusion imaging (MPI) uses the radioisotopes such as thallium, technetium sestamibi, and technetium tetrofosmin as flow tracers. In this modality, exercise and dobutamine are used to increase to target heart rate or adenosine and dipyridamole are administered for vasodilation. Under stress, myocardium supplied by normal or nonsignificantly diseased coronary arteries will receive adequate blood flow and tracer uptake will be uniform. Diseased coronary arteries are unable to increase blood flow to meet the increased demand. The myocardium beyond these diseased segments will have diminished tracer uptake and demonstrate a "perfusion defect."

There have been numerous studies reporting the prognostic value of MPI. De Lorenzo et al. (2002) evaluated 180 asymptomatic diabetes patients with exercise or dipyridamole technetium-99m sestamibi. In addition to finding silent ischemia in 21%, the study revealed a 2% annual death and MI rate for normal and 9% rate for abnormal MPI studies. The worst prognosis was seen in patients with "mixed" defects, indicating a combination of myocardial scar from a prior silent MI and ischemic tissue.

Berman et al. (2003) found a similarly higher event rate in patients with diabetes compared with nondiabetic subjects. In a study that compared 1,222 diabetes patients with 4,111 nondiabetic patients, a higher annual mortality rate in type 1 diabetes patients versus type 2 diabetes patients versus nondiabetic patients of 2.5%, 1.8%, and 0.6%, respectively, was reported for normal MPI studies. Higher cardiac mortality was also seen in abnormal scans with a 9% annual mortality for patients with type 1 diabetes compared with 4.6% and 4.7% annual mortality for nondiabetic patients and type 2 diabetes patients, respectively. In this cohort, type 1 diabetes patients were more likely to be younger, have had a prior MI, have undergone prior angioplasty and coronary artery bypass grafting surgery, and be diagnosed with hypertension.

For patients who cannot tolerate adenosine or dipyridamole infusion because of bronchospasm, allergy, or marked bradycardia, dobutamine stress MPI is a useful option with prognostic value in patients with diabetes. Schinkel et al. followed a cohort of 207 diabetes patients who underwent dobutamine stress MPI with technetium-99m sestamibi or tetrofosmin. This population had a higher degree of abnormal scans (64%) than other studies. Nevertheless, this cohort demonstrated a similar poor prognosis in patients with abnormal results, with a death or MI rate of ~10%, 22%, and 28% at 1, 3, and 5 years, respectively. The event rate was similarly low for normal perfusion studies and was ~0–1%, 3%, and 5% at 1, 3, and 5 years, respectively. As with other studies, prognosis was also correlated with the extent of ischemia.

Vanzetto evaluated 158 high-risk diabetes patients who were defined as having two or more risk factors (age >65 years, hypertension, tobacco abuse, peripheral vascular disease, microalbuminuria, elevated cholesterol, or abnormal resting ECG). These patients underwent exercise or dipyridamole thallium MPI. Although a low overall annual event rate (1.5%) was observed in patients with normal perfusion or ≤22% of myocardium with perfusion defects, a marked difference was again demonstrated between patients who could and could not exercise. The annual mortality was 0.7% for patients who could exercise and demonstrated normal or ≤22% abnormal perfusion area, compared with 4.6% in patients unable to exercise with similar perfusion. The annual rate for cardiac death was 11.6% for patients with >22% of myocardium with ischemia and 23.3% for combined cardiac death and MI. Giri et al. (2002) evaluated 929 diabetes patients and also found multivessel ischemia to be a powerful predictor for adverse outcomes. Women with diabetes are at higher risk for adverse events after abnormal MPI studies. In the cohort examined by Berman et al. (2003), female diabetes subjects had statistically higher annual mortality for all perfusion abnormalities compared with their male counterparts. Hachamovitch also demonstrated higher mortality in female diabetes subjects compared with male subjects for any given ischemic burden, regardless of therapy. Furthermore, it also appeared that despite the >50% reduction in mortality observed with revascularization in both sexes, women still had higher mortality.

ELECTRON BEAM COMPUTED TOMOGRAPHY

Coronary heart disease manifests with a significant amount of atherosclerotic plaque before the arterial lumen is compromised. This plaque, which is associated with the arterial intima, may calcify as a result of age, ongoing inflammation, or other unrecognized factors. Electron beam computed tomography (EBCT) quantitates the calcium level in the coronary arteries. Unfortunately, the arteries of patients with diabetes often have independent calcification of the arterial media (Monckeberg's calcinosis), which cannot be distinguished by EBCT. Although EBCT has prognostic value in certain populations and age-groups as a marker of atherosclerotic burden and subclinical coronary heart disease, it is not currently recommended by the American Heart Association for diagnosis or prognosis in patients with diabetes.

INVASIVE TESTING

The limitations of coronary angiography have been well shown by the use of intravascular ultrasound. Despite this, coronary angiography remains the gold standard for diagnosis and evaluation as well as clinical decision-making in current practice. Angiography is recommended for patients with noninvasive studies demonstrating multivessel disease or other high-risk findings. Subjects with symptoms and signs suggestive of a high pretest likelihood of disease should proceed to coronary angiography directly. Coronary angiography does have a small incidence of adverse events such as renal failure, stroke, MI, vascular access site injury, bleeding, and infection. The role of newer modalities such as multi-detector row CT (MDCT) angiography and magnetic resonance (MR) angiography is currently being explored.

BIBLIOGRAPHY

American Diabetes Association: Standards of medical care in diabetes (Position Statement). *Diabetes Care* 27:S15–S35, 2004

American Diabetes Association/American College of Cardiology: *Diabetes and Cardiovascular Disease Review*. Issue 5: Coronary Heart Disease in Women With Diabetes, 2003, pp. 1–8

Berman DS, Kang X, Hayes SW, Friedman JD, Cohen I, Abidov A, Shaw LJ, Amanullah AM, Germano G, Hachamovitch R: Adenosine myocardial perfusion single-photon emission computed tomography in women compared with men: impact of diabetes mellitus on incremental prognostic value and effect on patient management. *J Am Coll Cardiol* 41:1125–1133, 2003

De Lorenzo A, Lima RSL, Siqueira-Filho AG, Pantoja MR: Prevalence and prognostic value of perfusion defects detected by stress technetium-99m sestamibi myocardial perfusion single-photon emission computed tomography in asymptomatic patients with diabetes mellitus and no known coronary artery disease. *Am J Cardiol* 90:827–832, 2002

Giri S, Shaw LJ, Murthy DR, Travin MI, Miller DD, Hachamovitch R, Borges-Neto S, Berman DS, Waters DD, Heller GV: Impact of diabetes on the risk stratification using stress single-photon emission computed tomography myocardial perfusion imaging in patients with symptoms suggestive of coronary artery disease. *Circulation* 105:32–40, 2002

Hachamovitch R, Hayes SW, Friedman JD, Cohen I, Berman DS. Comparison of the short-term survival benefit associated with revascularization compared with medical therapy in patients with no prior coronary artery disease undergoing stress myocardial perfusion single photon emission computed tomography. *Circulation* 107:2900-2906, 2003

Kamalesh M, Matorin R, Sawada S. Prognostic value of a negative stress echocardiographic study in diabetic patients. *Am Heart J*. 143:163-168, 2002

Lee CD, Folsom AR, Pankow JS, Brancati FL; Atherosclerosis Risk in Communities (ARIC) Study Investigators: Cardiovascular events in diabetic and nondiabetic adults with or without history of myocardial infarction. *Circulation* 109:855–860, 2004

Lee DP, Fearon WF, Froelicher VF: Clinical utility of the exercise ECG in patients with diabetes and chest pain. *Chest* 119:1576–1581, 2001

Marwick TH, Case C, Sawada S, Vasey C, Short L, Lauer M: Use of stress echocardiography to predict mortality in patients with diabetes and known or suspected coronary artery disease. *Diabetes Care* 25:1042–1048, 2002

Redberg RF, Greenland P, Fuster V, Pyorala K, Blair SN, Folsom AR, Newman AB, O'Leary DH, Orchard TJ, Psaty B, Schwartz JS, Starke R, Wilson PW: Prevention Conference VI. Diabetes and Cardiovascular Disease Writing Group III: risk assessment in persons with diabetes. *Circulation* 105:e144–e152, 2002

Schinkel AFL, Elhendy A, van Domburg RT, Bax JJ, Vourouri EC, Sozzi FB, Valkema R, Roelandt JRTC, Poldermans D. Prognostic value of dobutamine-atropine stress myocardial perfusion imaging in patients with diabetes. *Diabetes Care* 25:1637-1643, 2002

Sozzi FB, Elhendy A, Roelandt JR, van Domburg RT, Schinkel AF, Vourvouri EC, Bax JJ, De Sutter J, Borghetti A, Poldermans D: Prognostic value of dobutamine stress echocardiography in patients with diabetes. *Diabetes Care* 26:1074–1078, 2003

Vanzetto G, Halimi S, Hammoud T, Fagret D, Benhamou PY, Gordonnier D, Bernard D, Machecourt J: Prediction of cardiovascular events in clinically selected high-risk NIDDM patients. *Diabetes Care* 22:19-26, 1999

Dr. Steinhoff is a Cardiologist at the Heart and Vascular Institute of Florida, Safety Harbor, FL. Dr. Menon is Assistant Professor and Dr. Smith is Professor of Medicine, and Director, Center for Cardiovascular Science and Medicine in the Division of Cardiology, University of North Carolina at Chapel Hill, Chapel Hill, NC.

51. Angina and Congestive Heart Failure in Patients with Diabetes

Anjli Maroo, MD, W. H. Wilson Tang, MD,
and James B. Young, MD, FACC

Diabetes mellitus is a well-established independent risk factor for cardiovascular disease in both men and women. Ischemic heart disease is a major source of morbidity and mortality, contributing to 75% of deaths in this patient population. Angina pectoris, a cardinal manifestation of ischemic heart disease, is extremely common in diabetic patients, with prevalence estimates approaching 40% of patients. However, many patients with diabetes experience episodes of silent ischemia and suffer a worse prognosis after the development of ischemic heart disease than their nondiabetic counterparts. Consequently, the diagnosis and treatment of ischemic heart disease and heart failure in the diabetic patient warrants special consideration.

PATHOPHYSIOLOGY AND CLINICAL PRESENTATION OF ANGINA

Angina is produced when myocardial oxygen demand outstrips myocardial oxygen supply, resulting in ischemia. The major determinants of oxygen demand and oxygen supply are shown in Table 51.1. Coronary atherosclerosis is the most common cause of inadequate myocardial oxygen supply. Numerous risk factors associated with the diabetic and pre-diabetic state may contribute to development of accelerated atherosclerosis and ischemia (Table 51.2). Increased myocardial oxygen demand, caused by conditions such as hypertension and left ventricular hypertrophy (LVH), can also produce ischemic symptoms.

Angina typically presents as a diffuse constant chest discomfort. Anginal pain can radiate to other areas of the body, such as the epigastric region, shoulders, arms, throat, neck, and lower jaw. It may be accompanied by shortness of breath, diaphoresis, nausea, or dizziness. Stable angina is usually precipitated by a predictable workload and is relieved by rest or nitroglycerine administration. In contrast, unstable angina is characterized by new-onset chest pain, accelerated symptoms, or symptoms at rest. Fixed atherosclerotic plaques large enough to compromise coronary blood flow during conditions of increased metabolic demand are usually responsible for symptoms of stable angina. Disruption of potentially smaller plaques with superimposed thrombosis and vasospasm can lead to unstable angina.

Table 51.1 Determinants of Myocardial Oxygen Supply and Demand

Myocardial oxygen supply	Myocardial oxygen demand
■ Oxygen-carrying capacity	■ Heart rate
■ Coronary artery blood flow	■ Left ventricular afterload (approximated
□ Artery diameter	by systolic blood pressure)
□ Vessel tone	■ Myocardial wall tension
□ Collateral blood flow	■ Myocardial contractility
□ Perfusion pressure	
□ Diastolic period	

SILENT ISCHEMIA IN DIABETIC PATIENTS

Although chest pain is one of the hallmark manifestations of ischemic heart disease, many patients with diabetes suffer from transient ischemic episodes that are clinically "silent." Silent ischemia can occur in patients who have never experienced prior anginal symptoms or in patients who also experience typical anginal symptoms from known coronary disease. The prevalence of silent ischemia in diabetic patients approaches 10–15%, which is significantly greater than that in their nondiabetic counterparts. Silent angina on ambulatory electrocardiography monitoring is predictive of multivessel coronary disease, increased adverse clinical outcomes, and poor survival.

The precise mechanism underlying ischemic chest pain is not well elucidated. Several theories explaining the phenomenon of silent ischemia have been proposed, including altered thresholds of pain sensitivity, autonomic neuropathy leading to sympathetic denervation, higher production of β-endorphins, and increased production of anti-inflammatory cytokines. Primary abnormalities of coronary

Table 51.2 Selected Atherogenic and Thrombogenic Risk Factors in Diabetes

- ■ Dyslipidemia
  - □ Elevated VLDL cholesterol
  - □ Low HDL cholesterol
  - □ Increased small LDL cholesterol
- ■ Endothelial dysfunction
- ■ Platelet abnormalities
  - □ Increased primary and secondary aggregation responses
  - □ Increased release of α granule contents
  - □ Increased thromboxane A_2 production
- ■ Coagulation abnormalities
  - □ Increased plasminogen activator inhibitor 1
  - □ Increased fibrinogen
- ■ Impaired coronary arterial remodeling
- ■ Impaired myocardial flow reserve

blood flow reserve, rather than increased myocardial oxygen demand, are believed to cause most episodes of silent ischemia, especially given that silent ischemia tends to occur at rest or with minimal exertion.

Silent ischemia can be detected by transient ST segment changes on exercise treadmill testing or ambulatory Holter monitoring, myocardial perfusion defects on nuclear imaging studies, or reversible regional wall motion abnormalities on stress or dobutamine echocardiography. ST segment changes suggestive of ischemia on exercise treadmill testing or Holter monitoring include flat or down-sloping ST depression of at least 1 mm, with a gradual onset and offset, lasting at least 1 min. Although exercise treadmill testing or ambulatory Holter monitoring are the most common modalities used for the diagnosis of silent ischemia, patients with abnormalities on baseline electrocardiogram such as LVH, left bundle branch block, pre-excitation, electronically paced ventricular rhythms, or digitalis effect, may require nuclear imaging or echocardiographic evaluation.

The decision to screen diabetic patients for silent ischemia is a difficult one (see Chapter 49). Patients with asymptomatic ischemia (often detected by exercise treadmill testing) have a higher risk of coronary events and sudden cardiac death. However, asymptomatic individuals often have a lower pretest probability of disease, which reduces the predictive accuracy of any screening test. The rate of false-positive tests may be lowered by selection of high-risk patients for screening. Nevertheless, there has been no consensus opinion from the American College of Cardiology or the American Heart Association regarding routine screening of asymptomatic individuals for silent ischemia.

DIAGNOSTIC TESTING FOR THE EVALUATION OF ANGINA

Noninvasive testing modalities for diabetic patients who experience angina are described in detail in Chapter 50. However, a number of factors specific to diabetic patients should be taken into account when performing noninvasive diagnostic tests for coronary artery disease. Hypertension, LVH, and increased left ventricular mass are common among individuals with diabetes. During exercise, these conditions can cause abnormal ST segment responses, wall motion abnormalities, and perfusion defects, leading to false-positive test results. Autonomic neuropathy can cause an abnormal chronotropic response to exercise. Triple-vessel or multivessel disease, which is more common in diabetic patients, can lower the sensitivity of pharmacological stress tests that rely on vasodilators such as adenosine or persantine.

Coronary angiography is recommended in patients with angina that is poorly controlled despite maximal medical therapy or in patients with abnormal or high-risk noninvasive test results. In addition, coronary angiography is indicated in diabetic patients with multiple risk factors and a high clinical suspicion of coronary artery disease, even with "normal" noninvasive test results. Diabetic patients with renal insufficiency warrant special consideration before angiography. The risks of progressive renal failure and dialysis should be clearly explained. Measures to prevent renal failure include periprocedural hydration, administration of *N*-acetylcysteine, and use of low osmolar, nonionic contrast. Diabetic patients who take metformin are at risk for lactic acidosis after catheterization. Metformin should be held on the day before and 2 days after the procedure to reduce the risk of lactic acidosis. Insulin and oral hypoglycemic medications should be held on the morning of the procedure.

MEDICAL THERAPY FOR ANGINA IN DIABETIC PATIENTS

Atherosclerotic coronary artery disease in individuals with diabetes is often a diffuse process, affecting proximal and distal coronary segments. In addition, diabetic patients often suffer from microvascular coronary disease. When percutaneous coronary intervention (PCI) or coronary artery bypass graft (CABG) surgery is not feasible, medications form the cornerstone of therapy for angina and for prevention of progression of atherosclerosis (Table 51.3).

Nitrates are first-line anti-anginal agents that decrease myocardial oxygen demand by reducing preload and afterload and increase myocardial oxygen supply by vasodilation of the coronary arteries. Nitrates are available in several formulations. Chronic therapy is associated with the phenomenon of nitrate tolerance. For this reason, many patients observe a 12- to 14-h nitrate-free period. Diabetic patients with autonomic neuropathy may develop marked orthostatic hypotension in response to nitrate therapy.

Table 51.3 Medical Therapy for Chronic Stable Angina

Drug	Starting Dosage	Major Side Effects
Nitrates		Headache, lightheaded-
Sublingual	0.3–0.4 mg	ness, flushing, orthostasis
Oral	10 mg t.i.d./30 mg q.d.*	
Transdermal	0.2 mg/h	
β-Blockers		Bradycardia, atrioventric-
β$_1$-selective		ular block, heart failure,
Metoprolol succinate	25 mg q.d.	fatigue, depression, erec-
Metoprolol tartrate	25 mg b.i.d.	tile dysfunction, exacer-
Atenolol	25 mg q.d./b.i.d.	bation of claudication,
Nonselective		bronchospasm, increased
Propranolol	40 mg b.i.d./q.i.d.	insulin-induced hypo-
		glycemia
CCBs		Bradycardia, AV block,
Verapamil	80 mg q.i.d./240 mg q.d.*	heart failure, flushing,
Amlodipine	5 mg q.d.	headache, constipation,
Nifedipine	20 mg q.i.d.	pedal edema
Diltiazem	60 mg q.i.d./240 mg q.d.*	
Aspirin	81–325 mg q.d.	Gastrointestinal ulcers, renal dysfunction, bronchospasm, rash

*Sustained release preparation.

β-Blockers alleviate anginal symptoms by reducing myocardial demand via a decrease in heart rate and cardiac contractility. Agents such as metoprolol and atenolol, which act selectively on the $β_1$-receptor, are preferred in diabetic patients because they do not interfere with peripheral vasodilation and glycemic control to the same extent as nonselective agents. In addition to being highly effective anti-anginal agents, β-blockers have been shown to prevent reinfarction and improve survival in patients who have already suffered a myocardial infarction (MI).

Calcium-channel blockers (CCBs) induce coronary and peripheral vasodilation, decrease heart rate, and reduce cardiac contractility. As a group, CCBs are effective anti-anginal agents that should be used as first-line agents if there is a contraindication to β-blockers or if significant side effects occur on β-blocker therapy. In addition, CCBs may be added to β-blockers or nitrates if these drugs provide inadequate symptom relief. The dihydropyridines (e.g., amlodipine) produce more peripheral vasodilation and have fewer negative chronotropic and inotropic effects than CCBs such as diltiazem and verapamil. Use of short-acting dihydropyridines (e.g., nifedipine) is discouraged because of the data suggesting an increased risk of MI. CCBs are the treatment of choice for Prinzmetal's (or variant) angina.

In the absence of contraindications, all patients with angina should receive low-dose enteric-coated aspirin (81–162 mg/day). Those with aspirin intolerance or allergy may be treated with clopidogrel (75 mg/day). In addition to anti-anginal therapy, diabetic patients with angina should undergo intensive cardiac risk factor modification to prevent progression of atherosclerosis. These therapies include treatment of hypertension (target blood pressure <130/85 mmHg), lipid-lowering therapies (target LDL cholesterol <100 mg/dl, triglycerides <150 mg/dl, and HDL >40 mg/dl), smoking cessation, glycemic control (target glycated hemoglobin A1C [A1C] <6.5%), and weight control. The role of angiotensin-converting enzyme (ACE) inhibitors in diabetic patients without MI, left ventricular systolic dysfunction, hypertension, or proteinuria is controversial. Although data from the Heart Outcomes Prevention Evaluation (HOPE) study support the use of the ACE inhibitor ramipril for primary prevention of coronary artery disease, it is possible that the derived benefit can be attributed to blood pressure–lowering effects alone.

The medical treatment of unstable angina in diabetic patients versus nondiabetic subjects is similar. Aspirin, heparin, nitrates, and β-blockers form the mainstay of therapy. Antiplatelet agents, including clopidogrel and intravenous glycoprotein IIb/IIIa (GP IIb/IIIa) inhibitors, should be used in high-risk individuals. Interestingly, the use of GP IIb/IIIa inhibitors may be particularly advantageous for diabetic patients with unstable angina in that the inhibitors confer a survival benefit.

CORONARY REVASCULARIZATION

Despite maximal medical therapy, many diabetic patients require coronary artery revascularization for relief of angina. Revascularization techniques include PCI, with or without stenting, and CABG. The initial management of acute coronary syndromes, including the decision to proceed with coronary angiography and revascularization, is similar in patients with and without diabetes.

After implantation of coronary stents, diabetic patients suffer from an increased rate of restenosis compared with nondiabetic subjects. Development of restenosis is a poor prognostic sign and is associated with increased long-term mortality. Intracoronary radiation may be used to treat in-stent restenosis in patients both with and without diabetes. The use of drug-eluting stents for prevention of restenosis has been shown to be efficacious in diabetic subgroups of the TAXUS IV and SIRIUS trials.

The indications for CABG, as opposed to PCI, are based on lesion number, location, and morphology. CABG is generally indicated when there is a large amount of myocardium at risk, for example with >50% stenosis of the left main coronary artery or severe triple-vessel disease. Although most trials comparing balloon angioplasty and CABG have demonstrated comparable outcomes, diabetic patients treated with insulin or oral hypoglycemic drugs have a higher survival rate if they undergo CABG for two- or three-vessel disease. Similarly, trials comparing coronary artery stenting versus CABG have demonstrated a higher 1-year event-free survival in diabetic patients who underwent CABG for multivessel disease, largely due to a higher rate of repeat revascularization procedures in the stent group. Further studies are needed to compare CABG with PCI with adjunctive GP IIb/IIIa inhibitor use and/or with drug-eluting stents.

CARDIOMYOPATHY AND HEART FAILURE IN DIABETIC PATIENTS

Heart failure is common in the diabetes population, with an overall prevalence of 12% from community-based studies. Patients with diabetes often experience a higher risk of developing congestive heart failure with or without MI. Overall, the annual estimated incidence of developing symptomatic heart failure is 8%. This risk is increased 2.4-fold in men with diabetes and 5-fold in women with diabetes when compared with matched control subjects, independent of coexisting hypertension or ischemic heart disease. According to the latest American College of Cardiology/ American Heart Association guidelines for the management of chronic heart failure, the presence of diabetes mellitus is regarded as stage A heart failure (patients at risk of heart failure) or stage B heart failure (patients with structural abnormalities such as LVH without overt cardiac dysfunction). Implementation of strategies to modify risk factors, including tight glycemic control and early medical therapy (such as ACE inhibitors), has led to significant reduction in cardiovascular morbidity and mortality attributable to heart failure in diabetic patients.

Although direct, concrete evidence is still lacking, most experts now acknowledge the existence of a distinct diabetic cardiomyopathy. Morphologic features associated with diabetic cardiomyopathy include myocyte hypertrophy, interstitial fibrosis, intramyocardial microangiopathy, and infiltration with periodic acid–Schiff-positive materials. However, many of these histological findings are often indistinguishable from other forms of nonischemic cardiomyopathies. A number of population-based studies have observed asymptomatic structural abnormalities (such as increased left ventricular mass and wall thickness) and functional alterations (such as diastolic dysfunction) in diabetic patients that long precede overt heart failure. These changes are not accounted for by age, sex, body habitus, race, or blood pressure differences. Some of these findings manifest only when provocative maneuvers (such as Valsalva) or special measurements (such as pulmonary venous flow patterns or tissue Doppler recordings) are performed. Other screening strategies such as plasma B-type natriuretic peptide assays may allow earlier recognition of cardiac abnormalities in diabetic patients, facilitating earlier preventive intervention.

In the setting of acute coronary syndrome, the incidence of heart failure is at least two times higher in patients with diabetes than in patients without diabetes. In addition, mortality from MI can be attributed to the development of heart failure in up to two-thirds of all patients with diabetes. Although the exact mechanism is unknown, metabolic perturbations may blunt the compensatory response of the diabetic myocardium in the setting of ischemia. Nevertheless, the higher incidence of post-infarction acute heart failure and poorer prognosis in diabetic patients cannot be explained by a larger degree of initial myocyte damage or long-term ventricular remodeling. What we know, however, is that tight control of glucose during the post-infarction period is an important component of the medical management. Even in patients without overt diabetes, peri-infarct hyperglycemia is associated with worse outcomes. The role of the glucose-insulin-potassium infusion in improving short- and long-term morbidity and mortality in the setting of acute MI has been established in the Diabetes Mellitus Insulin-Glucose Infusion in Acute Myocardial Infarction (DIGAMI) study. The DIGAMI regimen is an insulin and glucose infusion for tight glycemic control for at least 24 h during the acute event. This is followed by a 3-month subcutaneous insulin treatment to achieve tight glycemic control. Whether oral hypoglycemic agents can achieve the same effects is currently unknown.

Tight glycemic control is also an important component in the management of diabetic heart failure. Results from United Kingdom Prospective Diabetes Study (UKPDS) 35 have suggested that for every 1% decrement in A1C levels, there is a 16% relative reduction in the risk of developing heart failure. The safety and efficacy of newer oral agents that improve insulin sensitivity in this population are still unclear. Both the biguanides and the thiazolidinediones are still regarded as "relatively contraindicated" in diabetic patients with heart failure because of potential hepatotoxicity. In addition, there is concern that the use of thiazolidinediones may cause overt heart failure. However, thiazolidinedione-related fluid retention is largely restricted to the periphery, and the underlying mechanism remains unclear. However, it is apparent that these agents dramatically improve endothelial dysfunction and insulin resistance in diabetic patients with heart failure. Cautious use of these agents with careful monitoring can be safe and effective.

The management of patients with chronic heart failure and diabetes mellitus follows the same general approach used to treat these two syndromes individually, although special consideration should be given when using some heart failure drugs in the diabetic population (Table 51.4). Every effort should be made to maximize myocardial blood flow (either by percutaneous or surgical revascularization) in the failing heart to reverse the underlying hibernating myocardium. Anecdotal observations have suggested that high-dose thiazide diuretics may have an adverse effect on insulin sensitivity and therefore should be avoided unless clinically required. On the other hand, neurohormonal antagonists (such as ACE inhibitors

Table 51.4 Common Heart Failure Drugs with Special Considerations for Diabetic Patients

Drug Class (and common examples)	Start Dose (mg)	Target Dose (mg)	Special Considerations in Diabetic Patients
ACE inhibitors			Indicated for all heart failure patients unless contraindicated ($\downarrow$ blood pressure, $\uparrow$ potassium, $\uparrow$ creatinine [use hydralazine/ isosorbide dinitrate if creatinine >3 mg/dl], angioedema/cough)
Captopril	6.25–12.5	50 t.i.d.	
Enalapril	2.5–5	10 b.i.d.	
Lisinopril	2.5–5	10–20 q.d.	
Ramipril	1.25–2.5	5 b.i.d.	
β-Blockers			Indicated for all systolic heart failure patients unless con- traindicated ($\downarrow$ pulse rate, $\downarrow$ blood pressure, heart block, reactive airway disease)
Carvedilol	3.125–6.25	25 b.i.d.	
Metoprolol succinate	12.5–25	100 q.d.	
Bisoprolol	2.5–5	20 q.d.	
Spironolactone	12.5–25	NA	Indicated for advanced systolic heart failure (NYHA [New York Heart Association] III–IV), need to closely watch for $\uparrow$ potas- sium, $\uparrow$ creatinine in diabetic patients; no need for uptitration
Hydralazine/isosorbide dinitrate	25/10	100 t.i.d./ 40 q.i.d.	Indicated for ACE inhibitor/angiotensin II recep- tor blocker–intolerant patients and those with advanced renal insufficiency
Diuretics			Indicated for symptomatic relief from fluid retention; thiazides (but not loop diuretics) may attenuate insulin sensitivity
Furosemide	20–40	Titrate to	
Bumetanide	1–2	euvolemia	
Torsemide	1–10		
Metolazone	2.5–5		
Digoxin	0.125	NA	Indicated for advanced heart failure to prevent morbidity, particularly with concomitant atrial fibrillation; watch for toxicity, especially with amio- darone and renal insufficiency; prefer a lower dose (0.125 daily or every other day), especially in the elderly and in women; no need for uptitration
Angiotensin II receptor blockers			Indicated for ACE inhibitor– intolerant heart failure patients unless contraindicated ($\uparrow$ potassium, $\uparrow$ creatinine [use hydralazine/isosorbide dini- trate if creatinine >3 mg/dl], angioedema/cough)
Losartan	25	50 q.d.	
Valsartan	80	160 q.d.	
Candesartan	4	16 q.d.	

and β-blockers) that confer morbidity and mortality benefits in patients with heart failure are equally effective in diabetic subgroups. ACE inhibitors (or angiotensin II receptor antagonists if a patient is intolerant to ACE inhibitors) should be given at target doses to *every* diabetic patient with heart failure unless contraindicated. β-Blockers are well tolerated and clearly effective in diabetes subgroups in large-scale heart failure trials. Spironolactone may have important theoretical benefits in diabetic patients with advanced heart failure because of its ability to reduce myocardial fibrosis. However, spironolactone may significantly raise the risk of developing hyperkalemia and renal insufficiency in the diabetic population. Digoxin should be limited to individuals with symptomatic heart failure with recurrent hospitalizations or individuals with concomitant rapid atrial fibrillation. Digoxin toxicity is common in diabetic patients with concurrent renal insufficiency.

BIBLIOGRAPHY

Abizaid A, Costa MA, Centemero M, Abizaid AS, Legrand VM, Limet RV, Schuler G, Mohr FW, Lindeboom W, Sousa AG, Sousa JE, van Hout B, Hugenholtz PG, Unger F, Serruys PW: Clinical and economic impact of diabetes mellitus on percutaneous and surgical treatment of multivessel coronary disease patients: insights from the Arterial Revascularization Therapy Study (ARTS) trial. *Circulation* 104:533–538, 2001

Deedwania PC, Carbajal EV: Silent ischemia during daily life is an independent predictor of mortality in stable angina. *Circulation* 81:748–756, 1990

Devereux RB, Roman MJ, Paranicas M, O'Grady MJ, Lee ET, Welty TK, Fabsitz RR, Robbins D, Rhoades ER, Howard BV: Impact of diabetes on cardiac structure and function: the Strong Heart Study. *Circulation* 101:2271–2276, 2001

Hikita H, Etsuda H, Takase B, Satomura K, Kurita Λ, Nakamura H: Extent of ischemic stimulus and plasma beta-endorphin levels in silent myocardial ischemia. *Am Heart J* 135:813–818, 1998

Influence of diabetes on 5-year mortality and morbidity in a randomized trial comparing CABG and PTCA in patients with multivessel disease: the Bypass Angioplasty Revascularization Investigation (BARI). *Circulation* 96:1761–1769, 1997

Iribarren C, Karter AJ, Go AS, Ferrara A, Liu JY, Sidney S, Selby JV: Glycemic control and heart failure among adult patients with diabetes. *Circulation* 103:2668–2673, 2001

Kannel WB, McGee DL: Diabetes and cardiovascular disease: the Framingham study. *JAMA* 241:2035–2038, 1979

Langer A, Freeman MR, Josse RG, Armstrong PW: Metaiodobenzylguanidine imaging in diabetes mellitus: assessment of cardiac sympathetic denervation and its relation to autonomic dysfunction and silent myocardial ischemia. *J Am Coll Cardiol* 25:610–618, 1995

Mak KH, Moliterno DJ, Granger CB, Miller DP, White HD, Wilcox RG, Califf RM, Topol EJ: Influence of diabetes mellitus on clinical outcomes in the thrombolytic era of acute myocardial infarction: GUSTO-I Investigators: Global Utilization of Streptokinase and Tissue Plasmogen Activator for Occluded Coronary Arteries. *J Am Coll Cardiol* 30:171–179, 1997

Malmberg K, Ryden L, Efendic S, Herlitz J, Nicol P, Waldenstrom A, Wedel H, Welin L: Randomized trial of insulin-glucose infusion followed by subcutaneous insulin treatment in diabetic patients with acute myocardial infarction (DIGAMI study): effects on mortality at 1 year. *J Am Coll Cardiol* 26:57–65, 1995

Mazzone A, Cusa C, Mazzucchelli I, Vezzoli M, Ottini E, Pacifici R, Zuccaro P, Falcone C: Increased production of inflammatory cytokines in patients with silent myocardial ischemia. *J Am Coll Cardiol* 38:1895–1901, 2001

Moses JW, Leon MB, Popma JJ, Fitzgerald PJ, Holmes DR, O'Shaughnessy C, Caputo RP, Kereiakes DJ, Williams DO, Teirstein PS, Jaeger JL, Kuntz RE: Sirolimus-eluting stents versus standard stents in patients with stenosis in a native coronary artery. *N Engl J Med* 349:1315–1323, 2003

Nesto R: Screening for asymptomatic coronary artery disease in diabetes. *Diabetes Care* 22:1393–1395, 1999

Nesto RW, Phillips RT, Kett KG, Hill T, Perper E, Young E, Leland OS Jr: Angina and exertional myocardial ischemia in diabetic and nondiabetic patients: assessment by exercise thallium scintigraphy. *Ann Intern Med* 108:170–175, 1988

Sharaf BL, Williams DO, Miele NJ, McMahon RP, Stone PH, Bjerregaard P, Davies R, Goldberg AD, Parks M, Pepine CJ, Sopko G, Conti CR: A detailed angiographic analysis of patients with ambulatory electrocardiographic ischemia: results from the Asymptomatic Cardiac Ischemia Pilot (ACIP) study angiographic core laboratory. *J Am Coll Cardiol* 29:78–84, 1997

Stamler J, Vaccaro O, Neaton JD, Wentworth D: Diabetes, other risk factors, and 12-yr cardiovascular mortality for men screened in the Multiple Risk Factor Intervention Trial. *Diabetes Care* 16:434–444, 1993

Tang WHW, Young JB: Cardiomyopathy and heart failure in diabetes. *Endocrin Metab Clin N Am* 30:1031–1046, 2001

Dr. Maroo is a Fellow in the Department of Cardiovascular Medicine, Cleveland Clinic Foundation. Dr. Tang is Associate Staff, Section of Heart Failure and Cardiac Transplantation, Department of Cardiovascular Medicine, Cleveland Clinic Foundation and Assistant Professor of Medicine at the Cleveland Clinic Lerner College of Medicine. Dr. Young is Chairman of the Division of Medicine, and Medical Director of the George M. and Linda H. Kaufman Center for Heart Failure, Department of Cardiovascular Medicine, Cleveland Clinic Foundation, Cleveland, OH.

52. Myocardial Infarction

ERON D. CROUCH, MD, VENU MENON, MD, AND SIDNEY C. SMITH JR., MD

Although there has been a decline in the overall age-adjusted mortality rate among patients with known atherosclerotic coronary heart disease (CHD), there has been an increase in the mortality rate of diabetes patients with CHD. Currently, CHD accounts for 75% of all deaths in patients with diabetes. In addition, the incidence of death from cardiovascular causes in patients with diabetes and no history of CHD is similar to that observed in patients with known CHD and no diabetes. These observations highlight the prevalence of undiagnosed CHD in patients with diabetes and the gravity of myocardial infarction (MI) in this population.

FACTORS COMPLICATING MI IN PATIENTS WITH DIABETES

In general, diabetes patients with acute myocardial infarction (AMI) have a poorer prognosis than their nondiabetic counterparts. Studies have shown that the in-hospital death rate, after admission for AMI, is ~1.5–2.0 times higher in patients with diabetes than in nondiabetic individuals. Likewise, patients with diabetes who survive MI have a 40% higher risk of death after 6 years. AMI in diabetes patients may be complicated by several factors that contribute to this poorer short-term and long-term prognosis.

Accelerated Atherosclerosis

Several large autopsy registries have demonstrated increased coronary atherosclerotic burden in subjects with diabetes compared with their nondiabetic counterparts. Longstanding hyperglycemia, and subsequent hyperinsulinemia, leads to the development of microvascular disease, endothelial dysfunction, and increased transmigration of macrophages and other inflammatory cells into the subendothelium. Macrophages ingest modified LDL-cholesterol molecules, giving rise to foam cells, the hallmark of atherosclerosis. For uncertain reasons, among patients with diabetes, these atherosclerotic coronary arteries tend to remodel inwardly, further accelerating lumen occlusion. Subsequently, patients with diabetes have more pronounced and often multivessel coronary disease (including left main).

Prothrombotic State

Studies have also shown that diabetes patients with acute coronary syndrome (ACS) are more likely than nondiabetic subjects to present with intracoronary thrombi (94% versus 55%, respectively). These findings are probably related to the increased incidence of ulcerated intracoronary plaques (94% versus 61%, respectively) seen in the diabetes patients with ACS. In addition, the platelets of diabetes patients have an increased number of glycoprotein (GP) IIb/IIIa receptors and aggregate more readily than the platelets of nondiabetic patients. Furthermore, patients with diabetes have been shown to have increased levels of plasma fibrinogen and factor VII, which correlate with an increased risk of MI and sudden death.

Larger Myocardial Infarction Zone

Diabetes patients tend to have larger MIs than nondiabetic subjects. This is primarily because of more diffuse macrovascular and microvascular disease among patients with diabetes, which also contributes to more significant peri-infarct zone ischemia. Silent infarctions also plague up to 20–30% of all individuals with diabetes, leading to a significant number of delayed or missed diagnoses. A substudy of the Coronary Artery Surgery Study registry suggested that diabetes patients with silent ischemia had significantly lower survival than nondiabetic subjects with silent ischemia (59% versus 82%, respectively) at 6 years.

Autonomic Dysfunction

Autonomic dysfunction is an independent predictor of major cardiac events. It affects up to 50% of patients with diabetes and may contribute to lowering the threshold for a life-threatening arrhythmia by causing an imbalance in sympathovagal tone. Autonomic dysfunction also increases the risk of hemodynamic instability.

STRATEGIES TO PREVENT MI IN PATIENTS WITH DIABETES

As previously mentioned, it is well established that patients with diabetes, but no history of CHD, have a risk of cardiovascular death similar to nondiabetic patients with known CHD. As a result, the current American Heart Association (AHA) guidelines, American Diabetes Association (ADA) guidelines, and recommendations from the Adult Treatment Panel III (ATP III) of the National Cholesterol Education Program all suggest that risk factors in diabetes patients with no history of CHD should be modified as aggressively as in nondiabetic subjects with known CHD. The major modifiable risk factors are discussed below.

Glycemic Control

Although controlled clinical trials have not fully established the role of good glycemic control in preventing macrovascular disease, they have confirmed the benefit of good glycemic control in type 1 and type 2 diabetes patients with diabetes in the prevention of microvascular disease. The goal for glycemic therapy is to achieve a fasting glucose level between 90 and 130 mg/dl (5.0 and 7.2 mmol/l) and a glycated hemoglobin A1C level of <7%. Postprandial hyperglycemia may be an independent risk factor for CHD; however, there are currently no universally accepted guidelines to address this issue. The ADA recommends a 2-h postprandial glucose level of <180 mg/dl (<10 mmol/l).

Weight Reduction

The majority of type 2 diabetes patients are overweight (BMI 25–29.9 kg/m²) or obese (BMI ≥30 kg/m²). Excess body fat raises insulin resistance and may accelerate a decline in insulin secretion. Studies have shown that weight reduction can reduce insulin resistance and perhaps mitigate the metabolic risk factors associated with diabetes. For the optimal chance of maintaining weight loss, the goal should be to lose 10% of initial body weight gradually over 12 months.

Physical Activity

Physical inactivity contributes to the development of obesity; however, even patients with diabetes who are not obese can benefit from physical activity. Physical activity can improve insulin sensitivity; lower total cholesterol, LDL cholesterol, and triglycerides; raise HDL cholesterol; and further decrease the risk for CHD by improving overall cardiovascular fitness and function. Patients should receive a physical activity prescription based on the clinical judgment of the physician. The usually recommended prescription is ~30 min of moderate-intensity exercise daily; although, additional physical activity may be beneficial, if tolerable to the patient. The AHA provides an exercise prescription that can be recommended for clinical practice.

Lipid Control

The principle of managing patients with diabetes and no known CHD using target goals that are similar to those for the nondiabetic patient with known CHD can be extended to lipid management. Guidelines set by the National Cholesterol Education Program recommend that patients with diabetes maintain an LDL cholesterol of <100 mg/dl (<5.6 mmol/l), which is also supported by the ADA. For patients with triglyceride levels >200 mg/dl (>11.1 mmol/l), the target goal is a non–HDL cholesterol level (total cholesterol minus HDL cholesterol) of ≤130 mg/dl (≤7.2 mmol/l). It is also desirable to maintain an HDL cholesterol level >40 mg/dl (>2.2 mmol/l). These recommendations have been called into question by the Heart Protection Study (HPS), which demonstrated benefit from statin therapy among patients with diabetes and LDL cholesterol levels <100 mg/dl (<5.6 mmol/l). In this study, 20,536 patients with CHD, stroke, peripheral vascular disease, or diabetes were randomized to receive either 40 mg simvastatin daily or placebo for 5 years. Among the subgroup of patients with diabetes and known CHD, the event rate was 33% for the group treated with simvastatin versus 38% for the placebo group. In diabetes patients with no prior history of CHD, the event rate was 9% versus 14%, respectively. Overall, the mean LDL cholesterol level of the simvastatin-treated group was 77 mg/dl (4.3 mmol/l). The Pravastatin or Atorvastatin Evaluation and Infection Therapy (PROVE IT) trial enrolled 4,162 patients, including over 700 patients with diabetes who had been hospitalized for an acute coronary syndrome and compared 40 mg pravastatin daily (standard therapy) with 80 mg atorvastatin daily (intensive therapy). At 2 years, the PROVE IT trial demonstrated a significant reduction in events from using high-dose atorvastatin in patients with diabetes, which achieved a mean LDL cholesterol of 62 mg/dl (3.4 mmol/l), compared with using standard-dose pravastatin, with a mean LDL cholesterol of 95 mg/dl (5.3 mmol/l) [28.8% versus 34.6%, respectively]. Thus, many now feel that statin therapy is indicated for high-risk patients, such as those with diabetes, even when the LDL cholesterol level is less than the ATP III target level of 100 mg/dl (5.6 mmol/l).

Blood Pressure Control

Several controlled clinical trials have indicated that the risk of cardiovascular events and diabetes-associated death increases with increases in blood pressure and that lowering the blood pressure of patients with diabetes can significantly reduce this risk. The United Kingdom Prospective Diabetes Study illustrated that even modest blood pressure reduction in diabetes patients (10 mmHg systolic and 5 mmHg diastolic) can reduce the risk of developing congestive heart failure by 56%. The Heart Outcomes Prevention Evaluation (HOPE) trial randomized >9,000 patients with evidence of vascular disease or diabetes plus one other cardiovascular risk factor to the angiotensin-converting enzyme (ACE) inhibitor ramipril versus placebo. Overall, ramipril significantly reduced the composite end point of MI, stroke, or cardiovascular mortality to 14%, compared with 17.8% in the placebo group. In addition, the Microalbuminuria, Cardiovascular, and Renal Outcomes-HOPE (MICRO-HOPE) trial of 3,577 diabetes patients was terminated 6 months early because ramipril was shown to reduce the incidence of MI by 22%, stroke by 33%, cardiovascular death by 37%, and all-case mortality by 24% compared with placebo. For these reasons, the AHA recommends that in the absence of contraindications, ACE inhibitors be administered to all diabetes patients. The Joint National Committee (JNC)-7 on Prevention, Detection, Evaluation, and Treatment of High Blood Pressure, the ADA, and the National Kidney Foundation (NKF) all recommend that all patients with diabetes maintain a blood pressure of <130/80 mmHg. The NKF also recommends that diabetes patients with proteinuria >1 g/day lower their blood pressure goal to <125/75 mmHg.

Smoking Cessation

Because smoking is an independent risk factor for developing CHD, complete cessation should be the primary goal for all smokers, but especially those with diabetes. Counseling or referral to smoking-cessation programs should be offered to all diabetic smokers at every office visit. There are a variety of pharmacological therapeutic options (i.e., bupropion and nicotine-replacement products). Importantly, these options have been shown to be more effective when used in conjunction with a high-quality smoking cessation program. Bupropion should be used with precaution in patients with known or suspected ACS or heart failure because of its pro-arrhythmic potential. Patients that choose to quit without the help of a smoking-cessation program should have a follow-up within 2 weeks of their scheduled quit date and another after 1 month of abstinence.

INITIAL MANAGEMENT OF MI IN PATIENTS WITH DIABETES

Diagnosis

Up to one-third of patients with diabetes who present with AMI have symptoms other than the classic substernal chest pressure, radiating into the left arm, or they have no symptoms at all until the development of congestive heart failure. Atypical presentations, such as jaw or neck pain, epigastric pain associated with vomiting, isolated shortness of breath, and diabetic ketoacidosis, are common. Often, a high index of suspicion is needed to make the diagnosis. Up to 35% will not have characteristic electrocardiogram ST elevations or Q waves indicating myocardial injury or infarction, respectively. In addition, diabetes patients often have renal insufficiency, which may falsely elevate cardiac markers. Any one of the following AHA cardiac marker criteria can be used to assist in the diagnosis of AMI: *1)* serial increase, then decrease of plasma creatinine kinase subtype MB (CK-MB), with a change >25% between any two values; *2)* CK-MB >10–13 units/l or >5% of the total creatinine kinase activity; *3)* if only a single sample is available, CK-MB elevation more than twofold normal; or *4)* beyond 72 h of symptoms, a new isolated, elevated troponin T transthoracic echocardiography, looking for new regional wall-motion abnormalities, can also be helpful.

Management Strategies in ST-Segment Elevation Myocardial Infarction

Emergent target-vessel reperfusion with fibrinolytic therapy or primary percutaneous intervention (PCI) is the standard of care for the management of ST segment elevation myocardial infarction (STEMI). Although several large, randomized, clinical trials have demonstrated a survival benefit in using fibrinolytic therapy for STEMI, none have been specifically designed to evaluate its efficacy in patients with diabetes. A meta-analysis of nine large, randomized, clinical trials evaluating the use of fibrinolytic therapy for STEMI reviewed 58,600 patients, of which 4,529 (7.7%) had diabetes. In the subgroup of diabetes patients, fibrinolytic therapy significantly reduced overall mortality (13.6%) compared with the control group (17.3%) at 35 days. A slightly higher incidence of stroke was observed in the group receiving fibrinolytic therapy (1.9%) versus the control group (1.3%). Alteplase and reteplase should be used with adjunctive heparin, whereas the nonspecific fibrinolytic agents (such as streptokinase and urokinase) can be used without heparin. Additionally, adjunctive aspirin has demonstrated a 42% reduction in vascular mortality compared with streptokinase or aspirin alone (25%). When circumstances permit, a more aggressive reperfusion strategy using PCI is generally more beneficial than fibrinolytic therapy. A review of 11 clinical trials comparing primary PCI and fibrinolytic therapy in patients presenting with STEMI showed an overall decrease in the combined end point of mortality of nonfatal reinfarction at 30 days (7.0% versus 12.9%, respectively.) This benefit was more evident in the subgroup analysis of patients with diabetes, where a 30-day mortality or non-fatal reinfarction rate of 9.2% was observed for individuals who underwent primary PCI versus 19.3% for individuals treated with fibrinolytic therapy. When deemed appropriate by the interventionalist, PCI with coronary stenting is preferred over PCI alone. The Controlled Abciximab and Device Investigation to Lower Late Angioplasty Complications (CADILLAC) trial demonstrated that PCI with coronary stenting reduced the composite end point of death, reinfarction, disabling stroke, and need for revascularization compared with PCI alone (10.5% versus 18.0%, respectively) and was particularly beneficial in diabetes patients (9.2% versus 19.3%, respectively). Unfractionated heparin (UFH) or low-molecular-weight heparin (LMWH) should be given immediately. GP IIb/IIIa receptor antagonists can be given en route or in the catheterization laboratory.

Management Strategies in Non–ST Segment Elevation Myocardial Infarction

The initial management of non–ST segment elevation myocardial infarction (NSTEMI) is different from that of STEMI, owing to different pathophysiology. The target vessel in patients with NSTEMI is usually not completely occluded or supplies a small territory. The cornerstone of therapy is rapid platelet inhibition and plaque stabilization followed by medical management among low-risk patients and an early-invasive strategy for high-risk patients. Hemodynamically unstable patients with NSTEMI should receive emergent primary PCI. In the absence of contraindication, all patients with NSTEMI should receive either UFH or LMWH, although LMWH may be slightly more efficacious. The Efficacy and Safety of Subcutaneous Enoxaparin in Non–Q wave Coronary Events (ESSENCE) trial showed that enoxaparin significantly reduced the incidence of death, recurrent MI, and angina at 30 days when compared to UFH (16.6% versus 19.8%, respectively). The use of GP IIb/IIIa receptor inhibitors in the conservative management of patients with NSTEMI is controversial; however, there is evidence to support their use in patients in which an early invasive strategy is planned. A meta-analysis of six large-scale clinical trials enrolling a total of 23,072 patients admitted for NSTEMI/unstable angina, including 6,458 diabetes patients, found that 30-day mortality was significantly lower in diabetes patients using GP IIb/IIIa receptor inhibitors than in placebo subgroups (4.6% versus 6.2%, respectively). In addition, the 1-year mortality in patients with diabetes undergoing an early invasive strategy was significantly decreased by the use of abcixmab from 4.5% to 2.5%.

Surgical Revascularization

No clinical trials have evaluated outcomes of emergent coronary artery bypass graph (CABG) in the setting of AMI; however, an accumulating body of evidence points toward CABG as the preferred revascularization strategy in diabetes patients with unstable angina and multivessel coronary disease. The Bypass Angioplasty Revascularization Investigation (BARI) trial enrolled 1,829 patients, including 353 diabetes patients with angiographically documented multivessel coronary artery disease and either clinically severe angina or objective evidence of marked myocardial ischemia requiring revascularization. At 5 years, there was significantly increased all-cause mortality (35% versus 19%) and cardiac mortality (20.6% versus 5.8%) with multivessel PCI compared with surgical revascularization. The results of two other randomized trials comparing multivessel angioplasty to CABG are consistent with the BARI findings. These results raised concern about selection of angioplasty as a revascularization method in diabetes patients with multivessel coronary artery disease. Subsequent reports from the BARI investigators suggested that the survival benefit of CABG was limited to the 81% of diabetes patients receiving internal mammary grafts. Cardiac mortality was 2.9% when internal mammary grafts were used versus 18.2% when only saphenous vein graft conduits were used. The latter rate was similar to patients receiving percutaneous transluminal coronary angioplasty (20.6%). Some of the lingering questions regarding revascularization in diabetes patients with multivessel disease will be addressed in the ongoing BARI 2D study.

Glycemic Control

The role of tight glycemic control for diabetes patients in the setting of AMI is proven but infrequently practiced. The Diabetes Mellitus, Insulin, Glucose Infusion in Acute Myocardial Infarction (DIGAMI) study investigators randomized 620 patients with diabetes (83% with type 2 diabetes) with MI in 19 hospitals across Sweden to an experimental strategy of initial insulin glucose infusion followed by multidose insulin treatment for 3 months and compared that to a control strategy of insulin supplementation only if clinically indicated. The experimental treatment resulted in a dramatic reduction in mortality at 1 year (19% versus 26%, $P < 0.027$). This 30% reduction in mortality was maintained at 3.4 years of follow-up (33% versus 44%) and translated into a treatment effect of one life saved for every nine patients treated. On subgroup analysis, the maximum benefit was realized in low-risk patients without prior exposure to insulin with an absolute mortality reduction of 15%. The role of both high- and low-dose glucose-insulin potassium infusion has been studied with mixed results in the universe of patients presenting with acute MI. The recent Glucose-Insulin-Potassium Study (GIPS) randomized 940 patients receiving primary PCI for an STEMI to metabolic modulation with glucose-insulin-potassium (GIK) versus control. Whereas treatment with GIK did not decrease overall mortality in the trial, mortality among diabetes patients receiving GIK therapy ($n = 49$) was 4%, compared with 12% among control subjects with diabetes ($n = 50$). Further clinical research is clearly warranted in this area.

PERI-INFARCTION AND LONG-TERM MANAGEMENT GUIDELINES

Patients with diabetes surviving MI suffer from higher late mortality than their counterparts without diabetes. Late mortality is mainly related to recurrent MI and the development of heart failure. Peri-infarction and long-term management of diabetes patients consist of *1)* aggressively modifying risk factors (discussed in the previous section), *2)* optimizing medical therapy, and *3)* cardiac rehabilitation.

Aspirin

The AHA recommends (class I), in the absence of contraindications, a chewed 325-mg aspirin be administered as soon as possible after presentation and 75–162 mg/day aspirin be continued indefinitely.

Clopidogrel

The AHA recommends (class I) that 75 mg/day clopidogrel be administered to hospitalized patients who are unable to take aspirin because of hypersensitivity or major gastrointestinal intolerance. In hospitalized patients with NSTEMI in whom a conservative approach is planned, clopidogrel should be added to aspirin as soon as possible on admission and administered for at least 1 month and for up to 9 months. In patients for whom a PCI is planned, clopidogrel should be taken at least 1 month for bare metal stents and 3–6 months for drug-eluting stents and should be continued for at least 9 months in patients who are not at high risk for bleeding. In patients taking clopidogrel in whom elective CABG is planned, the drug should be withheld for 5–7 days.

UFH and LMWH

The AHA recommends (class I) that anticoagulation with subcutaneous LMWH or intravenous UFH be added to antiplatelet therapy with aspirin and/or clopidogrel. The AHA also acknowledges (class IIb) that the majority of the literature suggests that enoxaparin is superior to UFH as an anticoagulant in patients with unstable angina or NSTEMI, unless a CABG is planned within 24 hours.

GP IIb/IIIa Antagonists

The AHA recommends (class I) that a platelet GP IIb/IIIa antagonist be administered, in addition to aspirin (ASA) and heparin, to patients in whom catheterization and PCI are planned. The GP IIb/IIIa antagonist may also be administered just before PCI. The AHA also acknowledges (class IIb) that the majority of the literature suggests that eptifibatide or tirofiban can be administered, in addition to ASA and LMWH or UFH, to patients with continuing ischemia, with an elevated troponin, or with other high-risk features for which an invasive management strategy is not planned. In addition, the platelet GP IIb/IIIa antagonist can be administered to patients already receiving heparin, ASA, and clopidogrel in whom catheterization and PCI are planned. The GP IIb/IIIa antagonist may also be administered just before PCI.

β-Blockers

The AHA recommends (class I) that in the absence of contraindications, β-blockers be administered to all patients.

ACE Inhibitors

The AHA recommends (class I) that in the absence of contraindications, ACE inhibitors be administered to all patients with diabetes.

Statins and Other Lipid-Lowering Agents

The AHA recommends (class I) lipid-lowering agents and diet in all post-ACS patients, including post-revascularization patients, treating to a target LDL cholesterol level <100 mg/dl (<5.6 mmol/l). As noted earlier in this chapter, HPS and PROVE IT demonstrated benefit for patients treated with statin therapy whose LDL cholesterol levels were <100 mg/dl (<5.6 mmol/l). The AHA also acknowledges (class IIb) that the majority of literature suggests that a fibrate should be administered if HDL cholesterol is <40 mg/dl (<2.2 mmol/l), occurring as an isolated finding or in combination with other lipid abnormalities. In addition, fibrate therapy may be given to patients with HDL cholesterol <40 mg/dl (<2.2 mmol/l) and triglycerides of >200 mg/dl (11.1 mmol/l). Last, HMG-CoA reductase inhibitors and diet should begin 24–96 h after admission and continued after hospital discharge for all patients with LDL cholesterol >100 mg/dl (>5.6 mmol/l).

Nitroglycerin

The AHA recommends (class I) that anginal discomfort lasting more than 2 or 3 min should prompt the patient to discontinue the activity or remove himself or herself from the stressful event. If pain does not subside immediately, the patient should be instructed to take nitroglycerin. If the first tablet or spray does not provide relief within 5 min, then a second and third dose, at 5-min intervals, should be taken. Pain that lasts more than 15–20 min or persistent pain despite three nitroglycerin doses should prompt the patient to seek immediate medical attention by calling 9-1-1 and going to the nearest hospital emergency department, preferably via ambulance or the quickest available alternative.

Cardiac Rehabilitation

The AHA recommends (class I) considering the referral of postinfarction patients to an outpatient cardiac rehabilitation program.

SUMMARY

Patients with diabetes and underlying CHD have a more complex pathophysiology and worse prognosis. Optimal management of these patients begins with aggressive primary prevention strategies. In the setting of STEMI, emergent PCI is preferable over fibrinolysis, especially for those patients beyond the first 4 hours of symptoms. Most diabetes patients with NSTEMI will undergo coronary angiography and possibly primary PCI within the first 48 h of presentation. No clinical trials have evaluated outcomes of emergent CABG in the setting of AMI; however, an accumulating body of evidence suggests that CABG (with left internal mammary artery grafting) is superior to multivessel PCI in diabetes patients with unstable angina. Peri-infarction and long-term management of these patients requires aggressive risk factor modification, optimization of medical therapy, and cardiac rehabilitation. Because of their higher morbidity and mortality after MI, managing diabetes patients is challenging, and it is imperative that the clinician use comprehensive medical strategies for this population.

BIBLIOGRAPHY

American Heart Association Prevention Conference VI: Executive Summary: Diabetes and cardiovascular disease. *Circulation* 105:2231–2239, 2002

American Heart Association Prevention Conference VI: Writing Groups I-V: Diabetes and cardiovascular disease. *Circulation* 105:e132–e169, 2002

Aronson D, Rayfield E: Diabetes. In *The Textbook of Cardiovascular Medicine* (Online version) 2nd ed. Philadelphia, Lippincott, Williams & Wilkins, Available at http://pco.ovid.com/lrppco/index.html

Braunwald E, Antman EM, Beasley JW, Califf RM, Cheitlin MD, Hochman JS, Jones RH, Kereiakes D, Kupersmith J, Levin TN, Pepine CJ, Schaeffer JW, Smith EE 3rd, Steward DE, Theroux P, Gibbons RJ, Alpert JS, Faxon DP, Fuster V, Gregoratos G, Hiratzka LF, Jacobs AK, Smith SC Jr; American College of Cardiology; American Heart Association; Committee on the Management of Patients With Unstable Angina: ACC/AHA 2002 guideline update for the management of patients with unstable angina and non–ST-segment elevation myocardial infarction: summary article. *J Am Coll Cardiol* 40:1366–1374, 2002

Bypass Angioplasty Revascularization Investigation (BARI) Investigators: Influence of diabetes on 5-year mortality and morbidity in a randomized trial comparing CABG and PTCA in patients with multi-vessel disease. *Circulation* 96:1761–1779, 1997

CASS Principal Investigators and their Associates: Myocardial infarction and mortality in the Coronary Artery Surgery Study (CASS) randomized trial. *N Engl J Med* 310:750–758, 1984

Heart Outcomes Prevention Evaluation (HOPE) Study Investigators: Effects of an ACE inhibitor, ramipril, on cardiovascular events in high risk patients. *N Engl J Med* 342:145–153, 2000

Heart Protection Study Collaborative Group: MRC/BHF Heart Protection Study of cholesterol-lowering with simvastatin in 5963 people with diabetes: a randomized placebo-controlled trial. *Lancet* 361:2005–2016, 2003

HOPE Investigators: Effect of ramipril on cardiovascular and microvascular outcomes in people with diabetes mellitus: results of the HOPE study and MICRO-HOPE sub-study. *Lancet* 355:253–259, 2000

Klein L, Gheorghiade M: Management of the patient with diabetes mellitus and myocardial infarction: clinical trial update. *Am J Med* 116:47S–63S, 2004

Malmberg K: Prospective randomized study of intensive insulin treatment on long-term survival after acute myocardial infarction in patients with diabetes mellitus. *BMJ* 314:1512–1515, 1997

Mooradian AD: Cardiovascular disease in type 2 diabetes mellitus: current management guidelines. *Arch Intern Med* 163:33–40, 2003

Nesto RW: Treatment of acute myocardial infarction in diabetes mellitus. *Up To Date* Online Version 12.1, 2004 Available at www.uptodate.com

Pravastatin or Atorvastatin Evaluation and Infection Therapy: Thrombolysis in Myocardial Infarction 22 Investigators (PROVE IT): Comparison of intensive and moderate lipid lowering with statins after acute coronary syndromes. *N Engl J Med* 350:1495-1504, 2004

Dr. Crouch is a cardiology fellow; Dr. Menon is Assistant Professor of Medicine and Emergency Medicine and Director of Coronary Care Unit and Chest Pain Unit; and Dr. Smith is Professor of Medicine and Director of Center for Cardiovascular Science and Medicine, Division of Cardiology, University of North Carolina at Chapel Hill, Chapel Hill, NC.

53. Primary and Secondary Prevention: Lipid Outcome Studies in Diabetes

STEVEN HAFFNER, MD

DIABETES AND CORONARY HEART DISEASE: EXTENT OF DISEASE

Type 2 diabetes is associated with a two- to fourfold increased risk of cardiovascular disease. In addition, diabetes subjects have an increased case mortality rate after a myocardial infarction; therefore, diabetes subjects are at double jeopardy in terms of morbidity and mortality from coronary heart disease (CHD). In the general population, the incidence of CHD in diabetes subjects without preexisting cardiovascular disease is similar to the incidence of cardiovascular disease in nondiabetic subjects who have had previous cardiovascular disease. Nevertheless, there is heterogeneity of risk for cardiovascular disease among subjects with diabetes. Duration of diabetes has long been known to be a strong risk factor of cardiovascular disease; thus, newly discovered diabetes subjects with only mildly elevated glucose levels may have a lower risk of cardiovascular disease than subjects with more severe, longer-duration diabetes. In the United Kingdom Prospective Diabetes Study (UKPDS) 23, the baseline predictors of cardiovascular disease in order of entry into a Cox proportional hazards model were as follows: 1) LDL cholesterol, 2) low HDL cholesterol, 3) glycated hemoglobin A1C (A1C), 4) systolic blood pressure, and 5) cigarette smoking.

LIPOPROTEINS IN TYPE 2 DIABETES AND CLINICAL TRIALS

The characteristics of lipoproteins in patients with type 2 diabetes as compared with nondiabetic subjects are higher triglyceride levels and lower HDL cholesterol levels but relatively "normal" LDL cholesterol levels; however, the composition of the LDL particles is often altered in diabetes subjects so that it is smaller and denser and potentially atherogenic. Based on the observation that diabetes subjects had relatively "normal" LDL cholesterol levels but higher triglycerides and lower HDL cholesterol levels, in the past, diabetologists often began treating diabetes subjects with fibric acid such as gemfibrozil or fenofibrate. Indeed, gemfibrozil was shown to reduce CHD by ~60% in diabetes subjects in the Helsinki Heart Study, although the number of subjects was small ($n = 135$) and the results were not statistically significant. More recently, gemfibrozil was shown to reduce cardiovascular disease by 24% (*P* = 0.05) in a larger group of diabetes subjects (Veterans Affairs High-Density Lipoprotein Cholesterol Intervention Trial [VA-HIT])—a reduction similar to that seen in the nondiabetic subjects. The transition from this traditional view of fibric acid as initial therapy for diabetic dyslipidemia to the more recent view of statins as the initial drug of choice came from two types of observations: *1*) the observational data in UKPDS 23, which suggested that LDL was a very important risk factor for CHD, even in diabetes subjects with relatively low LDL cholesterol levels; and *2*) the extensive data that showed statins reduced CHD in diabetes subgroups by amounts equivalent to or, in some cases, greater than those seen in the fibric acid trial, such as the VA-HIT trial. The major primary prevention trials were the Air Force/Texas Coronary Atherosclerosis Prevention Study (TEX-CAPS/AFCAPS) and the recently published Heart Protection Study (HPS). The major secondary prevention trials were the 4S trial, the CARE trial, the Lipid trial, and the HPS. Of interest in the overall HPS, statin therapy was effective in reducing CHD, even in people who were below the conventional National Cholesterol Education Program Adult Treatment Panel III (NCEP ATP III) goals for diabetes and in CHD subjects with LDL levels <100 mg/dl. There is a paper currently under review suggesting that similar data exist for the diabetes subjects in the HPS, suggesting that the drug initiation levels in the most recent American Diabetes Association (ADA) guidelines on the management of dyslipidemia in adults with diabetes (American Diabetes Association [2003]) might be modified for diabetes subjects without vascular disease to initiate drug therapy at an LDL cholesterol level of 100 mg/dl (Table 53.1).

CURRENT ADA GUIDELINES

The ADA suggests as a matter of priority to focus initially on LDL cholesterol followed by an emphasis on HDL cholesterol and lastly a reduction of triglyceride levels (Table 53.2). This order of priorities was initially based on observational data from the UKPDS. The secondary goal for the NCEP is slightly different. If

Table 53.1 Treatment Decisions Based on LDL Cholesterol Level in Adults with Diabetes

	Medical Nutrition Therapy		Drug Therapy	
	Initiation level	LDL goal	Initiation level	LDL goal
With CHD, PAD, or CVD	≥100	<100	≥100	<100
Without CHD, PAD, and CVD	≥100	<100	≥130*	<100

Data are given in milligrams per deciliter. *For patients with LDL levels between 100 and 129 mg/dl, a variety of treatment strategies are available, including more aggressive medical nutrition therapy and pharmacological treatment with a statin; in addition, if the HDL level is ≤40 mg/dl, a fibric acid such as fenofibrate may be used in these patients. Medical nutrition therapy should be attempted before starting pharmacological therapy. CVD, cardiovascular disease; PAD, peripheral arterial disease. From the American Diabetes Association.

Table 53.2 Order of Priorities for Treating Diabetic Dyslipidemia in Adults*

Lowering LDL cholesterol*
  First choice
    HMG-CoA reductase inhibitor (statin)
  Second choice
    Bile acid binding resin (resin) or fenofibrate
Raising HDL cholesterol
  Behavioral interventions such as weight loss, increased physical activity, and smoking cessation
  Difficult except with nicotinic acid, which should be used with caution, or fibrate
Lowering triglyceride
  Glycemic control first priority
  Fibric acid derivative (gemfibrozil, fenofibrate)
  Statins are moderately effective at high doses in hypertriglyceridemic subjects who also have high LDL cholesterol
Combined hyperlipidemia
  First choice
    Improved glycemic control plus high-dose statin
  Second choice
    Improved glycemic control plus statin[†] plus fibric acid derivative[†] (gemfibrozil, fenofibrate)
  Third choice
    Improved glycemic control plus resin plus fibric acid derivative (gemfibrozil, fenofibrate)
    Improved glycemic control plus statin[†] plus nicotinic acid[†] (glycemic control must be monitored carefully)

*Decision for treating high LDL cholesterol before elevated triglyceride is based on clinical trial data indicating safety as well as efficacy of the available agents. [†]The combination of statins with nicotinic acid and especially with gemfibrozil or fenofibrate may carry an increased risk of myositis. Fibric acid therapy is recommended for patients with triglyceride levels >400 mg/dl.
From the American Diabetes Association.

subjects have a triglyceride level of ≥200 mg/dl after meeting LDL cholesterol goals, the secondary goal for non-HDL cholesterol is <130 mg/dl. As does the NCEP, the American Diabetes Association recommends an initial focus on LDL cholesterol with an LDL goal of <100 mg/dl. Because medical nutrition therapy is unlikely to lower the LDL cholesterol by >30 mg/dl, both the NCEP and the American Diabetes Association suggest that initial therapy for diabetes subjects who have an LDL cholesterol >130 mg/dl be both medical nutrition therapy and pharmacological therapy. There is a broader range of options for individuals who have an LDL cholesterol between 100 and 129 mg/dl. The ADA and NCEP suggest either further intensification of therapy with a statin or medical nutrition therapy, or possibly adding an agent for treatment of atherogenic dyslipidemia (fibric acid or nicotinic acid). After the publication of the HPS, it could be argued whether all diabetes subjects with LDL cholesterol ≥100 mg/dl might not receive statin therapy. There is currently interest in whether diabetes subjects who have CHD might be treated even more aggressively because diabetes subjects with prevalent CHD have a greater risk of future CHD than diabetes subjects without prevalent CHD (i.e., LDL cholesterol <75 mg/dl). There is currently no clinical trial data to support this recommendation. However, this hypothesis is being tested in diabetes subgroups in the treatment to new targets (TNT) and search trials.

COMBINATION THERAPY

The current recommendation of the ADA acknowledges the existence of combination therapy but does not make definitive recommendations about the use of combination therapy. This is because of the absence of evidence-based medicine from clinical trial as well as perceived safety concerns about some combination therapy. Currently, no clinical trial data have been published on diabetes subjects using a combination of statins and fibric acid or statins and nicotinic acid. The HATS regression trial data, which report on subjects with familial combined hyperlipidemia (Brown et al.), suggest that low-dose simvastatin (10–20 mg) plus high-dose nicotinic acid (3–4 g/day) reduced CHD by ~80% and slowed progression of atherosclerosis in a small group of 150 patients. Both subjects with diabetes and subjects with the metabolic syndrome were included in this population. Results were presented at the 2002 American College of Cardiology meeting on diabetes subjects from the HATS trial, but a full report has not been published. More definitive information on combination therapy may come from the Action to Control Cardiovascular Risk in Diabetes (ACCORD) trial, in which ~5,000 subjects with type 2 diabetes will be put on 20 mg simvastatin and then subjects will be randomized to placebo or 200 mg fenofibrate micronized.

Traditionally, physicians were concerned about the use of combination therapy because there may be an increased risk of myositis with statins and fibric acid or nicotinic acid. However, the actual risk of myositis with nicotinic acid in combination with statins is believed to be low. The risk of myositis with a combination of statins and fibric acid was accentuated by the increased mortality seen in subjects on gemfibrozil and cervistatin (Baycol). However, the risk of myositis of statins and fibric acids appears to be much less with other fibric acids and statins, particularly in subjects with normal renal function. A recent example of such an article is that by Athyros et al. on the combination of 200 mg fenofibrate micronized and 20 mg atorvastatin. Additional concerns with nicotinic acid relate to this possible effect on insulin resistance and increasing glucose intolerance. Older studies have suggested marked rises in A1C in subjects treated with 4 g nicotinic acid per day. However, more recent studies with smaller doses of nicotinic acid and careful attention to monitoring glycemic control have shown much smaller effects on A1C.

THE METABOLIC SYNDROME

Clustering of cardiovascular risk factors (hypertension, glucose intolerance, and dyslipidemia) has long been noted. Reaven postulated in his 1987 Banting lecture that insulin resistance might be the basis of this clustering of cardiovascular risk factors. Reaven further postulated that this syndrome could occur in nonobese subjects. Other authors have suggested that increased obesity and particularly visceral fat might be the most important etiology of this cluster of cardiovascular risk factors in Western society. Recently, a number of organizations have suggested criteria for defining the metabolic syndrome, including the World Health Organization (WHO) (in 1999) and the NCEP. It is not clear which of the two major criteria (NCEP or WHO) is superior at this time, although the NCEP definition is clearly simpler for the clinician in that it does not involve measurement of fasting insulin or urinary microalbuminuria or the performance of the oral glucose tolerance test. The NCEP criteria include waist circumference, high triglycerides, low HDL cholesterol, hypertension, or a fasting glucose ≥110 mg/dl (Table 53.3).

The prevalence of the metabolic syndrome in subjects with type 2 diabetes has been examined in several populations and appears to be ~80%. It is possible that the relatively unusual diabetes subject without the metabolic syndrome may be at lower risk of CHD and therefore may need less aggressive therapy, although this aspect needs to be studied further, particularly in prospective studies. The risk of CHD in nondiabetic subjects with the metabolic syndrome is of considerable interest. The ADA has recommendations for the treatment of impaired glucose tolerance but not for the metabolic syndrome. The NCEP suggests that the primary therapy of the metabolic syndrome should be behavioral (i.e., weight loss and increased physical activity). In addition, treatment of disorders associated with the metabolic syndrome, such as hypertension and dyslipidemia, should also be administered. These recommendations appear to be reasonable but are limited. The NCEP does not say, for instance, whether intensification of pharmacological therapy should be done in people with the metabolic syndrome above and beyond their global risk. One possibility would be to calculate global risk in all subjects rather than in those with just two or more major risk factors. If the global risk was 5–10% and the subject had the metabolic syndrome, the subject might be treated as if he or she had a global risk of ≥10%. Similarly, if the global risk was 15–20% and the subject had the metabolic syndrome, the subject might be

Table 53.3 NCEP ATP III: the Metabolic Syndrome*

Risk Factor	Defining Level
Abdominal obesity (waist circumference)	
Men	>102 cm (>40 inches)
Women	>88 cm (>35 inches)
Triglycerides	≥150 mg/dl
HDL cholesterol	
Men	<40 mg/dl
Women	<50 mg/dl
Blood pressure	≥130/85 mmHg
Fasting glucose	≥110 mg/dl

*Diagnosis is established when three or more of these risk factors are present. From the Expert Panel on Detection, Evaluation, and Treatment of High Blood Cholesterol in Adults.

treated as if he or she had a global risk of ≥20%. In this case, the subject might be considered to have a risk equivalent to CHD or diabetes subjects and have a suggested LDL cholesterol <100 mg/dl. Another potential limitation of the NCEP criteria is that no recommendation is made about insulin-sensitizing pharmacological therapies. Some of these therapies clearly improve lipoproteins (raise HDL cholesterol) and lower markers of subclinical inflammation (C-reactive protein); however, no randomized clinical trial exists showing the benefit of insulin-sensitizing therapies for reduction of cardiovascular disease.

The metabolic syndrome is likely to be an important focus for diabetologists in at least two ways. According to National Health and Nutrition Examination Survey (NHANES) data, there are at least 60% more subjects with the metabolic syndrome than there are subjects with type 2 diabetes. There is an increased attention to whether the metabolic syndrome itself should be treated. Furthermore, some cardiovascular predicting models have been shown to predict type 2 diabetes as well as impaired glucose tolerance. These subjects identified by a cardiovascular risk model are likely to have a higher risk of cardiovascular disease than subjects identified just by impaired glucose tolerance. Identifying groups using a predicting equation may be a more efficient way to prevent type 2 diabetes. Studies are underway to determine how well the metabolic syndrome predicts type 2 diabetes.

SUMMARY

Type 2 diabetes subjects have a marked increased rate of CHD. In both the ADA and the NCEP ATP III guidelines, diabetes is considered to be equivalent to CHD. The primary goal of lipid therapy for both of these organizations is the reduction of LDL cholesterol. The LDL goal is <100 mg/dl in both sets of recommendations. However, the secondary goal differs slightly. The ADA suggests a focus on raising HDL cholesterol and then lowering triglycerides, whereas the NCEP suggests lowering non-HDL cholesterol in subjects who have a triglyceride level of 200 mg/dl. These differences are relatively minor. In most diabetes subjects, the initial therapy will be a reduction of LDL cholesterol with statins and behavioral therapy. In some patients, fibric acids or nicotinic acid may be needed as additional therapy, although the circumstances in which these therapies will reduce CHD are not yet known. Recent attention has also focused on the existence of the metabolic syndrome. In nondiabetic subjects with the metabolic syndrome, behavioral intervention and possibly pharmacological therapy beyond what their global risk score might suggest should be considered.

BIBLIOGRAPHY

American Diabetes Association: Dyslipidemia management in adults with diabetes (Position Statement). *Diabetes Care* 27 (Suppl. 1):S68–S71, 2004

Athyros VG, Papageorgiou AA, Athyrou VV, Demitriadis DS, Kontopoulos AG: Atorvastatin and micronized fenofibrate alone and in combination in type 2 diabetes with combined hyperlipidemia. *Diabetes Care* 25:1198–1202, 2002

Brown BG, Zhao X-Q, Chait A, Fisher LD, Cheung MC, Morse JS, Dowdy AA, Marino EK, Bolson EL, Alaupovic P, Frohlich J, Serafini L, Huss-Frechette E, Wang S, DeAngelis D, Dodek A, Albers JJ: Simvastatin and niacin, anti-oxidant vitamins, or the combination for the prevention of coronary disease. *N Engl J Med* 345:1583–1592, 2001

Expert Panel on Detection, Evaluation and Treatment of High Blood Choles-terol in Adults: Executive Summary of the Third Report of the National Cholesterol Education Program (NCEP) Expert Panel on Detection, Evalu-ation and Treatment of High Blood Cholesterol in Adults (Adult Treatment Panel III). *JAMA* 285:2486–2497, 2001

Haffner SM: Management of dyslipidemia in adults with diabetes (Technical Review). *Diabetes Care* 21:160–178, 1998

Haffner SM, Lehto S, Ronnemaa T, Pyorala K, Laakso M: Mortality from coro-nary heart disease in subjects with type 2 diabetes and in nondiabetic subjects with and without prior myocardial infarction. *N Engl J Med* 339:229–234, 1998

Reaven GM: Insulin resistance and its consequences: non-insulin-dependent diabetes mellitus and coronary heart disease. In *Diabetes Mellitus: A Funda-mental and Clinical Text*. LeRoith D, Ed. Philadelphia, Lippincott-Raven, 1996, p. 509–519

Turner RC, Millns H, Neil HA, Stratton IM, Manley SE, Matthews DR, Holman RR: Risk factors for coronary artery disease in non-insulin dependent diabetes mellitus (UKPDS 23). *BMJ* 316:823–828, 1998

Dr. Haffner is Professor, Department of Medicine, University of Texas Health Science Center, San Antonio, TX.

54. ACE Inhibitors and Angiotensin II Receptor Antagonists as Reducers of Vascular Complications

SARAH CAPES, MD, MSc, FRCPC,
AND HERTZEL GERSTEIN, MD, MSc, FRCPC

Angiotensin-converting enzyme (ACE) inhibitors and angiotensin II receptor (A2) antagonists are drugs that have two main effects: promoting potentially beneficial metabolic changes in the vasculature and lowering blood pressure. The metabolic changes associated with both classes of drugs include reducing the effects of angiotensin II on target tissue, thereby decreasing vasoconstriction and decreasing stimulation of vascular smooth muscle growth. ACE inhibitors have the added effect of increasing levels of bradykinins (which promote vasodilation and increase insulin sensitivity), lowering levels of plasminogen activator inhibitor, and decreasing platelet aggregation. Equally important, the blood pressure–lowering effect of these and other classes of drugs has been shown in numerous clinical trials to translate into an improved cardiovascular prognosis for patients with diabetes. This chapter will summarize the evidence regarding the vascular benefits of ACE inhibitors and A2 antagonists in patients with diabetes.

METABOLIC EFFECTS OF ACE INHIBITORS AND A2 ANTAGONISTS

ACE Inhibitors Prevent Cardiovascular Events Independent of Their Blood Pressure–Lowering Effect

Cardiovascular disease affects >50% of all people with diabetes and is the major cause of death. At least four recent studies have explored the cardioprotective effects of ACE inhibitors in participants with either a history of cardiovascular disease or diabetes. The largest of these studies was the Heart Outcome Prevention Evaluation (HOPE) study. In the HOPE study, 3,577 people with diabetes were randomly assigned to treatment with 10 mg/day ramipril, versus placebo, in addition to their usual medications. Ramipril reduced the risk of the combined outcome of myocardial infarction (MI), stroke, or cardiovascular death by 25% over 4.5 years of follow-up (Table 54.1). About half of the diabetes patients had a diagnosis of hypertension at the time of randomization, and in those patients, the study drug (ramipril or placebo) was added to their usual antihypertensive medication (β-blocker in 28%, diuretic in 20%, and calcium-channel blocker in 44%). Ramipril had only

Table 54.1 Results of the HOPE Study in Patients with Diabetes

Outcome	Placebo Rate (%)	Relative Risk Reduction [% (95% CI)]	P
MI, stroke, or CV death	19.8	25 (12–36)	0.0004
MI	12.9	22 (6–36)	0.01
Stroke	6.1	33 (10–50)	0.0074
CV death	9.7	37 (21–51)	0.0001
Total death	14	24 (8–37)	0.004

CV, cardiovascular.

a modest blood pressure–lowering effect, and the reduced morbidity and mortality that was observed in patients treated with ramipril was shown to be independent of the change in blood pressure. Thus, the HOPE study clearly shows that ACE inhibitors have a cardioprotective effect over and above any antihypertensive effect. On the basis of this study, 22 high-risk, middle-aged people with diabetes would have to be treated with ramipril for 4.5 years to prevent one MI, stroke, or cardiovascular death. ACE inhibitors also improve outcome for patients with chronic congestive heart failure. Indeed, in the Studies of Left Ventricular Dysfunction (SOLVD) trial, enalapril reduced mortality and hospitalization for heart failure by 26% compared with placebo in patients with chronic congestive heart failure and reduced ejection fraction.

Although ACE inhibitors differ in structure and pharmacokinetic properties, all members of the class are likely to have similar cardioprotective effects. Notwithstanding this assumption, neither the optimal cardioprotective dose nor the comparable doses of each of the members of this class have been established. It is important to note, however, that higher doses of ACE inhibitors may be required for optimal cardioprotection. For example, in the Study to Evaluate Carotid Ultrasound Changes in Patients Treated with Ramipril and Vitamin E (SECURE) substudy of the HOPE study, there was evidence of a dose-response effect with slower progression of carotid atherosclerosis in patients treated with higher doses of ramipril (10 mg/day vs. 0 or 2.5 mg/day).

A2 Antagonists May Prevent Cardiovascular Events in Patients with Diabetes

The cardioprotective effects of A2 antagonists have been studied in select groups of individuals, and emerging evidence suggests that A2 antagonists may also have beneficial vascular metabolic effects. Studies in which patients with type 2 diabetes were treated with A2 antagonists are summarized in Table 54.2. Only one study has clearly demonstrated a reduction in cardiovascular events in diabetes patients using an A2 antagonist. This study, the Losartan Intervention for Endpoint Reduction in Hypertension (LIFE) study, only included people with significant hypertension and left ventricular hypertrophy. It showed the

Table 54.2 A2 Antagonists in Type 2 Diabetes

Study	n	% with Diabetes	Mean Age (yr)	Drug/Dose	Outcome	Results (A2 Antagonist vs. Comparator)	P
LIFE (diabetes, ↑BP, and left ventricular hypertrophy)	1,195	100	67	50–100 mg losartan vs. 50–100 mg atenolol	CV death, stroke, or MI	RRR = 0.24 (95% CI 0.02–0.42)	0.031
RENAAL study (diabetic nephropathy)	1,513	100	60	50–100 mg losartan vs. placebo	Doubling of serum creatinine, end-stage renal disease, or death	RRR = 0.16	0.02
					Fatal or nonfatal CV event	RRR = 0.1	0.26
					Myocardial infarction	RRR = 0.28	0.08
					First hospitalization for coronary heart failure	RRR = 0.32	0.005
CALM study (diabetes, ↑BP, and microalbuminuria)	199	100	60	16 mg candesartan vs. 20 mg lisiropril vs. combination of both drugs	Systolic and diastolic blood pressure, ACR	Combination reduced systolic and diastolic BP and urine ACR more than either drug alone	<0.05
IDNT study (diabetic nephropathy)	1,715	100	58–59	300 mg irbesartan vs. 10 mg amlodipine vs. placebo	Doubling of serum creatinine, ESRD, or death	RRR = 0.23 (vs. amlodipine) and 0.2 (vs. placebo)	0.006 / 0.02
IRMA study (diabetes and microalbuminuria)	590	100	58	150–300 mg irbesartan vs. placebo	Time to onset of diabetic nephropathy	RRR = 0.7 (95% CI 0.39–0.86) for 300 mg irbesartan; RRR = 0.39 (95% CI –0.08–0.66) for 150 mg irbesartan	<0.001 / 0.08

ACR, albumin-to-creatinine ratio; ↑BP, hypertension; CV, cardiovascular; CALM, Candesartan and Lisinopril Microalbuminuria; IDNT, Irbesartan Diabetic Nephropathy Trial; IRMA, Irbesartan in Patients with Type 2 Diabetes and Microalbuminuria; RRR, relative risk reduction.

benefit of losartan over atenolol within the group as a whole and the diabetes subgroup. Patients who were treated with 50–100 mg losartan had a significant 24% lower risk of cardiovascular death, stroke, or MI than those who were treated with 50–100 mg atenolol, despite equal lowering of blood pressure in both groups.

Other studies confined to patients with overt diabetic nephropathy have shown an improvement in renal outcomes, and some of these studies have also shown a trend toward improved cardiovascular prognosis. For example, in the Reduction of Endpoints in NIDDM with the Angiotensin II Antagonist Losartan (RENAAL) study, treatment with 50–100 mg losartan led to a significant 16% reduction in the primary endpoint of doubling of serum creatinine, end-stage renal failure, or death compared with placebo. The RENAAL study also showed a lower risk of first hospitalization for congestive heart failure and a trend toward reduced risk of fatal and nonfatal cardiovascular events in losartan-treated patients.

CARDIOPROTECTIVE EFFECTS OF BLOOD PRESSURE LOWERING

Systematic reviews and meta-analyses of the effects of various blood pressure–lowering agents have shown that lowering blood pressure by 10–12 mmHg systolic and 5–6 mmHg diastolic leads to as much as a 16% reduction in the risk of coronary artery disease and a 38% reduction in stroke risk. The beneficial effect of blood pressure lowering with ACE inhibitors was demonstrated in a meta-analysis performed by the Blood Pressure Lowering Treatment Trialists' Collaboration, which combined individual patient data from the HOPE study and three smaller studies in which ACE inhibitors were compared with placebo. The meta-analysis showed that high-risk patients (including those with diabetes) who were treated with an ACE inhibitor, compared with placebo, had significant 20–30% reductions in risk of stroke, coronary heart disease, major cardiovascular events, and cardiovascular death, as well as a reduction in total mortality (Fig. 54.1).

An overview of trials comparing blood pressure–lowering regimens based on different drugs did not find significant differences in cardiovascular outcomes among hypertensive patients treated with ACE inhibitors versus those treated with diuretic, β-blocker, or calcium antagonist–based regimens. The results of this overview were confirmed by the Antihypertensive and Lipid Lowering Treatment to Prevent Heart Attack Trial (ALLHAT). ALLHAT enrolled 42,418 hypertensive patients (about one-third of whom had diabetes) who were randomized to blood pressure regimens based on chlorthalidone, lisinopril, or amlodipine. All three regimens were equally effective in lowering the rate of the primary outcome of fatal coronary heart disease or nonfatal MI. Patients treated with chlorthalidone also had a lower risk of heart failure than individuals in the other two groups.

These studies reinforce the primary importance of good control of hypertension to prevent cardiovascular events in patients with diabetes. It is important to note that most hypertensive patients with diabetes will require more than one drug to adequately control their blood pressure. Indeed, in the United Kingdom Prospective Diabetes Study, 63% of patients required two or more antihypertensive agents

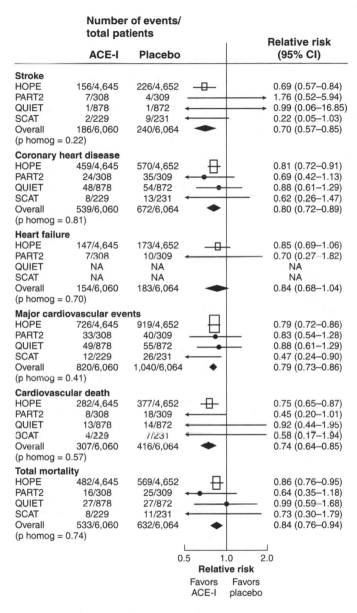

Figure 54.1 Comparisons of angiotensin-converting enzyme (ACE) inhibitor–based therapy with placebo. Boxes and horizontal lines represent relative risk and 95% CI for each trial. Size of boxes is proportional to inverse of variance of that trial result. Diamonds represent the 95% CI for pooled estimates of effect and are centered on pooled relative risk. ACE-I, ACE inhibitor; NA, data not available; PART2, Prevention of Atherosclerosis with Ramipril Trial; p homog, *P* value from the χ^2 text for homogeneity; QUIET, Quinapril Ischemic Event Trial; SCAT, Simvastatin/Enalapril Coronary Atherosclerosis Trial.

to achieve optimal blood pressure control. The results of ALLHAT and the overview performed by the Blood Pressure Lowering Treatment Trialists' Collaboration suggest that first treatment with a diuretic, ACE inhibitor, β-blocker, or calcium antagonist is appropriate (unless there is a specific indication for the use of one of these classes, such as ACE inhibitors for diabetes patients with microalbuminuria). For the majority of diabetes patients who require more than one drug to control their blood pressure, the results of the HOPE study strongly support the inclusion of an ACE inhibitor in the blood pressure–lowering regimen.

CONCLUSION

Blood pressure lowering is key to the prevention of cardiovascular events in hypertensive patients with diabetes. Diuretics, ACE inhibitors, β-blockers, and calcium antagonists provide similar benefits when used as initial blood pressure–lowering therapy. The large reduction in cardiovascular events in the face of a small reduction in blood pressure that was noted in the HOPE study suggests that ACE inhibitors have beneficial vascular effects that extend beyond their blood pressure–lowering effect. Although early data are suggestive, A2 antagonists have not yet clearly been proven to provide similar cardioprotection, and there is no evidence to support the combination of an ACE inhibitor and A2 antagonist at this time. We recommend that

- unless there is an indication for a specific class of drug, initial treatment of hypertension in diabetes patients may be with any one of a diuretic, ACE inhibitor, β-blocker, or calcium antagonist
- an ACE inhibitor should be included in the treatment regimen of hypertensive patients with diabetes who require more than one drug to control their blood pressure
- ACE inhibitors should also be considered in the treatment of normotensive individuals with diabetes at high risk of cardiovascular disease, to lower the risk of cardiovascular events

BIBLIOGRAPHY

ALLHAT Officers and Coordinators for the ALLHAT Collaborative Research Group: Major outcomes in high-risk hypertensive patients randomized to angiotensin-converting enzyme inhibitor or calcium channel blocker vs diuretic: the Antihypertensive and Lipid-Lowering Treatment to Prevent Heart Attack Trial (ALLHAT). *JAMA* 288:2981–2997, 2002

Blood Pressure Lowering Treatment Trialists' Collaboration: Effects of ACE inhibitors, calcium antagonists, and other blood-pressure-lowering drugs: results of prospectively designed overviews of randomised trials. *Lancet* 356:1955–1964, 2000

Brenner BM, Cooper ME, de Zeeuw D, Keane WF, Mitch WE, Parving HH, Remuzzi G, Snapinn SM, Zhang Z, Shahinfar S, for the RENAAL Study Investigators: Effects of losartan on renal and cardiovascular outcomes in patients with type 2 diabetes and nephropathy. *N Engl J Med* 345:861–869, 2001

Heart Outcome Prevention Evaluation (HOPE) Study Investigators: Effects of ramipril on cardiovascular and microvascular outcomes in people with diabetes mellitus: results of the HOPE study and the MICRO HOPE substudy. *Lancet* 255:253–259, 2000

Lindholm LH, Ibsen H, Dahlof B, Devereux RB, Beevers G, de Faire U, Fyhrquist F, Julius S, Kjeldsen SE, Kristiansson K, Lederballe-Pedersen O, Nieminen MS, Omvik P, Oparil S, Wedel H, Aurup P, Edelman J, Snapinn S: Cardiovascular morbidity and mortality in patients with diabetes in the Losartan Intervention for Endpoint Reduction in Hypertension Study (LIFE): a randomised trial against atenolol. *Lancet* 359:1004–1010, 2002

Dr. Capes is Assistant Professor, Department of Medicine, McMaster University, Hamilton, Ontario, Canada. Dr. Gerstein is Professor, Department of Medicine, McMaster University, Hamilton, Ontario, Canada.

Dr. Gerstein holds the McMaster University Population Health Institute Chair in Diabetes Research (sponsored by Aventis).

55. Peripheral Arterial Disease

GARY GIBBONS, MD, AND CHRISTOPHER LOCKE, DPM

L ower-extremity peripheral arterial disease (PAD) is among the most important reasons for nonhealing ulceration, pain, and amputation in individuals
with and without diabetes. The incidence of PAD in patients with diabetes is
at least four times that of nondiabetic individuals and increases with age and duration of diabetes. In population-based studies, pulse deficits were found in ~10% of
diabetes subjects and absent pulses were found in ~20–30%. Critical ischemia has
been found to be associated with 62% of cases where there was nonhealing ulceration and to be a causal factor in 46% of amputations. PAD results in decreased
arterial perfusion to the lower extremity and the foot. It contributes to limb ulceration and impaired wound healing and decreases the ability to fight infection by
delaying or preventing the delivery of oxygen, nutrients, the components of a
proper immune response, and antibiotics to the infected area. Revascularization
procedures offer great hope to diabetes patients with limb-threatening ischemia
and should be considered before any thought of amputation.

RISK FACTORS AND PREVENTION

Whereas diabetes is an important risk factor for PAD, hypertension, smoking,
hyperlipidemia, obesity, and family history are well-established risk factors and
contribute additional risk for patients with diabetes.

Prevention of or delaying the onset of PAD is best achieved by the elimination
of risk factors including cigarette smoking, good control of diabetes, control of
hypertension and hyperlipidemia, maintaining ideal weight, and routine and
proper exercise. Periodic clinical arterial examination, including noninvasive
testing when appropriate, identifies patients at risk so they can be observed more
carefully or referred to a arterial specialist.

PATHOPHYSIOLOGY

Diabetic PAD is more common, occurs at a younger age, and advances more
rapidly with a roughly equal male-to-female ratio compared with nondiabetic PAD.
Whereas the pathology of atherosclerosis is similar in patients both with and without diabetes, there are several distinguishing features characterizing diabetic PAD.

In the patient with diabetes, there is a predilection for peripheral arterial occlusive disease to primarily involve the tibial and peroneal arteries, but the foot arteries (dorsalis pedis, posterior tibial, and plantar) are usually spared. There is no occlusive microarterial disease of the diabetic foot that precludes revascularization. This misconception leads to inappropriate arterial care extended to many diabetes patients. Because there is sparing of the foot vessels, tissue perfusion in the ischemic diabetic foot can be restored with appropriate arterial reconstructions.

Patients with diabetes frequently develop microarterial dysfunction—a non-occlusive impairment involving arterioles and capillaries that begins early in the life of a diabetes patient. There is increased microarterial pressure and flow leading to endothelial injury with sclerosis (basement membrane thickening). The result is a limited capillary capacity with loss of autoregulatory function including the abolition of a vasoconstrictor response. Leukocyte migration is impeded and oxygen defusion is impaired, resulting in decreased oxygen use. Increased arteriovenous shunting associated with autonomic neuropathy, an impaired hyperemic response to heat and inflammation, the loss of a postural vasoconstrictor response, increased capillary permeability leading to edema formation, and a diminished or loss of other neurogenic regulatory responses all alter the diabetes patient's ability to respond to injury with a proper and orderly sequence of wound healing.

CLINICAL PRESENTATION

The clinical presentation of patients with major artery occlusions or hemodynamically significant stenosis varies depending on their activity level and the adequacy of collateral pathways. Claudication, the inability to walk a given distance (usually described in blocks) because of an ache or pain in the muscles of the leg, is the earliest symptom of PAD. The stenosis or blockage can usually be determined by the group of muscles involved and is generally one level above. Patients with significant foot pain while walking generally have tibial/peroneal arterial disease, patients with calf claudication usually have superficial femoral artery disease, and patients who describe buttock, hip, or thigh claudication have disease involving the aorta and iliac arteries. Establishing the diagnosis of ischemia in the diabetes patient is made more difficult by the presence of peripheral sensory and autonomic neuropathy. Because of neuropathy, diabetes patients may not be able to adequately describe pain and state that they just have to stop.

As PAD progressively worsens, rest pain occurs and is usually described as a deep aching of the muscles in the foot that is present at rest or at night. Patients often get relief by hanging their feet dependently or walking around, especially at night. If the disease progresses further, tissue ulceration and/or gangrene can develop. Because of neuropathy, especially with the loss of sensation, diabetes patients may present with tissue loss or gangrene as the first sign of severe PAD.

Clinical evaluation, judgment, and experience remain the most important means for determining the degree of arterial compromise in the diabetic lower extremity (Table 55.1). Noninvasive testing by whatever means is only complementary to a clinical evaluation (Table 55.2). A rule of thumb is that arterial consultation and arteriography/magnetic resonance angiography (MRA) are indicated when there is a question of ischemia complicating a diabetic foot problem.

Table 55.1 Signs and Symptoms of PAD

- Intermittent claudication
- Feet cold to touch
- Nocturnal and rest pain relieved with dependency
- Absent pulses
- Blanching on elevation
- Delayed venous filling after elevation (>25 s)
- Dependent rubor
- Atrophy of subcutaneous fatty tissue
- Shiny skin
- Loss of hair on feet and toes
- Thickened nails, often with fungal infection
- Gangrene or nonhealing ulcer or surgical procedure
- Miscellaneous: blue toe syndrome, acute arterial occlusion

ARTERIOGRAPHY

Precision arteriography visualizing the foot vessels remains the most cost-effective means for definitive evaluation of diabetic lower-extremity ischemia. More than 90% of diabetes patients presenting with ischemic foot ulcerations/gangrene have demonstrated surgically correctable occlusive disease with current arteriographic techniques, especially digital subtraction arteriography. Although there is an increased risk of contrast-induced renal insufficiency, proper hydration remains the best means for preventing or minimizing this complication. Metformin should be discontinued at least 24 h before arteriography, as should other nephrotoxic medications. Further advances in MRA may make it the procedure of choice in the future, especially in patients with renal compromise.

TREATMENT

The treatment of diabetic PAD depends on

- its severity
- the patient's presentation
- the potential for rehabilitation
- an appropriate conduit

Table 55.2 Noninvasive Arterial Tests

- Doppler systolic pressure measurements
- Doppler ankle pressure measurements and ankle:brachial index
- Doppler waveform analysis
- Pulse volume recordings
- Toe pressures
- Transcutaneous oxygen pressure
- Duplex color flow scanning
- MRA

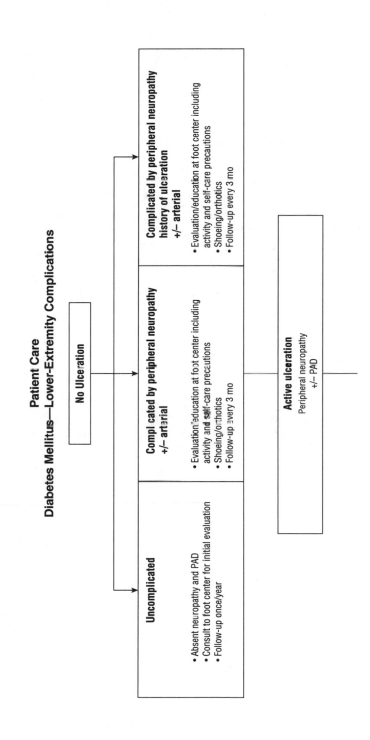

Patient Care
Diabetes Mellitus—Lower-Extremity Complications

No Ulceration

Uncomplicated

- Absent neuropathy and PAD
- Consult to foot center for initial evaluation
- Follow-up once/year

Complicated by peripheral neuropathy
+/– arterial

- Evaluation/education at foot center including activity and self-care precautions
- Shoeing/orthotics
- Follow-up every 3 mo

Complicated by peripheral neuropathy
history of ulceration
+/– arterial

- Evaluation/education at foot center including activity and self-care precautions
- Shoeing/orthotics
- Follow-up every 3 mo

Active ulceration
Peripheral neuropathy
+/– PAD

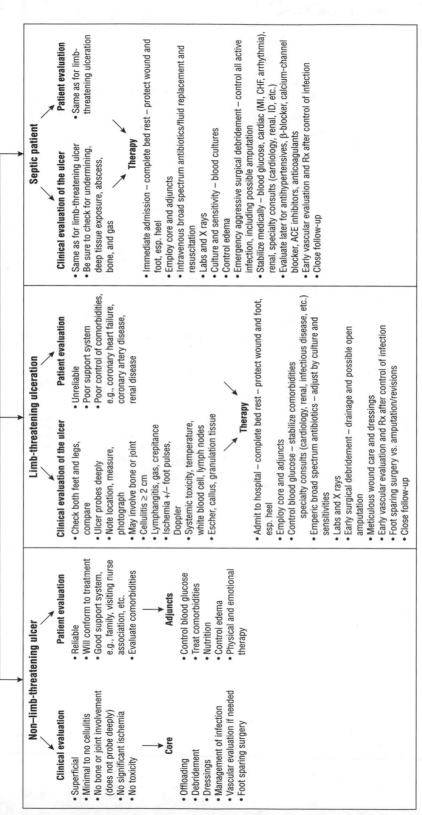

Figure 55.1 Patient care algorithm. ©Foot Care Specialists at Boston Medical Center, Boston, MA.

Mild to moderate claudication (more than two blocks) is best treated by controlling risk factors through smoking cessation, weight reduction, control of lipid levels and hypertension, good diabetes control, and an active and aggressive exercise program. Protective footwear and inspection are important during exercise. Individuals with diabetes can live with significant PAD without a problem until some type of traumatic event initiates an ulcer. Vasodilator therapy has generally been ineffective, as has sympathectomy. Antiplatelet agents (aspirin, Plavix, Pletal) are frequently used, but their efficacy has not been confirmed in clinical trials. The use of hemorheologic agents (pentoxifylline) to reduce blood viscosity has not been generally successful for dramatically improving walking distance. Pletal is a newer vasodilator plus antiplatelet agent that has been shown to improve walking distance. It is generally well tolerated, with the major side effects being dizziness, tachycardia, or gastrointestinal upset. It is contraindicated for any patient with a history of congestive heart failure.

Indications for arterial reconstruction include

- disabling claudication
- ischemic rest pain
- night pain
- tissue ulceration
- gangrene
- inability of a surgical procedure to heal because of associated ischemia

If a health care professional believes that ischemia is complicating wound management, then the patient should be referred to a arterial surgeon knowledgeable about diabetic arterial disease and its treatment.

ENDOVASCULAR PROCEDURES

The success of endovascular procedures (balloon angioplasty, atherectomy, laser angioplasty) has been more limited in diabetes patients because PAD tends to be more diffuse and preferentially involves the smaller distal arterial tree. Also, the atherosclerotic lesions tend to be longer and more heavily calcified. The best results are achieved with balloon angioplasty of short isolated aorta/iliac artery stenoses or occlusions. Angioplasty involving the popliteal to tibial or peroneal arteries is generally contraindicated because of the high early failure rate and a higher rate of restenosis or occlusion. Routine use of stents requires further clinical studies. Gene therapy may hold promise for the future but is yet unproven for routine use.

REVASCULARIZATION PROCEDURES

Diabetes patients tolerate revascularization extremely well, with excellent outcomes and morbidity and mortality rates equal to those of nondiabetic individuals and no greater than amputation.

Aortoiliac (inflow) procedures are similarly performed in patients with and without diabetes and require the use of synthetic grafts.

Distal revascularization techniques (outflow) have demonstrated excellent outcomes with patency and limb salvage equal to or better than that achieved in nondiabetic patients. We have learned that to achieve the most rapid and durable healing of an open foot ulcer, a pulse must be restored to the foot via a distal revascularization to a vessel with direct continuity to the dorsalis pedis, posterior tibial, or plantar arteries themselves. The autologous vein is the conduit of choice, and a flexible approach tailors the revascularization procedure to an individual patient's needs. At 3 years, graft patency is 87% and limb salvage is 92%. Early recognition and aggressive surgical drainage of foot sepsis is critical, followed by prompt and thorough evaluation and treatment of ischemia. Our multidisciplinary algorithm (Fig. 55.1) has resulted in primary healing or reconstructive foot surgery replacing the need for amputation at any level. From the patients' perspective, this aggressive approach relieves their pain, heals their wounds, and expedites return to function and well-being.

BIBLIOGRAPHY

Caputo GM, Cavanaugh PR, Ulbrecht JS, Gibbons GW, Karchmer AW: Assessment and management of foot disease in patients with diabetes. *N Engl J Med* 33:854–860, 1994

Gibbons GW: Vascular evaluation and long-term results of distal bypass surgery in patients with diabetes. *Clin Pod Med Surg* 12:129–140, 1995

Gibbons GW, Burgess AM, Guadagnoli E, Pomposelli FB Jr, Freeman DV, Campbell DR, Miller A, Marcaccio EJ Jr, Nordberg P, LoGerfo FW: Return to well-being and function after infrainguinal revascularization. *J Vasc Surg* 21:35–44, 1995

Gibbons GW, Habershaw GM: Special consideration for the diabetic foot. In *Peripheral Arterial Disease Diagnosis and Treatment*. Vol. 15. Coffman JD, Eberhardt RT, Eds. Totowa, NJ, Humana Press, 2002, p. 265–280

Gibbons GW, Habershaw GM: The septic diabetic foot "foot sparing surgery." In *Advances in Vascular Surgery*. Vol. 4. Ernst CB, Ed. Chicago, Mosby-Year Book, 1995, p. 211–226

Gibbons GW, Marcaccio E Jr, Freeman DV, Campbell DR, Miller A, LoGerfo FW: Improved quality of diabetic foot care 1984 vs 1990: reduced length of stay and costs, insufficient reimbursement. *Arch Surg* 128:576–581, 1993

Pecoraro RE, Reiber GE, Burgess EM: Pathways to diabetic limb amputation: basis for prevention. *Diabetes Care* 13:513–521, 1990

Pomposelli FB Jr, Jepsen SJ, Gibbons GW, Campbell DR, Freeman DV, Gaughan BM, Miller A, LoGerfo FW: A flexible approach to infrapopliteal vein grafts in patients with diabetes mellitus. *Arch Surg* 126:724–729, 1991

Dr. Gibbons is a Professor of Surgery at Boston University School of Medicine as well as Executive Director and Foot Care Specialist at Boston Medical Center, Boston, MA. Dr. Locke is an Assistant Professor of Surgery at Boston University School of Medicine as well as a Podiatrist and Foot Care Specialist at Boston Medical Center, Boston, MA.

56. Foot Ulcers and Infections

GARY GIBBONS, MD, AND CHRISTOPHER LOCKE, DPM

PATHOPHYSIOLOGY

Minor trauma leading to cutaneous ulceration is the precipitating event for diabetic foot problems. The presence of neuropathy, vascular insufficiency, and an altered response to infection makes the patient with diabetes uniquely susceptible to foot problems. Neuropathy includes sensory, motor, and autonomic loss. Sensory neuropathy leads to loss of protective sensation. Motor neuropathy can affect the intrinsic muscles of the foot and can lead to characteristic deformities (i.e., digit contractures). An apropulsive (steppage) gait may develop. Autonomic neuropathy results in a falsely warm foot secondary to altered blood flow. Reduction in sweating causes abnormally dry skin that fissures and cracks easily, opening the foot up to bacterial invasion.

Peripheral vascular occlusive disease has important distinctions in patients with diabetes. The intima and media of diabetic arteries frequently contain extensive calcium (Monckeberg's sclerosis), making them rigid and noncompressible. Results of noninvasive vascular laboratory tests are thus often incorrect or misleading. Surgical manipulation of these calcified vessels is delicate, and laser therapy of distal calcified vessels is contraindicated. Development of collateral circulation around occlusions and stenoses is poor, especially in diabetes patients who smoke, with resulting limb-threatening consequences (rest pain or tissue loss). Diabetic macrovascular disease frequently involves the tibial/peroneal vessels between the knee and the foot. However, the foot vessels are usually spared; thus, modern treatment approaches to ischemic diabetic foot ulcers should no longer be based on the concept of small-vessel disease. Bypass grafts to the distal tibial and dorsalis pedis arteries will restore excellent tissue perfusion. All patients presenting with foot ulcerations should be evaluated for an ischemic component.

Infections are often undetected until limb and sometimes life are threatened. Diabetes patients do not feel the progression of ulceration, and the signs and symptoms of infection (i.e., temperature, tachycardia, elevation of leukocyte count) are not manifest until late. The first sign of serious infection may be loss of blood glucose control or a flu-like syndrome. Any patient reporting this must be carefully evaluated for infection.

PREVENTION

Patient education is essential. The following instructions may help patients avoid foot ulcers and infections.

Shoes

- Wear well-fitting shoes even if they are not stylish.
- Change shoes during the day to relieve pressure areas.
- Try running or walking shoes for everyday wear.
- Select dress shoes of soft leather and have them fitted carefully.
- Use orthotics to help accommodate the foot.
- Break in new shoes slowly.
- Shake shoes out and inspect them before wear for areas that might cause blisters or rubbing.

Foot Hygiene

- Wash feet daily with mild soap. Rinse and dry thoroughly, especially between the toes.
- Apply moisture-restoring creams once or twice daily except between the toes.
- Wear clean intact socks appropriate for the shoes being worn.
- Avoid astringents and all over-the-counter preparations for calluses, corns, nails, etc.
- Trim nails with a slightly rounded edge.
- Avoid "self-bathroom surgery." Seek a qualified professional for treatment of all foot problems.
- Do not use foot soaks.
- Do not use heating pads or sleep next to space heaters or stoves; hot or cold sensations in the feet result from neuropathy not poor circulation.
- Wear socks if feet feel cold.
- Never go barefoot.

Problems to Report to Doctor

- Report cuts or breaks in the skin.
- Report ingrown nails.
- Report changes in color or discoloration of the foot.
- Report pain or loss of sensation.
- Report change in architecture of the foot.

CLINICAL MANAGEMENT

It is important for patients to control weight and blood pressure, eliminate smoking, and exercise daily. Careful evaluation for infection is mandatory in diabetes patients who suddenly lose control of their blood glucose levels.

Table 56.1 Clinical Evidence of Arterial Insufficiency

- Diminished or absent pulses
- Absent hair from forefoot or toes
- Cornification of nails
- Atrophic skin and subcutaneous tissue
- Decreased skin temperature
- Pallor on elevation
- Dependent rubor
- Venous filling time >25 s

The patient's legs and feet, including the heels and the areas between the toes, should be examined at regular intervals, and neurological and vascular examinations should be conducted. Table 56.1 lists the clinical signs of vascular insufficiency, and these signs indicate the need for noninvasive testing and a consultation with a vascular specialist.

Skin changes, callus formation, or foot deformities should be evaluated, and shoes should be inspected for appropriateness, excessive wear, and foreign bodies. Patients at high risk for developing foot ulcers may need to be seen more frequently or referred to a specialist for particular problems (Table 56.2).

Table 56.2 Patients at High Risk for Ulceration

- History of previous ulcer
- Neuropathy: sensory, motor, autonomic
- Peripheral arterial disease
- Structural changes:
  - Hammertoes
  - Bunions
  - Charcot's foot
  - Pes cavus or planus
  - Other pathological changes in shape
- Callus formation
- Bleeding into callus or under a nail
- Skin changes
  - Dyshidrosis
  - Ingrown nails
  - Mycotic toenails
  - Evidence of poor hygiene
  - Fissuring
  - Chronic tinea pedis
  - Chronic skin infections
- Abnormal gait
- Abnormal patterns of wear on shoes

MANAGEMENT

The severity of the infected foot ulcer will determine the proper course of treatment. A major decision is whether the patient can be initially treated as an outpatient or needs to be admitted to the hospital. Early superficial ulcers with minimal (<2 cm) cellulitis may be treated at home if there is no evidence of systemic toxicity and the patient is compliant, reliable, and has a vigilant support system. Hospitalization is indicated if there is no significant improvement within 24–48 h.

Inspection of the wound to determine the extent of tissue destruction and sepsis is the first step. Carefully cleanse the area with an antiseptic solution, and, with a sterile probe, forceps, and scissors, unroof all encrusted areas. Inspect the wound to determine the extent of tissue destruction and possible bone and joint involvement. Little or no anesthesia is required because most of these patients have neuropathy. Our multidisciplinary algorithm (see Fig. 55.1 [p. 508]) contains proven effective protocols for treating superficial uncomplicated ulcers and deep ulcers with limb-threatening potential.

Treatment of Superficial Uncomplicated Ulcers and Infections

In addition to the guidelines found in Fig. 55.1, the following guidelines apply:

- Debride ulcers of any necrotic, fibrotic, or hyperkeratotic tissue to a clean bleeding granular base.
- Apply plain gauze sponges wetted with saline solution (wet to moist dressings) to open the ulcer once or twice a day. New technology wound products may be used depending on wound environment.
- Treat fissures or cracks in the skin with an antibiotic ointment and a plain gauze outer dressing.
- Treat athlete's foot (with superficial bacterial superinfection) with local antifungal cream or solution on plain gauze and an oral antibiotic. Keep the region dry with lambs wool and change socks frequently.
- Weight bearing is avoided until healing is ensured and then resumed gradually. If weight bearing progresses too rapidly, acute Charcot's foot (neuropathic joint disease) may result. Special devices may be used to help offload plantar ulcerations.
- Footwear should be modified to protect sensitive high-risk areas.

Once healed, these patients are regarded as high risk, and careful follow-up, including modification of footwear and orthotics, is recommended.

Treatment of Limb-Threatening Infections

The treatment of limb-threatening infections is also outlined in Fig. 55.1 (p. 508). Surgical intervention, especially in a patient with systemic toxicity, should not be delayed even if the patient has not yet been stabilized medically and blood glucose is not controlled. Blood glucose control often requires the use of insulin and careful inpatient monitoring.

Proper antibiotic therapy and wound care are essential to limb salvage. Whenever possible, deeply infected tissue or bone should be cultured. Initial use of intravenous broad-spectrum antibiotics is justified by the polymicrobial nature of these infections. Absorption of oral antibiotics may be inhibited by associated gastroenteropathy, especially in hyperglycemic, seriously ill patients.

Choice of an initial antibiotic or combination depends on

- local bacterial resistance patterns
- prior antibiotic history
- gram stain of deep exudate
- appearance of wound and pus
- allergies
- associated renal, hepatic, and cardiac impairment
- cost and individual health maintenance organization or hospital formulary

Changing antibiotics and the duration of therapy depends on bacterial sensitivities and the response of the wound to surgical management.

To determine the extent of tissue destruction or bone or joint involvement, plain X rays (plus/minus magnification views) are helpful initially but are not definitive. Scans and magnetic resonance may be useful in the differential diagnosis of osteomyelitis versus acute Charcot's disease. In difficult cases, consult with an experienced radiologist. Often, clinic examination and wound inspection with sterile probing will provide the most beneficial information.

Surgical management of potentially serious foot ulcers in diabetes patients requires debridement that is extensive enough to ensure there is no undrained pus or necrotic tissue left. It is a misconception that treatment of infections in diabetes patients should be limited to antibiotics and small incisions for drainage. Diabetes patients do not tolerate undrained infection, but they heal well if the infection is completely resolved and circulation is adequate.

Dressings are begun with the initial surgical management and should consist of diluted isotonic antiseptic solutions or saline applied to plain gauze and packed into the wound one to three times per day. Soaks, heat, whirlpools, astringents, full-strength solutions, or harsh medicines should be avoided. Standard wet-to-moist dressings are the most effective means for mechanically debriding the wound and permitting continual wound observation.

Assessment of the vascular status of the involved extremity is needed once sepsis is controlled. Because of the peculiarities of diabetic peripheral arterial disease, noninvasive laboratory testing plays only a complementary role to clinical evaluation and judgment. No one should accept the notion of small-vessel disease in the diabetic foot, and complete up-to-date arteriography should be done. This procedure should include visualization of the foot vessels in patients who are definitely ischemic or in cases where there is question. Vascular reconstruction, especially pedal artery bypass grafting, is successful in almost 90% of extremities with limb-threatening ischemia. After revascularization, revisions or more distal forefoot-saving amputations can be carried out, with the ultimate achievement of limb salvage.

Once wounds are adequately drained and debrided of necrotic tissue, there are many adjunctive therapies that can be used to prepare the wounds for closure: skin substitutes and living skin equivalents seeded with dermal cells. When placed over a clean wound bed, these living cells can stimulate the formation of granulation tissue and neoepithelialization by acting as a local factory for the necessary growth factors and wound-healing adjuncts. Negative pressure wound therapy (i.e., vacuum-assisted closure) can be used on certain wounds to help manage wound exudate and promote wound closure. No randomized control trial demonstrates the benefit of hyperbaric oxygen therapy (HBO) for routine management of diabetic lower-extremity wounds. It is expensive, and if the wound is ischemic, vascular evaluation and treatment remains the standard of care. Local limb HBO chambers are contraindicated because they are not really HBO, and there are no trials documenting success.

Adjunctive treatments can provide the proper conditions for healing in appropriately selected patients. First and foremost to this is the tight control and maintenance of blood glucose. Other adjunctive measures include evaluation and treatment of comorbidities, control of edema, nutrition evaluation and treatment, and physical and emotional therapy as needed.

BIBLIOGRAPHY

Gibbons GW: The diabetic foot: amputation and drainage of infection. *J Vasc Surg* 5:791–793, 1987

Gibbons GW, Eliopoulos G: Infections of the diabetic foot. In *Management of Diabetic Foot Problems.* Kozak GP, Hoar CS Jr, Rowbotham JL, Wheelock FC Jr, Gibbons GW, Campbell DR, Eds. Philadelphia, Saunders, 1984, p. 191

Gibbons GW, Habershaw GM: Special consideration for the diabetic foot. In *Peripheral Arterial Disease Diagnosis and Treatment.* Vol. 15. Coffman JD, Eberhardt RT, Eds. Totowa, NJ, Humana Press, 2002, p. 265–280

Gibbons GW, Habershaw GM: The septic diabetic foot "foot sparing surgery." In *Advances in Vascular Surgery.* Vol. 4. Ernst CB, Ed. Chicago, Mosby-Year Book, 1995, p. 211–226

Gibbons GW, Marcaccio EJ Jr, Burgess AM, Pomposelli FB Jr, Freeman DV, Campbell DR, Miller A, LoGerfo FW: Improved quality of diabetic foot care: 1984 vs. 1990: reduced length of stay and costs, insufficient reimbursement. *Arch Surg* 128:573–581, 1993

LoGerfo FW, Gibbons GW, Pomposelli FB Jr, Campbell DR, Freeman DV, Miller A, Quist WC: Evolving trends in the management of the diabetic foot. *Arch Surg* 127:617–621, 1992

Dr. Gibbons is a Professor of Surgery at Boston University School of Medicine as well as Executive Director and Foot Care Specialist at Boston Medical Center, Boston, MA. Dr. Locke is an Assistant Professor of Surgery at Boston University School of Medicine as well as a Podiatrist and Foot Care Specialist at Boston Medical Center, Boston, MA.

Index

About the American Diabetes Association

The American Diabetes Association is the nation's leading voluntary health organization supporting diabetes research, information, and advocacy. Its mission is to prevent and cure diabetes and to improve the lives of all people affected by diabetes. The American Diabetes Association is the leading publisher of comprehensive diabetes information. Its huge library of practical and authoritative books for people with diabetes covers every aspect of self-care—cooking and nutrition, fitness, weight control, medications, complications, emotional issues, and general self-care.

To order American Diabetes Association books:
Call 1-800-232-6733. Or log on to http://store.diabetes.org

To join the American Diabetes Association:
Call 1-800-806-7801. www.diabetes.org/membership

For more information about diabetes or ADA programs and services:
Call 1-800-342-2383. E-mail: Customerservice@diabetes.org or log on to www.diabetes.org

To locate an ADA/NCQA Recognized Provider of quality diabetes care in your area: www.ncqa.org/dprp

To find an ADA Recognized Education Program in your area:
Call 1-888-232-0822. www.diabetes.org/recognition/education.asp

To join the fight to increase funding for diabetes research, end discrimination, and improve insurance coverage: Call 1-800-342-2383. www.diabetes.org/advocacy

To find out how you can get involved with the programs in your community: Call 1-800-342-2383. See below for program Web addresses.

- *American Diabetes Month:* Educational activities aimed at those diagnosed with diabetes—month of November. www.diabetes.org/ADM
- *American Diabetes Alert:* Annual public awareness campaign to find the undiagnosed—held the fourth Tuesday in March. www.diabetes.org/alert
- *The Diabetes Assistance & Resources Program (DAR):* Diabetes awareness program targeted to the Latino community. www.diabetes.org/DAR
- *African American Program:* Diabetes awareness program targeted to the African American community. www.diabetes.org/africanamerican
- *Awakening the Spirit: Pathways to Diabetes Prevention & Control:* Diabetes awareness program targeted to the Native American community. www.diabetes.org/awakening

To find out about an important research project regarding type 2 diabetes:
www.diabetes.org/ada/research.asp

To obtain information on making a planned gift or charitable bequest:
Call 1-888-700-7029. www.diabetes.org/ada/plan.asp

To make a donation or memorial contribution:
Call 1-800-342-2383. www.diabetes.org/ada/cont.asp